Veterinary Oncology

Robert Klopfleisch
Editor

Veterinary Oncology

A Short Textbook

Springer

Editor
Robert Klopfleisch
Institut für Tierpathologie
Freie Universität Berlin
Berlin
Germany

ISBN 978-3-319-41122-4 ISBN 978-3-319-41124-8 (eBook)
DOI 10.1007/978-3-319-41124-8

Library of Congress Control Number: 2016954239

Printed on acid-free paper

This Springer imprint is published by Springer Nature
The registered company is Springer International Publishing AG Switzerland
The registered company address is Gewerbestrasse 11, 6330 Cham, Switzerland

Contents

Contributors

Editor

Robert Klopfleisch, DACVP
Institut für Tierpathologie
Freie Universität Berlin
Berlin, Germany

Authors

Natali Bauer
Abteilung klinische Laboratoriumsdiagnostik und klinische Pathophysiologie,
Klinikum Veterinärmedizin
Justus-Liebig-Universität Gießen
Giessen, Germany

Angele Breithaupt, DiplECVP
Institut für Tierpathologie
Freie Universität Berlin
Berlin, Germany

Mathias Brunnberg, Dipl. ECVS, MSc (Small Animal)
Klinik für kleine Haustiere
Freie Universität Berlin
Berlin, Germany

Manfred Henrich, DECVP
Institut für Veterinär-Pathologie
Justus-Liebig-Universität Giessen
Giessen, Germany

Olivia Kershaw, DECVP
Institut für Tierpathologie
Freie Universität Berlin
Berlin, Germany

Stephanie Plog, DECVP
IDEXX Laboratories Ltd.
Wetherby, United Kingdom

Melanie Wergin, PhD (Radiation-Oncology)
Abteilung Onkologie/Strahlentherapie
Medizinische Kleintierklinik,
Ludwig-Maximilians-Universität München,
Munich, Germany

Basic Principles of Carcinogenesis

Robert Klopfleisch

R. Klopfleisch (ed.), *Veterinary Oncology*, DOI 10.1007/978-3-319-41124-8_1

1.1 Hallmarks of Cancer

As our knowledge of carcinogenesis advances, it is becoming increasingly evident that it is an overwhelmingly complex process. Moreover, in many ways carcinogenesis does not seem to follow a predictable pattern; often the process is quite unique. But we can identify several universal features of this process, as presented in the hallmark model by Hanahan et al. (2011). According to this model, tumors are characterized by the following *main hallmarks of cancer*:

- Genome instability, mutation, and epigenetic change
- Sustained proliferation and evasion of growth suppression
- Evasion of apoptosis
- Deregulation of energy metabolism
- Induction of angiogenesis
- Invasion and metastasis

Genome Instability, Mutation, and Epigenetic Change

The first step of carcinogenesis is the development of genetic aberrations in the potential tumor cells. These aberrations are mainly *mutations* with actual changes in the nucleotide sequence of the cell. Mutations are caused either by carcinogenic noxa (described in Sect. 1.4) or by other stimulants and mistakes in DNA replication. The latter become more frequent with acquired or inherited inefficiency of the DNA repair systems. In addition, gene activity may also be permanently influenced by *epigenetic changes* in the form of DNA methylation and histone modifications.

Regardless of whether mutations are caused by obligate carcinogens or impaired DNA repair mechanisms, most of the acquired mutations are thought to be either lethal or irrelevant for the fitness of the affected tumor cell. Very few of the acquired mutations seem to be initial "driver mutations" for tumor progression, invasion, and finally metastasis. The identification of driver genes and mutations is a major goal of cancer research. This research has been driven by the search for "the one" mutation initiating and driving carcinogenesis for any given tumor type. Just recently, however, *global cancer genome analysis* has shown that carcinogenesis is a complex process involving several mutations and changes in multiple signaling cascades. Cancer genome analysis has also shown that clinically and morphologically similar tumors may have a high grade of *inter-tumor genetic heterogeneity* (Fig. 1.1). For instance, cancer genome sequencing of 510 human breast cancer tumor samples found 30,626 somatic mutations, of which mutations in only three genes, P53, PIK3CA, and GATA3, were present in 10–45 % of all tumors. A similar variability in the "genome landscape" has also been identified in other tumor types, and it is now assumed that *most somatic mutations are only present in <5 % of tumors of a specific type.*

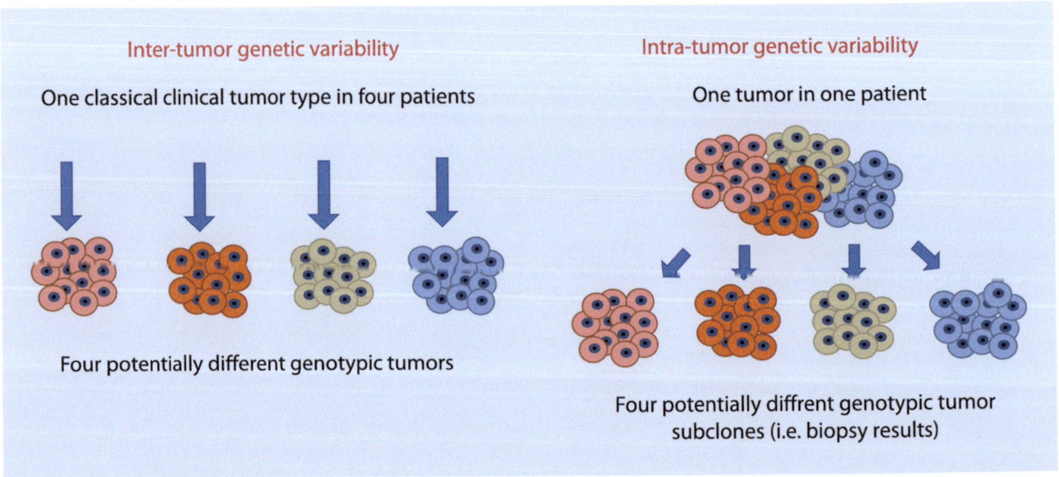

Fig. 1.1 Inter- and intra-tumor genetic heterogeneity. Cancer genome analysis has revealed that tumors, which were once classified phenotypically by their clinical behavior or pathomorphological appearance, might significantly differ in their genotypes (inter-tumor genetic variability). Furthermore, genome analysis of tissue samples taken from one tumor also revealed a high intra-tumor genetic variability

Cancer genome analysis has also found that most tumors are additionally characterized by a high grade of *intra-tumor genetic heterogeneity*. This heterogeneity of tumor cells within one tumor is the result of disruption of the pathways responsible for genomic stability like nucleotide excision or double-strand break repair in tumor cells. This leads to a constant accumulation of random mutations in different tumor cells. Intra-tumor heterogeneity is a *challenge for diagnostics* in daily practice (◘ Fig. 1.1). For instance, a comparison of the genome of numerous biopsies from different human clear cell renal carcinomas showed that biopsies from different tumors may be more similar than biopsies from one tumor and that biopsies from one tumor can be very distinct from one another. These results raise questions of how to define the genetic status of tumors for therapeutic classification.

Despite the overwhelming complexity and variability of the genetic changes associated with carcinogenesis, only few genes seem to be affected by driver mutations. Deeper pan-tumor analysis of the cancer genome project data shows that only approximately 120–140 genes and their different mutations might be relevant for the initiation and progress of carcinogenesis. Of these, approx. 70 genes have been identified as *tumor suppressors*, which are "brakes of carcinogenesis," and approx. 50 genes are *proto-oncogenes*, which are "accelerators of carcinogenesis." These driver mutations are present in variable combinations in different tumors irrespective of histological types. However, Vogelstein et al. (2013) have proposed that all identified *driver mutations have a major impact on carcinogenesis by influencing a select few* (*no more than 12*) *signaling pathways*, which contribute to three core cellular functions: cell fate, cell survival, and genome maintenance. If this is true, the complexity of tumor genomes can be reduced to a target few and thus potentially treatable genetic aberrations.

The theory that *genomic instability is* a major driver of carcinogenesis is supported by the high number of documented driver mutations in genes involved in genome stability and the massive changes in gene copy number and genome sequence in most tumors. Defects in genome maintenance and repair can therefore be considered to be an *important initial factor in carcinogenesis*, since they predispose pre- and neoplastic cells to acquire genotypes that enable them to develop all other hallmarks of cancer. Of the several genes involved in genome maintenance, so-called caretakers or guardians of the genome, P53 and the BRCA genes have been most intensely studied. For instance, BRCA1 is a major cause of the *hereditary breast-ovarian cancer syndrome of women*, which impressively depicts the relevance of impaired DNA repair mechanisms on carcinogenesis and genome instability. BRCA1 protein is part of a DNA repair complex, which repairs the continuously occurring, multicausal DNA double-strand breaks and erroneous DNA insertions and deletions. Disabling BRCA1 mutations in women leads to an increased risk of up to 80 % for developing breast cancer and a risk of up to 50 % for developing ovarian cancer. Unfortunately, similar syndromes are suspected but yet not proven in nonhuman species.

Due to the difficulties of directly observing or experimentally inducing the process in vivo, several questions on the chronological sequence of genomic alteration during carcinogenesis remain. It is assumed that many tumors evolve from dysplasia to benign to malignant tumors by acquiring a set of more or less specific mutations. This hypothesis of a gradual malignant transformation has been mainly developed based on the findings in human colorectal cancer and is summarized in the *Vogelstein* (*multistep carcinogenesis*) *model* (◘ Fig. 1.2). In colorectal cancer a *first "gatekeeping" mutation in the APC gene* is considered to be the initial step in the carcinogenesis process with the development of a *small, slow-growing* (*micro*)*adenoma*. Subsequently, mutations of KRAS, CDC4, and CIN are required for the development into a *large, advanced adenoma*. Finally, several mutations including p53, PTEN, BAX, SMAD4, and other genes are required for transition into a *metastatic carcinoma*. This *process can be stretched over several years*. For colorectal cancer it has been shown to take 6 years to develop a small adenoma, another 17 years for an early carcinoma, and another 5 years for the development of metastases.

The Vogelstein model may however not fully reflect the carcinogenetic process of other tumor types, especially those which do not have observable benign forms, like pancreatic and prostate carcinomas. In these cases it could be hypothesized that a preceding accumulation of relevant mutations before the actual gatekeeper mutation or a generally faster transformation process in a small number of initial tumor cells takes place.

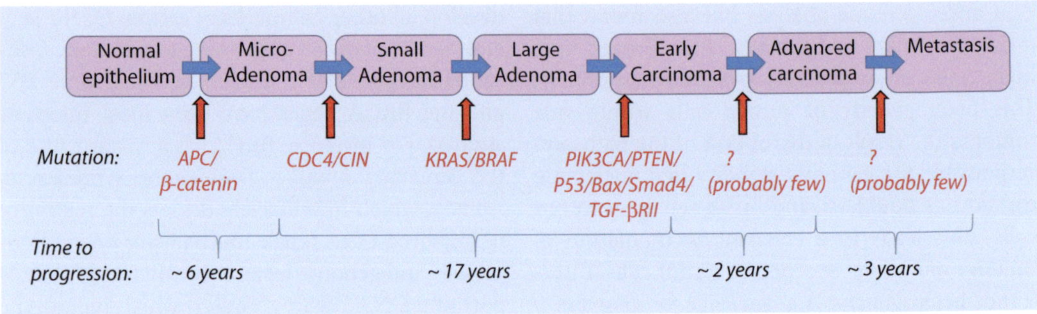

Fig. 1.2 Vogelstein model of multistep carcinogenesis (Modified from Jones et al. 2008). In this model, originally describing tumor progression of colorectal cancer, carcinogenesis is driven by a stepwise accumulation of mutations, which can be stretched over years and decades. In other tumor types, the process can however be shorter without detectable benign tumor interstages

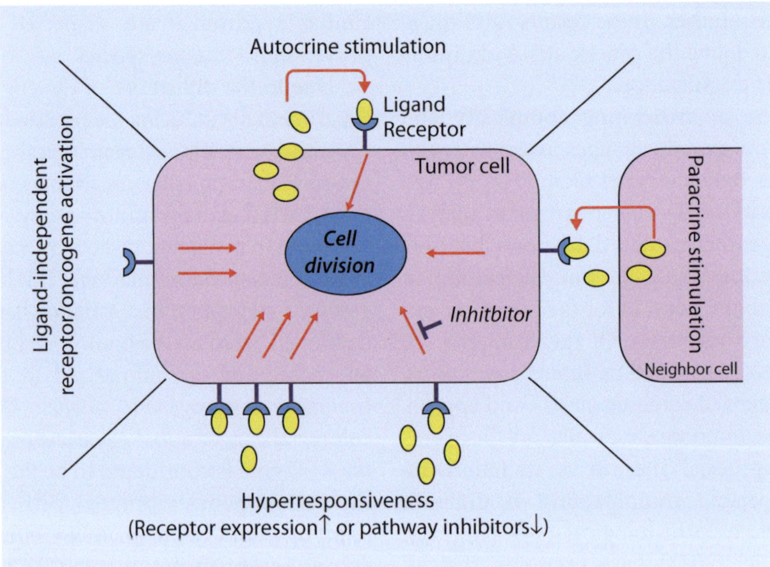

Fig. 1.3 Mechanisms of increased proliferation stimulation in tumor cells

Sustained Proliferation and Evasion of Growth Inhibition

Increased, sustained, and unregulated cell division is another very basic hallmark of cancer, which is caused by internal and/or external growth signals and evasion of growth inhibition. External and internal growth stimuli may be perceived by at least four mechanisms (Fig. 1.3):

- Autocrine stimulation by excessive synthesis of growth factors by the tumor cells themselves
- Paracrine stimulation by tumor-induced growth factors secreted by stromal cells in the microenvironment
- Hyperresponsiveness to normal levels of growth hormones due to increased receptor expression or loss of receptor pathway inhibitors
- Ligand-independent, constitutive receptor activation due to mutations

For instance, canine mast cell tumors display at least three of these mechanisms. A de novo expression of the pro-proliferative interleukin-2 receptor and its ligand interleukin-2 on neoplastic but not on normal mast cells has been described, which constitutes an *increased autocrine stimulus*. In addition, approx. 30 % of most malignant canine mast cell tumors contain a tandem duplication in exon 11 of the KIT gene, a tyrosine kinase receptor. This mutation induces a ligand-independent, *permanent activation of KIT signaling* and hence leads to increased proliferation and survival of neoplastic canine mast cells. The switch from external to *autonomous internal growth stimulation* due to downstream activation of signaling cascades seems to be a very common step during carcinogenesis. For instance, high-grade, malignant canine mast cell tumors show significantly lower membrane-bound KIT receptor expression than low-grade mast cell tumors. Similarly, metastatic canine mammary carcinomas usually have decreased or no estrogen and progesterone receptor expression compared to adenomas.

The sustained proliferation of cancer cells is even more impressive, considering how intensely guarded cell cycle progression is in normal cells. Tumor cells develop mechanisms which allow for *evasion of growth inhibition* programs that normally inhibit unregulated cell proliferation. These programs are normally dependent on central *tumor suppressors* that function in diverse ways to suppress cell growth and proliferation:

- Specific and direct negative-feedback mechanisms of proliferative signaling cascades
- Central tumor suppressors ("guardians") of cell cycle progression
- Contact inhibition by adjacent cells

For instance, nonneoplastic cells possess several *negative-feedback mechanisms to attenuate pro-proliferative signaling*. A prominent example is the *PTEN phosphatase*, which counteracts PI3-kinase by degrading its product, phosphatidylinositol trisphosphate (PIP3). Loss of PTEN expression due to mutations promotes proliferation and carcinogenesis. Accordingly, loss of PTEN has been identified as a prognostic factor for canine and feline mammary tumors, which is correlated with an increased risk for distant metastases, tumor recurrence, and shorter survival.

Two prototypical tumor suppressors are usually used to explain the principle of *central guardians of cell cycle progression*. The *retinoblastoma-associated protein* (*RB*) plays a central role in the integration of mostly extracellular growth stimuli. Phosphorylation of RB by diverse cyclin-dependent kinases (CDKs) enables RB to release the transcription factor E2F and to progress from the G1 phase to the S phase of the cell cycle. Genetic defects of RB and/or functional changes induced by viral proteins are common features of human tumor cells. Similarly, *canine and feline papillomaviruses* associate with and may induce degradation of *RB* to induce cell proliferation in fibroblasts and squamous cell carcinomas. Genetic or at least functional RB insufficiency is also suspected for diverse canine and feline tumors, including hemangiosarcomas, but this is not fully proven yet. In contrast to RB, *p53-mediated growth inhibition* is mainly based on intracellular signals such as DNA damage or stress-associated metabolic changes. According to the type, intensity, and persistence of these signals, p53 either temporarily halts the cell cycle or triggers apoptosis. *Mutations of p53* have been identified in a small fraction of canine brain, skin, bone, and mammary tumors. This identification has also been made in similar feline tumors, although it is much more rare. The relevance of both proteins should however not be overstated, since several mechanisms functionally redundant to p53 and RB seem to be present in cells and may compensate for loss of their function.

Cell-to-cell contact is another important mechanism to preserve tissue homeostasis by growth inhibition. This *contact inhibition* is lost in some cancer types. A prototypical example is the *E-cadherin-/beta-catenin-mediated contact inhibition*. When E-cadherin on an epithelial cell is bound to its counterpart on the neighboring cell, its cytoplasmic tail binds beta-catenin. Loss of E-cadherin expression frees beta-catenin. Beta-catenin then travels to the nucleus and activates expression of several pro-proliferative pathways. Aberrant E-cadherin expression is a typical finding in malignant canine mammary, prostate, and squamous cell carcinomas. Another mechanism currently in focus is the *merlin-cadherin-transmembrane growth factor receptor complex*. This complex strengthens the cadherin-mediated cell-to-cell attachments, sequesters growth factor receptors, and thereby restricts their growth signals to the cell limits. Loss of the complex loosens the cell adhesion, increases growth factor signaling, and induces cell proliferation.

■ Apoptosis Evasion

As mentioned before, DNA damage, overwhelming proliferation signaling, increased cell stress, and metabolic imbalances can lead either to a temporary halt of cell proliferation or *induction of programmed cell death by apoptosis*. In tumor cells, this mechanism is obviously disturbed, since genomic instability, metabolic stress, and excessive proliferation are hallmarks of cancer. Two methods of apoptosis induction exist: the extrinsic method, induced by extracellular signaling by immune cells, and the intrinsic method, induced by several intracellular signals like DNA or mitochondrial damage. *Disturbance of the intrinsic apoptosis pathway* is considered more relevant for carcinogenesis. P53 and the anti-apoptotic Bcl-2 protein family are the most intensely analyzed apoptosis-associated proteins with influence on carcinogenesis. *Bcl-2 proteins* inhibit apoptosis by binding and suppressing the proapoptotic proteins Bax and Bak. Increased Bcl-2 protein expression has been found in canine mast cell tumors, hemangiosarcomas and melanomas, and in feline lymphomas and skin tumors. In addition, *loss of p53 expression* or its function is also associated with a failure to transcribe the detection of DNA damage into apoptotic death.

▪ Deregulation of Energy Metabolism

The sustained and massive proliferation of tumor cells also represents a challenge for energy metabolism. Normal cells satisfy their energy demand under aerobic conditions by mitochondrial oxidative phosphorylation to produce ATP. Generating ATP under anaerobic glycolysis has only 1/18th the efficiency of aerobic glycolysis and produces large amounts of lactate under hypoxic conditions. Most cancer cells as well as normal proliferating cells nevertheless use anaerobic glycolysis as their major pathway to obtain ATP regardless of the availability of oxygen, a phenomenon termed *aerobic glycolysis or* "the Warburg effect." Initially it was thought that cancer cells have a mitochondrial defect and thus fail to use aerobic respiration, an idea that has been omitted in recent years. It is now hypothesized that cancer metabolism focuses on *facilitating biomass generation* rather than efficient ATP production. In addition, efficient ATP production is only required when resources are scarce for the single cell or the complete organism. Local energy deficiency is usually not a problem for well-vascularized tumors. In any case tumors lose every aspect of their "sense of social responsibility" in terms of energy saving for the sake of the rest of the body. Notably, tumors have been shown to develop subclonal cell populations, which utilize the lactate produced by aerobic glycolysis as their main energy source.

▪ Induction of Angiogenesis

Despite their predominant reliance on anaerobic glycolysis ("Warburg effect"), tumors also require *nutrients and oxygen supply* and the removal of metabolic end products and carbon dioxide. This is only possible if the tumor cell is in proximity to a functional vessel not further than 100–200 µm away. Tumors therefore have to be able to induce *angiogenesis* to survive and grow. In normal tissues, the microvasculature is largely quiescent, and angiogenesis is "switched on" only during wound healing. In contrast, tumor masses are usually characterized by highly active angiogenesis. The induction of angiogenesis is based on the secretion of proangiogenic growth factors and inhibition of anti-angiogenic pathways. The best analyzed prototypes of proangiogenic factors are vascular endothelial growth factor (*VEGF*) and fibroblast growth factor (*FGF*). VEGF is either secreted by the tumor cells or is freed from the extracellular matrix-bound form by tumor-associated activation of matrix metalloproteases. In addition, bone marrow-derived macrophages, neutrophils, mast cells, and progenitor cells may infiltrate the tumor margins; the associated peritumoral inflammation also supports the induction of angiogenesis. VEGF expression levels within the tumor mass and VEGF serum levels are also positively correlated with increased angiogenesis and occasionally with increased malignancy in diverse canine tumor types.

▪ Invasion and Metastasis

Metastasis is defined as a spread of cancer from one organ or organ part to another organ or organ part. Dissemination of cancer cells throughout the body occurs through one or more of *three routes of metastasis*:

- Lymphogenic spread via lymph vessels mainly to lymph nodes
- Hematogenic spread via blood vessels to distant organs
- Transcoelomic spread via direct contact to other serosal surfaces in the abdominal cavity

Lymphogenic dissemination of cancer cells includes the invasion of lymph vessels and the transport in the lymphatic system to regional lymph nodes and to distant organs. It is usually combined with hematogenic spread. For *hematogenic spread,* tumor cells have to invade adjacent blood vessels to gain access to the circulation and are then transported with the bloodstream to distant sites. Only a few tumors like canine osteosarcomas seem to metastasize exclusively hematogenously and usually do not develop lymph node metastases. Pancreatic and ovarian cancer and mesotheliomas often spread by *transcoelomic metastasis* mostly in combination with the two other routes of metastasis. Transcoelomic metastasis includes breaching of the serosal surface and direct implantation of tumor cells on the serosal surface of adjacent organs.

Distant metastasis, which is based on hematogenic and often on preceding lymphogenic spread, can be described as a *metastatic cascade*, which is composed of five major steps (◘ Fig. 1.4):

- Loosening of contact to adjacent cells
- Invasion of the surrounding extracellular matrix (ECM) and vessels, often associated with epithelial-mesenchymal transition (EMT)
- Survival in the bloodstream as circulating tumor cells (CTC)
- Extravasation and formation of micrometastasis
- Development of a macro-metastasis

The *first step of the metastatic cascade* is the separation of a potentially metastatic cell from the adjacent cells. This is often associated with a *downregulation of cell adhesion proteins*, such as E-cadherin and *loss of cell-contact inhibition* (as described above). In contrast, proteins necessary for invasion and migration through the ECM are upregulated. These include factors like CD44 and focal adhesion kinase (FAK) for cell matrix interaction as well as various *matrix metalloproteinases for ECM digestion and loosening*. Neoplastic epithelial cell separation from neighboring cells and ECM invasion are often associated with a change in neoplastic epithelial cell shape from typical polygonal to more mesenchymal spindloid, which is called *epithelial-mesenchymal transition* (*EMT*). It is now accepted that this permanent or intermittent EMT is associated with or even a prerequisite for epithelial cells to separate, invade, resist apoptosis, and metastasize. Several transcription factors are involved and used as *markers of EMT, including Snail, Slug, and Twist*. It is currently unclear, if mesenchymal sarcoma cells are experiencing a similar transition but without recognizable changes in their shape or if they use different mechanisms. The invasive process seems to also be influenced by the surrounding stromal stem cells and macrophages, which may contribute important factors like matrix metalloproteinases.

After invasion of the vasculature, tumor cells are transported individually or in small clusters by the bloodstream and referred to as *circulating tumor cells* (*CTC*). There is much effort to develop

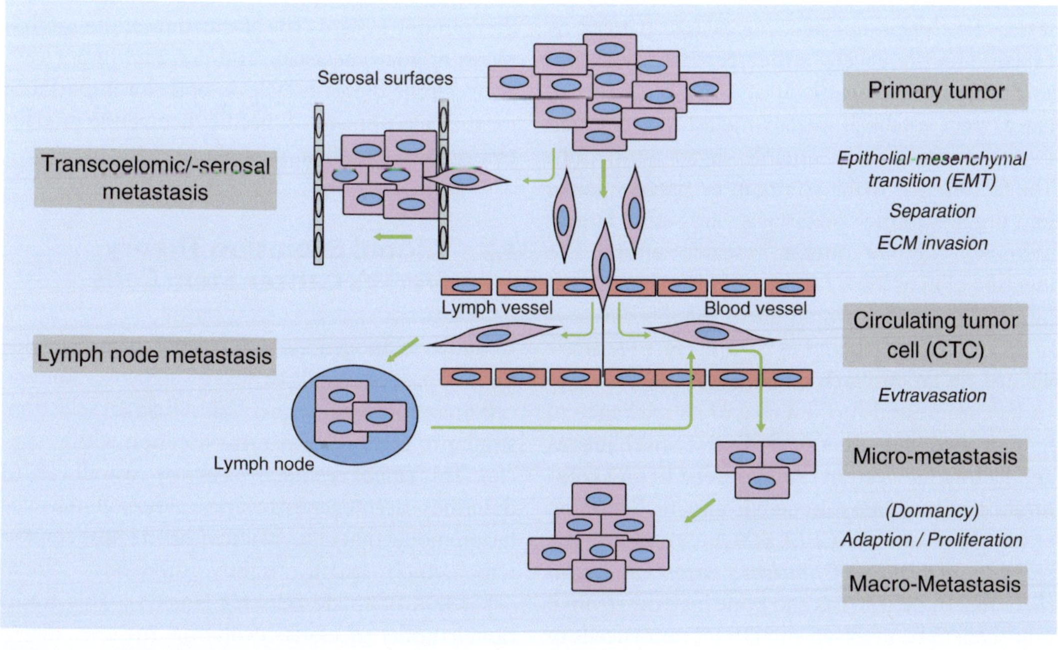

◘ **Fig. 1.4** The metastatic cascade and forms of metastatic spread

"*liquid biopsy*" methods for detection of CTC in blood samples of patients with potentially metastatic tumors, which would be less invasive and more informative about the actual disease status than tissue biopsies of the primary tumor. First studies indicate that *canine mammary tumor CTC* can be detected in the peripheral blood using the markers *CLDN7, CRYAB, ATP8B1, and EGFR* in the peripheral blood of dogs with canine mammary tumors. Their presence is specifically and sensitively correlated with the development of metastatic disease in dogs. Although primary tumors may shed thousands or millions of tumor cells into the circulation, they are usually present in very low numbers of *<10 CTC per milliliter blood* and thus per millions of peripheral blood leukocytes. In addition, not all the circulating tumor cells are of clinical relevance. It is assumed that <0.1 % of CTC are able to establish macro-metastatic disease, and their total number in the blood is not necessarily correlated with the development of metastasis.

The question of why and where *CTC extravasate and form metastases* is still largely unknown. It is nevertheless clear that metastatic tumors of different cellular origin have a typical organ-specific metastasis pattern. For instance, canine mammary tumors and osteosarcomas most commonly metastasize to the lung, while feline pulmonary carcinomas often metastasize to the distal phalanges. On the other hand, certain organs like the heart or the skin are only rarely affected by metastases. The organ-specific metastasis pattern is explained with Paget's rather general "seed and soil" *theory* of metastasis. It says that a tumor cell (seed) will establish macro-metastases or even micrometastases in a suitable organ (soil) only. The factors that make an organ or tissue suitable for organ-specific metastasis are still largely unknown, despite intense research effort. The identification of these factors is however of utmost interest, since they would allow for the development of targeted therapies to prevent metastatic disease. So far, research on bone-specific metastasis has progressed furthest due to its relevance to human medicine. There are diverse mechanisms and factors involved in tumor spread to and colonization of the bone microenvironment. Secretion of the *chemokines CXCL12, CXCL13*, etc., and the *receptor activator of nuclear factor-kB ligand* (*RANKL*) by osteoblasts and bone marrow stromal cells seem to be involved and attract cancer cells to the bone marrow. In addition, certain bone sialoproteins and collagens facilitate bone marrow invasion by binding to integrins commonly present on cancer cells.

Establishment of micrometastases is the next step after extravasation of CTC. *Micrometastases* are much more common than the clinically detectable macro-metastases. They are very small groups of often dormant or only slowly growing tumor cells, which are not detectable by common clinical imaging technologies. In the next step, micrometastatic tumor cells have to adapt to the tissue microenvironment at the new location to develop into *macro-metastases*, a process called colonization. *Colonization* seems to be very difficult for tumor cells in many respects beyond physical dissemination. It is assumed that most metastatic tumors disseminate millions of tumor cells into the circulation, of which only a fraction is able to establish micrometastases. Most of these micrometastases however stay in a state of dormancy. *Dormancy* is defined as a condition in which cancer cells do not divide or proliferate; during dormancy they stay in the G0 or G1 stage of the cell cycle and wait for appropriate, mostly unknown, signals to proliferate again. Dormant cancer cells as micrometastases or in the form of *minimal residual disease* (*MRD*) in the location of the resected primary tumor are the major cause of tumor relapse. It is known that dormancy can be caused by either inability to activate angiogenesis, nutrient starvation, systemic factors shed by the primary tumor, antigrowth signals embedded in the tissue extracellular matrix, or tumor-suppressing actions of the immune system. The elucidation of the mechanisms of micrometastatic and dormant tumor cells to overcome these obstacles is of major importance for the development of specific therapeutic modalities for long-term treatment of metastatic tumors.

1.2 Clonal Evolution Theory Versus Cancer Stem Cells

Initially, carcinogenesis was thought to be an evolutionary process that is driven by stepwise, somatic cell mutations with sequential, subclonal selection, similar to Darwinian natural selection within species. This *clonal evolution model* by Nowell (1976) describes carcinogenesis using a cancer clonal evolution model that takes place within a tissue ecosystem, which usually tightly suppresses clonal expansion of single cells (◘ Fig. 1.5). This traditional model of clonal evolution suggests that a series of clonal expansions and competitions leads to a dominance of one or few clones within the neo-

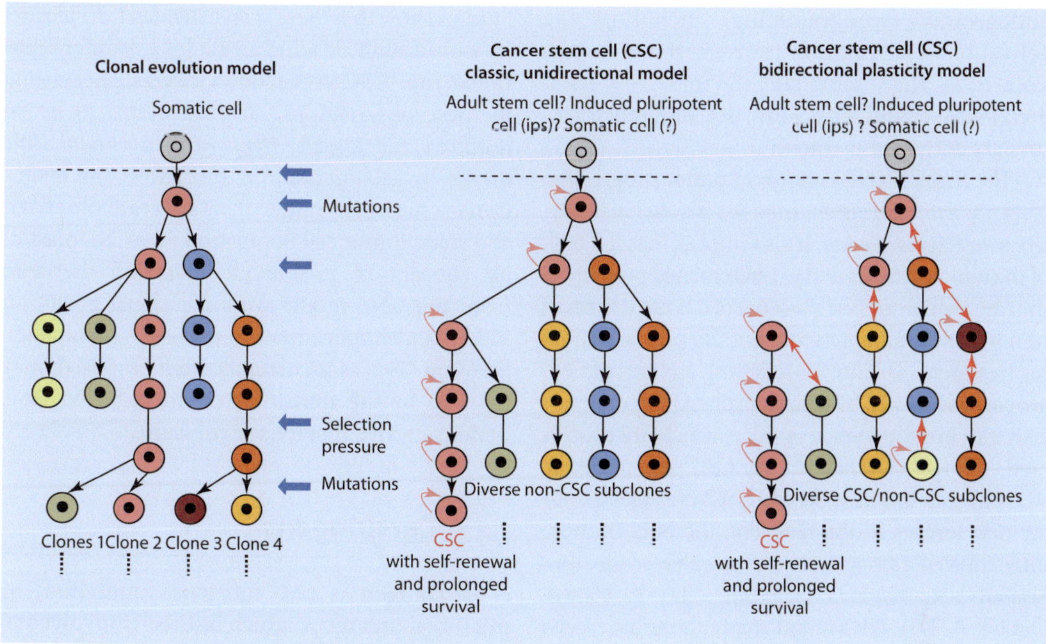

Fig. 1.5 Three main models of tumor progression

plasm. All of these clones are able to contribute to progression. Carcinogenesis in this model involves the *sequential accumulation of mutations and selection of the fittest variants*, i.e., tumor clones with the most profitable mutations in the current environment. These clones evolve by the interaction of advantageous "driver" *mutations* including the subgroup of "mutator" *mutations*, i.e., mutations increasing genomic instability, per se neutral "passenger" *mutations,* and disadvantageous or "fatal" *mutations*, respectively. This process leads to a unique cancer, which is built of impermanent subclones of cancer cells. The time frame of a clonal evolution to the level of metastasis can be anywhere from a few months to decades. What this time frame will be depends on the level of *genetic instability* in tumor cells and *epigenetic changes*, which contribute to the evolutionary process much faster than genetic changes do. There is an ongoing debate over whether malignant clones evolve gradually through a sequence of genetic alterations and clonal expansions or if a few highly relevant punctuated genetic alterations by an acute single insult directly and indirectly dramatically change the genome.

The original clonal evolution model proposed that basically all tumor cells contribute to the process of clonal evolution by acquiring mutations, by cell division, and by propagation of this mutation to its progeny. This idea has been challenged and is now complemented by the *cancer stem cell (CSC) model* (Fig. 1.5). The classical CSC concept assumes that tumor proliferation, similar to nonneoplastic tissue proliferation, is driven by the small subset of stem cells. CSC have the ability to *divide asymmetrically*, allowing *self-renewal* and differentiation into non-CSC progeny. The progeny then lack tumor-initiating capabilities. There are three main hypotheses on the *origin of CSC*, which are still under debate:

1. Malignant transformation of normal adult stem cells into CSC
2. Dedifferentiation of mature cancer cells into CSC
3. Induction of pluripotent cancer cells (iPS)

The *first hypothesis* of a transformation of adult stem cells into CSC is based on the observation that CSC have a self-renewal capacity similar to normal stem cells. In addition, transformation into a malignant tumor cell may take several years, a time span that is only survived by adult stem cells. *The second hypothesis* of CSC development by dedifferentiation of mature tumor cells into CSC is based on the recent observation of CSC plasticity, which is described in the paragraph below. Finally, *the third hypothesis* on the origin of CSC is related to the recent identification of induced pluripotent stem cells (iPS). iPS are normal somatic cells which are transformed into CSC by endogenous reprogramming, including the activation of at least four transcriptional factors known as the "Yamanaka factors": OCT3/4, Sox2, c-Myc, and Klf4. How the Yamanaka factors are activated is unclear.

The classical CSC concept of tumor progression is seen as a *unidimensional and unidirectional hierarchy with CSC at the top*. It also implies that the bulk of the tumor consists of the differentiated progeny of the CSC, which are just passengers but not drivers of tumor growth and therefore not the primary target for treatment. The tumor-initiating abilities of CSC are currently tested by xenotransplantation of tumor cells into immunodeficient mice, which are considered the *gold standard for CSC identification*. According to this model, only CSCs are able to initiate new tumors in the recipient; the bulk of more differentiated tumor cells are not able to do this. Several *CSC markers* including CD133, Nanog, Oct3/4, ALDH, CD44, and many more have been identified in the CSC of animal assays and are now used as antibody-based surrogate markers. The actual *frequency of CSC in the blood of cancer patients* is still under debate. Current xenotransplantation studies found CSC to be rare, with a share of only <2 % of all tumor cells. This number may however underestimate the number of CSC cells due to substantial skepticism about the value of xenotransplantation studies. It is argued that xenotransplantation may select only CSC that are able to grow in a mouse and not necessarily all CSC that are able to contribute to tumor progression in other microenvironments in the actual tumor host.

The recent progress in cancer genome sequencing has revealed high inter-tumor heterogeneity, i.e., heterogeneity between tumors of different individuals, and intra-tumor heterogeneity, i.e., heterogeneity between tumor cells of the same tumor. The tremendous *intra-tumor heterogeneity* has especially challenged the unidimensional, unidirectional, and hierarchical structure of the classical CSC model with one prototypic stem cell at the top. It is now assumed that CSC may be the actual cell accumulating somatic mutations and thus underlying a clonal evolution. This implies a *multidimensional hierarchical structure* with several different tumor subclones with different CSC at the top (◘ Fig. 1.5).

The unidirectional character of the CSC model cascade with an asymmetrical CSC division resulting in a terminally differentiated non-CSC daughter cell has also been challenged recently. Studies show that there is an *extended CSC plasticity* within a tumor, which includes a dedifferentiation of non-CSC to CSC and vice versa. According to these observations, *stemness seems to be an acquired and losable, temporary functional state* driven by accumulation of mutations and evolutionary pressures rather than a feature of a fixed and static tumor cell population. The CSC plasticity concept of phenotypic reversion therefore fuses the CSC model with the clonal evolution model and implies that an exclusive therapeutic focus on CSC, as is currently often proposed, may fail due to the transition of non-CSC to CSC under selective therapeutic pressure.

1.3 Carcinogens

A carcinogen is any substance, radiation, or microbial organism, which is directly involved in the initiation of cancer. This is usually due to its ability to directly damage the genome or to indirectly influence the genome by interruption of cellular metabolic processes which then induce genetic or epigenetic changes. Tables 1.1 and 1.2 list and summarize some common examples of the 116 group 1 carcinogens with proven carcinogenic effect for humans as defined by the *International Agency for Research on Cancer* (*IARC*, ► http://monographs.iarc.fr/). Their carcinogenic effect has not been proven for all domestic animals but is most likely transferable. Table 1.3 summarizes the most important biologic carcinogens for domestic animals.

1.4 Clinically Relevant Tumor Effects

▪ Mass Effect of the Primary Tumor and Metastasis

The term "*mass effect*" describes the increasing space occupation of the growing tumor or its metastases. Constant tumor-associated compression on neighboring structures leads to atrophy of the adjacent cells and functional disturbances of adjacent nerves. For example, brain tumors inevitably exert a fatal mass on surrounding tissues due to the restricted space in the cranial cavity, causing increased intracranial pressure and brain damage.

Table 1.1 Common group 1 carcinogens for human as defined by the International Agency for Research on Cancer (IARC): chemicals, metals, arsenic, dusts, and fibers

	Tissues affected	Carcinogenic mechanism
Chemicals		
Aromatic amines (incl. 4-aminobiphenyl, benzidine, 2-naphthylamine, anilines)	Urinary bladder	Direct genotoxicity
Polycyclic aromatic hydrocarbons (PAHs) (incl. benzo[a]pyrene)	Lung, skin, urinary bladder	Direct genotoxicity
Aflatoxins	Liver	Direct genotoxicity
Benzene	Hemato-lymphatic organs	Direct genotoxicity
1,3-Butadiene	Hemato-lymphatic organs	Direct genotoxicity
Dioxin	Soft tissue, lung	Direct genotoxicity
Formaldehyde	Nasopharynx, hemato-lymphatic	Direct genotoxicity
Sulfur mustard	Lung	Direct genotoxicity
Vinyl chloride	Liver, vessels	Direct genotoxicity
Arsenic compounds	Lung, skin, urinary bladder	Oxidative DNA damage, epigenetic effects
Metals		
Beryllium and beryllium compounds	Lung	Chromosome aberrations, aneuploidy, DNA damage
Cadmium and cadmium compounds	Lung	DNA repair inhibition, genomic instability
Chromium (VI) compounds	Lung	Direct DNA damage, genomic instability, aneuploidy
Nickel compounds	Lung, nasal cavity, and paranasal sinuses	DNA damage, chromosome aberrations, genomic instability, DNA repair inhibition, epigenetic alteration, histone modification
Fibers and dusts		
Asbestos	Lung, pleura, larynx, ovary	Macrophage activation, inflammation, generation of reactive oxygen and nitrogen species, genotoxicity, aneuploidy, epigenetic alteration, activation of signaling pathways
Erionite	Pleural scrosa	Genotoxicity
Silica dust, crystalline in the form of quartz or cristobalite	Lung	Macrophage activation, persistent inflammation

Table 1.2 Common group 1 carcinogens as defined by the (IARC): pharmaceuticals

	Tissues affected	Carcinogenic mechanism
Pharmaceutica		
Diethylstilbestrol	Breast	Estrogen receptor mediated, genotoxicity, epigenetic change
Estrogen/progestagen contraceptives	Breast, cervix, liver, endometrium	Estrogen receptor mediated, genotoxicity
Tamoxifen	Endometrium	Estrogen receptor-mediated events, genotoxicity
Alkylating agents (busulfan, chlorambucil, cyclophosphamide, lomustine treosulfan)	Hemato-lymphatic organs	Genotoxicity
Chlornaphazine	Urinary bladder	Genotoxicity
Cyclosporine	Hemato-lymphatic organs, skin, diverse	Immunosuppression
Phenacetin	Renal pelvis, ureter	Genotoxicity, cell proliferation

Table 1.3 Microbial agents with proven carcinogenic effect in domestic animals

	Tissues affected	Carcinogenic mechanism
Papillomaviruses (several species)	Diverse, mainly skin and gastrointestinal tract	Viral proteins induce proliferation, immune evasion
Retroviruses (feline/bovine leukemia virus (FeLV, BLV), jaagsiekte sheep retrovirus (JSRV), enzootic nasal tumor virus 1 (ENTV1))	Hemato-lymphatic organs, nasal mucosa, type II pneumocytes	Insertion-based activation/inactivation of host cell oncogenes/tumor suppressor genes, introduction of new oncogenes
Spirocerca lupi (nematode)	Esophageal soft tissue (dog)	Chronic inflammation suspected

Table 1.4 Common tumor-specific paraneoplastic syndromes in veterinary oncology

Paraneoplastic syndrome	Tumor type	Carcinogenic Mechanism
Acromegaly	Somatotrophic pituitary tumors	Growth hormone secretion-induced IGF-1 secretion
Erythrocytosis	Renal tumors, lymphoma	Secretion of erythropoietin or HIF-1
Gastrointestinal ulceration	Mast cell tumor, gastrinoma	Hyperhistaminemia, hypergastrinemia
Glomerulonephritis/nephrotic syndrome	Leukemia, myeloma	Mainly antibody secretion
Hyperadrenocorticism	Pituitary corticotropic tumors, adrenocortical tumors	Secretion of ACTH, cortisol
Hyperaldosteronism	Adrenocortical tumors	Aldosterone secretion
Hypercalcemia of malignancy	Lymphoma, myeloma, anal sac apocrine gland adenocarcinoma, parathyroid tumors	Hyperparathyroidism, secretion of parathormone-related peptide, bone lysis, diverse cytokines
Hyperestrogenism	Ovarian tumors, Sertoli cell testicular tumors	Estrogen secretion
Hypergammaglobulinemia	Myeloma, lymphoma	Antibody secretion
Hyperglycemia	Glucagonoma, cortisol-secreting tumors	Glucagon secretion, cortisol-induced peripheral insulin resistance
Hyperthyroidism	Thyroid tumors	Thyroid hormone secretion
Hypertrophic osteopathy	Primary lung tumors, urinary bladder rhabdomyosarcoma, esophageal tumors	Unknown
Hypoglycemia	Insulinoma, hepatic/salivary tumors, lymphoma	Insulin secretion, tumor utilization of glucose, decreased hepatic glycogenolysis or gluconeogenesis, IGF-1/IGF-2 secretion
Hypothyroidism	Thyroid tumors	Thyroid gland destruction

Thrombocytopenia	Hemangiosarcoma, lymphoma	Platelet destruction/consumption, decreased platelet production
Myasthenia gravis	Thymoma, lymphoma,	Antibodies against nicotinic acetylcholine receptors
Necrolytic migratory erythema/superficial necrolytic dermatitis	Glucagonoma	Exact mechanisms unclear, glucagon secretion
Nodular dermatofibrosis	Renal cystadenoma/cystadenocarcinoma, uterine tumors	Unknown
Peripheral neuropathy	Lung tumors, leiomyosarcoma, multiple myeloma, lymphoma, insulinoma	Hypoglycemia, unknown
Thymoma-associated exfoliative dermatitis	Thymoma	Unknown

ACTH adrenocorticotropic hormone, *IGF* insulin-like growth factor, *HIF* hypoxia-induced factor

Paraneoplastic Syndromes

Paraneoplastic syndromes (*PNS*) are tumor-associated clinical signs, which are not the consequence of the mass effect of the primary tumor or its metastases. PNS are usually reversible and successful treatment leads to alleviation of their clinical signs. Knowledge of paraneoplastic signs is often helpful in tumor diagnosis, since they are often the first clinical sign, and for many tumors, like endocrine tumors, they can be more relevant than the local mass effect of an otherwise non-problematic tumor. PNS are usually mediated by humoral factors. The more general paraneoplastic syndromes like cancer cachexia, hyperthermia, and anemia and numerous major tumor-specific paraneoplastic syndromes are listed in Table 1.4.

Cancer Cachexia

Cancer cachexia is a very common *paraneoplastic clinical sign* in many cancer patients. It is a multifactorial and often irreversible syndrome of loss of skeletal muscle (*sarcopenia*) and body fat. Cachexia is assumed to be the cause of death in up to 20 % of human cancer patients. Comparable epidemiologic data are lacking for veterinary oncology. The pathogenesis of tumor cachexia is still not fully elucidated. *Several mechanisms are involved* in the increased energy wasting in cancer patients, including changes in the mitochondrial metabolism, lipolysis in adipocytes and an increased fraction of thermogenically active brown adipose tissue, chemokine-associated (IL-1, IL-6, TNFα) metabolic changes and upregulation of the ubiquitin-proteasome pathway in skeletal muscle metabolism, systemic inflammation, and many more.

Anemia

Anemia is also a very common PNS in veterinary oncology. There is a long list of potential causes for tumor-associated anemia including anemia of chronic disease, acute and chronic hemorrhage, or microangiopathic hemolytic anemia. *Anemia of chronic disease* is mainly caused by chronic increase in IL-6-induced hepcidin serum levels, which negatively influence iron metabolism. In addition, mainly inflammatory cytokines but also many hormones secreted by endocrine tumors may *suppress bone marrow erythropoiesis*, influence the release of renal erythropoietin, or reduce the life-span of erythrocytes. Mainly hemangiosarcomas, but also gastrointestinal tract tumors, may cause *severe acute or mild chronic hemorrhage* and potentially microcytic and hypochromic anemia. Hemangiosarcomas are also the cause for *microangiopathic hemolytic anemia*, which involves shearing of erythrocytes at fibrin deposition and/or damaged endothelium. Another more uncommon cause of tumor-associated anemia is bone marrow suppression due to *hyperestrogenism*. Sertoli cell testicular tumors and granulosa cell ovarian tumors in dogs are the most common cause of tumor-derived hyperestrogenism.

Hyperthermia (Fever)

The incidence of fever as a PNS in veterinary medicine is unknown but is a moderately common paraneoplastic syndrome in human patients. Cancer-associated hyperthermia is caused by excess secretion of the cytokines IL-1, IL-6, TNF-α, and prostaglandins. Cancer-associated fever is nevertheless often caused by cancer-associated infections rather than the cancer itself.

Cancer-Type-Specific Paraneoplastic Syndromes

Common tumor-specific paraneoplastic syndromes are listed in Table 1.4.

Suggested Reading

Argiles JM, Busquets S, Stemmler B, Lopez-Soriano FJ (2014) Cancer cachexia: understanding the molecular basis. Nature reviews. Cancer 14:754–762

Bergman PJ (2012) Paraneoplastic hypercalcemia. Top Companion Anim Med 27:156–158

Cancer Genome Atlas Network (2012a) Comprehensive molecular portraits of human breast tumours. Nature 490(7418):61–70

Cancer Genome Atlas Network (2012b) Comprehensive genomic characterization of squamous cell lung cancers. Nature 489(7417):519–525

Cancer Genome Atlas Network (2012c) Comprehensive molecular characterization of human colon and rectal cancer. Nature 487(7407):330–337

Cancer Genome Atlas Network, Weinstein JN, Collisson EA, Mills GB, Shaw KR, Ozenberger BA, Ellrott K, Shmulevich I, Sander C, Stuart JM (2013) The Cancer Genome Atlas Pan-Cancer analysis project. Nat Genet 45(10):1113–1120 da Costa A, Oliveira JT, Gartner F, Kohn B, Gruber AD, Klopfleisch R (2011) Potential markers for detection of circulating canine mammary tumor cells in the peripheral blood. Vet J 190:165–168

da Costa A, Lenze D, Hummel M, Kohn B, Gruber AD, Klopfleisch R (2012) Identification of six potential markers for the detection of circulating canine mammary tumour cells in the peripheral blood identified by microarray analysis. J Comp Pathol 146(2–3):143–151

da Costa A, Kohn B, Gruber AD, Klopfleisch R (2013) Multiple RT-PCR markers for the detection of circulating tumour cells of metastatic canine mammary tumours. Vet J 196(1):34–39

Freeman LM (2012) Cachexia and sarcopenia: emerging syndromes of importance in dogs and cats. J Vet Intern Med/Am Coll Vet Intern Med 26:3–17

Greaves M, Maley CC (2012) Clonal evolution in cancer. Nature 481:306–313

Hanahan D, Weinberg RA (2011) Hallmarks of cancer: the next generation. Cell 144(5):646–674

Jiang WG, Sanders AJ, Katoh M, Ungefroren H, Gieseler F, Prince M, Thompson SK, Zollo M, Spano D, Dhawan P, Sliva D, Subbarayan PR, Sarkar M, Honoki K, Fujii H, Georgakilas AG, Amedei A, Niccolai E, Amin A, Ashraf SS, Ye L, Helferich WG, Yang X, Boosani CS, Guha G, Ciriolo MR, Aquilano K, Chen S, Azmi AS, Keith WN, Bilsland A, Bhakta D, Halicka D, Nowsheen S, Pantano F, Santini D (2015) Tissue invasion and metastasis: molecular, biological and clinical perspectives. Semin Cancer Biol 35:S244–S275

Jones S, Chen WD, Parmigiani G, Diehl F, Beerenwinkel N, Antal T, Traulsen A, Nowak MA, Siegel C, Velculescu VE et al (2008) Comparative lesion sequencing provides insights into tumor evolution. Proc Natl Acad Sci U S A 105(11):4283–4288

Kandoth C, McLellan MD, Vandin F, Ye K, Niu B, Lu C, Xie M, Zhang Q, McMichael JF, Wyczalkowski MA et al (2013) Mutational landscape and significance across 12 major cancer types. Nature 502(7471):333–339

Klopfleisch R, Lenze D, Hummel M, Gruber AD (2010) Metastatic canine mammary carcinomas can be identified by a gene expression profile that partly overlaps with human breast cancer profiles. BMC Cancer 10:618

Klopfleisch R, Lenze D, Hummel M, Gruber AD (2011) The metastatic cascade is reflected in the transcriptome of metastatic canine mammary carcinomas. Vet J 190(2):236–243

Klopfleisch R, Meyer A, Schlieben P, Bondzio A, Weise C, Lenze D, Hummel M, Einspanier R, Gruber AD (2012) Transcriptome and proteome analysis of tyrosine kinase inhibitor treated canine mast cell tumour cells identifies potentially kit signaling-dependent genes. BMC Vet Res 8:96

Klopfleisch R (2013) Personalized medicine in veterinary oncology: minimal residual disease and circulating tumour cells in dogs. Vet J 195(3):263–264

Klopfleisch R (2015) Personalised medicine in veterinary oncology: one to cure just one. Vet J 205(2):128–135

Klose P, Weise C, Bondzio A, Multhaup G, Einspanier R, Gruber AD, Klopfleisch R (2011) Is there a malignant progression associated with a linear change in protein expression levels from normal canine mammary gland to metastatic mammary tumors? J Proteome Res 10(10):4405–4415

Meyer A, Gruber AD, Klopfleisch R (2013) All subunits of the interleukin-2 receptor are expressed by canine cutaneous mast cell tumours. J Comp Pathol 149:19–29

Nowell PC (1976) The clonal evolution of tumor cell populations. Science 194:23–28

Pang LY, Argyle DJ (2014) The evolving cancer stem cell paradigm: implications in veterinary oncology. Vet J 205:154–160

Ressel L, Millanta F, Caleri E, Innocenti VM, Poli A (2009) Reduced PTEN protein expression and its prognostic implications in canine and feline mammary tumors. Vet Pathol 46:860–868

Turek MM (2003) Cutaneous paraneoplastic syndromes in dogs and cats: a review of the literature. Vet Dermatol 14:279–296

Vander Heiden MG, Cantley LC, Thompson CB (2009) Understanding the Warburg effect: the metabolic requirements of cell proliferation. Science 324:1029–1033

Vogelstein B, Papadopoulos N, Velculescu VE, Zhou S, Diaz LA Jr, Kinzler KW (2013) Cancer genome landscapes. Science 339(6127):1546–1558

Basic Principles of Cancer Diagnostics

Robert Klopfleisch and Natali Bauer

R. Klopfleisch (ed.), *Veterinary Oncology*, DOI 10.1007/978-3-319-41124-8_2

2.1 Diagnostic Cancer Imaging

Diagnostic cancer imaging refers to all noninvasive techniques used to visualize internal tumors and their metastases. It is an essential prerequisite for initial diagnosis, for generating a treatment plan, and for evaluating the success of treatment. The modalities most commonly used in veterinary oncology are ultrasound, x-ray radiography, computed tomography (CT), and magnetic resonance imaging (MRI). Each method has its advantages and disadvantages and is of value for specific diagnostic questions (◘ Table 2.1).

2.1.1 Ultrasound

Diagnostic ultrasound uses ultrasound waves for visualization of tumors in internal organs. It is based on the *reflection of sound waves* from the border between two tissues with different acoustic impedance. The acoustic impedance depends on the physical density of the tissue and the achievable velocity of the sound waves sent from the transducer into the tissue. The higher the difference in acoustic impedance, the more sound is reflected at the border between two tissues, and the more sound is detected by the transducer. If the sound wave hits a gas-filled space or a solid bone, almost all the acoustic energy is reflected back toward the transducer. This means the structures behind the border (between, e.g., the bone and muscle) cannot be seen.

Compared with the other diagnostic imaging modalities, ultrasound has the advantages of fast real-time imaging, a comparably low cost, and the lack of x-ray exposure. Disadvantages are limited imaging of the bone and air-filled spaces, comparably low image resolution, and restricted body penetration (◘ Table 2.1). Ultrasound is commonly used as a first-line diagnostic tool for the evaluation of body cavity effusion and abdominal tumors.

2.1.2 Radiography

Radiography is still the predominant first-line imaging modality for many questions in veterinary oncology. It is often used as a comparatively inexpensive and easily accessible screening test, which can be supplemented with the higher resolution of CT or MRI, if necessary. Radiography uses electromagnetic x-rays to visualize internal body structures based on variations in their opacity. Opacity is the ability of a structure to absorb x-rays. A photographic film or a digital detector captures the nonabsorbed x-rays after passage

◘ **Table 2.1** Advantages and disadvantages of commonly used imaging methods in veterinary oncology

Imaging method	Advantage	Disadvantage
Ultrasound	Low cost Fast High sensitivity Real-time results Fast and inexpensive abdominal imaging	Often limited image resolution Difficult to analyze gas-filled body cavities Limited use for bone imaging Limited penetration Extensive training required
Radiography	Low cost Excellent bone imaging Easy global screening, especially for small animals Standard method, relatively easy to read	Superimposition of overlying structures Low soft tissue detail Low sensitivity for small tumors X-ray exposure
Computed tomography (CT)	No superimposition of overlying structures High sensitivity for small tumors Better bone imaging than MRI	High cost High x-ray exposure General anesthesia required Extensive training required
Magnetic resonance imaging (MRI)	Excellent (soft) tissue differentiation High resolution Excellent brain imaging	High cost General anesthesia required Extensive training required

through the body. The more a structure absorbs an x-ray, the more radiopaque (white) the structure will appear on a radiograph. Conversely, the less a structure absorbs an x-ray, the more x-ray is able to pass through onto the film, and the less radiopaque it will appear (darker).

The major advantages of radiographs are the comparatively low cost, the easy global depiction of large body parts (in small animals), and the excellent bone imaging capacity. The disadvantages are the superimposition of overlying structures due to the summation of the opacity of all structures in the path of the ray, the low detail of soft tissue structures, and the cell-damaging x-ray exposure (◘ Table 2.1). For these reasons, radiographs are commonly used as a screening tool for detecting tumor masses anywhere in the body except for the cranial cavity.

2.1.3 Computed Tomography

Computed tomography is an enhancement of classic radiography. It is based on the same mechanism of x-rays passing through structures of varying opacity. However, CT is a composite of numerous radiographs taken from different angles and integrated by computer processing. This approach produces cross-sectional, i.e., tomographic, slice images of the body and thus avoids superimposition of different tissues.

Other advantages of CT include higher sensitivity for detecting small tumors, improved bone imaging compared to MRI, and the possibility of CT-guided biopsies if ultrasound cannot be used. The main disadvantages are higher cost and higher x-ray exposure compared to radiographs. Accordingly, CT is commonly used to detect small tumors or metastases, for planning surgical approaches, or for radiotherapy.

2.1.4 Magnetic Resonance Imaging

Magnetic resonance imaging also produces three-dimensional pictures of the body based on a stack of cross-sectional imaging slices, similar to CT. However, whereas CT uses x-rays to produce images, MRI uses a strong magnetic field and the movement of hydrogen atoms based on their polarity to produce images. The obvious advantage to this approach is that it does not require radiation exposure. However, the use of incredibly high-powered magnets is not without its own dangers, and care must be taken to ensure no metal objects are brought into the MRI chamber.

Advantages of MRI include excellent (soft) tissue differentiation, a general high resolution of small tissue structures, and excellent brain imaging. The disadvantage is that an MRI scan takes longer than a CT scan (requiring longer anesthesia) and that it is more expensive. MRI is the method of choice for detecting central nervous system tumors; it is also increasingly the imaging modality of choice for analyzing the extent of soft tissue invasion of osteosarcomas.

2.2 Basic Principles of Cancer Cytology

Natali Bauer

Cancer cytology uses microscopy to examine a small amount of tumor cells on a stained slide. It is an initial diagnostic tool used to type tumors for therapeutic and prognostic purposes. Cytology has several *advantages* over more invasive biopsy techniques: it is rapid, is minimally invasive, generally does not require anesthesia, carries a lower risk of hemorrhage, and is relatively inexpensive and owners are likely to approve the procedure without much concern. Thus, it is often the first diagnostic step when cancer is suspected. More invasive biopsies are taken when cytology does not result in a definite diagnosis or when further differentiation is required (i.e., the subtype of lymphoma or a definite differentiation between mesothelioma and carcinoma). There are *a few contraindications* to taking a cytology sample. Invasive biopsy techniques are also contraindicated in these cases, and removal of the whole tumor or organ is preferred. *It is not recommended* as a sampling method of cavernous lesions in organs such as the liver and spleen (e.g., when hemangiosarcoma is suspected). The risks of hemorrhage or metastasis are higher than the benefits of diagnostic accuracy. *Cytology and/or biopsy is also not recommended* as a technique for differentiating between adenoma and carcinoma in mammary tumors. These tumors are usually a mixture of benign and malignant neoplasia, and complete surgical excision with radical mastectomy and removal of associated lymph nodes is the treatment of choice.

2.2.1 Cytology Technique: General Considerations

Additional information can improve the accuracy of cytological diagnosis. Information on the signalment and history of the patient can narrow down the most likely differentials. Understanding the biological behavior of the tumor (growth rate, size) can improve interpretation of cytological results. Appropriate aspiration technique, preparation of high-quality smears, and good staining procedures are required for the cytologist to adequately assess the sample.

The following *general rules for taking of cytological specimens* should be followed:

1. Signalment of the patient and behavior of the tumor should be included with the sample.
2. The more slides and the higher the quality of the cytological specimen, the better the diagnosis.
3. Samples taken from the margins of the tumor provide the most information, especially in cystic or necrotic masses.
4. If possible, samples should be taken from the projected site of surgical excision to avoid seeding tumor cells into healthy tissue.
5. Fine needle aspirates are more likely to represent deeper layers of tissue than fluids or superficial imprints of a mass.
6. The more vascularized the mass, the smaller the needle and the quicker aspiration should be.
7. Aspirated material cannot always be visualized in the syringe.
8. Use frosted slides labeled with a pencil.
9. Cytological specimens should not have contact with formalin fumes.

2.2.2 Cytology Technique: Specific Methods

2.2.2.1 Sampling Techniques and Preparation of Cytology Specimens

Very little material is required to prepare cytological specimens; the procedure can be performed in any veterinary practice or clinic. Materials include *glass slides* with frosted end, a *21- or 22-gauge needle*, and a *5-cc or 10-cc syringe*. Smaller needles are used for soft, vascularized masses or organs; larger needles are used for firm masses. Slides should always be labeled with a pencil because the alcohol in the staining solution dissolves ink.

Samples for cytological evaluation can be obtained by fine needle aspiration, by imprints from biopsies or masses, or by aspiration of body cavity fluids. Which method is appropriate depends on the type and localization of the tumor.

■ **Fine Needle Aspiration (FNA)**

FNA is commonly used to take samples from organs or solid masses. There are two main methods of FNA sampling: the aspiration technique and the non-aspiration technique.

The *aspiration technique* (◘ Fig. 2.1) is especially useful for firm masses. The needle with the attached syringe is inserted into the mass. The syringe is aspirated to approximately ¾; negative pressure will draw up small amounts of tissue. The needle can be moved slightly while aspirating (if the mass is large enough) to obtain cellular material from several areas. The negative pressure on the needle is gently released before the needle is removed from the mass. The needle is carefully removed from the syringe. Air is aspirated into the syringe without the needle attached. The needle is reattached. The aspirated material in the hub of the needle is then expelled onto a glass slide by rapidly depressing the plunger of the syringe.

The *non-aspiration technique* (◘ Fig. 2.2) is especially useful for highly vascularized tissues as it helps to avoid contaminating the sample with blood. Either the needle is inserted into the tissue without a syringe attached or air is drawn into the syringe prior to inserting the needle into the tissue. The needle is moved back and forth rapidly in several directions approximately ten times to obtain tissue cells which are drawn into the needle with capillary action alone. The needle is then removed from the tissue. The material at the hub is rapidly expelled on a glass slide with the method described above.

Smears are now prepared using a second glass slide. The sample material can either be spread evenly across the slide using the same technique used to *prepare a blood smear* (45° angle), or the so-called *squash preparation technique* (*or slide-over-slide technique*) is used (◘ Fig. 2.3). In the squash preparation technique, the smear is created without an angle.

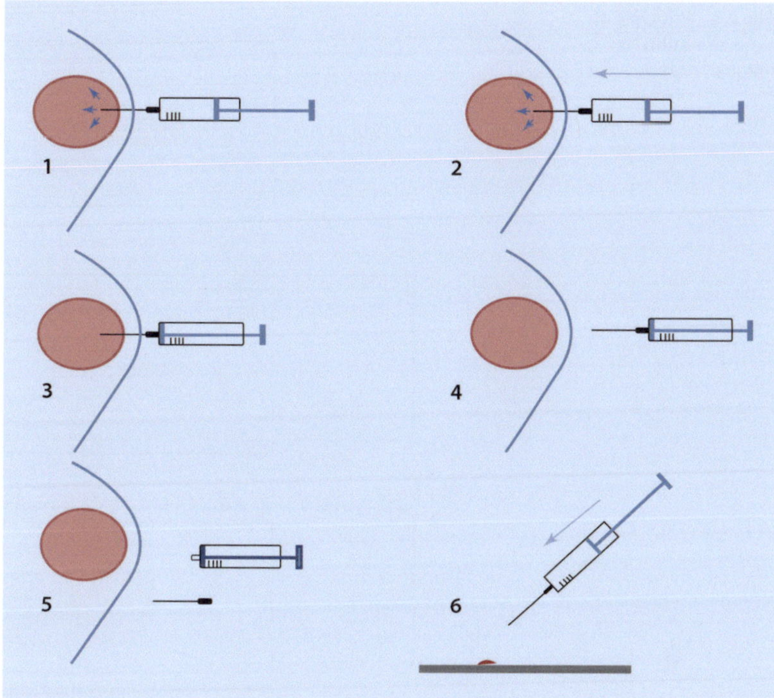

■ **Fig. 2.1** Principle of fine needle aspiration, aspiration technique

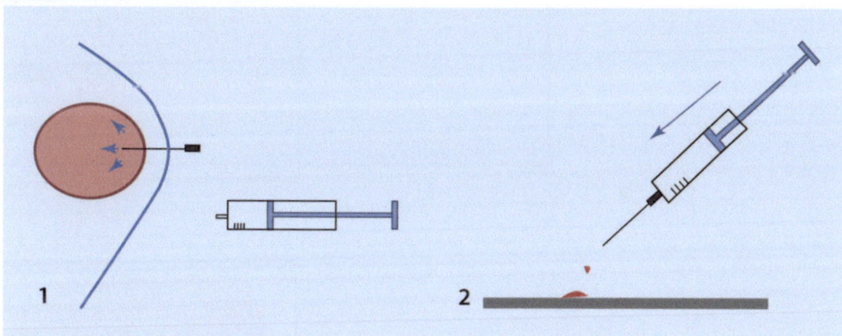

■ **Fig. 2.2** Principle of fine needle aspiration, non-aspiration technique

■ Imprint Smears

Imprints can be easily obtained from biopsies, surgically removed tissues, or the surface of ulcerated masses. Excess fluid or blood should be removed with blotting paper prior to preparing an imprint smear to avoid diluting or contaminating cellular material. The clean tissue is gently pressed against the glass slide several times, if possible (■ Fig. 2.4a). FNA should be performed in addition to impression smears to assess deeper tissue layers.

■ Evaluation of Fluids

Fluids such as *thoracic or abdominal effusions, urine* (e.g., for diagnosis of a transitional cell carcinoma), *bronchoalveolar lavage* (BAL), *cerebrospinal fluid* (CSF), or *synovial fluid* can also be evaluated to diagnose a neoplastic process.

Direct smears are usually prepared from fluid samples to assess cellularity, with the exception of CSF and BAL fluid, which usually don't contain enough cells. An evaluation of cells and even a differential cell count can also be performed on cellular fluids ($>20 \times 10^9$/L cells) without prior preparation of a sediment smear.

A *sediment smear or cytospin* can be performed on fluids with a lower cell count. Sediment can be obtained with a sedimentation chamber prepared with a syringe attached to a slide (■ Fig. 2.4b). Cells settle directly on the slide. Low-force centrifugation similar to preparation of urine sediment can also be used, but generally the results

2

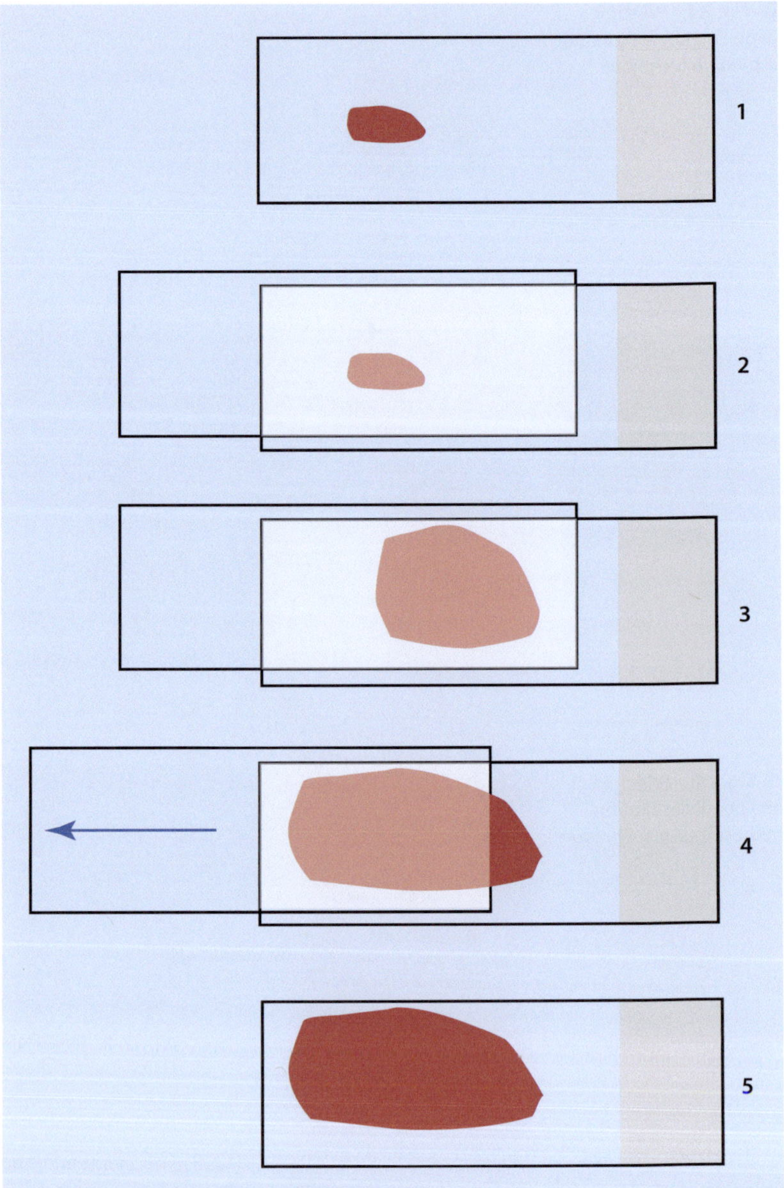

Fig. 2.3 Principle of smear preparation technique

are not as good because more cells are destroyed by mechanical force. Smears are prepared as described above

2.2.2.2 Staining Techniques

Romanowsky-type stains such as *May-Grünwald-Giemsa, Wright,* or *Diff-Quik* are the standard stains for cytological specimens in oncology. Cytological specimens should not come in contact with formalin fumes as they can markedly impair the staining quality. Immunocytological stains can be performed for classification of atypical cell populations; however, these procedures are relatively time-consuming and expensive and are therefore not routinely offered.

May-Grünwald-Giemsa or Wright Stain

The May-Grünwald-Giemsa and Wright stains are commonly performed in larger veterinary laboratories. Their *advantage* is that they provide a standardized staining result and excellent visualization of chromatin structure and nucleoli (Fig. 2.5a). Their *disadvantage* is that they take longer (i.e., approximately 30 min versus approximately 5 min for Diff-Quik).

Fig. 2.4 Principles of smear preparation. (**a**) Imprint smear. (**b**) Material and assembly of a self-made sedimentation chamber. Approximately 200 μL of fluid are filled in the chamber, the cells are allowed to settle on the slide for 1 h, and the supernatant is then removed thoroughly

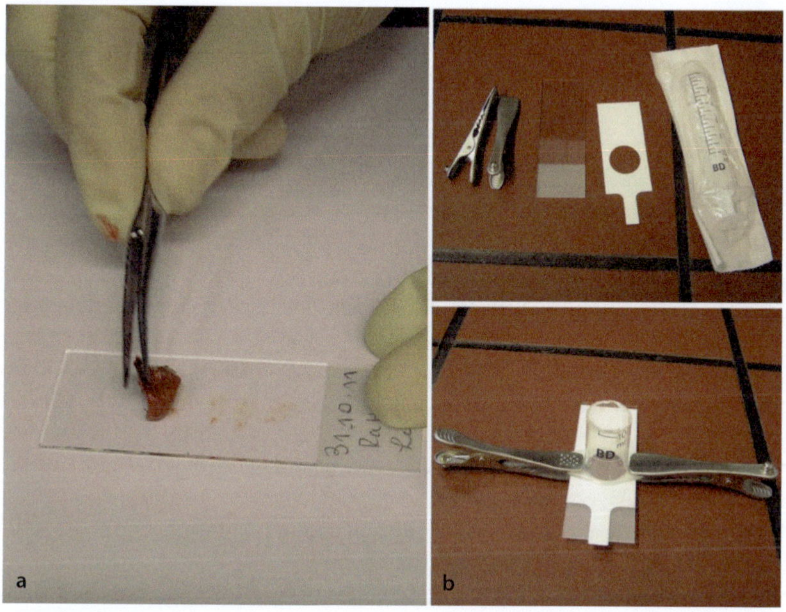

Fig. 2.5 Staining characteristics and differences in staining quality of May-Grünwald-Giemsa stain (**a**) and Diff-Quik stain (**b**), large granular lymphoma, abdominal lymph node, cat, 1000×. Note the lymphatic blasts with the clumped chromatin pattern (*red arrow*, **a**) and the large azurophilic intracytoplasmic granules (*black arrow*, **a**) seen in the May Grünwald-Giemsa-stained slide compared to the relatively indistinct chromatin structure (*red arrow*, **b**) and the weakly stained intracytoplasmic azurophilic granules (*black arrow*, **b**) observed in the Diff-Quik-stained smear

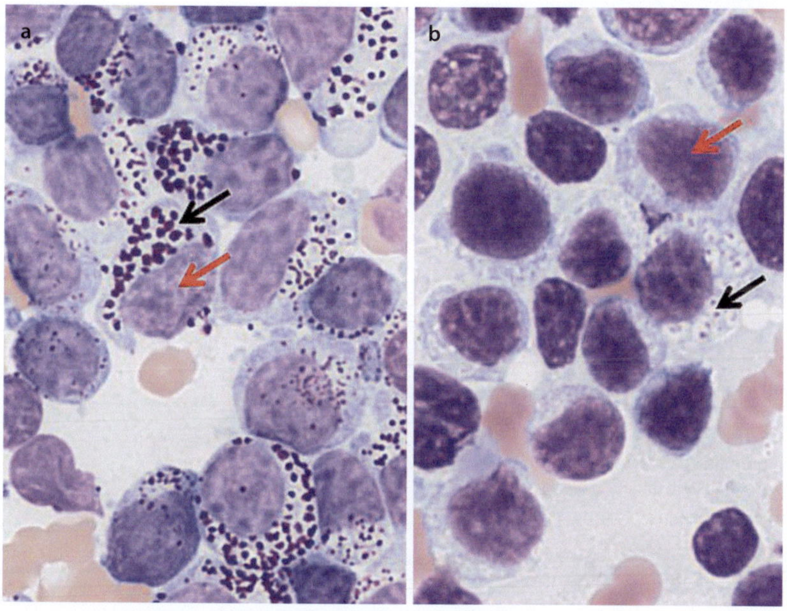

Fast Stains

Fast stains such as *Diff-Quik* are commonly performed in veterinary practices or during emergency duty. The *disadvantage* of fast stains is that the results are not standardized. Moreover, the chromatin structure and nucleoli are less distinct compared to the May-Grünwald-Giemsa or Wright stain, which makes the signs of malignancy more difficult to evaluate (Fig. 2.5b). In addition, *mast cell* granules and *granules of large granular lymphocytes* (Fig. 2.5b) do not always take up Diff-Quik stains. A second slide with May-Grünwald-Giemsa or Wright may be required to identify atypical round cells.

2.2.3 Analysis and Diagnosis of Cytological Specimens

The *major advantage* of cytology over histopathology is the ability to evaluate single-cell morphology. Some details such as intracytoplasmic granules in large granular lymphoma (◘ Fig. 2.5) or intracytoplasmic vacuoles in B-cell lymphoma with Mott cell differentiation cannot be visualized on histopathology. Cytology provides a fast and minimally invasive accurate diagnosis, especially in tumors which are classified by cellular details such as intracytoplasmic granules (◘ Fig. 2.6).

The *major limitation* of cytology is that tissue architecture cannot be evaluated. This means well-differentiated tumors cannot be discerned from hyperplastic or dysplastic tissue. Moreover, small focal processes might be easily missed by fine needle aspiration (◘ Fig. 2.7). Punch biopsies or incisional biopsies are good alternatives. Core biopsies have no advantage over cytology.

▪ Microscopic Evaluation of Cytological Specimen

Before evaluating a slide under the microscope, it is helpful to macroscopically assess their overall quality and identify regions with potential tissue cells rather than aspirated blood.

Under the microscope, the slide is first thoroughly evaluated at a low magnification (100×) without oil to assess the stain quality and preparation of the smear; the background and the overall cellular picture including the predominating cellular population; the presence of potential focal processes (e.g., clusters of metastasized cells); signs of malignancy such as high cellularity, macrocytosis, anisocytosis, anisokaryosis, and pleomorphism; and the presence of mitotic figures. The area where cells are spread in a monolayer is identified to be assessed later at a higher magnification (◘ Fig. 2.8a).

In the next step, the cellular detail is evaluated at a high magnification (600× or 1000×) with oil immersion. Here, the color and structure of cytoplasm and nuclear chromatin as well as the morphology of nucleoli are assessed (◘ Fig. 2.8b).

2.3 Basic Principles of Cancer Biopsies

A biopsy is a tissue fraction of a tumor taken for diagnosis, grading, and therapy considerations. There are several *advantages* of full-tissue biopsies compared to fine needle aspiration and cytology. Biopsies allow a more comprehensive

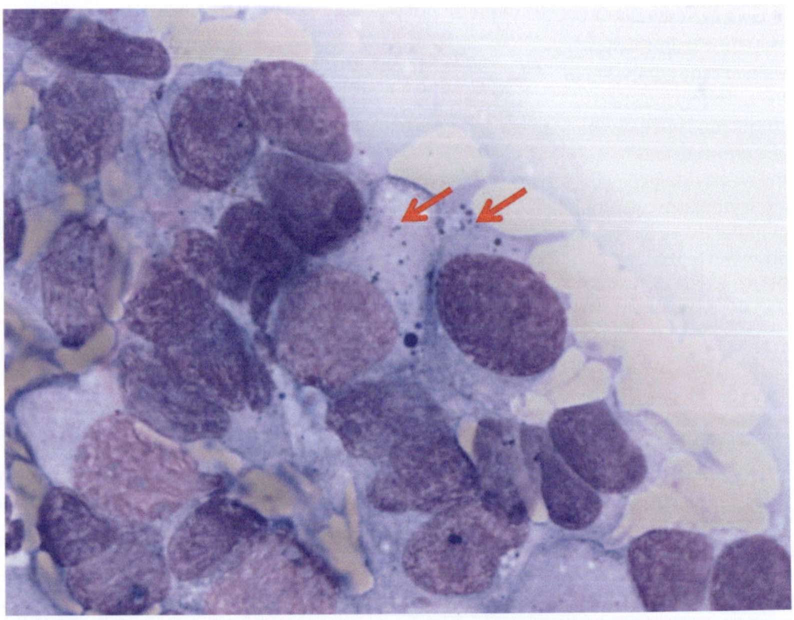

◘ **Fig. 2.6** Poorly differentiated melanoma, dog, May-Grünwald-Giemsa, 1000×. Note the spindle-shaped poorly pigmented melanocytes with a few dustlike intracytoplasmic melanin granules (*red arrow*), which can be excellently seen in cytological specimens. This is a nice example of the *advantage* of cytology as a diagnostic tool in evaluating single-cell morphology histopathologic and eventually immunohistochemical analysis of tumor cells in situ: the general tumor texture can be evaluated; the amount of necrosis and fibroplasia can be determined; the position of tumor cells relative to each other can be assessed; and the loss of cell adhesion can be assessed in epithelial tumors. When performed correctly, tissue biopsies also allow for the evaluation of tumor margins and confirm the presence or absence of tumor cells in intra- or peritumoral lymph or blood vessels. The *disadvantages* of tissue biopsies are that they are in general more elaborate, time-consuming, and costly than cytology; they may also require anesthesia and induce larger wounds.

Pretreatment biopsies are highly relevant for planning and executing of a treatment protocol once cancer has been diagnosed. They are used when cytology is not sensitive and specific enough

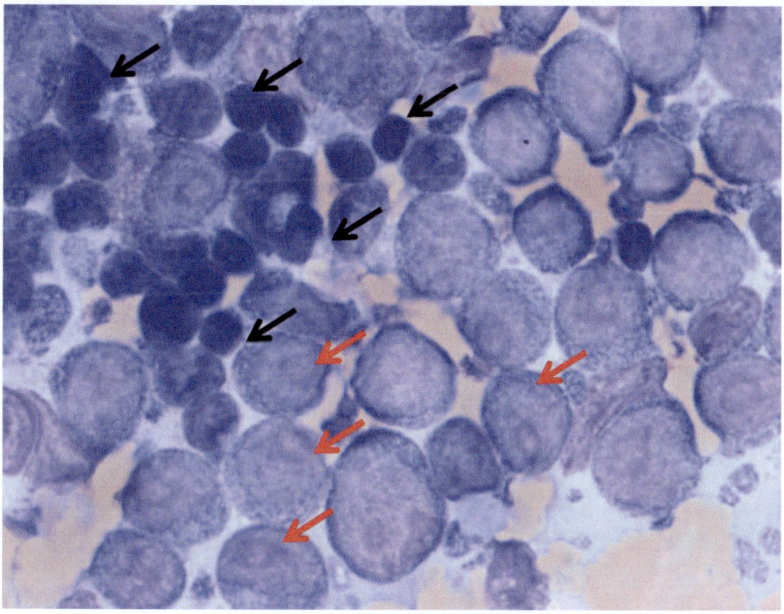

Fig. 2.7 Limitations of cytology, fine needle aspirate of the spleen, dog, May-Grünwald-Giemsa, 1000×. Note the small region with predominance of lymphatic blasts (*red arrow*) surrounded by normal splenic tissue represented by small mature lymphocytes (*black arrow*). Histopathology is required to evaluate the architecture of the splenic tissue and differentiate focal lymphoma from splenic lymph follicles

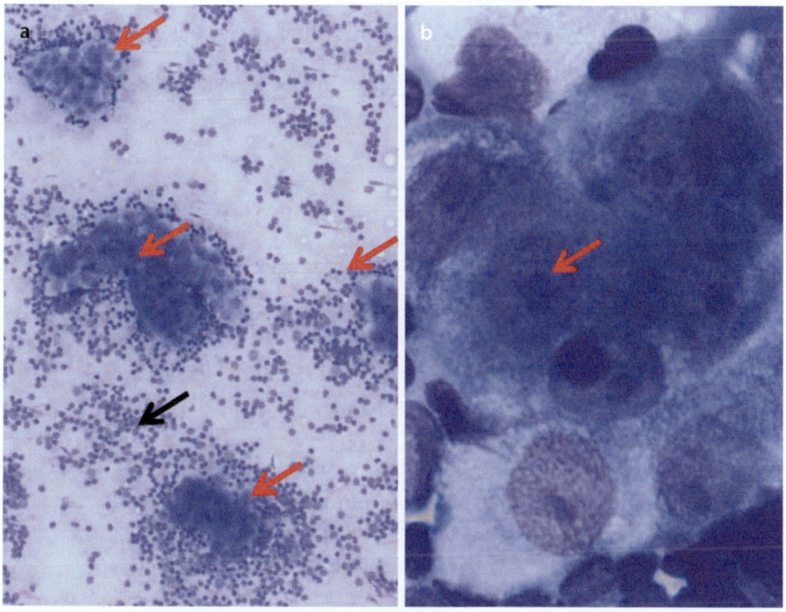

Fig. 2.8 Technique of microscopy, metastasized carcinoma in the mandibular lymph node, cat, May-Grünwald-Giemsa, 100× (**a**), 1000× (**b**). (**a**) First, the slides are evaluated at a 100× magnification to detect the overall cell population (here: small- and medium-sized mature lymphocytes, *black arrow*) and potential focal processes (here: clusters of atypical epithelial cells, *red arrow*). (**b**) Then, interesting areas are examined at a 1000× magnification to evaluate cellular details (here: finely stippled chromatin structure and macronucleoli in the carcinoma cells, *red arrow*)

for a definite tumor diagnosis. Specific indications for a pretreatment biopsy are:

2

1. Uncertainty of the neoplastic (vs. inflammatory) character of a mass
2. Uncertainty of the tumor type
3. A major impact of the tumor type/subtype on the therapy protocol (e.g., required tumor margins, presurgical chemo-/radiotherapy, euthanasia due to poor prognosis, etc.)

Postsurgical biopsies of resected tumors are also commonly submitted for histopathologic evaluation for the following indications:

1. Confirmation of the pretreatment diagnosis obtained from a small biopsy or cytological specimen
2. Evaluation of the surgical margins for evidence of incomplete resection

2.3.1 Biopsy Technique: General Considerations

Proper biopsy location within a tumor and adequate tissue preservation once the biopsy has been taken are both fundamental for the quality of the histopathologic diagnosis. (A common saying of pathologists is "Garbage in, garbage out." Or a poorly performed biopsy gives poor histopathology results.)

The preferable *location of a tumor biopsy* depends on the type, stage, and location of the tumor and is therefore often not perfectly predictable. Biopsies taken from the *tumor center* of a malignant, fast-growing neoplasia may only contain necrotic tissue (due to hypoxia as vascularization moves outward toward the tumor periphery where active cell division is taking place). Biopsies taken from the *tumor periphery* are very helpful in the evaluation of tumor margins and vascular invasion but may only contain cells from the tumor capsule or inflamed peripheral nonneoplastic tissue if the biopsy is not large enough. Under best possible conditions, *several biopsies from different areas* of the tumor center and tumor margins are taken for maximal representation.

An accurate histopathologic diagnosis of a biopsy is only possible if the *tissue handling* preserves the original morphology of the cells and tissue structure. Autolysis due to *insufficient or delayed formalin fixation*, tissue and cell destruction due to *unnecessary mechanical forces from coarse forceps*, or thermal *destruction of cell nuclei due to electrocautery* are common avoidable artifacts. The following *general rules for taking a biopsy* should therefore be considered:

1. The larger the biopsy, the better the diagnosis.
2. The larger the biopsy, the more fixative is required (tissue: fixative ratio of 1:10).
3. Tumor margins are usually the most informative area for pathologists (except for bone tumors).
4. Surgical instead of coarse anatomical forceps avoid unnecessary mechanical trauma.
5. Avoid seeding tumor cells in the biopsy channel or body cavities.
6. Avoid electrocautery and associated thermal tissue destruction.
7. Fix biopsies immediately in 4 % formaldehyde to prevent autolysis and reduction of countable mitotic figures.

2.3.2 Biopsy Technique: Specific Methods

Core Needle Biopsy

Core needle biopsies (*CNB*) use a cutting-edge biopsy needle with a hollow core (Fig. 2.9). A small cylinder-shaped tissue sample, *usually 14 gauge/1 mm in diameter and 1 cm long*, is obtained. CNB is used for external skin masses and masses in internal organs. Bone tumor biopsies are

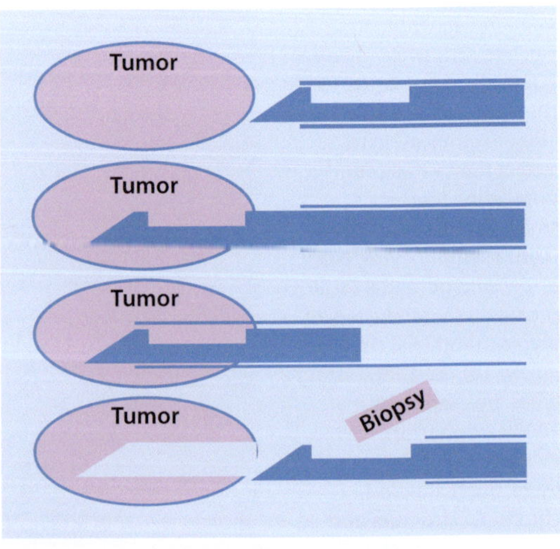

Fig. 2.9 Principle of core needle biopsy

obtained using more stable *hollow core drill needles*, trocars, or regular core needles in cases of accessible, superficial bone tumors. In contrast to other tumors, *bone tumor biopsies should be taken from the center* of the tumor to avoid peripheral reactive nonneoplastic bone tissue.

Computed tomography or ultrasound guidance is usually necessary to get a sufficiently accurate biopsy for diagnostic evaluation when taking core needle biopsies of internal organs and bone tumors. *Local anesthesia* and a small skin cut are necessary to avoid unnecessary pain and blunting of the needle. *Several needle cores* of different areas of the tumor may be obtained through one skin incision to increase the representativeness of the biopsy. CNB is *more accurate than cytological samples* but less accurate than excisional or incisional biopsies, which are usually larger.

Punch Biopsy

A *punch biopsy* removes a round cutaneous tissue sample using a sharp hollow cutting punch with a *diameter of 3–7 mm* (Fig. 2.10). It was *originally designed for obtaining skin biopsies* and allows the excision of wider but shorter tissue samples than core needle biopsies. For deeper subcutaneous tumors, the skin has to be incised first to reach the actual tumor mass. The base of the core is cut off using scissors, and the wound has to be closed using one or two sutures or staples. Anesthesia is necessary similar to core needle biopsies.

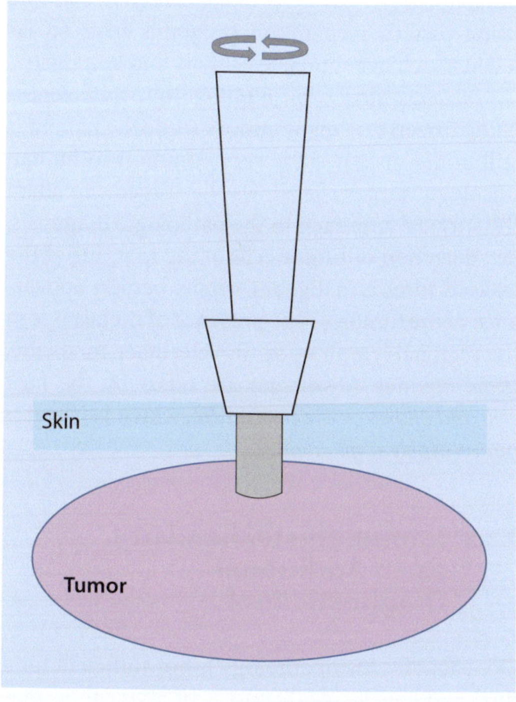

Fig. 2.10 Principle of punch biopsy

Incisional Biopsy

An *incisional biopsy* is a wedge-shaped segment of tissue excised using a scalpel (Fig. 2.11). *Tumor samples are larger* using this method, which allows for a *more accurate diagnosis*. Incisional biopsies *are recommended if*:

1. Both core needle and punch biopsies failed to obtain a representative tissue sample.
2. A larger tissue sample is required from a necrotic/ulcerated tumor.
3. An exploratory laparotomy allows the removal of a larger tumor piece.

Anesthesia and wound closure with sutures or staples are necessary. Electrocautery should not be used prior to complete removal of the tissue biopsies to avoid thermal artifacts.

Excisional Biopsy

Excisional biopsy includes the *complete excision of the tumor* without presurgical analysis of the tumor type (Fig. 2.12). It is the *method of choice for small, slowly growing cutaneous tumors, splenic tumors, and pulmonary tumors*. These tumors are treated with standard protocols, regardless of the specific tumor type. For all other tumor types, non-excisional biopsies should be considered first because histopathologic tumor classification may allow for a customized treatment protocol based on a pretreatment diagnosis.

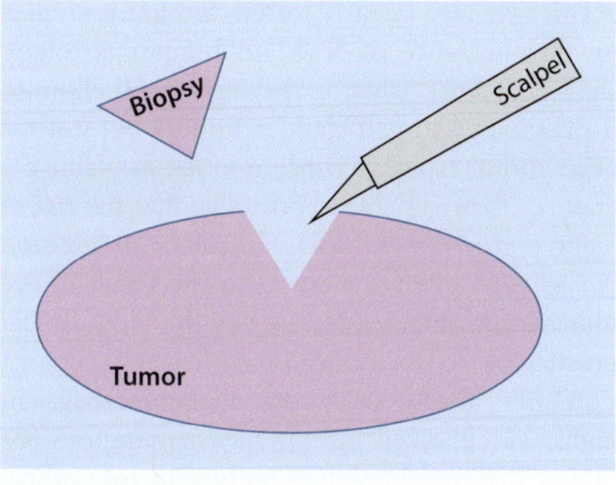

Fig. 2.11 Principle of incisional biopsies

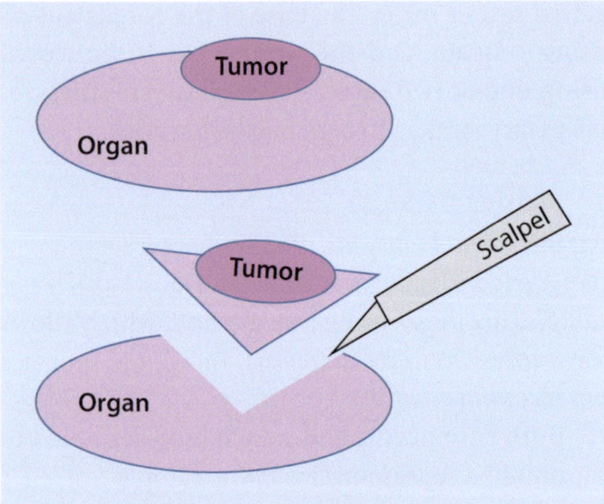

■ **Fig. 2.12** Principle of excisional biopsies

2.3.3 Biopsy-Associated Risks

There is a significant body of literature that warns clinicians about the *risk of seeding tumor cells* (*needle tract metastasis, NTM*) or even inducing distant metastasis by taking biopsies in companion animals. A recently published meta-analysis found that although *NTM is a very rare event,* biopsy-induced seeding of tumor cells into the biopsy tract may be a potential risk. There is *no evidence that supports the hypothesis of biopsy-induced malignancy* in the available literature on human or veterinary oncology. There are only seven reported cases in the literature of needle tract metastases or tumor seeding in companion animals. Five cases of *transcutaneous fine needle aspirations of canine transitional cell carcinomas* of the urogenital tract have been reported in the literature. One case of *canine prostate carcinoma* and one case of *pulmonary adenocarcinoma* with NTM have also been reported. Similarly, studies on the incidence of NTM in human oncology show some risk when biopsying mesotheliomas, melanomas, and gall bladder tumors but not for other tumor types. According to the available literature, it's reasonable to postulate that the *risk of biopsy-induced metastasis and tumor progression is negligible* when compared to the value of the information obtained by biopsies for daily clinical practice.

Other biopsy risks include hemorrhage in highly vascularized tumors like hemangiosarcomas or the introduction of pathogens into otherwise sterile structures like the globe of the eye.

2.3.4 Histopathologic Analysis and Diagnosis of Tissue Biopsies

The *major advantage of histopathologic evaluation* of biopsies over cytology is the possibility to evaluate tumor cells in their structural context. For instance, biopsies of tumor margins can be used to evaluate invasiveness, to assess whether the tumor capsule is intact, and to look for anaplastic epithelial tumor cells.

The basic and most commonly used method for histopathologic evaluation of tumor samples is the hematoxylin-eosin (H/E) stain of formalin-fixed and paraffin-embedded biopsies (■ Fig. 2.13). The major principle of paraffin embedding, microtome sectioning, and H/E staining is illustrated in Fig. 2.13a–e.

Veterinary oncology bases its tumor classification system on the *WHO Histological Classification of Tumors of Domestic Species* (publisher Armed Forces Institute of Pathology and World Health Organization, ■ Figs. 2.14 and 2.15). The WHO classification is supplemented by relevant scientific reports on the clinicopathologic features of animal tumors. Histopathologic diagnoses are currently still based on *trained human skills for pattern recognition* and experience. *Attempts to substitute human histopathologic skills by image analysis software* using pattern recognition programs have so far failed to achieve similar sensitivity and specificity.

Intraoperative consultation by pathologists using frozen section of tumors while the patient is still under anesthesia is very common in human oncologic surgery. It allows the surgeon to adapt the surgical approach to the pathologic diagnosis, i.e., detection of tumor cells at the margins of the excised tumor, malignant versus benign appearance of the tumor, or the presence of metastases in the regional lymph node. In veterinary medicine, these obvious advantages are offset by the *high cost and efforts* of the procedure, which is why it *is not routinely implemented.*

2.3.5 Immunohistochemistry as an Additional Diagnostic Tool

Occasionally, histopathology is not sufficient for a final and conclusive diagnosis of atypical or anaplastic epithelial or stromal tumors. In addition,

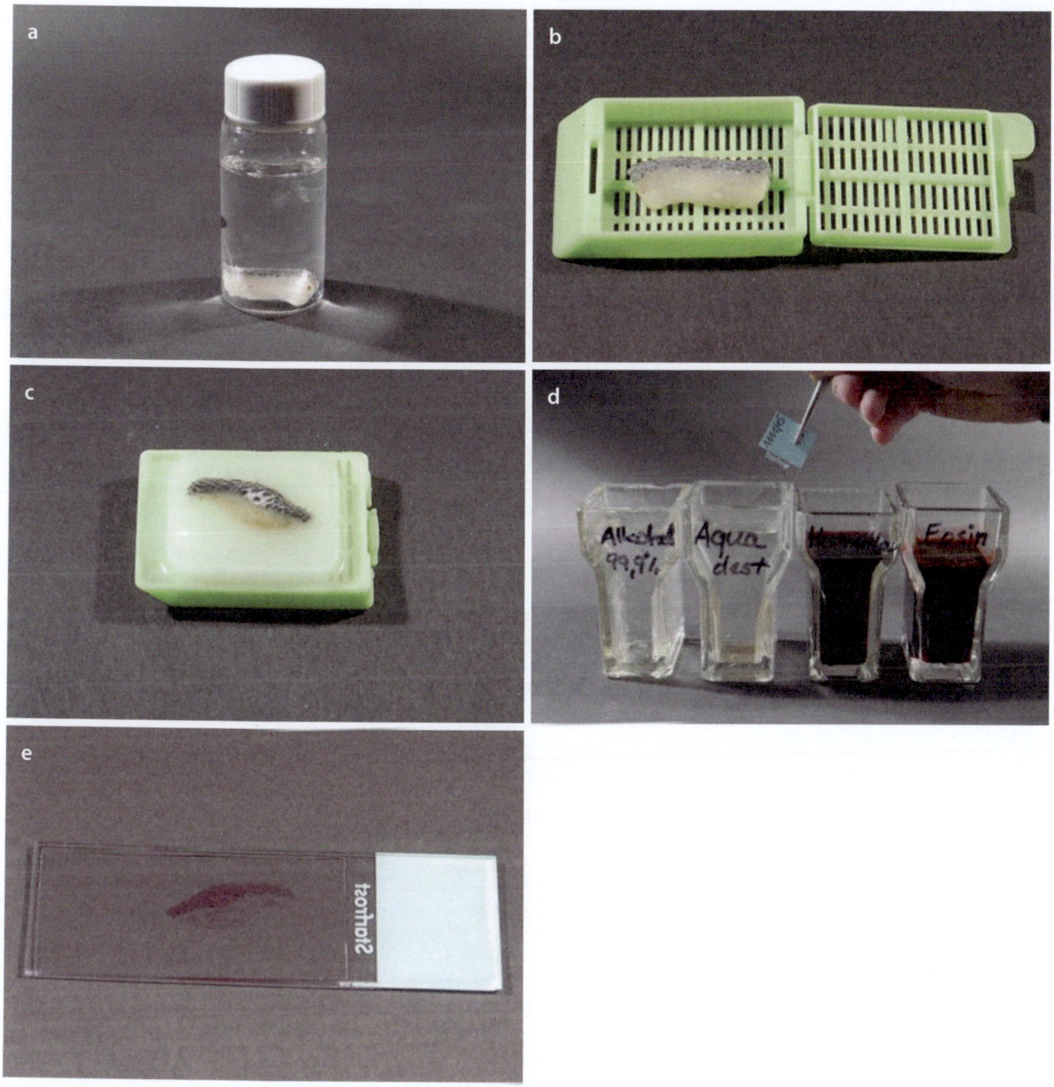

Fig. 2.13 Principle of hematoxylin-eosin staining of formalin-fixed and paraffin-embedded tissue biopsies. (**a**) Formalin-fixed biopsies are cut into several mm-thick tissue slices and (**b**) put into histology cassettes. (**c**) Subsequently, tissue samples are embedded in paraffin and cut with a microtome into histologic sections a few µm thick. (**d**, **e**) Finally, sections are deparaffinized, stained with hematoxylin and eosin, and placed on cover-slipped slides

2

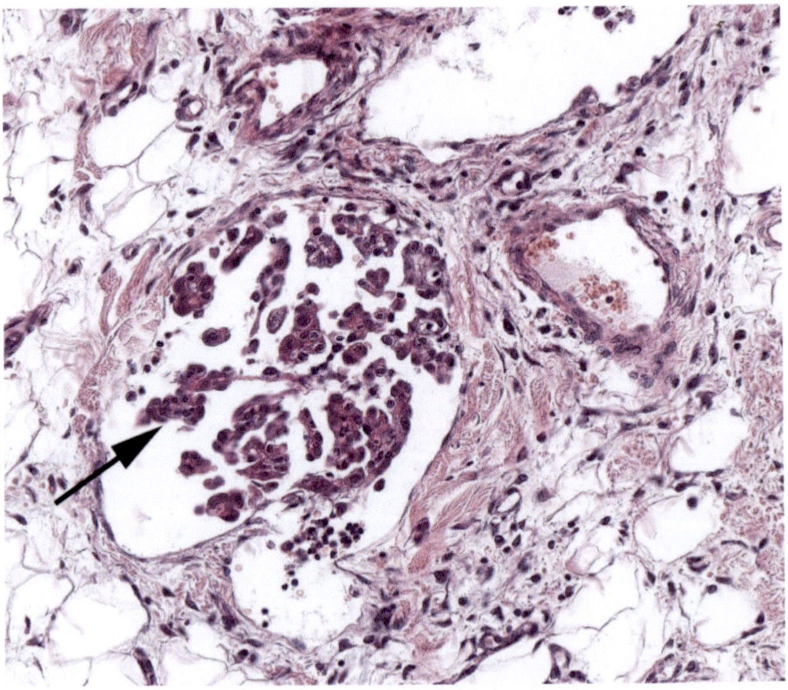

Fig. 2.14 Hematoxylin-eosin (H/E) stain of intravascular metastatic tumor cells of a canine mammary carcinoma (*arrow*). Cell nuclei are *blue* while the cytoplasm and most other structures are *purple*

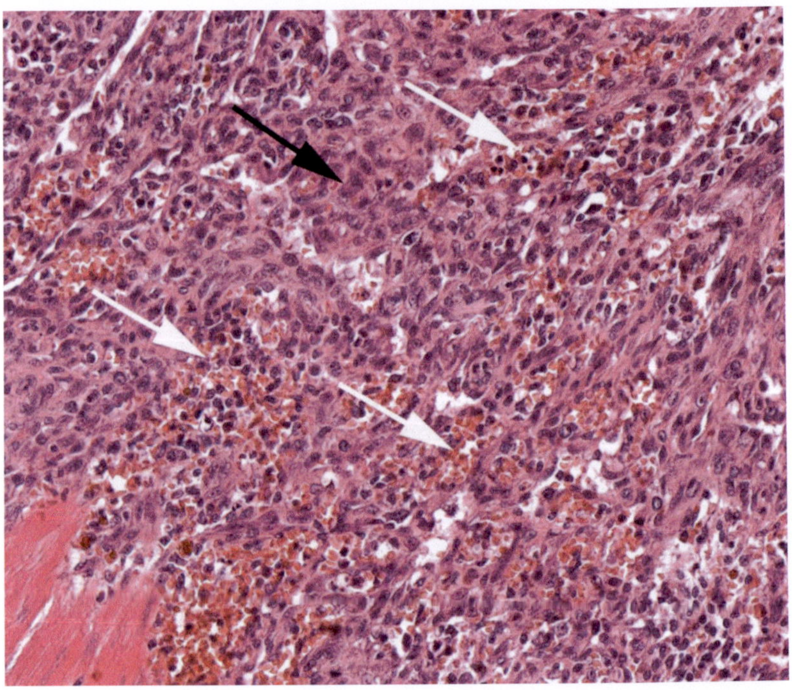

Fig. 2.15 Hematoxylin-eosin (H/E) stain of an almost solid canine hemangiosarcoma. A few erythrocytes and vessel-like cavities (*white arrows*) are interspersed between abundant mostly plump neoplastic endothelial cells (*black arrows*)

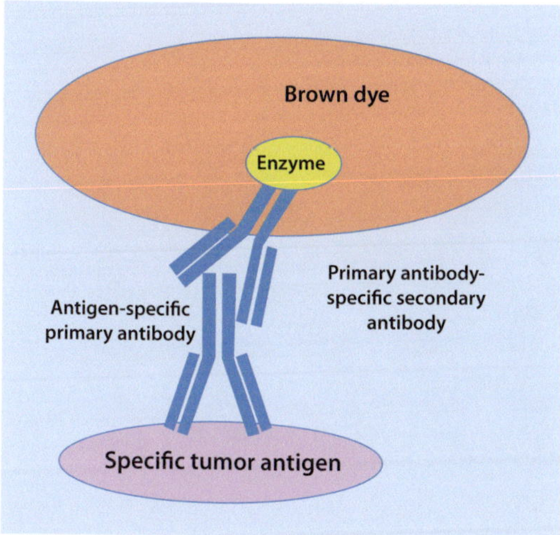

Fig. 2.16 Principle of indirect immunohistochemistry: the tumor is marked with an antigen-specific primary antibody; the primary antibody is marked with a primary antibody-specific secondary antibody; the secondary antibody is conjugated with an enzyme; the bound enzyme converts a colorless medium into a brown dye

hematopoietic round cell tumors like B-cell or T-cell lymphoma are not finely discernable by their histopathologic features in H/E-stained slides. *Immunohistochemistry* (*IHC*) for the detection of tumor-specific proteinaceous markers is a common method to supplement histopathology. IHC is based on the high sensitivity of antibodies for specific epitopes in and on the cells in histopathologic sections (Fig. 2.16). Enzymatic reactions with dyes of different colors are stably incorporated into the tissue around the antibody binding site, which can then be visualized. Table 2.2 summarizes the most commonly used IHC markers in veterinary oncology.

Table 2.2 Common immunohistochemical tumor markers in veterinary oncology

Tumor marker	Detected cell type	Typical staining pattern
CD3	T-lymphocyte origin	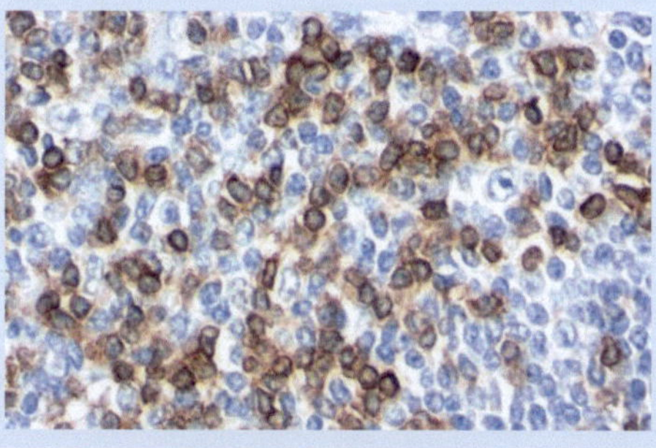
PAX5	B-lymphocyte origin	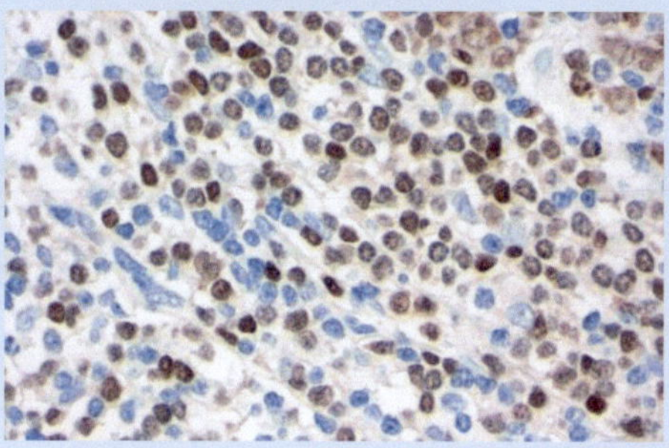

(continued)

2

Table 2.2 (continued)

Tumor marker	Detected cell type	Typical staining pattern
CD45R, CD79	B-lymphocyte origin	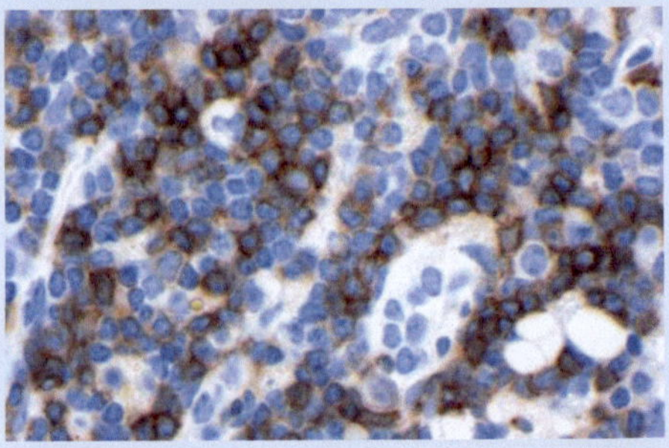
KIT (CD117)	Diverse, mainly mast cell origin, gastrointestinal stromal tumors (GIST)	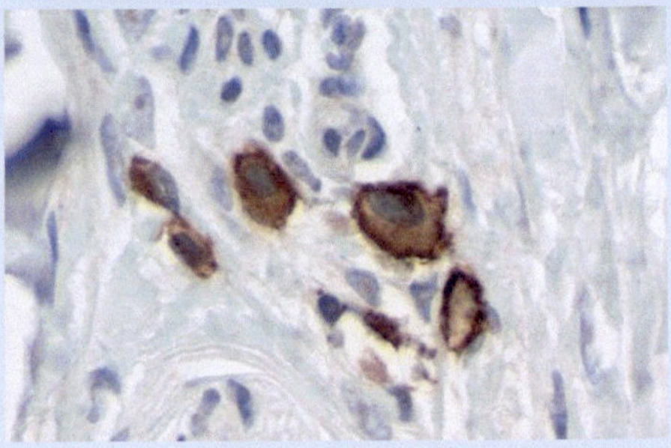
Vimentin	Mesodermal (stromal) cell origin	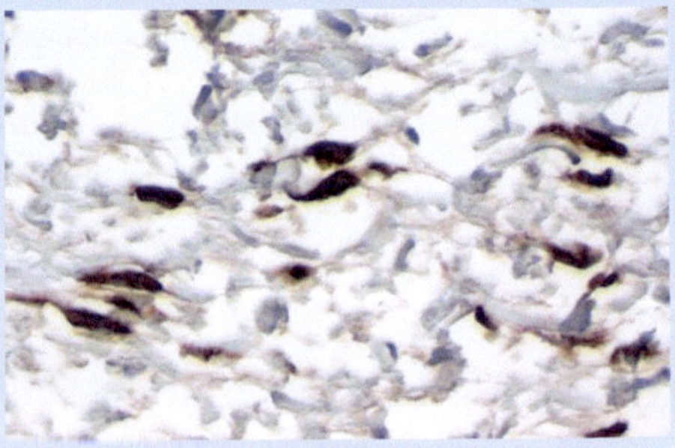
Pan-cytokeratin	Epithelial cell origin	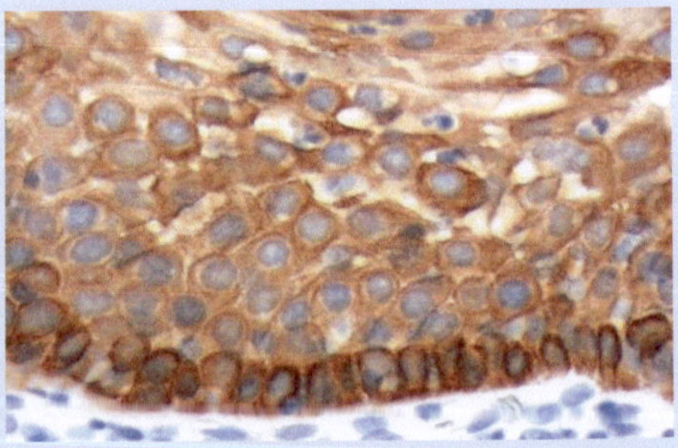

Table 2.2 (continued)

Tumor marker	Detected cell type	Typical staining pattern
Smooth muscle actin (SMA)	Smooth muscle cell origin	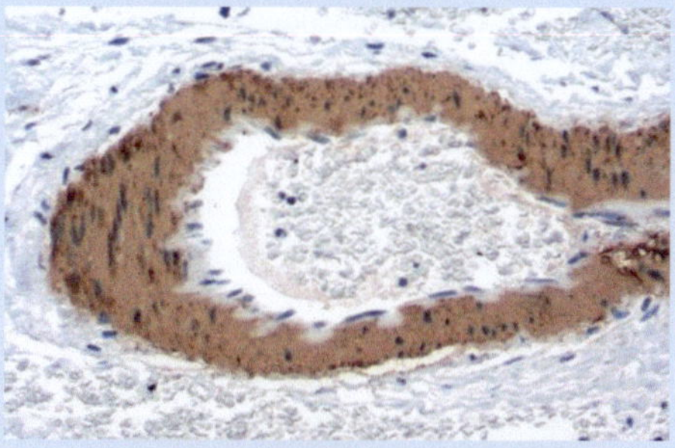
Melan A	Neuroectodermal (melanocyte) cell origin	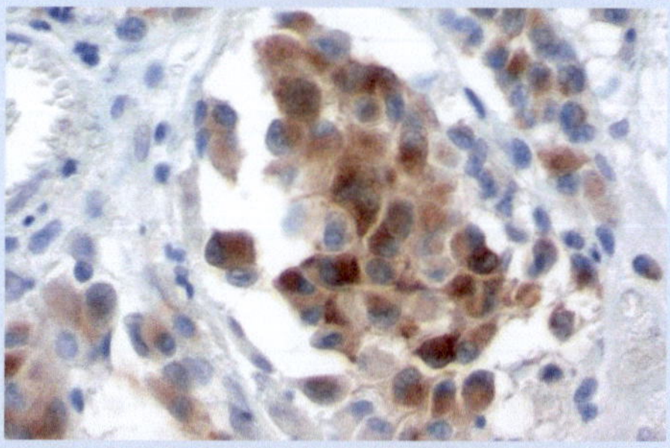
S100	Neuroectodermal cells	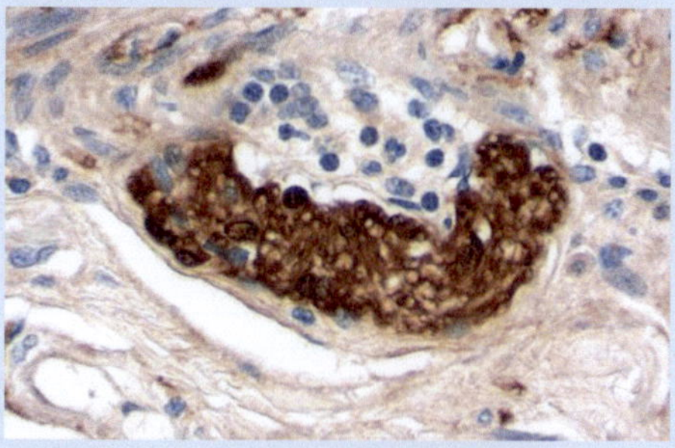
Synaptophysin	Neuroendocrine cell origin	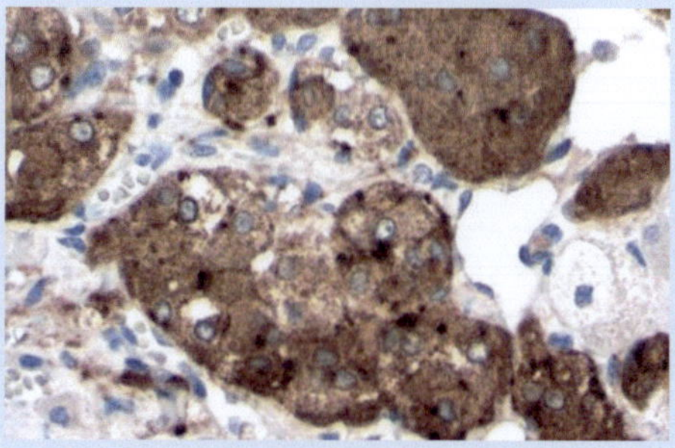

(continued)

Table 2.2 (continued)

Tumor marker	Detected cell type	Typical staining pattern
Chromogranin	Neuroendocrine cell origin	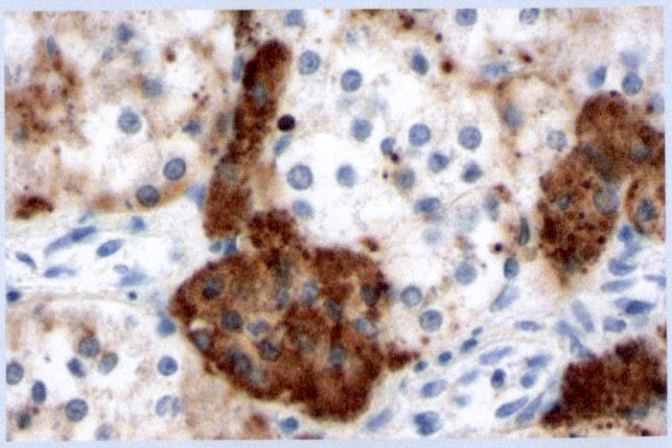
Von Willebrand factor (vWF)	Endothelial cell origin	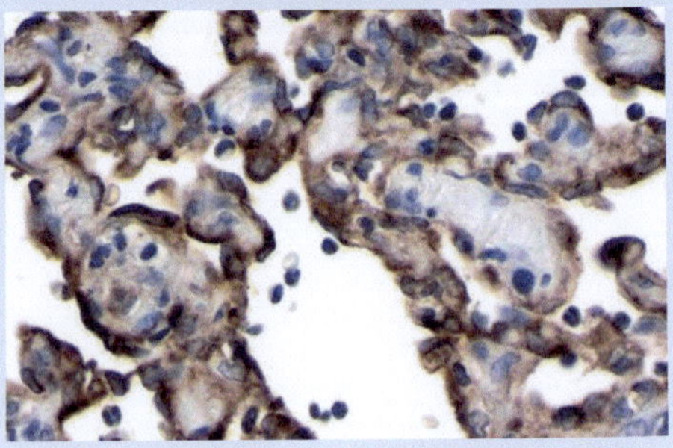
CD31	Endothelial cell origin	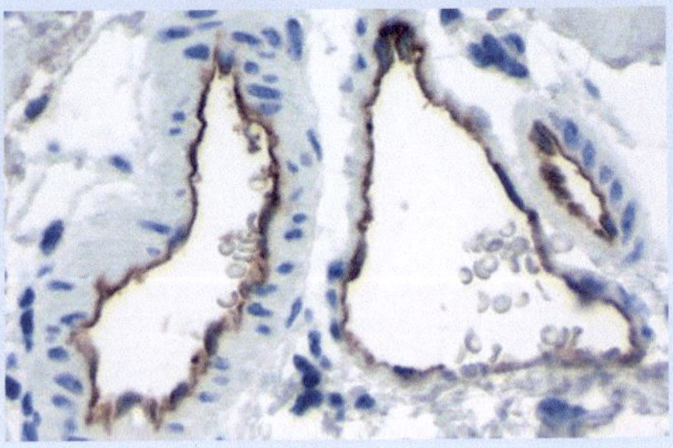

Basic Principles of Cancer Therapy

Mathias Brunnberg, Robert Klopfleisch, and Melanie Wergin

R. Klopfleisch (ed.), *Veterinary Oncology*, DOI 10.1007/978-3-319-41124-8_3

Therapeutic treatment of cancer often depends in large part on finances in veterinary oncology. While surgery is still the most commonly used treatment option, chemotherapy, radiotherapy, and imaging modalities such as PET scans used in human medicine are prohibitively expensive in veterinary medicine. However, new state-of-the-art treatment centers are being built in most countries, which make cutting-edge diagnostics and therapy available to veterinary patients. Although still a sobering diagnosis, cancer is no longer the death sentence that it once was, and treatment options in veterinary oncology are evolving rapidly.

The most common therapeutic modalities in veterinary oncology are *surgery, chemotherapy, and radiotherapy, each* applied with variable success. Selection of the treatment option and success of treatment, both very much depend on the tumor type, the stage of tumor development, and the location of the tumor. Defining *some of the common terms and definitions used in veterinary oncology* will help us in our discussion in the following chapters on general and specific aspects of cancer therapy.

Curative therapy aims at and anticipates the complete removal or killing of all tumor cells and thus the complete cure of the patient.

Palliative therapy, in contrast, aims at palliation of unpleasant symptoms associated with the neoplastic disease. Cure is neither achievable nor expected.

The *definition of the extent of remission* during or after therapy is defined by the *Response Evaluation Criteria In Solid Tumors* (*RECIST*). Remission is difficult to differentiate in its stages and to define in veterinary medicine. In human medicine, PET scans are often used as the imaging modality of choice to detect the presence of neoplastic cells after therapy and determine remission status. This is not commonly available in veterinary medicine due to cost considerations.

Complete remission (*CR*) is the complete disappearance of the tumor during or after therapy. The tumor is no longer detectable by physical examination, imaging, or hematologic or biochemical analysis.

Partial remission (*PR*) is defined as a 30 % decrease in the sum of the largest diameters of two neoplastic lesions in one organ or five lesions in the whole body. Computed tomography (CT) and magnetic resonance imaging (MRI) are the preferred methods for diameter measurement.

Progressive disease (*PD*) is defined as a 20 % increase in the sum of the largest diameters of the lesions after or during therapy.

Stable disease (*SD*) is defined as being neither in remission nor in progression.

Median survival is the length of time after initial therapy at which 50 % of the patients have died and 50 % of the patients are alive.

Disease-free interval (*DFI*) is defined as the time between complete remission and local recurrence or development of metastases.

Progression-free interval/survival (*PFI/PFS*) is defined as the time period after therapy during which stable disease (SD) was achieved.

3.1 Oncologic Surgery

M. Brunnberg

"Surgery is the oldest treatment for cancer and, as a single modality, cures more animals and people with cancer than any other treatment"(VSSO). Surgery plays a key role in most treatment plans for small animal cancer patients. Oncologic surgery describes the use of surgery as sole treatment. In contrast, the term surgical oncology is usually used to describe surgical procedures performed in conjunction with other treatments like chemotherapy or radiation therapy.

Typical surgical procedures in oncology include complete resection with a curative intention, palliative procedures to alleviate pain and improve quality of life, and diagnostic surgeries including biopsies and cytoreductive or debulking surgeries. Numerous factors influence which type of surgery is appropriate in a given case, including tumor type, the presence of local or distant metastasis, patient health status, patient age, and owner expectations. The surgeon should be well informed on these factors prior to surgery in order to choose the most appropriate treatment. A multidisciplinary approach to patient assessment, with collaboration between pathologists, radiologists, oncologists, and internists, is required to evaluate the need and the invasiveness of the surgery, the resectability of the tumor, as well as the determination of possible pre-, intra-, and postoperative complications.

3.1.1 Patient Preparation

Evaluating the patient's status prior to surgery using diagnostic imaging, fine needle aspirates or biopsies, and laboratory tests is important for two reasons. First, an initial *tumor characterization* has to be performed to estimate factors like tumor type, dimensions, stage, vascularization, and lymph node involvement. Those factors have a direct influence on the choice of surgical procedures. Second, veterinary cancer patients are usually older animals and often suffer from several *comorbidities*, which put them at a higher risk of intra- or postoperative complications. For instance, oncology patients are often cachectic which might complicate wound healing. Since most oncology surgeries are elective procedures, treatment of comorbidities and stabilization of the patient can and should be initiated prior to surgery.

Reconstructive techniques for wound closure need to be carefully considered before surgery when treating large skin tumors or undertaking widespread resections. The widest possible surgical field is clipped, sterilized, and draped, keeping in mind that it might be necessary to increase the operating field during surgery or change the type of resection intraoperatively. Perioperative antibiotic treatment is usually indicated.

3.1.2 General Aspects of Oncologic Surgery

The *basic surgical instrument* set includes atraumatic forceps and variable numbers of traumatic and atraumatic tissue clamps. Direct manipulation of the mass should be avoided. Instruments and gloves should be changed after direct tumor contact since repeated contact increases the risk of tumor seeding. Electrosurgery, laser surgery, and cryosurgery tend to cause severe tissue degeneration at the line of incision, which can impede proper margin assessment by the pathologist. Although these are useful tools, they may not be the most appropriate choice for oncologic surgery.

Most general surgical principles are also valid for oncologic surgery. This includes the fact that the first procedure is the most likely to succeed. With each successive procedure, the chances for a curative outcome are reduced. It is also important to follow *Halsted's principles*, which include gentle tissue handling, control of hemorrhage, strictly aseptic technique, preservation of blood supply to tissues, elimination of dead space, and accurate tension-free wound closure. Halsted's principles are particularly important when treating skin tumors. Surgical *tumor removal approaches* can be characterized as intralesional, marginal, and wide or radical resection. The type of resection should be selected based on the tumor type, location, and further comorbidities (▫ Table 3.1).

The *skin incision* is usually performed with a scalpel blade. Scalpel incisions provide the clearest margins for histopathological diagnosis. A combination of sharp and blunt dissection along tissue planes is usually performed with scissors. Direct manipulation of the mass with forceps or other graspers can lead to fragmentation of the mass and subsequent tumor seeding. In general the surgery should be as atraumatic as possible.

During surgery the following *important tumor zones* have to be considered: the tumor mass, the pseudocapsule, the reactive zone, and the surrounding healthy tissue (▫ Fig. 3.1). If the goal of the surgery is complete removal of the mass, then the intralesional pseudocapsule zones should be resected. Marginal resection has to be avoided whenever possible due to the risk of leaving tumor cells behind. Vessels supplying or draining the tumor should be ligated early during surgery to avoid tumor cell migration during manipulation.

Wound closure with a monofilament suture material close to the tumor bed is recommended to minimize the risk of tumor cell trapping. Wound lavage or body cavity lavage in oncologic surgery is controversial. On the one hand, lavage might induce tumor cell migration, but on the other hand, removal of blood clots and foreign material and hydration of tissue are strongly recommended to avoid complications in wound healing.

3

Table 3.1 Technique and indication for different resection types in oncologic surgery

Type of resection	Technique	Indication
Intralesional	Intracapsular piecemeal removal of the mass Most of the tumor not removed	Benign lesions Cytoreductive surgery Debulking surgery
Marginal	Extra- or pseudocapsular dissection through the reactive zone Microscopic satellite tumors not removed	Benign tumors (e.g., lipomas) Prior to radiation therapy
Wide	Intended to remove all tumor cells With additional tumor type/grade-dependent margin of healthy tissue	Curative intent surgery Most solid tumors
Radical	Removal of the tumor with the entire compartment including abundant healthy tissue	Bone tumors Highly malignant tumors

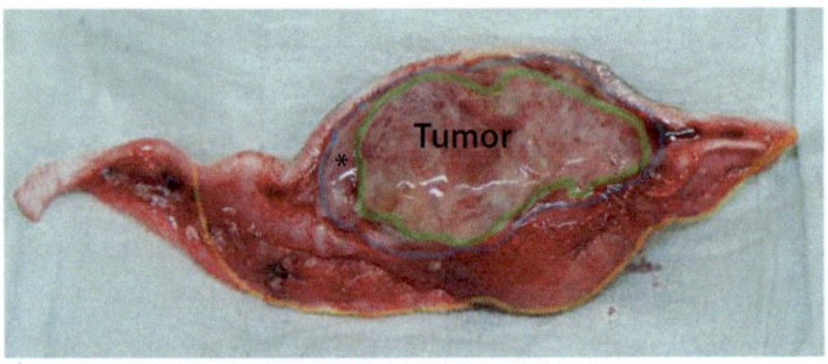

Fig. 3.1 Carpal neurofibrosarcoma mass of a 7-year-old male Staffordshire terrier. The pseudocapsule/reactive zone (*star*) and resection margins (*green* intralesional, *blue* marginal, *orange* wide) are indicated

The use of *drains* is generally not indicated in oncologic surgery. In case of seroma formation drains can be used after margin assessment of the mass. If postoperative external beam therapy is planned, it is useful to mark the wound bed and the tumor margins to determine the extent of the radiation field. For histopathologic margin assessment, the margins should be labeled with sutures, ink, or other marking techniques. Most *common mistakes* in oncologic surgery include incomplete resection, intraoperative tumor seeding, and the use of inappropriate suture material and instruments as well as traumatic techniques.

3.1.3 Oncologic Surgery of Bone Tumors

Osteosarcomas is the most common bone tumor in dogs and cats. It is often metastatic, and hence screening of the entire patient and tumor staging should be performed. Advanced diagnostic tools like scintigraphy might also be indicated. Surgical treatment is usually curative in cats but is considered palliative in dogs.

The most common types of surgery in bone tumors are radical resections (amputations) and wide resections. Prior to limb amputation, the animal should be examined for orthopedic or neurologic diseases of the contralateral limb, which influence postoperative functionality and quality of life. Furthermore, the owner should be thoroughly informed of what to expect after amputation. Radical amputations, including scapulectomy for treating tumors of the forelimb and femur osteotomy for treating tumors of the hind limb, are both controversial procedures. Subtotal amputations offer some degree of lateral protection of the thorax or caudal abdomen and are often easier to perform. However, subtotal amputations also leave additional dead weight in the form of nonfunctional stumps in the place of the limbs. This additional weight can have an impact on postoperative gait mechanics. Total limb amputations have the advantage of removing this dead weight.

Tumors of the phalanx and digits are usually treated by amputation of the digit or phalanx only. Limb-sparing surgeries (Fig. 3.2) or osteosynthesis of pathologic fractures are less commonly performed. Possible tumor locations for limb-sparing surgeries are shown in Table 3.2.

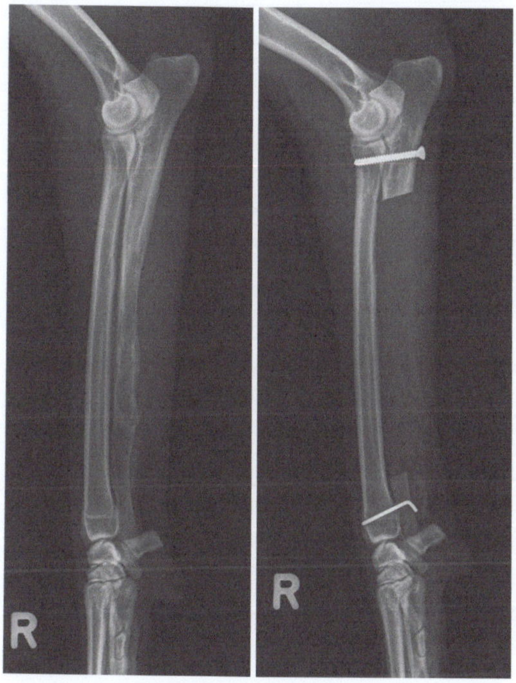

Fig. 3.2 Radiograph of the right front limb of a flat-coated retriever with an appendicular osteosarcoma before (*left*) and after (*right*) partial ulnar resection

Although wide and radical resections are described as the treatment of choice in appendicular bone tumors, there are cases where osteosynthesis of tumor-associated pathologic fractures makes sense. Neurologic or orthopedic disease of the contralateral limb, as well as cosmetic concerns, might be good reasons not to amputate. Most discussions in the literature mention plate osteosynthesis as the method of choice for pathologic fracture stabilization, but all stabilization methods commonly used for traumatic fractures can also be used for pathologic fractures as long as stable fixation of the implant can be achieved.

Bone tumors of the head or the axial skeleton usually cannot be treated by wide or radical resections. Instead debulking procedures or surgeries with marginal resections are performed. Advanced imaging techniques like computer tomography (CT) or MRI should be performed prior to surgery to evaluate the dimensions of the tumor and possible intradural or intraaxial involvement. Mandibular or maxillary tumors in dogs can be treated with good success rates with varying degrees of mandibulectomies or maxillectomies, respectively.

3.1.4 Oncologic Surgery of Skin Tumors

Primary wound closure can be sacrificed for the purpose of achieving appropriate margins in oncologic surgery. Understanding open wound management, tension-relieving techniques, skin grafting, and reconstruction techniques is therefore essential for oncologic surgery. Body wall reconstructive techniques might be necessary if the body wall is involved.

Various local or subdermal plexus skin flaps can be used for small- or moderate-sized skin defects. Preservation of the local blood supply to the flap is the key to flap survival. Skin defects on the lower extremities are treated with tension-relieving techniques like relaxing incisions or free skin grafts. Axial pattern flaps are used for large skin defects. They contain a cutaneous artery and vein, which allows preparation of larger flaps and a better flap survival compared to free grafts. Different skin-closing techniques and common axial pattern flaps are listed in Table 3.3.

3.1.5 Oncologic Surgery of Central Nervous System Tumors

Tumors of the nervous system can be differentiated into intracranial, spinal, and peripheral tumors. There are some case reports of successful treatment of intra- and extra-axial tumors, although brain surgery in small animal patients is still in its infancy. Surgery should only be undertaken for primary brain tumors. Due to the high risk of intra- and postoperative complications, a state-of-the-art anesthesiology including detailed monitoring of the patient and an intensive care unit is mandatory for intracranial oncologic surgery. Studies with significant case numbers in veterinary medicine of surgical treatment of intracranial neoplasia are only available for feline meningioma. Tumors of the peripheral nervous system are most commonly peripheral nerve sheath tumors. Tumors that are limited to the

3

Table 3.2 Limb-sparing surgeries of appendicular bone tumors

Location	Options	Remarks
Scapula	Partial scapulectomy	Preservation of the mid-scapula Dorsal scapular tumors No soft tissue involvement
	Subtotal scapulectomy	Preservation of the glenohumeral joint Mid-distal scapular tumors No soft tissue involvement
Radius	Radial resection and substitution: Cortical allografts Endoprosthesis Pasteurized autografts Vascularized ulnar transposition Bone transport osteogenesis	Involvement of the radius ≤50 % Combined with pancarpal arthrodesis
Ulna	Partial ulnar resection	Only ulnar tumors below the elbow
Pelvis	Hemipelvectomy Total hemipelvectomy Mid-caudal hemipelvectomy Mid-cranial hemipelvectomy	Based on the location at the pelvis Includes amputation of the hind limb
	Hemipelvectomy Caudal hemipelvectomy	Only limb-sparing hemipelvectomy The acetabulum is preserved

Table 3.3 Examples of common skin wound-closing techniques

Technique	Type	Approximate defect size/localization	Remarks
Direct closure		<5 cm diameter	
Tension-relieving techniques	Undermining	>5 cm diameter	Risk of seroma formation
	Walking sutures	>5 cm	
	Relaxing incisions	>5–10 cm lower extremities	Cosmetic appearance
Local plexus flap	Advancement flap	>10–15 cm	a.k.a. single pedicle flap
	Rotation flap	>10–15 cm	
	Transposition flap	>10–15 cm	
	Interpolation flap	>10–15 cm	Bridging incision necessary
	Skin fold flap	>10–30 cm	Elbow fold flap Flank fold flap
Axial pattern flaps	Thoracodorsal	Thorax, shoulder, forelimb, axillary defects	
	Omocervical	Facial, ear, cervical, shoulder, axillary defects	
	Caudal superficial epigastric	Caudal abdominal, inguinal, flank, perineal, thigh defects	

periphery are usually treated by amputation with a curative intent, while central nervous nerve sheath tumor surgery is usually only palliative.

3.1.6 Oncologic Surgery of Tumors of Viscera/Internal Organs/Body Cavities

Surgery of tumors located in the body cavities can be challenging. Obvious masses that seem to be limited to one organ during preoperative staging might turn out to involve other organs as well (◘ Fig. 3.3). Therefore, in-depth knowledge of surgical techniques for partial or complete resection of visceral organs is mandatory if these procedures are to be undertaken. An understanding of temporary vascular occlusion and vascular surgical techniques is also necessary in certain circumstances (e.g., liver tumors, adrenal gland tumors). In addition to basic surgical instruments, advanced surgical equipment like staplers, vascular clips, vessel-sealing devices, harmonic scalpels, and others might be required. Tumors located in the abdominal or thoracic cavity have a higher risk for seeding tumor cells than tumors located elsewhere. Therefore, final tumor staging and surgical planning is performed intraoperatively once access to the body cavity is established and the entire body cavity has been explored.

Separation of adjacent tissues or organs with laparotomy sponges can reduce the risk of tumor seeding. Partial or complete resection of the tumor is usually possible, depending on the organ involved. Autotransfusion of blood from abdominal or thoracic effusion is contraindicated in neoplastic disease. Lavage of the abdominal or thoracic cavity is indicated in case of a ruptured neoplasia. Gloves and instruments are changed after mass removal and cavity lavage.

Manipulation of abdominal viscera can lead to cardiac arrhythmias, which can progress to life-threatening dysrhythmias that require treatment. Therefore, EGC-monitoring is indicated both intraoperatively and postoperatively for 3 days.

3.1.7 Postoperative Patient Care

Postoperative patient care is based on the organ system involved, the general health status of the patient, and the tumor type and localization. Patients with tumors removed from the thoracic or abdominal cavity usually require intensive care and continuous monitoring for several days. If primary wound closure was not possible, daily wound treatment might be indicated.

3.2 Cancer Chemotherapy

R. Klopfleisch

One classical feature of tumors is their proliferative character, i.e., the high fraction of mitotically active cells in a tumor. *Classical cancer*

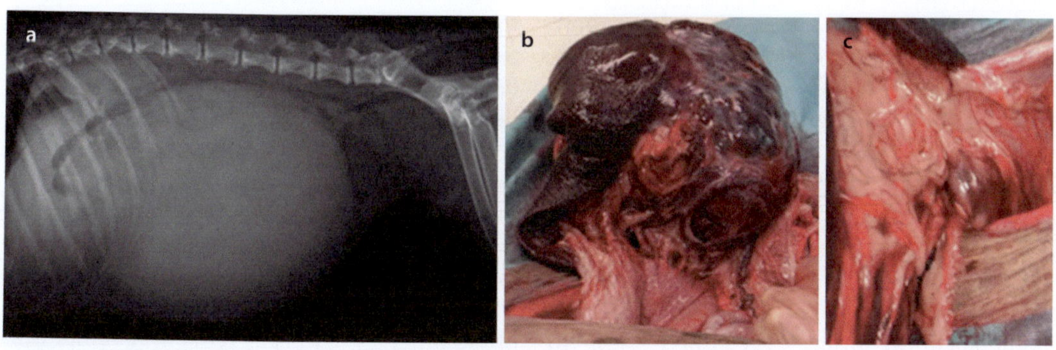

◘ **Fig. 3.3** 11 year old male mix breed dog. (**a**) Lateral radiograph of the abdomen with obvious mass effect. (**b**) Intraoperative view of the spleen with mass. (**c**) Additional at the base of the greater omentum *chemotherapy drugs* take advantage of this by targeting *mitotically active cells*. Unfortunately, the processes targeted by these drugs are also present in nonneoplastic dividing cells such as the bone marrow, intestinal epithelium, and skin. This is why myelosuppression, leukopenia, and cutaneous and gastrointestinal tract toxicity are the *most common side effects of cancer chemotherapy*.

One major goal of research on new chemotherapeutic compounds is the identification of unique signaling cascades, metabolic processes, or tumor markers expressed only by neoplastic cells. *Newly developed cancer chemotherapy drugs* focus on these more specific features. One recent example is the mutational activation of pro-proliferative signaling cascades like KIT tyrosine kinase receptor signaling in canine mast cells, which can be inhibited by *tyrosine kinase inhibitors*. *Monoclonal antibodies* with or without attached toxic proteins are also used to specifically target surface receptors on human tumors like the HER/NEU receptor on human breast cancer or the interleukin-2 receptor on human T-cell lymphoma. Therapeutic monoclonal antibodies are currently not used for routine treatment of tumors in domestic animals, mostly due to their high costs.

Classical chemotherapy drugs targeting dividing cells are thus still by far the most important group of drugs used in veterinary chemotherapy. Their efficacy very much depends on the fraction of dividing cells, which is much less constant during tumor growth than one may intuitively assume. The growth curve of most tumors is similar to what has been described for the human population by the *Gompertzian growth curve*. Growth of both tumor cells and human populations is characterized by an *initial slow growth phase*, which develops into a fast *exponential growth phase* when a sufficient nutrient supply is available. Finally, it reaches a *plateau phase* when space, nutrients, and oxygen are limited. In the plateau phase a large fraction of the tumor's cells are in the *nondividing G0 phase* of the cell cycle and therefore not possible targets for classical chemotherapeutical drugs. The tumor size to growth phase correlation is most probably tumor type specific and very much depends on the ability of the tumor to induce vascularization. However, an often postulated maximal tumor size at which the tumor may switch into the plateau phase is a volume of 1 cm^3. According to Gompertzian kinetics, chemotherapy is thus most efficient when the tumor is small, which is unfortunately often before it is clinically detectable.

3.2.1 General Forms of Chemotherapy Protocols

The term *primary chemotherapy* defines a therapy plan, which is based solely on chemotherapy without other tumor-directed therapy modalities. It is applied when the tumor is primarily systemic as is often the case for hematopoietic leukemic tumors.

Curative chemotherapy is applied with the intention to cure neoplastic disease or at least to allow for prolonged survival of more than 2 years. Unfortunately, very few tumors can be successfully cured by this definition with chemotherapy alone. One example would be low-stage canine B-cell lymphoma.

Palliative chemotherapy, in contrast, is given to alleviate tumor-associated symptoms and to slow down tumor growth but not to cure neoplastic disease.

Monochemotherapy is a treatment protocol that includes only one drug. The advantage of this approach is to offer palliative care at an accessible cost for patients that might otherwise be euthanized.

Polychemotherapy is a treatment protocol, which includes a combination of more than one drug. Polychemotherapy protocols have a higher treatment efficacy in most cases. The protocols aim for a synergistic therapeutic effect, targeting a broader range of heterogeneous tumor cells and decreasing the risk of chemotherapy resistance development.

Neoadjuvant chemotherapy is defined as a chemotherapy given prior to surgery or radiotherapy. Its rationale is to shrink the tumor so that less extensive surgery or radiotherapy is required.

Adjuvant chemotherapy is given after surgery or radiotherapy to kill any remaining tumor cells in the surgical or radiation fields. In addition, it is used to prevent or at least slow down growth of distant micrometastases outside the treatment field.

Induction chemotherapy describes the first more intense phase of chemotherapy protocols when higher doses or more complex drug combinations are given at shorter intervals. The rationale is to kill as many fully sensitive tumor cells *before resistance* can develop.

Consolidation chemotherapy is less aggressive and applied after initiation therapy if complete remission is not achieved.

Maintenance chemotherapy is an even less intense protocol initiated after complete remission by induction or consolidation therapy. The rationale here is to prevent growth of potentially residual tumor cells. There is an ongoing discussion about whether maintenance chemotherapy should be replaced by more intense short-term protocols in dogs with complete remission.

Metronomic chemotherapy is most often defined as a long-term, low-dose chemotherapy protocol, which is of minimal toxicity. The goal is to specifically target the endothelium and thus prevent intra-tumor angiogenesis and subsequently tumor growth.

First-line or standard chemotherapy is a protocol which has been selected by empirical evidence or by prospective studies to have the highest probability of successful treatment of a given tumor type.

Second-line/rescue therapy chemotherapy is the switch to a second protocol when first-line standard chemotherapy fails to achieve the expected results. Again, empirical evidence or scientific studies are used to identify these rescue protocols or drugs.

3.2.2 Chemotherapeutic Agents

▪ Alkylating Agents

Alkylating agents are a large group of cytostatic drugs that work by attaching an alkyl group to cellular DNA (◘ Table 3.4). This alkylation induces *cross-linking of the DNA double helix strands.* Cross-linking inhibits uncoiling and separation and thus duplication of the DNA strands, which in turn inhibits cell division. The cytostatic effect of alkylating agents is not restricted to tumor cells. They are also *cytotoxic or even carcinogenic for nonneoplastic cells.*

▪ Platinum-Containing Drugs

Platinum complexes are cytotoxic via several mechanisms. They induce *cross-linking of the DNA* double strand and thereby prevent cell division, *induce point mutations*, and *inhibit DNA repair mechanisms*, all of which finally trigger apoptosis (◘ Table 3.5).

▪ Antitumor Antibiotics

Antitumor antibiotics are produced by fungi of the *Streptomyces* genus. They have *multiple toxic effects on dividing cells*, which include intercalation with the DNA double strands, induction of DNA double-strand breaks, and inhibition of topoisomerase II. They thus prevent cell division and induce apoptosis in dividing cells (◘ Table 3.6).

▪ Antimicrotubule Agents

Antimicrotubule agents are plant-derived alkaloids. Of these, vinca alkaloids and taxanes are the two most important drug groups. All

◘ **Table 3.4** Alkylating agents and their most common indications in veterinary oncology

Alkylating agent	Indication
Cyclophosphamide	Lymphoma, carcinoma, sarcoma
Chlorambucil	Lymphoma, myeloma, mast cell tumor
Ifosfamide	Lymphoma
Lomustine	Lymphoma, mast cell tumor
Carmustine	Lymphoma, brain tumors
Streptozocin	Insulinoma

◘ **Table 3.5** Platinum-containing drugs and their most common indication in veterinary oncology

Platinum drug	Indication
Cisplatin	Carcinoma, sarcoma, mesothelioma, transitional cell carcinoma
Carboplatin	Similar to cisplatin but not nephrotoxic and more expensive

3

Table 3.6 Antitumor antibiotics and their most common indications in veterinary oncology

Antibiotic	Indication
Doxorubicin	Carcinoma, sarcoma, lymphoma
Mitoxantrone	Lymphoma, transitional cell carcinoma
Actinomycin	Lymphoma
Bleomycin	Squamous cell carcinoma

Table 3.7 Antimicrotubule agents and their most common indications in veterinary oncology

Antimicrotubule agent	Indication
Vincristine	Lymphoma, canine transmissible venereal tumor, mast cell tumor
Vinblastine	Lymphoma, mast cell tumor
Vinorelbine	Mast cell tumor, lung tumor

antimicrotubule drugs *cause microtubule dysfunction*, which is not understood in all aspects. They are believed to inhibit both the formation and disassembly of microtubules, which ultimately prevents the completion of mitosis (Table 3.7).

Antimetabolites

Antimetabolites are *highly similar to endogenous nucleotides like purines and pyrimidines* required for DNA synthesis. Antimetabolites block the enzymes involved in DNA synthesis. They work either by competitive binding or by incorporating into newly synthesized but fragile DNA strands. Both mechanisms inhibit cell division and are believed to induce apoptosis (Table 3.8).

Tyrosine Kinase Inhibitors

The tyrosine kinase inhibitors *masitinib* and *toceranib* have been tested for the treatment of several canine tumor types but seem to have the highest efficacy in the treatment of canine mast cell tumors. They inhibit several tyrosine kinase receptors including the stem cell factor receptor *KIT*, the platelet-derived growth factor receptor (*PDGFR*), the vascular endothelial growth factor-2 (*VEGFR2*), and several others.

Table 3.8 Antimetabolites and their most common indications in veterinary oncology

Antimetabolite	Indication
Methotrexate	Lymphoma
Cytosine arabinoside	Lymphoma
5-Fluorouracil, 5-FU	Carcinoma

Prednisolone and L-Asparaginase

Prednisone non-specifically inhibits DNA synthesis and cell division. It is inexpensive and comparatively well tolerated. It is commonly used in the treatment of lymphomas, plasma cell tumors and, mast cell tumors. The usefulness of prednisone in the treatment of canine lymphoma has been questioned by recent studies.

L-Asparaginase is a bacterial enzyme that degrades the amino acid asparagine. It is thought to induce a systemic asparagine deficiency, which mostly affects proliferative cells. However, increased asparagine synthesis by increased asparagine synthetase activity is a commonly observed resistance mechanism in tumor cells treated with L-asparaginase.

3.2.3 Mechanisms of Chemotherapy Resistance

As described above, multiple drug protocols play a key role as neoadjuvant or adjuvant treatment in veterinary oncology. Unfortunately most tumors do not respond to the majority of anticancer drug groups and are therefore *intrinsically resistant*. Other tumors are initially sensitive but develop an *acquired resistance* during treatment. Resistance, whether acquired or intrinsic, is often the reason chemotherapy ultimately fails. The exact mechanisms behind intrinsic and acquired chemotherapy resistance in the tumors of veterinary patients are unknown. There is nevertheless an increasing understanding of the mechanisms of resistance in human tumors; the first drugs to overcome or prevent chemotherapy resistance are now on the market. Tumors in human patients and in veterinary patients in veterinary medicine share some clinical behaviors and responses to chemotherapeutic drugs so it is not unreasonable to hope that these drugs will also be of use in veterinary oncology.

Box 3.1. Most Important Mechanism of Chemotherapy Resistance in Tumors

1. Increased efflux by ABC transporter proteins
2. Drug inactivation in tumor cells
3. Changes in drug targets
4. Increased DNA damage repair
5. Apoptosis evasion
6. Cancer stem cells and quiescence

Six main mechanisms of chemotherapy resistance have been postulated and are discussed briefly in this chapter: ABC transporter proteins, drug inactivation, drug target change, DNA repair, apoptosis evasion, and tumor stem cells.

▪ Increased Efflux by ABC Transporter Proteins

Drug efflux from the cell is executed mainly by membrane transporter proteins known as ATP-binding cassette (ABC) transporters. There are at least 49 ABC transporters, of which the *multidrug resistance protein 1* (*MDR1*, P-glycoprotein (PGP), ABCB1), the *MDR-associated protein 1* (*MRP1*, ABCC1), and the breast cancer resistance protein (BCRP, ABCG2) have been the most intensely investigated. All ABC transporters can eliminate hydrophobic chemotherapy drugs from cells, including antimetabolites, platinum compounds, microtubule inhibitors, and tyrosine kinase inhibitors (TKI). MDR1 is overexpressed in tumors prior to chemotherapy and thus contributes to intrinsic resistance. It may also increase in expression during chemotherapy and would therefore contribute to acquired resistance. *MDR1*, *MRP1*, *and BCRP expressions* are also detectable in several canine tumors; their expression level may be *correlated with the efficacy and outcome of chemotherapy protocols* or intrinsic resistance of canine lymphomas and mammary tumors. In addition, MDR1 expression in feline tumors is thought to contribute to resistance in this species. Three generations of ABC transporter modulators/inhibitors have been developed to address this problem. Only the first-generation *MDR1 inhibitors verapamil and cyclosporine A* have been successfully tested, both in canine mammary tumors and cutaneous mast cell tumor cells. In addition, *tyrosine kinase inhibitors* including masitinib seem capable of reversing acquired doxorubicin resistance in canine lymphomas.

▪ Drug Inactivation in Tumor Cells

Most research on chemotherapeutic resistance is focused on intracellular drug activation and inactivation in tumor cells, although all phases of drug metabolism in the body, i.e., absorption, distribution, hepatic metabolism, and excretion, probably contribute to resistance. The most important pathways of drug activation and inactivation include the cytochrome P450 (CYP) system, the glutathione S-transferase (GST) superfamily, and uridine diphospho-glucuronosyltransferase (UGT) superfamily.

The *cytochrome P450* (*CYP*) *system* is the major enzyme involved in drug metabolism and therefore of importance for chemotherapy resistance in cancer. Many genetic polymorphisms in the CYP system have been identified in tumors compared to nonneoplastic cells. However, the relevance of these polymorphisms for tumor resistance mechanisms in veterinary patients is unknown.

Glutathione of the GST superfamily and metallothionein are metabolic pathways that contribute to resistance to doxorubicin, alkylating agents, and platinum drugs. Expression of both glutathione and metallothionein has been identified in several canine and feline tumors. Increased GST expression is associated with increased risk of lymphoma development and resistance to chemotherapy protocols in canine lymphomas.

The *uridine diphospho-glucuronosyltransferase* (*UGT*) *superfamily* of enzymes catalyzes glucuronidation and is thus involved in the inactivation of hydrophilic glucuronides used by cytotoxic drugs. A downregulation of UGT transcription has been described in human tumors, but its relevance for chemotherapy resistance in animals is not clear.

▪ Changes in Drug Targets

Quantitative and qualitative changes of drug targets represent well-known mechanisms of chemotherapy resistance in human oncology. For one quantitative change can occur, such as *decreased or lost expression of the target gene product* by the tumor cells. Tumor cells can also be selected for bearing a qualitatively different mutated drug target, which causes a change in the drug-binding site. For instance, prolonged treatment of canine mast cell tumor cells with *tyrosine kinase inhibitors (TKI)* leads to overexpression or de novo *expression of alternative proliferative pathways or to the selection of tumor cell subclones with mutations in the KIT gene*, which may cause ineffective TKI binding to KIT.

▪ Increased DNA Damage Repair

Insufficient DNA damage repair systems are major mechanisms of carcinogenesis in several tumor types. For instance, dysfunctional p53 activity is suspected in some canine and feline tumors. Although intact *DNA damage response (DDR)* is desirable in health, its desirability is questionable in terms of chemotherapy resistance. Induction of DNA damage and subsequent *cell death by apoptosis* is the main mechanism of action for platinum-based drugs and alkylating agents. This requires *apoptosis induction via DNA damage sensors and p53*. If these pathways are dysfunctional due to mutations, the drugs are ineffective. Highly effective DDR is also a cause of resistance because it allows tumor cells to repair and survive chemotherapy-induced DNA damage. Application of DDR inhibitors together with DNA-damaging agents is a promising although somewhat counterintuitive therapy strategy. The most prominent DDR inhibitors, such as olaparib, interfere with the single-strand break DNA repair enzyme *poly-ADP-ribose polymerase (PARP1)*. Unfortunately, there are no studies available on the efficacy of PARP1 inhibitors in tumors of veterinary patients.

▪ Apoptosis Evasion

Evasion of chemotherapy-induced apoptosis is another common mechanism of resistance to chemotherapy. The best understood mechanism of apoptosis evasion by tumor cells is based on *overexpression of apoptosis genes*, of which Bcl-2 and TNF related apoptosis-inducing ligand (TRAIL) are the most intensely studied. Compounds like navitoclax are able to antagonize *Bcl-2 overexpression*, while recombinant TRAIL and TRAIL receptor (TrailR)-activating antibodies have been successfully tested in stimulating apoptosis induction in combination with classic chemotherapeutic drugs. Unfortunately there is little available data on apoptosis evasion in veterinary oncology. However, it is known that overexpression of the anti-apoptotic proteins *survivin* and *myeloid cell leukemia sequence 1 (MCL1)* is a negative prognostic factor for early treatment of canine lymphoma with a CHOP-based protocol.

▪ Cancer Stem Cells and Quiescence

There is increasing evidence that *cancer stem cells (CSC) are of central relevance for chemoresistance*. It has been repeatedly shown that CSC have highly active drug efflux pumps, increased detoxification enzyme levels, enhanced DNA repair efficacy, and apoptosis resistance, all of which are mechanisms of chemotherapy resistance. In addition, CSC are able to switch into a *state of quiescence or dormancy* and therefore can evade the effects of classical chemotherapeutic drugs, which are usually only effective on proliferating cells. *Therapy modalities directly targeting CSC* or quiescent CSC are therefore a major focus in tumor research. Activity of a few signaling pathways, namely, WNT, Notch, and Hedgehog (HH), contributes to the CSC phenotype. Application of *bone morphogenetic protein (BMP)*, a WNT signaling inhibitor; *cyclopamine*, a nHHS pathway inhibitor; or *antibodies against Notch pathway proteins* has been used to directly target CSC in human breast cancer and glioblastoma CSC.

3.3 Radiation Oncology in Veterinary Medicine

M. Wergin

Radiation treatment of human and veterinary patients has seen tremendous progress in the past few decades. Common research topics included fractionation schemes, dosing, and improvements in technical equipment.

3.3.1 Biology of Radiation Therapy

In ionizing radiation, incoming rays have enough energy to eject an orbital electron from an atom or molecule. *Ionizing radiation* used in radiotherapy is divided into x-radiation (x-ray) and gamma radiation (γ-radiation). By consensus, the term *x-ray* refers to ionizing radiation with energy of up to 200 KeV, an energy range that is used primarily in diagnostic imaging. *γ-radiation* is an ionizing radiation with energy between 200 KeV and 26 MeV. The energy absorbed by tissues is given in *gray* (*Gy*). One gray corresponds to an energy deposit of 1 J/kg.

Energy is absorbed as the rays slow down and pass through tissue, establishing energy deposits. These deposits can eventually lead to direct or indirect damage. The *direct damage* is caused by the initiation of DNA double-strand breaks (DSB). These DSB lead to chromosomal aberrations, which can simultaneously affect many genes and cause mutation, malfunction, and cell death. Ionizing radiation causes mainly *indirect damage*. Energy absorption by the water molecules in the tissue causes *hydroxyl radicals* (*·OH*) to form. These free radicals have unpaired electrons, which can cause DNA damage. Another indirect effect of ionizing radiation is the production of *reactive oxygen species* (*ROS*). ROS can only be built when oxygen is present in the cell. Tumors are often hypoxic due to their abnormal and chaotic vasculature. Hypoxia causes radioresistance to ionizing radiation, because ROS cannot be built. It has been shown that ionizing radiation must be 2.9 times higher to kill hypoxic tumor cells than to kill well-oxygenated tumor cells.

Many tumors can be treated with a curative intent with doses between 30 and 55 Gy. When radiation is applied, the dose must be *fractionated* into multiple small doses. The *4R's of radiation* explain the need for fractionation: repair, reoxygenation, radiosensitivity, and repopulation. *Repair* of radiation-induced damage is possible in normal cells when radiation is given in small doses. Normal cells can repair the damage within 6 h, but the repair capacity of tumor cells is significantly reduced. *Reoxygenated* tumor cells are easier to kill. When radiation is given in multiple fractions, some tumor cells are killed during the course of fractionation. This reduces the volume of the tumor. When the volume of the tumor is reduced, the oxygenation of the remaining tumor is increased. Reoxygenated tumor cells need a smaller dose to be killed, and radiation is more effective. The *radiosensitivity* of cells depends on the cell cycle. Cells are more radiosensitive during mitosis and in the G2 phase. The redistribution of cells from more resistant cell cycle phases to sensitive phases can increase the effect of radiation. The *fourth R* is *repopulation*. Tumor cells can divide and repopulate the tumor if the course of radiation is interrupted for too long. The time between radiation fractions should therefore not be prolonged, especially for fast dividing tumors like squamous cell carcinomas.

3.3.2 Indications for Radiation Therapy

Radiation therapy is applied for different tumor types (◘ Table 3.9).

The *total dose and the fractionation scheme* depends on the radiosensitivity of the tumor. It is restricted by the radiosensitivity of normal tissue within the treatment field. The skin and underlying muscle are more radiation resistant than neural tissues like the brain or the spinal cord.

Radiation can be given as a single, *primary treatment*, for example, in brain tumors, squamous cell carcinoma of the nasal planum in cats (◘ Fig. 3.4), or nasal tumors. In addition to primary radiation, radiotherapy can be adjunctive to surgery and/or chemotherapy. *Adjuvant radiation* means that surgery or chemotherapy is given before radiation treatment. This option is chosen if the tumor can be removed surgically (◘ Fig. 3.5). If the tumor is too big to be removed, a *neoadjuvant radiotherapy* can be advantageous. Neoadjuvant radiation means that radiation is given before surgery and/or chemotherapy. Radiation can reduce the tumor burden, making the tumor more amenable to surgery.

The typical radiation treatment in veterinary medicine is given four to five times a week until the total dose is reached. *Hypofractionation* is when radiation is given only two to three times a week. This is usually done for palliative care. An exception is the curative treatment of oral malignant melanoma. If tumors have a rapid tumor doubling time, then an *accelerated protocol* can be used to reduce the repopulation during treatment. This protocol is, for example, used to treat squamous cell carcinoma of the nasal planum and the eyelid in cats.

Before starting radiation, the *goal of the treatment* should be determined. Often many factors need to be taken into consideration to choose the best treatment for an individual patient. A *curative treatment* is chosen if a cure or a long-term tumor control can be achieved and if the patient

3

Table 3.9 Current radiotherapy protocols for common tumors and associated prognosis

Tumor localization	Tumor type	Radiotherapy protocol	Prognosis	References
Skin and subcutis	Sarcoma (dog)	Curative	S: 70 months	Forrest et al. (2000), McKnight et al. (2000)
		Palliative	S: 12 months	Plavec et al. (2006)
	Injection site sarcoma (cat)	Curative	S: 36 months	Eckstein et al. (2009)
		Palliative	S: 10 months	Eckstein et al. (2009)
	Mast cell tumor	Curative	Depending on grade: grade 2 MCT, cure in 90 %	Frimberger et al. (1997), Poirier et al. (2006a, b)
		Palliative		Thamm et al. (2006)
Oral tumors	Malignant melanoma	Palliative	S: 10 months	Proulx et al. (2003), Freeman et al. (2003)
	Squamous cell carcinoma	Curative	S: 12–36 months	LaDue-Miller et al. (1996), Théon et al. (1993, 1997a, b)
	Sarcoma	Curative	S: 12–24 months	Théon et al. (1993), Poirier et al. (2006a, b)
		Palliative	S: 10 months	Théon et al. (1993)
	Acanthomatous epulis	Curative	Curative in 80–90 %	Théon et al. (1997b)
Nasal tumors	Carcinoma sarcoma lymphoma	Curative	S: 12–24 months	Théon et al. (1993), Adams et al. (2005)
		Palliative	S: 10 months S: cat with nasal lymphoma, 24 months	Buchholz et al. (2009), Haney et al. (2009)
Tumors of the nasal planum	Squamous cell carcinoma (cat)	Curative	70 % cure rate	Melzer et al. (2006)
Brain tumors	Meningioma	Curative	S: 30 months	Rohrer Bley et al. (2003, 2005), Théon et al. (2000a)
	Glioma	Curative	S: 30 months	Rohrer Bley et al. (2003, 2005)
	Pituitary tumor	Curative	S: 24–48 months	RohBley et al. (2005), Kent et al. (2007)
Thyroid tumors	Carcinoma	Curative	12–36 months	Théon et al. (2000b)
		Palliative	12–24 months	Brearley et al. (1999)
Mediastinum	Thymoma	Curative or palliative	Cat: 24 months Dog: 8 months	Smith et al. (2001)

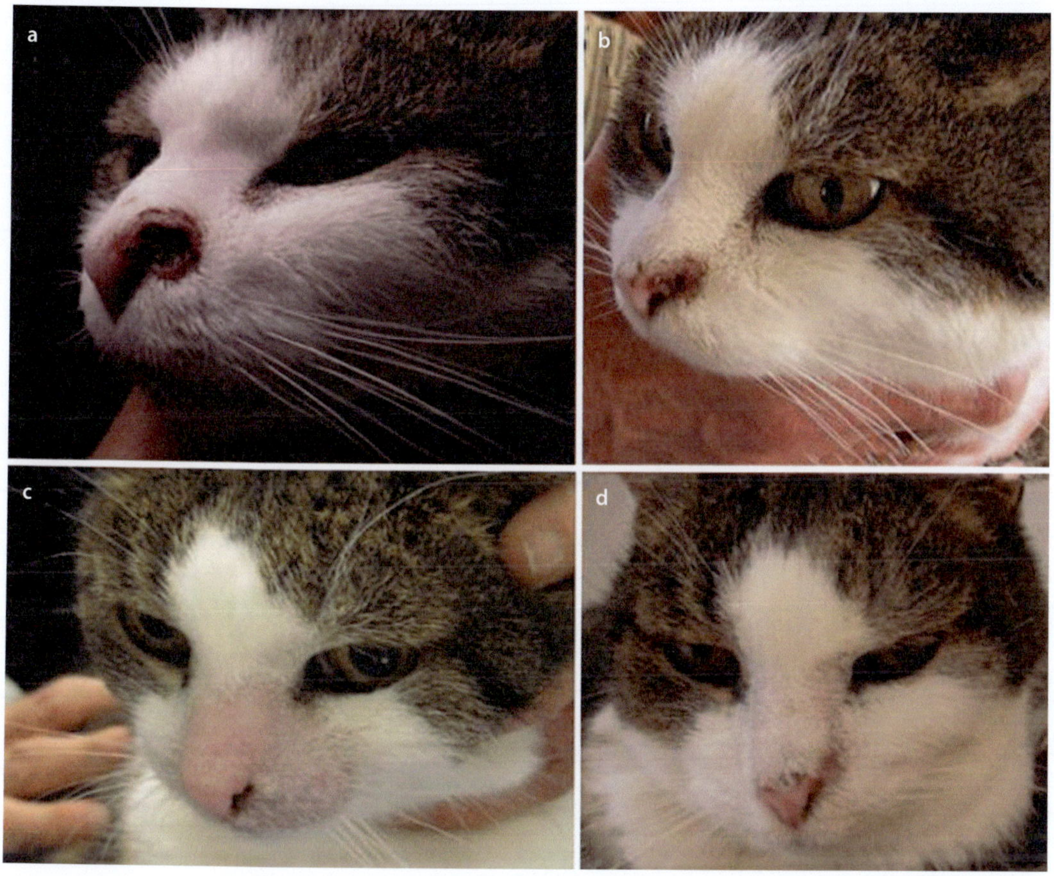

Fig. 3.4 Radiation of an SCC of the nasal planum of a cat. Primary radiation of a squamous cell carcinoma (*SCC*) of the nasal planum of a cat. Radiation was applied as the sole treatment option. An accelerated protocol with ten fractions twice daily was used. (**a**) The SCC before radiation. (**b**) The SCC at the end of radiation: the tumor already appears smaller. (**c**) 3 weeks after completion of therapy. The tumor is healed and the hair has fallen off. (**d**) The tumor has been cured and the hair has grown back 3 months after radiation

has no other life-threatening disease. A curative radiation protocol is usually given within 14–20 fractions of 2.5–4 Gy. The radiation is given 4–5 days a week. In general, a curative protocol is more strenuous and is accompanied by more severe side effects.

Palliative radiation is used to improve quality of life when the patient cannot be cured due to several reasons, for example, risk of developing distant metastasis or presence of distant metastasis at the time of diagnosis. Another reason to choose palliative treatment might be age of the patient or overall health. Palliative treatment is also used to reduce pain in both neoplastic and benign disease processes. The protocols for palliative radiation should be designed to slow tumor growth or to reduce tumor volume with only mild to no acute radiation side effects. The higher the radiation dose per fraction, the more severe are the late reactions developing. In a palliative approach, the life expectancy of the treated patients is so short that late reactions will most likely not develop. Radiation to control pain in patients with osteosarcoma contains 2–5 fractions with 6–10 Gy per fraction. One study showed that treatment with two fractions of 8 Gy was sufficient to treat bone pain in these dogs. Pain control starts approximately 3 weeks after finishing radiation. The pain can be controlled for 2–4 months with radiation. Palliative radiation can also be used to treat pain in benign disease such as arthrosis.

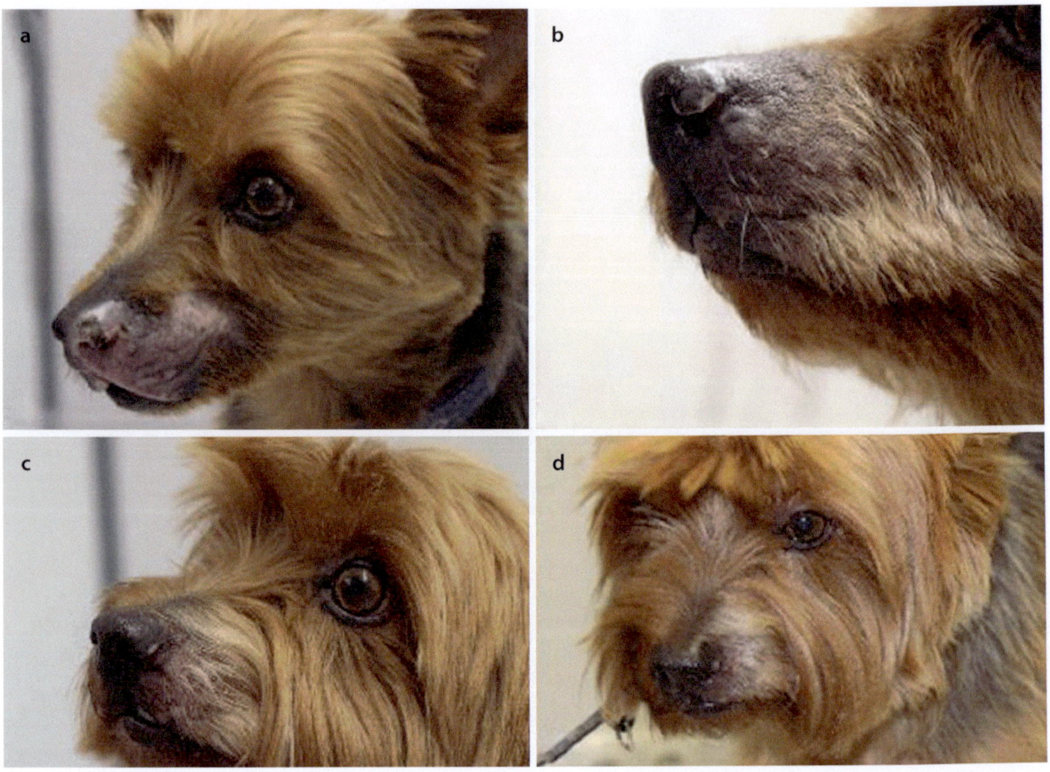

Fig. 3.5 Adjuvant treatment of a dog with a mast cell tumor. An adjuvant curative radiation treatment was chosen for this dog with a Grade II mast cell tumor. The tumor was removed 2 weeks before radiation. (**a**) The skin has healed 2 weeks after completion of therapy. (**b**) The hair has not regrown at the 3-month recheck, (**c, d**) but at the 6-month recheck, the hair has grown back in white (leukotrichia)

3.3.3 Adverse Side Effects of Radiation

The side effects of radiation depend on the type of healthy tissue in the field of radiation and on the applied dose. The skin or mucosa or surgical scars, in the case of adjuvant radiation, are most frequently affected. Side effects of radiation are divided into acute and late reactions.

Acute reactions are typically affecting the *skin* and mucosa but can also affect other tissues within the radiation field. The irradiated skin develops a moist desquamation comparable to a sunburn. Necrosis and hyperemia (also called mucositis) of irradiated mucosa can also be observed (Fig. 3.6). Self-mutilation of affected skin areas is another common problem. An Elizabethan collar should be used, if necessary. Bandaging is not recommended because irradiated skin is very delicate. Antibiotics, steroids, or NSAIDs are commonly used to support the healing process. The severity of radiation reaction depends on the localization of radiation, the volume of irradiated skin, and the individual radiation sensitivity. In general, the skin of dogs is more radiation sensitive than the skin of cats. Leukotrichia, white hair, is typically seen when haired skin was in the radiation field (Fig. 3.7).

Late reactions may develop months to years after radiation. Late reactions are more common when hypofractionated, high-dose per fraction protocols are applied. Keratoconjunctivitis sicca, cataracts, and retinopathy are common late reactions to radiation. Cataracts develop over years and are usually not clinically relevant. Irradiation can also be carcinogenic, but this is a long-term effect that is of minor relevance in veterinary medicine due to shorter patient life span. The risk of developing irradiation-induced tumors 5 years after radiation has been calculated to be 3.5 %.

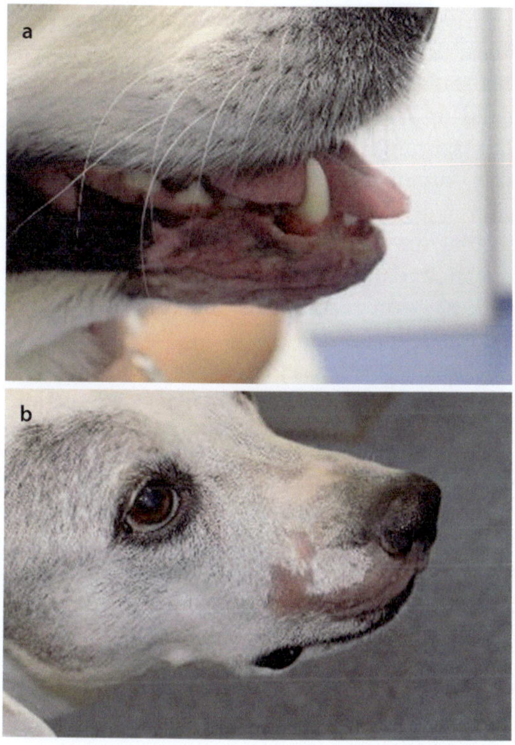

■ **Fig. 3.6** (**a**) Acute side effects of radiation of moist desquamation of the skin and mucositis of the oral mucosa at the end of curative radiation. (**b**) Skin reactions at the end of curative radiation. A rapid healing of affected skin within 3 weeks is usually seen

3.3.4 Radiation Treatment Devices

Ionizing radiation can be applied in different ways:

- External beam radiation
- Internal radiotherapy
- Particle therapy
- Therapy with nuclides

External beam radiation, also called teletherapy, is the most common form of radiation therapy in human and veterinary medicine. The patient is positioned, and an external source is pointed at the target tissue. For external beam radiation, different sources can be used:

- Superficial x-rays: 50–200 keV
- Orthovoltage x-rays: 200–500 keV
- Supervoltage x-rays: 500–1000 keV
- Megavoltage x-rays: 1–25 MeV

Megavoltage x-rays are the most common; in veterinary medicine the use of 3–9 MeV is sufficient for the treatment of small animals. Superficial x-rays and orthovoltage x-rays can only be used for skin-associated tumors, because the energy is too weak for a deeper penetration. The maximum dose of energy is deposited at the skin surface, and only 10 % of the energy reaches a 2 cm depth. Severe cutaneous side effects are the result.

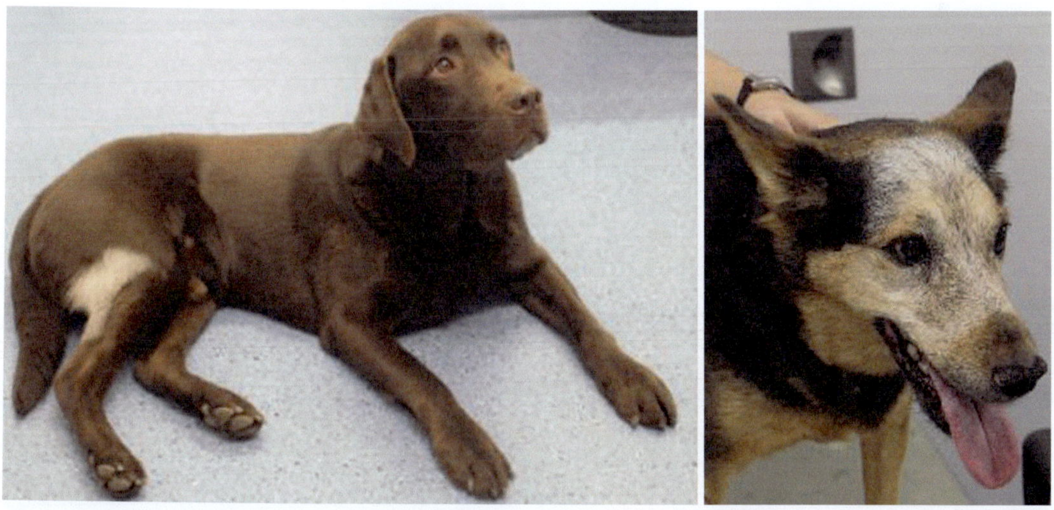

■ **Fig. 3.7** Leukotrichia (regrowth of white hair) is a typical observation in irradiated skin. Both dogs received curative radiation. No further late reactions are present

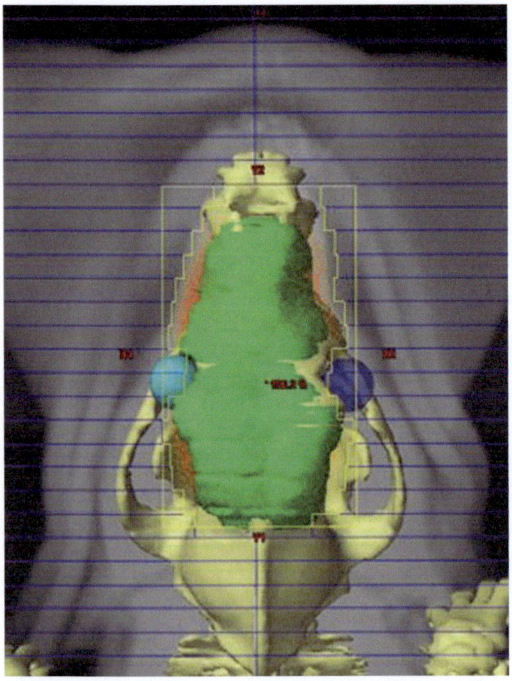

■ **Fig. 3.8** Multileaf collimator. A coronal CT scan of the head of a dog with a nasal adenocarcinoma is shown. Primary curative radiation was planned. To protect the eyes (*dark blue* and *light blue color*), a multileaf collimator (*MLC*) was used for treatment planning. The MLC is shown by the *blue lines*, and the individually shaped field is shown

Megavoltage irradiation is mainly given with linear accelerators (Linac). Linacs utilize x-rays, also called photons or electron beams. Photons build up in tissue by depth. This buildup has a skin-sparing effect. Electrons can be used to treat skin tumors and subcutaneous tumors. The advantage of electrons is the limited penetration so that the underlying tissue is protected from radiation damage. The source-to-skin distance with electron radiation is 100 cm allowing big fields to be irradiated.

Linacs provide very clear margins of the treatment field, allowing high-precision radiation. They are also equipped with a multileaf collimator (MLC), which allows the radiation field to be shaped individually (■ Fig. 3.8). Usually, photon irradiation is given with multiple beams to achieve a homogenous dose distribution within the treatment field. For complex planning a specific planning software is used (■ Fig. 3.9).

3.3.5 Therapy Planning

The first step in therapy planning is to define the fractionation scheme of radiation. The second step is to define the treatment volume. Planning

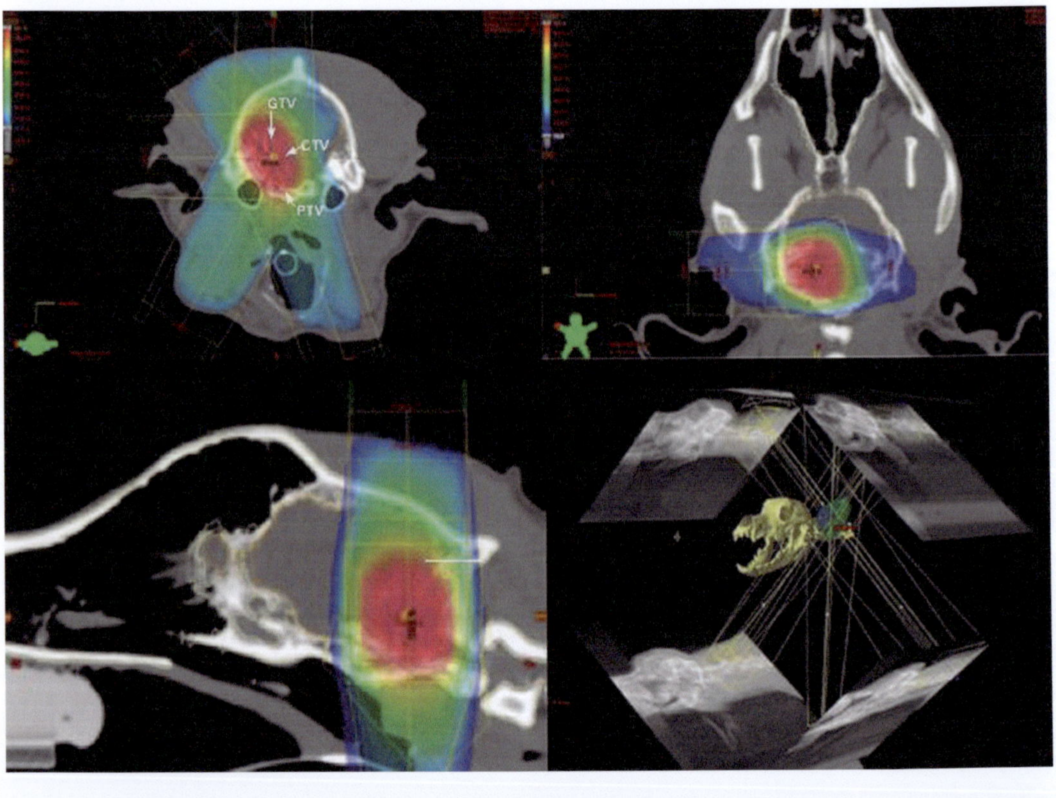

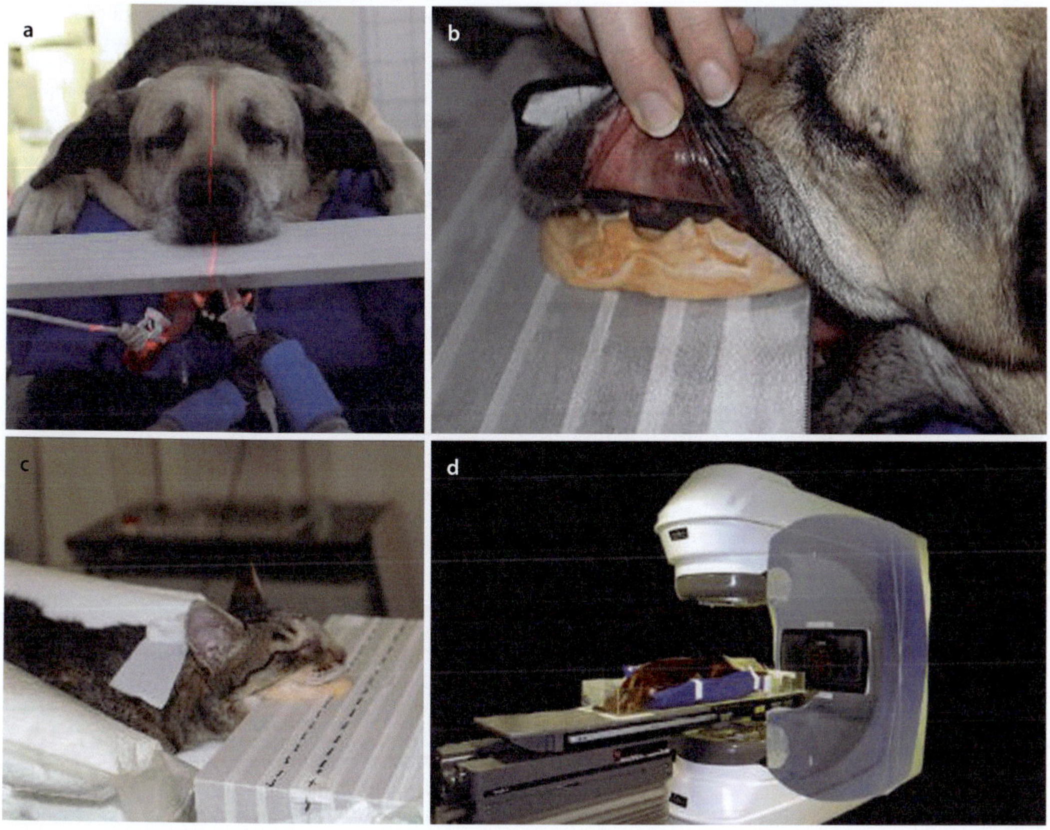

Fig. 3.10 Positioning devices. (**a**) Dog is placed in a Plexiglas box with a vacuum cushion. The cushion helps to keep the body in the same position for every treatment. The box has a bridge to place the head. (**b**) A bite block is placed on the bridge. (**c**) The same system is used for cats. (**d**) The box is placed on the treatment table, and the position of the box and of the patient in the box is checked before every single treatment

software is used to achieve the optimal dose distribution within the treatment volume. A computer tomography (CT) is needed for planning. Before the CT scan, a positioning device is adapted to the patient. Precise positioning assures that the treated volume is as small as possible, and high-risk organs are protected. A bite block of the upper jaw can be used for positioning (Fig. 3.10). The planning must assure that the dose within the tumor is 95–105 % of the prescribed dose. The tumor volume must be determined by diagnostic imaging. MRI is more precise than CT in determining the tumor volume. Modern tumor planning software allows CT and MRI to be overlaid, to precisely determine the radiation volume. The gross tumor volume (GTV) is the visible tumor seen by CT and/or MRI. The clinical tumor volume (CTV) is defined by the visible tumor volume and healthy tissue most likely being invaded by tumor cells. The planning tumor volume (PTV) adds the positioning inaccuracy to the CTV. The more precise the positioning device, the smaller the PTV (Fig. 3.9).

Fig. 3.9 Radiation therapy planning for teletherapy. A transversal, coronal, and sagittal image of a CT scan is shown. The dog had a brain tumor and received curative radiation. The dose distribution within the tissue is shown. *Red color* indicates a high dose (100 %) and the *blue* and *green colors* show a low dose. Note that the tumor volumes are given on the transversal view: gross tumor volume (*GTV*), clinical tumor volume (*CTV*), and the planning tumor volume (*PTV*). The tumor was treated with 95–105 % of the prescribed dose, and non-effected parts of the brain were largely protected from radiation

3.3.6 Internal Beam Radiation

Internal beam radiation, also called *brachytherapy*, is a less commonly used approach. Brachytherapy is delivered from a short distance. The radiation source is placed directly into or next to the tumor using small pellets, seeds, or wire. The insert can be either temporary or permanent. *Iridium-192* is the most commonly used radioactive substance. Iridium can be inserted directly into the tumor. However, the delivered dose cannot be planned as accurate as external beam radiation. The *afterloading technique* is a newer treatment approach. With this technique, one or multiple catheters are inserted into the tumor, and the radiation source is placed in the catheter. The advantage of this system is that medical staff is exposed to lower radiation doses. Newer planning systems are available in human medicine to assure an accurate dose delivery, but these systems are not yet used in veterinary medicine.

Suggested Reading

Adams WM, Bjorling DE, McAnulty JE et al (2005) Outcome of accelerated radiotherapy alone or accelerated radiotherapy followed by exenteration of the nasal cavity in dogs with intranasal neoplasia: 53 cases (1990–2002). J Am Vet Med Assoc 227:936–941

Brahme A (ed) (1988) Accuracy requirements and quality assurance of external beam therapy with photons and electrons. Acta Oncol, 4th edn (Suppl 1)

Brearley MJ, Hayes A, Murphy S (1999) Hypofractionated radiation therapy for invasive thyroid carcinoma in dogs. J Small Anim Pract 40:206–210

Bristow RG, Hill RP (2004) Molecular and cellular basis of radiotherapy. In: Tannock IF, Hill RP, Bristow RB, Harrington L (eds) The basic science of oncology, 4th edn. McGraw Hill Companies, New York, pp 273–279

Buchholz J, Hagen R, Leo C et al (2009) 3D conformal radiation therapy for palliative treatment of canine nasal tumors. Vet Radiol Ultrasound 50:679–683

Eckstein C, Guscetti F, Roos M et al (2009) A retrospective analysis of radiation therapy for the treatment of feline vaccine-associated sarcoma. Vet Comp Oncol 7:54–68

Forrest LJ, Chun R, Adams WM et al (2000) Postoperative radiotherapy for canine soft tissue sarcoma. J Vet Intern Med 14:578–582

Freeman KP, Hahn KA, Harris FD et al (2003) Treatment of dogs with oral melanoma by hypofractionated radiation therapy and platinum-based chemotherapy (1987–1997). J Vet Intern Med 17:96–101

Frimberger AE, Moore AS, LaRue SM et al (1997) Radiotherapy of incompletely resected, moderately differentiated mast cell tumors in the dog: 37 cases (1989–1993). J Am Anim Hosp Assoc 33:320–324

Gillette EL, LaRue SM, Gillette SM (1995) Normal tissue tolerance and management of radiation injury. Semin Vet Med Surg (Small Anim) 10:209–213

Hall EJ (2000) Time, dose, and fractionation in radiotherapy. In: Hall EJ, Giaccia AJ (eds) Radiobiology for the radiologists, 6th edn. Lippincott William & Wilkins, Philadelphia, pp 378–397

Haney SM, Beaver L, Turrel J et al (2009) Survival analysis of 97 cats with nasal lymphoma: a multi-institutional retrospective study (1986–2006). J Vet Intern Med 23:287–294

Harris D, King GK, Bergman PJ (1997) Radiation therapy toxicities. Vet Clin North Am Small Anim Pract 27:37–46

Hill RP, Bristow RG (2004) The scientific basis of radiotherapy. In: Tannock IF, Hill RP, Bristow RB, Harrington L (eds) The basic science of oncology, 4th edn. McGraw Hill Companies, New York, p 305

History of radiation oncology, University of Alabama at Birmingham Comprehensive Cancer Center. Archived from the original

Kent MS, Bommarito D, Feldman E et al (2007) Survival, neurologic response, and prognostic factors in dogs with pituitary masses treated with radiation therapy and untreated dogs. J Vet Intern Med 21:1027–1033

Klopfleisch R, Kohn B, Gruber AD (2016) Mechanisms of tumour resistance against chemotherapeutic agents in veterinary oncology. Vet J 207:63–72

LaDue T, Klein MK (2001) Toxicity criteria of the veterinary radiation therapy oncology group. Vet Radiol Ultrasound 42:475–476

LaDue-Miller T, Price GS, Page RL et al (1996) Radiotherapy of canine non-tonsillar squamous cell carcinoma. Vet Radiol Ultrasound 37:74–77

Mayer MN, Grier CK (2006) Palliative radiation therapy for canine osteosarcoma. Can Vet J 47(7):707–709

McKnight JA, Mauldin GN, McEntee MC et al (2000) Radiation treatment for incompletely resected soft tissue sarcomas in dogs. J Am Vet Med Assoc 217:205–210

Melzer K, Guscetti F, Rohrer Bley C et al (2006) Ki67 reactivity in nasal and periocular squamous cell carcinomas in cats treated with electron beam radiation therapy. J Vet Intern Med 20:676–681

Northrup NC, Roberts RE, Harrell TW, Allen KL, Howerth EW, Gieger TL (2004) Iridium-192 Interstitial Brachytherapy as Adjunctive Treatment for Canine Cutaneous Mast Cell Tumors. J Am Anim Hosp Assoc 40(4):309–315

Pioneer in X-Ray therapy (1957) Science 125(3236):18–19

Plavec I, Kessler M, Kandel B et al (2006) Palliative radiotherapy as treatment for non-resectable soft tissue sarcomas in the dog – a report of 15 cases. Vet Comp Oncol 4:98–103

Poirier VJ, Adams WM, Forrest LJ et al (2006a) Radiation therapy for incompletely excised grade 2 canine mast cell tumors. J Am Anim Hosp Assoc 42:430–434

Poirier VJ, Rohrer Bley C, Roos M et al (2006b) Efficacy of radiation therapy for the treatment of macroscopic canine oral soft tissue sarcoma. In Vivo 20:415–420

Pommer A (1958) X-ray therapy in veterinary medicine. In: Brandly CA, Jungher EL (eds) Advances in veterinary science. Academic, New York

Proulx DR, Ruslander DM, Dodge RK et al (2003) A retrospective analysis of 140 dogs with oral melanoma treated with external beam radiation. Vet Radiol Ultrasound 44:352–359

Rich T, Allen RL, Wyllie AH (2000) Defying death after DNA damage. Nature 96:643–649

Rohrer Bley C, Blattmann H, Roos M, Sumova A, Kaser-Hotz B (2003) Assessment of a radiotherapy patient immobilization device using a single plane port radiographs and a remote computed tomography scanner. Vet Radiol Ultrasound 44:470–475

Rohrer Bley C, Sumova A, Roos M et al (2005) Irradiation of brain tumors in dogs with neurological signs: a retrospective survival analysis of 46 cases (1997–2003). J Vet Intern Med 19:849–854

Ruppert R, Seegenschmied MH, Sauer R (2004) Radiotherapy of osteoarthritis. Indication, technique and clinical results. Orthopade 33:56–62

Schwyn U, Crompton NE, Blattmann H, Hauser B, Klink B, Parvis A, Ruslander D, Kaser-Hotz B (1998) Potential tumour doubling time: determination of Tpot for various canine and feline tumours. Vet Res Commun 22(4):233–247

Smith AN, Wright JC, Brawner WR Jr et al (2001) Radiation therapy in the treatment of canine and feline thymomas: a retrospective study (1985–1999). J Am Anim Hosp Assoc 37:489–496

Thamm DH, Turek MM, Vail DM (2006) Outcome and prognostic factors following adjuvant prednisone/vinblastine chemotherapy for high risk canine mast cell tumour: 61 cases. J Vet Med Sci 68:541–548

Théon AP, Madewell BR, Harb MF et al (1993) Megavoltage irradiation of neoplasms of the nasal and paranasal cavities in 77 dogs. J Am Vet Med Assoc 202:1469–1475

Théon AP, Rodriguez C, Madewell BR (1997a) Analysis of prognostic factors and patterns of failure in dogs with malignant oral tumors treated with megavoltage irradiation. J Am Vet Med Assoc 210:778–784

Théon AP, Rodriguez C, Griffey S et al (1997b) Analysis of prognostic factors and patterns of failure in dogs with periodontal tumors treated with megavoltage irradiation. J Am Vet Med Assoc 210:785–788

Théon AP, Le Couteur RA, Carr EA et al (2000a) Influence of tumor cell proliferation and sex-hormone receptors on effectiveness of radiation therapy for dogs with incompletely resected meningiomas. J Am Vet Med Assoc 216:701–707

Théon AP, Marks SL, Feldman ES et al (2000b) Prognostic factors and patterns of treatment failure in dogs with unresectable differentiated thyroid carcinomas treated with megavoltage irradiation. J Am Vet Med Assoc 216:1775–1779

Thrall DE (1997) Biologic basis of radiation therapy. Vet Clin North Am Small Anim Pract 27:21–35

Turrel JM, Koblik PD (1983) Techniques of afterloading Iridium- 192 interstitial brachytherapy in veterinary medicine. Vet Radiol 24:278–283

Skin Tumors

Robert Klopfleisch

R. Klopfleisch (ed.), *Veterinary Oncology*, DOI 10.1007/978-3-319-41124-8_4

4.1 Skin Tumors of the Dog

There is a wide variety of skin tumors in the dog; tumors derive from the epithelial cells of the epidermis and adnexa, the melanocytes, dermal stromal cells, subcutaneous adipocytes, or infiltrating hematopoietic cells. Mast cell tumors are the most common canine skin tumor. Soft tissue sarcomas including (i.e., lipomas, subcutaneous peripheral nerve sheath tumors, fibrosarcomas) histiocytomas, squamous-cell carcinomas, melanomas, hair follicle tumors, and cutaneous glandular tumors are other common tumors, which all have a similar but lower incidence.

4.1.1 Canine Epithelial Tumors

4.1.1.1 Canine Hair Follicle Tumors

Box 4.1. Canine Hair Follicle Tumors in Three Facts

1. Mostly benign or merely locally invasive.
2. Surgery mostly curative.
3. Subclassification into histologic subtypes is of minor clinical relevance.

Epidemiology and Pathogenesis

Hair follicle tumors are common skin tumors of the dog. They are divided into three main tumor types according to their histopathologic appearance, which are nevertheless very similar in their clinical appearance and biologic behavior.

Trichoblastomas are benign tumors, which are currently believed to arise from epidermal basal cells or follicular stem cells. The tumor was previously called a basal cell tumor but has been renamed recently and is now known as trichoblastoma in the dog. Trichoblastomas are tumors of middle-*aged* to older dogs. A breed disposition for some terrier breeds may be present.

Trichoepitheliomas are also benign tumors, which present with histologic growth patterns resembling hair follicles. They are tumors of middle-*aged* to older dogs. A *breed* disposition may be present for retrievers and poodles. An invasive and metastatic malignant form of the tumor has been described but is very rare.

Pilomatricomas are benign tumors, which are thought to arise from cells of the hair bulb. They are more common in middle-aged dogs than in older dogs. There is no confirmed *breed* disposition. Malignant pilomatricomas are rarely observed and are characterized by local infiltration, tumor satellites, and metastasis into the lung, bone, and less commonly into other organs.

Clinical Appearance

The three main types of canine hair follicle tumors cannot be separated by their clinical appearance. All present as solid, well-circumscribed, <5 cm in diameter large, partly cystic, slowly growing tumors. They may be ulcerated and hairless. Pilomatricomas may be firmer due to calcification and rare ossification. All three tumors are mostly benign but the surrounding skin and the regional lymph nodes should be checked for tumor satellites or regional metastasis.

Cytology and Histopathology

Cytology of hair follicle tumors presents with relatively well-differentiated squamous epithelial cells admixed with mostly large amounts of cellular debris or keratin (Figs. 4.1, 4.2, and 4.3). *Histopathology* is necessary to identify the specific tumor type and invasive character and to analyze the surgical margins.

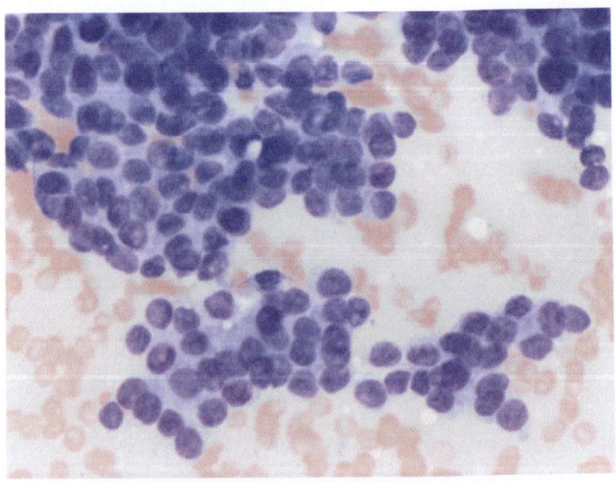

Fig. 4.1 Cytology, trichoblastoma, dog, May-Grünwald-Giemsa, 500×. Note the clusters of small basaloid epithelial cells showing a typical "ribbonlike" growth pattern (Photo: with permission of Dr. N. Bauer, Faculty of Veterinary Medicine, Justus-Liebig-University, Giessen, Germany)

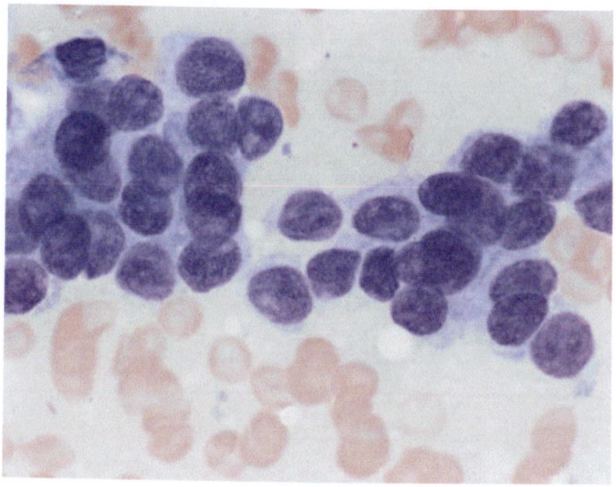

Fig. 4.2 Cytology, trichoblastoma, dog, May-Grünwald-Giemsa, 1000×. Note the clusters of small, uniform cuboidal to slightly spindle-shaped basaloid epithelial cells with round nuclei and fine chromatin pattern (Photo: with permission of Dr. N. Bauer, Faculty of Veterinary Medicine, Justus-Liebig-University, Giessen, Germany)

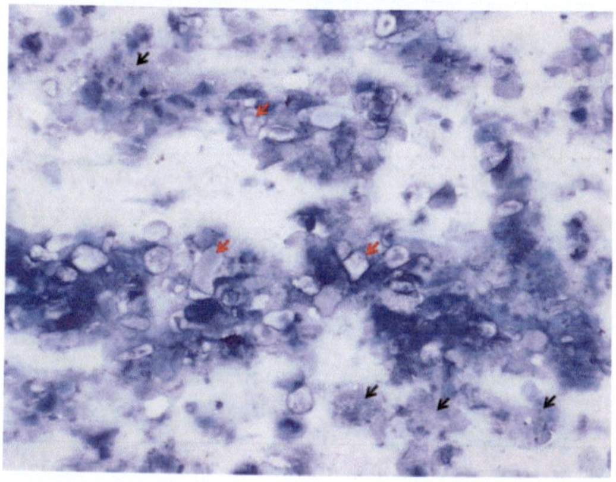

Fig. 4.3 Cytology, cystic mass with keratinized debris indicative of epidermal inclusion cyst or hair follicle tumor that look similar in cytological specimens, dog, May-Grünwald-Giemsa, 100×. Note numerous anuclear keratinocytes (*red arrow*) between large amounts of amorphous keratinized debris (*black arrow*) (Photo: with permission of Dr. N. Bauer, Faculty of Veterinary Medicine, Justus-Liebig-University, Giessen, Germany)

Therapy

Surgery with appropriate tumor margins is usually curative.

Suggested Reading

(Abramo et al. 1999; Brachelente et al. 2013; Carroll et al. 2010; Hoshino et al. 2012; Masserdotti and Ubbiali 2002)

4.1.1.2 Canine Squamous Cell Carcinomas

Box 4.2. Canine Cutaneous Squamous Cell Carcinomas in Five Facts

1. Rather rare tumors.
2. UV light may be involved in carcinogenesis.
3. Mostly flat, ulcerated plaques.
4. Rarely metastasize but grow invasively.
5. Surgery with wide margins is the therapy of choice.

Epidemiology and Pathogenesis

Squamous cell carcinomas (SCC) of the skin are rather *rare tumors* in dogs. There is no *breed* or *age* predisposition. Actinic damage due to UV light plays a role in carcinogenesis in light-colored dogs or body areas. Rare, multicentric, noninvasive SCC are potentially induced by *Papillomavirus infection* and called *Bowen's disease* based upon the feline disease. Black-coated dogs are predisposed to develop *subungual SCC* at the digits.

Clinical Appearance

SCC usually presents as ulcerated, invasive *plaque-like lesions*; only rarely do they present as prominent, cauliflower-like actual masses (Fig. 4.4). *Metastasis is uncommon* but the regional lymph node should be palpated or biopsied, and lung metastases should be excluded radiographically in animals with large tumors. Advanced *SCC of the nasal planum* has a more guarded prognosis due to the aggressive invasive character and the difficulties associated with surgery in this location.

Cytology and Histopathology

Cytology of SCC usually presents with variably differentiated epithelial cells, keratin, and signs of secondary inflammation due to a superficial infection of ulcerated tumors (Figs. 4.5 and 4.6). *Histopathology* of an incisional biopsy or of the excised tumors is necessary for final diagnosis and evaluation of surgical margins. SCC is characterized by variably differentiated epithelial tumor cells, with typical keratinization and keratin pearls. Stromal proliferation and secondary inflammation due to ulceration are common.

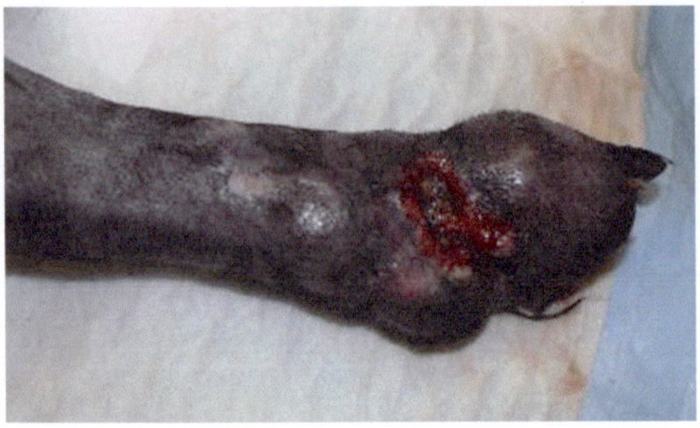

Fig. 4.4 Subungual squamous cell carcinoma (relapse after amputation of one digit) with invasion of the bone and osteolysis, dog. Ulcerated flat mass at the right hind paw of an 11-year-old Giant Schnauzer (Photo: with permission of Prof. M. Kramer, Faculty of Veterinary Medicine, Justus-Liebig-University, Giessen, Germany)

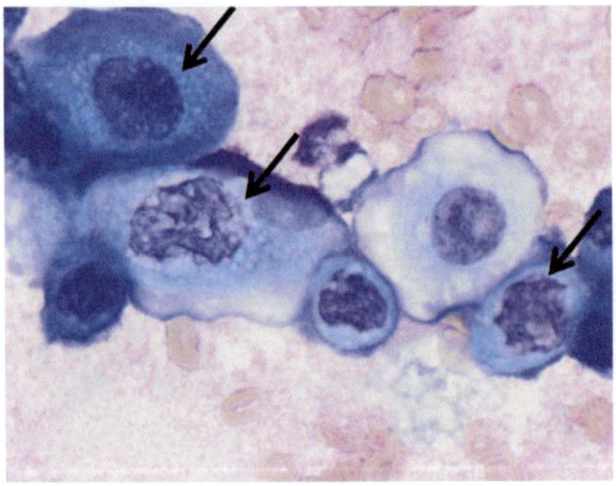

Fig. 4.5 Cytology, squamous cell carcinoma, Giant Schnauzer (the same dog as in Fig. 4.4), May-Grünwald-Giemsa, 1000×. Marked anisocytosis, anisokaryosis, and pleomorphism of epithelial cells as well as marked variation in maturation reflected by a high variation in nuclear-to-cytoplasm ratio and increased, highly variable cytoplasm basophilia. Often, multiple perinuclear vacuoles containing colorless keratohyalin (*arrows*) are seen also strongly suggestive of squamous-cell carcinoma (Photo: with permission of Dr. N. Bauer, Faculty of Veterinary Medicine, Justus-Liebig-University, Giessen, Germany)

Therapy

Surgery with wide margins is the treatment of choice for SCC. Tumor-free margins are strongly correlated with a good prognosis, while metastasis or nonsurgical treatment is associated with a poor prognosis.

The efficacy of *radiotherapy* is not tested for cutaneous SCC of the dog. However, SCC in other locations is usually sensitive to radiation.

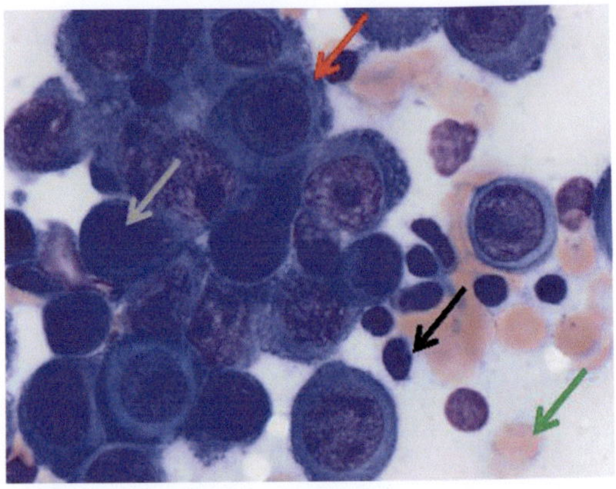

Fig. 4.6 Cytology, metastatic squamous cell carcinoma, lymph node, dog, May-Grünwald-Giemsa, 1000×. Note the large cluster of round to cuboidal epithelial cells (*red arrow*) with moderate anisocytosis, anisokaryosis, pleomorphism, and variation of nuclear-to-cytoplasm ratio. The epithelial cells possess one to several prominent nucleoli, often macronucleoli (*gray arrow*, i.e., nucleoli with a diameter >5 μm and thus approximately of the size of an erythrocyte). They are surrounded by few small mature lymphocytes (*black arrow*) representing the lymphoid tissue (*green arrow*) (Photo: with permission of Dr. N. Bauer, Faculty of Veterinary Medicine, Justus-Liebig-University, Giessen, Germany)

Chemotherapy using 5-fluorouracil, doxorubicin, cisplatin, mitoxantrone, or Cox-2 inhibitors has been applied intralesionally or systemically for tumors where excision was impossible. Short-term reduction of tumor size was observed in these cases but relapsed tumor growth will occur.

Suggested Reading

(Belluco et al. 2013; Langova et al. 2004; O'Brien et al. 1992; Thomson 2007; Waropastrakul et al. 2012; Webb et al. 2009)

4.1.1.3 Canine Tumors of the Sebaceous and Apocrine Skin Glands

Box 4.3. Canine Tumors of the Sebaceous and Apocrine Glands in Three Facts

1. Usually benign tumors.
2. Wide surgical excision curative.
3. Carcinomas very rarely metastasize.

Epidemiology and Pathogenesis

Sebaceous gland adenomas are benign tumors of sebaceous gland origin. They are commonly found on the head, limbs, and trunk; a *breed* predisposition exists for cocker spaniels, poodles, miniature schnauzers, and terriers at the *age* of 10 years. *Sebaceous gland carcinomas* are very rare tumors with low-grade malignancy commonly found on the head and neck. Adenomas show a *sex* predisposition for males; carcinomas have a *breed* predisposition for cocker spaniels and terriers.

Apocrine gland adenomas are fairly common tumors of the head and neck of longhaired dog *breeds* and cocker spaniels. They have an almost similar incidence to *apocrine gland carcinomas,* which are more common in golden retrievers and are often found on the front legs. Both benign and malignant tumors are mostly diagnosed in dogs between the *ages* of 8 and 10 years.

Eccrine gland adenomas and *carcinomas* are rare tumors of the sweat glands of the footpad.

▪ Clinical Appearance

Sebaceous gland adenomas usually present as rather small, slowly growing, multiple papilloma-like nodules. They may have a sebaceous surface and are often inflamed due to secondary bacterial infection. Adenomas are usually well circumscribed and do not metastasize. *Sebaceous gland carcinomas* are fast and invasively growing tumors, which are often ulcerated and inflamed.

Apocrine gland adenomas are usually solitary, well-circumscribed, and sometimes cystic tumors. *Apocrine gland carcinomas* are fast-growing often-ulcerated tumors with invasion of the surrounding tissues and sometimes lymph and blood vessels. Regional or distant metastasis is nevertheless very uncommon.

▪ Cytology and Histopathology

Cytology is only occasionally able to differentiate benign from malignant gland tumors. *Sebaceous gland tumors* present cytologically with large, uniform single cells and cell groups with a foamy (sebaceous) cytoplasm (◘ Fig. 4.7). Basal cells without foamy cytoplasm are usually concurrent findings in cell groups. *Apocrine gland tumors* are characterized by mostly uniform to pleomorphic epithelial cells (◘ Fig. 4.8).

Histopathology of incision or excision biopsies is necessary to confirm malignancy of the tumors. While *sebaceous gland adenomas* present as an accumulation of well- to moderately well-differentiated proliferations of sebaceous glands with well-defined tumor borders, *sebaceous gland carcinomas* are characterized by loss of differentiation and invasive growth into surrounding tissues. Similarly, *apocrine gland carcinomas* are differentiated from adenomas by an increased cellular pleomorphism and infiltrative growth at the tumor borders. *Apocrine gland mixed tumors* present very much like mixed mammary gland tumors, with intratumoral cartilage.

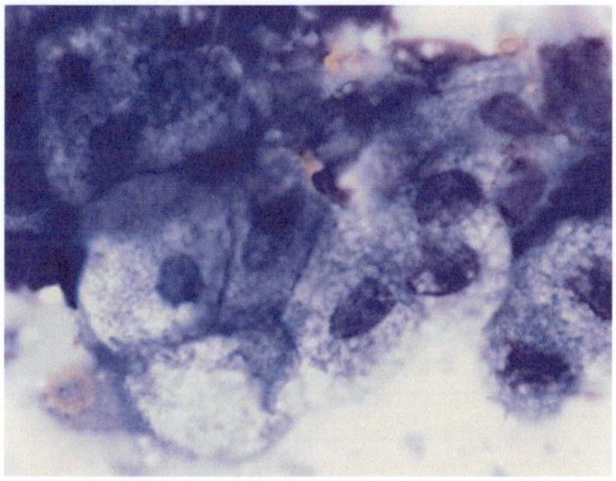

◘ **Fig. 4.7** Cytology, sebaceous gland adenoma, dog, May-Grünwald-Giemsa, 1000×. Note the round to cuboidal uniform epithelial cells with centrally located nuclei, fine chromatin pattern, and abundant amounts of basophilic cytoplasm containing multiple, clearly circumscribed vacuoles (Photo: with permission of Dr. N. Bauer, Faculty of Veterinary Medicine, Justus-Liebig-University, Giessen, Germany)

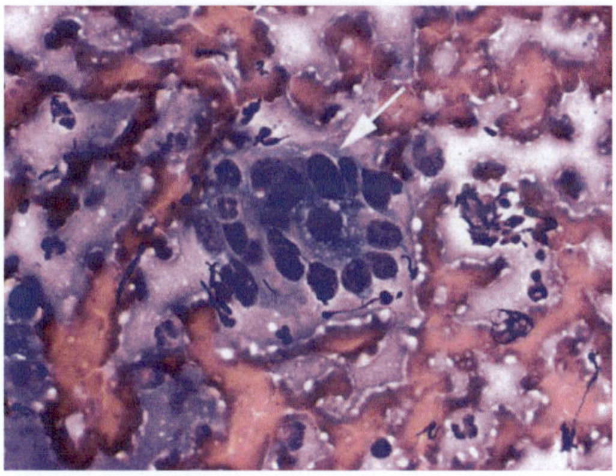

◘ **Fig. 4.8** Cytology, apocrine gland adenoma, dog, May-Grünwald-Giemsa, 400×. Note the clusters of epithelial tumor cells (*arrow*) surrounded by erythrocytes (red) and degenerate neutrophilic granulocytes

▪ Therapy

Surgery with wide tumor margins is usually curative. Reports on the application of chemotherapy or radiotherapy are not available.

4.1.1.4 Canine Perianal Gland Tumors

4

Box 4.4. Canine Perianal Gland Tumors in Four Facts

1. Mostly benign, testosterone-dependent hepatoid gland adenomas.
2. Less often malignant hepatoid gland carcinomas or anal sac apocrine gland adenocarcinomas.
3. One-third of dogs with apocrine gland adenocarcinomas with PTHrP-induced hypercalcemia.
4. Cytology is usually not able to conclusively confirm malignancy.

▪ Epidemiology and Pathogenesis

Two types of glands commonly develop neoplasms in the perianal area of dogs: the nonsecretory, sebaceous hepatoid glands and the apocrine glands of the anal sac.

Hepatoid gland adenomas are the most common tumors of the perianal region and represent up to 90 % of all perianal tumors. *Old intact male dogs, male dogs with testicular interstitial cell tumors,* and *ovariohysterectomized female dogs* with a deceased estrogen to testosterone ratios are predisposed. The development of these benign tumors is therefore thought to be testosterone dependent. This assumption is also supported by the observation that castration of male dogs is usually therapeutic. Cocker spaniels, Beagles, Bulldogs, and Samoyeds may have a *breed* predisposition. The mean age of affected animals is 10 years old.

Hepatoid gland carcinomas are rare tumors of the perianal glands with an incidence of <10 % of all perianal tumors. Affected dogs are on average 11 years old. These tumors occur in intact and castrated males and females, indicating a decreased developmental dependency on hormonal factors. There is a mild predisposition for large-breed males.

Apocrine gland adenocarcinomas of the anal sacs are rather rare but highly malignant perianal tumors. They develop from the apocrine glands around the anal sacs, which are located ventrolateral to the anus. Cocker spaniels seem to have a breed predisposition. There is no gender predisposition. The medium age of dogs with apocrine gland adenocarcinoma is 10 years.

▪ Clinical Appearance

Hepatoid gland adenomas are slow and expansively growing benign tumors. They usually appear as pain-free *single or multiple nodules* of up to 4 cm around the anus but may also be present on the prepuce, scrotum, or tailhead. Occasionally, they may ulcerate and become infected; they are rarely adherent or fixed to deeper structures.

Hepatoid gland carcinomas are malignant, invasive, and fast-growing tumors with a *metastatic rate of 15–50 %*. The regional sublumbar and pelvic lymph are commonly affected; distant metastases to the lungs, liver, kidney, and bone are rather rare. Macroscopically, the tumors look similar to adenomas but they are usually faster growing and more often fixed to the underlying tissues (▫ Fig. 4.9). *Obstruction of the pelvic canal* by sublumbar/pelvic lymph node metastasis occasionally leads to clinical signs of rectal obstipation, dyschezia, or perianal pain. Ultrasound is commonly used to evaluate the status of the regional lymph nodes. If lymph node metastasis is detected, thoracic radiographs should be taken to evaluate the presence of lung metastases. Histology of tissue biopsies is required to confirm the diagnosis.

Apocrine gland adenocarcinomas of the anal sacs are highly malignant usually unilateral tumors. Metastatic rates of 50–90 % have been

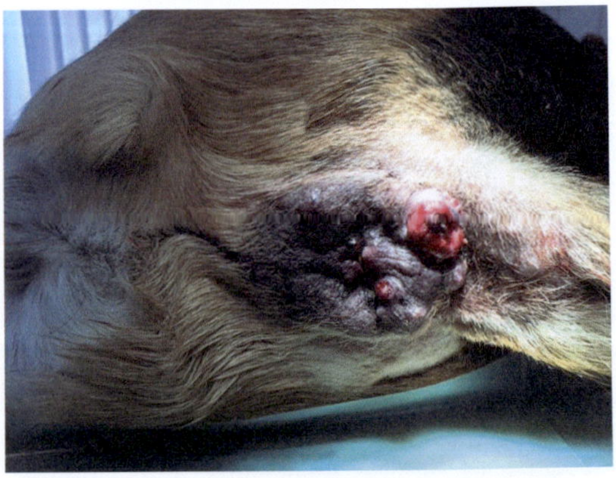

▫ **Fig. 4.9** Ulcerated, multinodular hepatoid gland carcinoma in a dog (Photo: with permission of Dr. O. Beger, Small Animal Practice, Cossebaude, Germany)

described. The regional sublumbar lymph nodes and pelvic nodes are affected in most cases at the time of the initial diagnosis. Distant lung, liver, spleen, and bone metastases usually develop at later stages of the diseases. A paraneoplastic hypercalcemia of malignancy, due to the release of *parathyroid hormone-related peptide (PTHrP)*, is present in one-third of the animals. Clinical signs of dogs with apocrine gland adenocarcinoma are either related to the mass effect of the primary tumors and its metastases, including perianal discomfort, dyschezia, tenesmus, or constipation, or due to paraneoplastic hypercalcemia. Concurrent clinical signs often include polyuria/polydipsia, anorexia, lethargy, bradycardia, and paresis. Abdominal radiographs, ultrasound, and magnetic resonance imaging are commonly used to identify lymph node or distant metastasis.

▪ Cytology and Histopathology

Cytology is usually not able to differentiate benign from malignant hepatoid gland tumors. Apocrine gland adenocarcinomas are characterized cytologically by polyhedral cells with a blue-gray, granular cytoplasm.

Histopathology of tissue biopsies is needed to evaluate the invasiveness of the tumor at the borders and to confirm malignancy of the *primary hepatoid tumor*. In addition, malignant tumors also show a less orderly arrangement of the epithelial cells and an increased number of mitotic figures. *Apocrine gland adenocarcinomas* are histologically characterized by solid sheets of tumor cells, rosette formation, or a tubular arrangement of the tumor cells. The tumors cells are usually highly monomorphic despite their malignant behavior.

▪ Therapy

Castration is the treatment of choice for *hepatoid gland adenomas*. Complete regression and a lack of recurrence are common after castration. In cases with lack of or incomplete regression in female dogs, surgical excision is recommended.

Hepatoid gland adenocarcinomas usually do not respond to castration. *Aggressive surgery* with appropriate margins is therefore indicated. Recurrence after extensive surgery is a negative prognostic indicator that is unfortunately relatively common. *Postsurgical radiotherapy* may improve the long-term outcome but there is a lack of reliable data. Tumors with a diameter of < 5 cm are in general associated with an improved 2-year disease-free interval. The prognosis for dogs with metastatic disease is poor.

Apocrine gland adenocarcinomas are usually treated with *aggressive surgery*. However, complete resection is often not possible, and more than 50 % of the animals develop metastatic disease at the time of initial diagnosis. Removal of affected lymph nodes may have a palliative effect. Survival times of 6–18 months have been reported for dogs with apocrine gland adenocarcinomas treated with surgery. *Chemotherapy and RT* are recommended as standard adjuvant treatment options for anal sac adenocarcinoma in the literature. However, clinical data on the success of these modalities are scarce. Chemotherapy using carboplatin, cisplatin, and actinomycin D has been reported. A few reports on the efficacy of curative and palliative radiotherapy of the primary tumors and affected lymph nodes weakly indicate a potential clinical effect for both approaches. Metastatic disease and, to a lesser extent, hypercalcemia have been described as negative prognostic indicators for survival.

▪ Suggested Further Reading

(Anderson et al. 2015; Bennett et al. 2002; Bergman 2012; Bowlt et al. 2013; de Swarte et al. 2011; Emms 2005; Hobson et al. 2006; Polton 2007; Polton and Brearley 2007; Ross et al. 1991; Vail et al. 1990)

4.1.1.5 Canine Cutaneous Papillomas

> **Box 4.5. Canine Cutaneous Papillomas in Four Facts**
>
> 1. Induced by canine papillomaviruses.
> 2. Mostly young dogs.
> 3. Immunosuppression/deficiency predisposes to infection.
> 4. Spontaneous remission within weeks is common.

▪ Epidemiology and Pathogenesis

Papillomas are rare *Papillomavirus-induced benign tumors* of the skin and the oral cavity (see Chap. 9) of juvenile and *young dogs*. In older dogs, a virus-associated etiology is not always confirmed. Canine papillomaviruses infect and stimulate proliferation in differentiated keratinocytes. These proliferation and neoplastic transformation are mainly induced by the *Papillomavirus* proteins E6 and E7, which destabilize p53 and inhibit the retinoblastoma protein. An association has been suggested between *Papillomavirus* infection and the development of *squamous-cell carcinomas (SCCs)* due to the detection of *Papillomavirus* protein and DNA in SCC. *Immunosuppression* or deficiency is thought to be an important factor for acute and persistent *Papillomavirus* infection. Infected dogs usually develop immunity against new infections.

4

▪ Clinical Appearance

Papillomas are single or multiple, *prominent or pedunculated, superficially frayed tumors.* Inverted papillomas are a rare benign variant, which grows into the subcutaneous tissue rather than externally. Spontaneous regression within weeks or a few months is commonly observed.

▪ Cytology and Histopathology

Cytology may present with a dominance of proliferating spindle cells from the tumor base and center and is rather unspecific. *Histopathology* is necessary to confirm the diagnosis and to exclude other epithelial skin tumors. The presence of a strong mesenchymal proliferation at the base of the tumor leads to the diagnosis of a *fibropapilloma.*

▪ Therapy

Surgical excision is curative but due to the usual spontaneous remission often not necessary. A local application of 5-fluorouracil on papillomas has been described but is associated with side effects that override the benefits of the treatment.

▪ Current Trends in Research

Research is ongoing on the identification of new emerging canine *papillomaviruses*, their potential association with other tumors like SCC, and the cellular immune response to papillomaviral infection.

▪ Suggested Further Reading

(Beckwith-Cohen et al. 2014; Lange and Favrot 2011; Luff et al. 2012; Munday et al. 2011; Munday et al. 2015)

4.1.2 Canine Cutaneous Melanomas

Box 4.6. Canine Cutaneous Melanomas in Five Facts

1. Cutaneous melanomas mostly benign and pigmented.
2. Surgery mostly curative.
3. Amelanotic tumors and malignant tumors develop rarely.
4. Digital melanomas often metastatic, even after early amputation of the digit.
5. Immunohistochemistry occasionally necessary to confirm diagnosis in amelanotic melanomas.

▪ Epidemiology and Pathogenesis

Melanomas are tumors of the melanin-producing melanocytes, which are derived from the neural crest and thus are not mesenchymal or epithelial tumors. Common locations are the oral cavity (see chapter GIT), the skin, and the digits and intra- or periocular (see Chap. 6). In contrast to the mostly malignant melanomas of the oral cavity and the digit, cutaneous melanomas of other skin regions are *usually benign* with a minority of malignant cutaneous melanomas. There is a predisposition of dark-coated *breeds* for cutaneous and digital melanomas. Melanomas may occur at any age but are most commonly found at the *age* of 9–10 years. The *etiology* of melanomas in the dog is unclear; a contribution of UV-light exposure to carcinogenesis as in human melanomas is not confirmed, and specific driver mutations are not identified.

▪ Clinical Appearance

Cutaneous melanomas are usually presenting as slow-growing, small, solitary, pigmented, well-circumscribed masses anywhere in the skin (◘ Fig. 4.10). *Amelanotic cutaneous melanomas,* common in the oral cavity, are the exception but are possible. In contrast, *digital melanomas* are usually fast-growing, ulcerated, not necessarily pigmented tumors. Metastasis of digital melanomas to the regional lymph node and the lung is common and often apparent at the time of diagnosis.

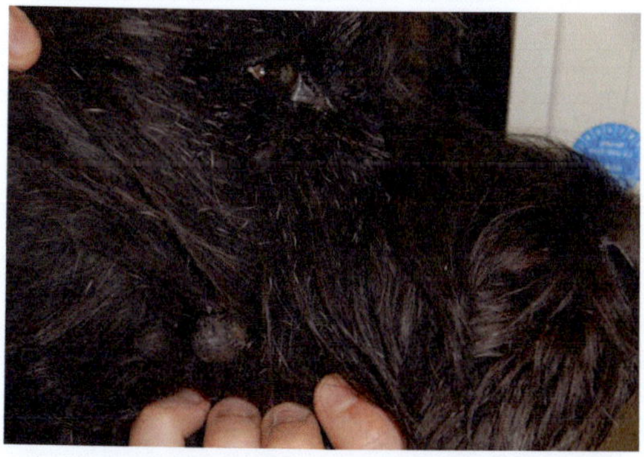

■ **Fig. 4.10** Poorly differentiated melanoma (confirmed with histology), dog. Pigmented dermal mass at the jaw of a 12-year-old Giant Schnauzer (Photo: with permission of the Faculty of Veterinary Medicine, Justus-Liebig-University, Giessen, Germany)

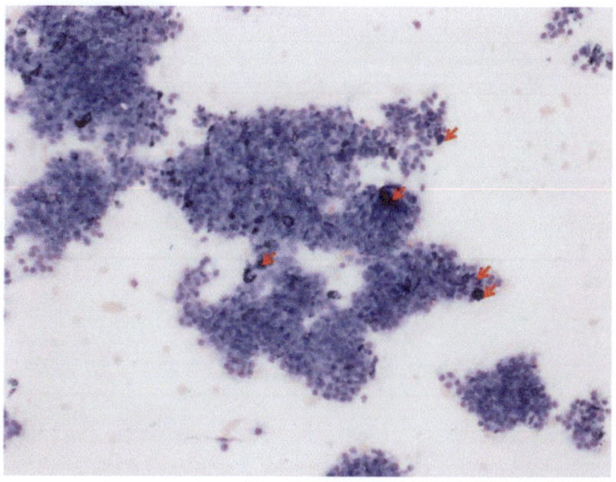

■ **Fig. 4.11** Cytology, poorly differentiated, mostly amelanotic melanoma, dog (the same dog as in ■ Fig. 4.10), May-Grünwald-Giemsa, 100×. Note the clusters of cohesive, spindle shaped to polygonal mainly poorly pigmented melanocytes with few scattered pigmented melanocytes/melanophages (*red arrows*) (Photo: with permission of Dr. N. Bauer, Faculty of Veterinary Medicine, Justus-Liebig-University, Giessen, Germany)

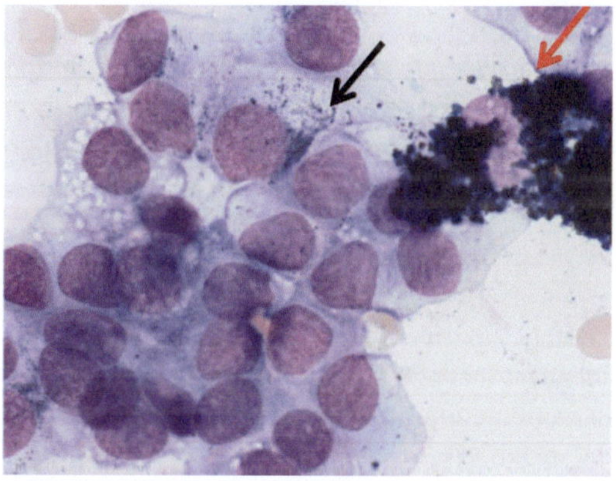

■ **Fig. 4.12** Cytology, poorly differentiated, mostly amelanotic melanoma, dog (the same dog as in ■ Fig. 4.10), May-Grünwald-Giemsa, 1000×. Note the spindle shaped to polygonal mainly poorly to nonpigmented melanocytes with few dustlike melanin granules (*black arrow*). In contrast, melanophages contain numerous round, markedly bigger granules of engulfed melanin (*red arrow*) (Photo: with permission of Dr. N. Bauer, Faculty of Veterinary Medicine, Justus-Liebig-University, Giessen, Germany)

■ Cytology and Histopathology

Cytology of pigmented melanomas is usually straightforward due to the cytoplasmic dark brown to black granules (■ Figs. 4.11, 4.12, 4.13, and 4.14). Amelanotic tumors are however more difficult to diagnose by cytology due to the highly diverse histologic appearance of melanomas. This is also true for the *histopathology*. Detection of melanin cells in pigmented tumors allows for diagnosis of a melanoma. Cellular and nuclear pleomorphism, a high number of mitotic figures, and invasive behavior at the tumor borders are associated with malignant behavior. *Amelanotic tumors* are, however, challenging due to their pleomorphic appearance. They may show spindle cell, epitheloid, or even round cell-like growth patterns. Immunohistochemical markers may help for a conclusive classification of these tumors, however challenging due to their pleomorphic appearance. Immunohistochemical markers may help for a conclusive classification of these tumors.

■ Therapy

Surgery with wide margins is the treatment of choice for both cutaneous benign and malignant melanomas. Surgery alone is associated with a good prognosis and cure of the majority of benign cutaneous, non-digital melanomas. Surgical excision of malignant cutaneous and digital melanomas is however often associated with *recurrence*. Most dogs with *digital melanomas* are euthanized within 1 or 2 years after digit amputation due to distant metastases.

Chemotherapy using doxorubicin, cisplatin, and other anticancer drugs has been described preferentially for the treatment of oral melanoma and may be a potential adjunctive treatment option.

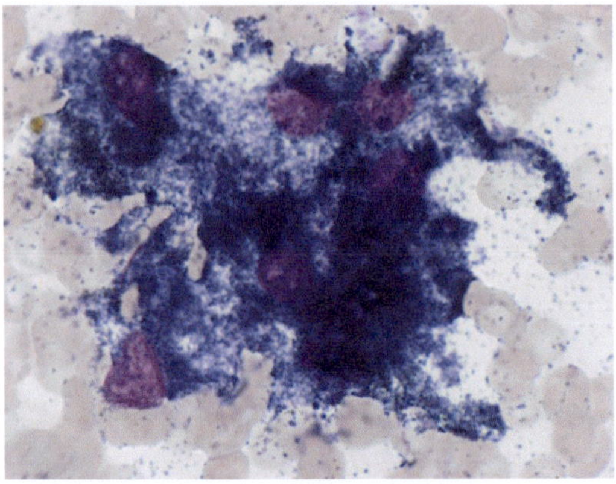

Fig. 4.13 Cytology, well-differentiated, melanotic melanoma, dog, May-Grünwald-Giemsa, 1000×. Pigmented melanocytes are usually easy to diagnose due to the presence of abundant and typical dark blue melanin granules. However, melanoma cells are often fragile in cytological specimens. Cellular borders therefore tend to be indistinct and ruptured and free melanin granules are often present (Photo: with permission of Dr. N. Bauer, Faculty of Veterinary Medicine, Justus-Liebig-University, Giessen, Germany)

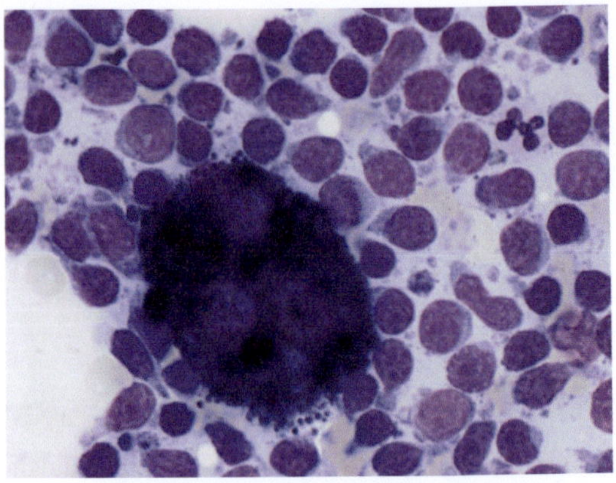

Fig. 4.14 Cytology, lymph node metastasis, melanoma, dog (the same dog as in Fig. 4.10), May-Grünwald-Giemsa, 1000×. Note the group of highly pigmented melanocytes with numerous melanin granules almost masking the nucleus (Photo: with permission of Dr. N. Bauer, Faculty of Veterinary Medicine, Justus-Liebig-University, Giessen, Germany)

Radiotherapy is an important therapy option for oral melanomas but not for a common approach for the treatment of the mostly benign cutaneous melanomas.

Prognostic Factors and Markers

Melan-A, S100, PNL2, CSPG4, and *tyrosinase* are variably specific and sensitive immunohistochemical markers for cells of melanocytic origin. In combination they are however very helpful in the diagnosis of amelanotic and pleomorphic malignant melanomas. Prognostic factors for canine cutaneous melanomas are presented in Table 4.1.

Current Trends in Research

There is ongoing research on the use of vaccination against melanoma-specific antigens in melanoma-bearing dogs. Chondroitin sulfate proteoglycan-4 (CSPG4), tyrosinase, and disialoganglioside GD3 have been tested for their value as vaccination targets for canine melanoma with variable success.

Suggested Further Reading

(Abramo et al. 1999; Brockley et al. 2013; Herzog et al. 2013; Lange and Favrot 2011; Ottnod et al. 2013; Smedley et al. 2011; Spangler and Kass 2006; Waropastrakul et al. 2012)

Table 4.1 Prognostic factors for canine cutaneous melanoma

Factor	Influence on prognosis
Distant metastasis	Negative
Tumor size	Possibly negative
Histologic classification as malignant	Variably negative
Nuclear atypia	Negative
Mitotic index	Negative
Lack of pigmentation	Negative
Ulceration	Negative
(Vascular) infiltration	Negative
High Ki67 index	Negative
DNA ploidy	Negative

4.1.3 Canine Soft Tissue Sarcomas

Canine malignant mesenchymal tumors of all body areas are commonly designated as *soft tissue sarcomas (STS)* due to their similar clinical behavior and response to treatment. Commonalities of this *heterogeneous tumor group* are highly invasive growth, high rate of recurrence, low-to-moderate frequency of local and distant metastases, and a similar response to treatment. The term STS embraces tumors of different histogenesis such as fibrosarcomas, rhabdomyosarcomas, leiomyosarcomas, peripheral nerve sheath tumors, perivascular wall tumors, and liposarcomas. Synovial cell sarcomas, hemangiosarcomas, and osteosarcomas are sometimes but not consistently also included into the STS group. This chapter covers in its first part the current general ideas on diagnosis, therapy, and prognosis of STS which are also correct for non-cutaneous STS. In the remaining chapter, there is a more detailed description of cutaneous liposarcomas, fibrosarcomas, and subcutaneous peripheral nerve sheath tumors (PNST) since they are unequivocally specific tumor entities, although their specific characteristics are currently clinically irrelevant. Cutaneous vascular tumors including hemangiosarcomas, hemangiomas, and perivascular wall tumors are described in more detail in Chap. 15.

STS are relatively common tumors of *middle-aged to old dogs*. There is no confirmed sex or breed predisposition.

▪ Clinical Appearance

Soft tissue sarcomas are mostly solitary, slowly but infiltratively growing tumors which can arise in every anatomic location. Due to their *infiltrative growth*, they are usually not freely moveable on palpation. The minority of STS develops *metastases*. The clinical symptoms associated with the tumors almost completely depend on the location and the mass effect of the tumor on the affected and adjacent organs. Cytology, histopathology (biopsies), and imaging are necessary for the final diagnosis, complete staging, and therapy planning of STS.

Computed tomography (CT) and *magnetic resonance imaging (MRI)* with or without the use of contrast agents are necessary to perceive the full extension of the usually highly infiltrative STS. Palpation and sight are often underestimating the full extension of STS. A staging system has been developed for all tumors falling into the category of canine STS independent from their histogenesis (◘ Table 4.2).

▪ Cytology and Histopathology

Fine-needle aspirates of STS are characterized by the presence of cells with a more or less spindloid cell shape, indistinct cellular borders, and often an eosinophilic, sometimes fibrillary, matrix between the cells. Depending on the histotype, i.e., lipo-, rhabdomyo-, or fibrosarcomas, etc., several other features may also be present. *Histologically*, all STS are characterized by the presence of more or less spindloid tumors cells. In addition, every STS subtype may show other features like adipocyte- or rhabdomyocyte-like appearance. *STS grade* is of higher clinical relevance than histotype (◘ Table 4.3). Immunohistochemical markers (see Dennis et al. 2011) can be used to further differentiate the histologic type/origin of STS if standard histopathology is not sufficiently typical.

▪ Therapy

Surgical resection with 2–3 cm lateral margins in the normal tissue and at least one fascial plane into the deep is recommended to decrease the recurrence rate. This may also include amputation. Confirmed or assumed incomplete resection with smaller margins in difficult anatomic locations requires adjuvant radiotherapy and chemotherapy.

Radiotherapy is an important adjuvant therapy for STS. It is associated with 3-year survival rates of up to 70 % of patients. Coarse fractionated radiotherapy and hypofractionated radiotherapy are most commonly recommended. Of note, one study found that radiation within the first month after surgery was associated with a higher risk for recurrence than radiation after 1 month.

Adjuvant, metronomic chemotherapy, i.e., the administration of low doses of, for instance, cyclophosphamide with an increased frequency and may be for longer periods, is currently seen as a promising approach to prevent intratumoral angiogenesis and tumor growth. In addition, classical *non-adjuvant, doxorubicin-based chemotherapy* protocols are considered to be promising for the treatment of non-resectable STS.

▪ Prognosis

The prognosis for STS is good, if local tumor control is achieved. Thus, incomplete resection and recurrence (recurrent tumors are usually more difficult to be treated) but also tumor grade are the most important prognostic factors.

Table 4.2 Staging system for canine soft tissue sarcomas (Liptak and Forrest 2012)

Stage	Tumor size	Lymph node metastases	Metastasis	Histologic grade
1	T_{any} (any r size)	N0 (none)	M0 (none)	I–II
II	T_{1a} (<5 cm, superficial) T_{1a} (<5 cm, deep) T_{2a} (>5 cm, superficial)	N0 (none)	M0 (none)	III
III	T_{2b} (>5 cm, deep)	N0 (none)	M0 (none)	III
IV	T_{any} (any r size) T_{any} (any r size)	N1 (present) N_{any}	M_{any} M1 (present)	I–III

Table 4.3 Grading system for soft tissue sarcomas (Dennis et al. 2011)

Histologic criteria	Points	Features
A. Differentiation	1	Resembles normal adult mesenchymal tissue
	2	Specific histologic subtype but poor differentiation
	3	Undifferentiated, unknown histotype
B. Necrosis	1	None
	2	≤50 % necrosis
	3	>50 % necrosis
C. Mitoses per 10 HPF (400×)	1	0–9 mitoses/10 HPF
	2	10–19 mitoses/10 HPF
	3	>19 mitoses/10 HPF
Total score (A+B+C)	≤3	*Grade I*
	4–5	*Grade II*
	≥6	*Grade III*

▪ Suggested Reading

(Bacon et al. 2007; Baker-Gabb et al. 2003; Burton et al. 2011; Demetriou et al. 2012; Dennis et al. 2011; Dernell et al. 1998; Elmslie et al. 2008; Hohenhaus et al. 2016; Kung et al. 2014; Kuntz et al. 1997; Lawrence et al. 2008; Liptak and Forrest 2012; Matz 2015; Ogilvie et al. 1989; Prpich et al. 2014; Rassnick 2003)

4.1.3.1 Canine Lipomas and Liposarcomas

Box 4.7. Canine Cutaneous Lipomas in Four Facts

1. Benign, slowly growing tumors.
2. Cytologically not differentiated from normal adipose tissue.
3. Surgery curative.
4. Malignant tumors often recur even after aggressive surgery.

▪ Epidemiology and Pathogenesis

Lipomas, benign tumors derived from the subcutaneous adipocytes, are very common tumors of the canine skin. Other adipocytic tumors of the skin include the less common semimalignant *infiltrative lipomas* and the rare malignant *liposarcomas*. Lipomas are more common in older dogs and females and commonly appear at the trunk. They belong to the group of soft tissue sarcomas (STSs).

▪ Clinical Appearance

Lipomas are single, cutaneous, small to very large lesions. They are soft to the touch and are not associated with alopecia or ulceration. *Infiltrative lipoma* and *liposarcoma* are firmer on palpation and less movable due to their infiltrative growth into the surrounding tissues. The common staging system for canine soft tissue sarcoma is used for liposarcoma (Table 4.2).

▪ Cytology and Histopathology

Cytology of lipomas and in most cases of infiltrative lipomas presents with well-differentiated adipocytes, which cannot be differentiated from normal adipocytes of the skin (◘ Figs. 4.15, 4.16, and 4.17).

Histologically, lipoma tumor cells cannot be differentiated from normal adipocytes in expansively growing tumors. Similarly, infiltrative lipomas are also composed of differentiated adipocytes, which nevertheless are growing invasively into adjacent muscles and fascia. The common grading system for canine soft tissue sarcoma is used for liposarcomas (◘ Table 4.3).

▪ Therapy

Surgery is curative for *lipoma*. Even very aggressive surgery *sometimes does not prevent local recurrence of infiltrative lipoma or liposarcoma*.

Postsurgical *radiotherapy* may prolong the time to recurrence of infiltrative lipoma but there is a lack of sufficient data; it has not been described for liposarcoma.

▪ Suggested Further Reading

(McEntee et al. 2000; Bacon et al. 2007; Baker-Gabb et al. 2003; Burton et al. 2011; Demetriou et al. 2012; Dennis et al. 2011; Dernell et al. 1998; Elmslie et al. 2008; Hohenhaus et al. 2016; Kung et al. 2014; Kuntz et al. 1997; Lawrence et al. 2008; Liptak and Forrest 2012; Matz 2015; Ogilvie et al. 1989; Prpich et al. 2014; Rassnick 2003)

4.1.3.2 Canine Cutaneous Fibromas and Fibrosarcomas

Box 4.8. Canine Fibrosarcomas in Three Facts

1. Benign fibromas are cured by surgical resection.
2. Fibrosarcomas are invasively growing and often recurring after surgery.
3. Adjuvant radiotherapy is reducing the recurrence rate.

▪ Epidemiology and Pathogenesis

Cutaneous fibrosarcomas are moderately common malignant tumors derived from subcutaneous fibrocytes. They belong to the group of soft tissue sarcomas (STS) in the dog. They are more common in *older dogs*, but are particularly *aggressive in young dogs*. The etiology is unclear. *Fibromas* are rather rare benign tumors of the subcutaneous fibrocytes. They are more common in older dogs.

▪ Clinical Appearance

Fibromas are small, solitary, soft to firm, well-circumscribed nodules, which can be ulcerated in mechanically stressed areas of the skin. *Fibrosarcomas* are fast-growing, locally invasive, usually large tumors and may be soft and firm on palpation due to necrotic and cystic tumor areas. Metastasis is common in

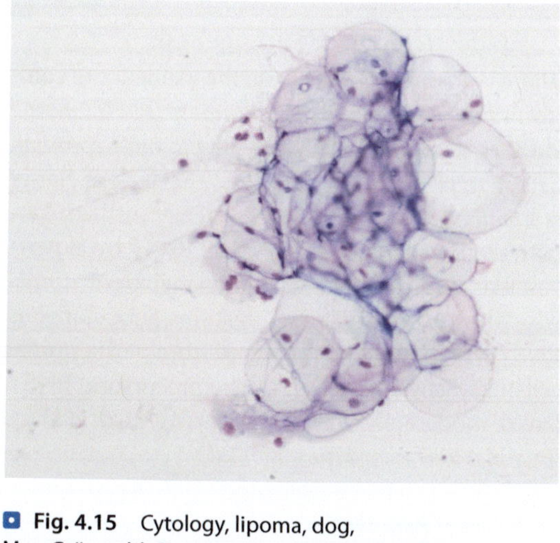

◘ **Fig. 4.15** Cytology, lipoma, dog, May-Grünwald-Giemsa, 100×. Note the cluster of well-differentiated adipocytes with eccentrically located oval nuclei and abundant amounts of a clear cytoplasm (Photo: with permission of Dr. N. Bauer, Faculty of Veterinary Medicine, Justus-Liebig-University, Giessen, Germany)

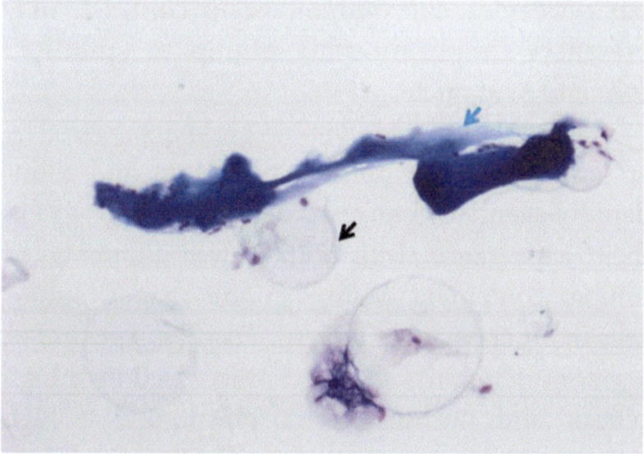

◘ **Fig. 4.16** Cytology, infiltrative lipoma, dog, May-Grünwald-Giemsa, 100×. Note the differentiated adipocytes (*black arrow*) closely associated with clusters of striated muscle tissue (*blue arrow*) indicative of infiltrative lipoma. However, a definite diagnosis cannot be made based on cytology alone (Photo: with permission of Dr. N. Bauer, Faculty of Veterinary Medicine, Justus-Liebig-University, Giessen, Germany)

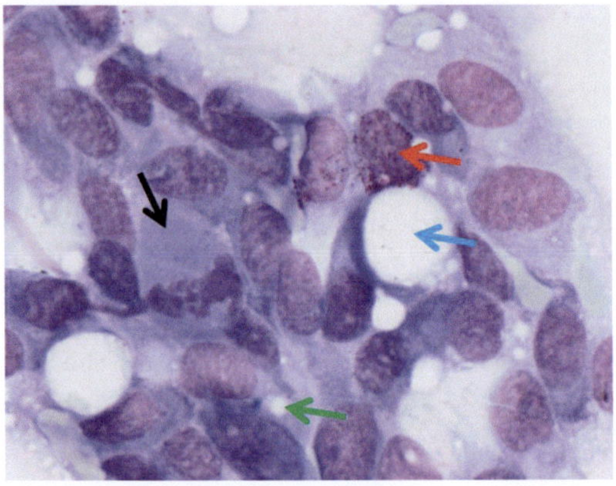

Fig. 4.17 Cytology, liposarcoma, dog, May-Grünwald-Giemsa, 1000×. Note the clusters of moderately cohesive spindle shaped to plump cells with oval nuclei, fine to granular chromatin pattern, and moderate amounts of lightly basophilic cytoplasm occasionally containing clearly circumscribed vacuoles (fat). The spindle cell population is intermixed with fatty vacuoles (*blue arrow*). There are several mitotic figures and occasional well-differentiated mast cells (*red arrow*) (Photo: with permission of Dr. N. Bauer, Faculty of Veterinary Medicine, Justus-Liebig-University, Giessen, Germany)

approximately 20% of cases. The common staging system for canine soft tissue sarcoma is used for fibrosarcomas (Table 4.2).

Cytology and Histopathology

Cytology may present with well-differentiated spindle cells in fibromas, which are sometimes difficult to discriminate from normal subcutaneous fibrocytes. Fibrosarcomas, in contrast, may present with pleomorphic plump to spindloid cells and oval nuclei.

Histopathologically, fibromas are characterized by an accumulation of uniform fibroblasts and abundant collagen. *Fibrosarcomas* may be very variable in their appearance with rather well-differentiated tumors containing plump spindle-shaped tumor cells in a herringbone pattern. *Poorly differentiated, aggressive fibrosarcomas* are characterized by a high cellular and nuclear pleomorphism and a high mitotic rate. The common staging system for canine STS is used for fibrosarcomas (Table 4.3).

Therapy

Surgery is curative for fibromas. In contrast, early resection of fibrosarcomas, while the best treatment option, still has a guarded prognosis. Up to two-thirds of the tumors develop recurrence, which is associated with a poor prognosis. Since fibrosarcomas belong to the group of STS, *adjuvant radiotherapy, doxorubicin-based chemotherapy protocols,* and *metronomic therapy* can reduce the risk of recurrence.

Suggested Further Reading

(Beckwith-Cohen et al. 2014) (Bacon et al. 2007; Baker-Gabb et al. 2003; Burton et al. 2011; Demetriou et al. 2012; Dennis et al. 2011; Dernell et al. 1998; Elmslie et al. 2008; Hohenhaus et al. 2016; Kung et al. 2014; Kuntz et al. 1997; Lawrence et al. 2008; Liptak and Forrest 2012; Matz 2015; Ogilvie et al. 1989; Prpich et al. 2014; Rassnick 2003)

4.1.3.3 Canine Cutaneous Peripheral Nerve Sheath Tumors (PNST)

Box 4.9. Canine Cutaneous Peripheral Nerve Sheath Tumors in Five Facts

1. Derived from perineuronal Schwann cells or their precursors.
2. Difficult to be separated from perivascular wall tumors.
3. Surgery with wide margins often curative.
4. Recurrence nevertheless common.
5. Adjuvant radiotherapy or chemotherapy may reduce the risk of recurrence.

Epidemiology and Pathogenesis

There is an ongoing debate on the incidence of *cutaneous peripheral nerve sheath tumors (PNST)*. Some authors state that PNST *may be the most common STS subtype of the skin/subcutis*. This lack of clarity is mainly based on the inconsistency in the histopathologic criteria to differentiate PNST from perivascular wall tumors and hemangiopericytoma, which have similar histologic features. Subcutaneous PNSTs are thought to be derived from perineuronal cells like Schwann cells or their precursors. PNST have a moderately to highly *invasive growth character and a low metastatic potential.*

Clinical Appearance

PNST are usually solitary, *slow but infiltratively growing* masses. They can occur in the subcutis of any body part with a *predisposition for the limbs.* The common staging system for canine soft tissue sarcoma is used for PNST (Table 4.2).

Cytology and Histopathology

Cytology may present with well-differentiated spindle cells, presence of more or less spindloid cell shape, indistinct cellular borders, and often an eosinophilic, sometimes fibrillary, matrix between the cells. *Histopathologically,* PNST are graded according to the common grading system for canine STS (◻ Table 4.3). They present as well-circumscribed tumors with moderate cellularity, spindle to ovoid cells with occasional presence of Antoni A/B pattern, and palisading nuclei (Verocay-like bodies). Cells are often arranged in whorls around the capillaries or collagen island, which makes them difficult to be separated from perivascular wall tumors.

Therapy

Surgery can be curative when performed with sufficiently large margins into the normal tissue (2–3 cm). Since PNST belong to the group of STS, *adjuvant radiotherapy, doxorubicin-based chemotherapy protocols,* and *ametronomic therapy* can reduce the risk of recurrence.

Suggested Further Reading

(Brehm et al. 1995; Chijiwa et al. 2004; Klopfleisch et al. 2013; Meyer and Klopfleisch 2014; Suzuki et al. 2014)

4.1.4 Canine Cutaneous Hematopoietic Tumors

Mast cell tumors are the most common hematopoietic tumor of the canine skin. Cutaneous histiocytomas and plasmacytomas are less common. Cutaneous lymphomas are rarely observed and are described in Chap. 6.

4.1.4.1 Canine Cutaneous Mast Cell Tumors

Box 4.10. Canine Cutaneous Mast Cell Tumor in Seven Facts

1. The most common cutaneous tumor of the dog.
2. KIT receptor signaling major proliferative stimulus for mast cells.
3. Activating mutations in the KIT gene are present in 30 % of the tumors.
4. Two currently applied histologic grading systems.
5. Surgery is often curative for low-grade mast cell tumors.
6. Surgery and irradiation are the treatment of choice for tumors in difficult locations.
7. Tyrosine kinase inhibitors have strong but short-term effects on tumor regression.

Epidemiology and Pathogenesis

Canine mast cell tumors (MCT) are the *most common cutaneous tumor* of the dog, representing approximately 20 % of all skin tumors. They may occur at any age but are most common in older dogs with a mean *age* of 9 years; there is no *gender* predilection. There seems to be a genetic basis for MCT because a *breed predisposition* exists for boxers, retrievers, pug-dogs, Boston terriers and Stafford terriers, and Rhodesian ridgebacks. However, tumors in these breeds are generally of low malignancy and favorable prognosis. In contrast, *Shar-Pets* are also predisposed to develop MCT but these are often high-grade tumors with a poor prognosis.

The *molecular pathogenesis* and *etiology* of canine MCT are mostly unknown. Chronic inflammation, a viral etiology or mutations or abnormal expression of relevant tumor suppressors like p53, p21, or p27 as potential causes have been tested but disproven as direct causes. The only potential factor currently under review in the carcinogenesis of canine MCT is the *stem cell factor receptor (KIT* or *CD117).* Binding of its ligand stem cell factor (SCF) leads to activation of its tyrosine kinase domain and promotes proliferation, differentiation, and survival of nonneoplastic mast cells. KIT is expressed in both nonneoplastic and neoplastic mast cells. Expression may however change from normal membrane-bound expression to cytoplasmic KIT expression in neoplastic mast cells, indicating abnormal function. Several somatic, not inherited, *KIT mutations* in exons 8, 9, 11, and 12 of the gene have been identified, of which a tandem duplication of a part of exon 11 has been best analyzed. This mutation leads to a permanent and unregulated activation of KIT signaling and increased risk of local recurrence, metastasis, and worse prognosis. Activating KIT mutations are present in up to 30 % of the high-grade tumors, which indicates that other mechanisms of carcinogenesis have to be relevant in the majority of tumors. Another potential mechanism of MCT carcinogenesis may be de novo expression of all subunits of the *interleukin-2 receptor (IL-2R),* a major proliferation stimulus for lymphocytes, and its ligand IL-2. Both are expressed in almost all low-grade and a fraction of high-grade MCT cells and activated nonneoplastic mast cells but never in resting, nonneoplastic mast cells.

▪ Clinical Appearance

MCT are *solitary lesions* in 90 % of cases. They are mostly found on the trunk or the limbs, less often on the head and neck, and even less often on the mucous membranes. A *visceral form*, called systemic mastocytosis or gastrointestinal MCT, may occur; this is described in the chapter on hematopoietic cancer and GIT cancer, respectively (see Chaps. 6 and 9). MCTs are always considered *potentially malignant*. Nevertheless, well-differentiated tumors have a metastatic rate of less than 10 %. High-grade MCTs are locally invasive and develop *metastases* with a rate ranging from 50 % to almost 100 % depending on the studies. The first step in metastasis is usually metastasis to the local lymph nodes and then to the spleen, liver, and other visceral organs. Lung involvement is uncommon.

Low-grade MCT may be slow growing and present for years. In contrast, *high-grade MCT* may be ulcerated and rapidly growing with smaller surrounding satellite nodules and massive inflammation and edema due to the release of vasoactive amines like histamine. Degranulation of histamine-containing mast cell granules during examination may induce *Darier's signs*, which consist of rapid swelling and wheal formation, often described by owners as "growing and shrinking" of the tumors. Release of histamine by the cutaneous tumors frequently leads to a *gastrointestinal paraneoplastic syndrome.* Stimulation of *gastric histamine receptors* leads to massive hydrochloric acid secretion with vomiting, *gastric ulceration,* and abdominal pain. Only dogs with massive tumor burden and a sudden massive histamine release are at risk of developing a hypotensive anaphylactic reaction.

Several, often extensive, *diagnostic workup schemes* for accurate diagnosis of canine MCT are available. However, MCT diagnosis is usually based on FNA, although it is not sufficient for proper tumor grading (see the next chapter). In a next step, *clinical staging* is performed according to a World Health Organization (WHO) system (▪ Table 4.4). Due to the overlapping clinical behavior and the strong influence of therapy and histologic grading on prognosis, the staging system is of reduced clinical value and repeatedly criticized.

A *standard workup scheme for* canine cutaneous MCT has been developed by Thamm and Vail. Any suspicious ultrasound findings in the liver and spleen should be analyzed by fine-needle aspirates. Screening of buffy coat smears of centrifuged blood for mast cells, ultrasound of the primary tumor, or thoracic radiographs are not considered to be of significant prognostic value. Histopathologic grading and analysis of

▪ Table 4.4 Staging system for canine mast cells tumors (WHO)

Stage	Tumor	Lymph node metastases	Systemic signs	Prognosis
0–1 0–2	One tumor, incompletely excised	No No	No Yes	Better than III/IV
I–1 I–2	One tumor in the dermis	No No	No Yes	Better than III, IV
II–1 II–2	One tumor in the dermis	Yes Yes	No Yes	Similar to II in most treatment protocols
III–1 III–2	Multiple or large or infiltrating tumors	Yes/No Yes/No	No Yes	Worse than I/II
IV	Any tumor	Yes	Yes	Worse than I/II

surgical margins and eventually of suspicious lymph nodes or hepatic and spleen lesions are necessary for a final decision on the appropriate therapy option.

Cytology and Histopathology

Fine-needle aspiration (FNA) of an MCT is a very helpful and easy method to make a presurgical diagnosis of this tumor type (Figs. 4.18, 4.19, 4.20, 4.21, and 4.22). Its sensitivity and specificity for tumor grading are, however, low compared to histopathology of biopsies. There is a single study that refuses this finding. Identification of lymph node metastasis (>3 % mast cells) is also difficult using FNA due to the presence of similar numbers of mast cells in lymph nodes of healthy dogs.

Histopathologic analysis using tissue biopsies is the definitive technique to diagnose and grade canine MCT and to evaluate tumor borders. Besides the standard hematoxylin and eosin (H&E) stain, toluidine stain is also used to increase sensitivity due to the specifically eosin- or purple-stained metachromatic granules in well- to moderately differentiated mast cells. Variable amounts of concurrently present eosinophilic granulocytes dispersed between the MCT cells also help in the diagnosis of MCT. Two concurrent grading systems are currently available for canine MCT (Table 4.5). The classic *3-tier Patnaik grading* has been used for decades but is increasingly criticized for classifying 40 % of tumors as intermediate grade, without specifying clinical or therapeutic criteria for malignancy or benign classification. A new *Kiupel 2-tier grading system* avoids these problems and separates MCT in only two groups, low- and high-grade MCT.

Therapy

Surgery, radiotherapy, and chemotherapy with different drug classes can be used for the treatment of MCT. Their application and combination very much depend on tumor staging and grading.

Exclusive surgery is the treatment of choice for localized, low- and intermediate-grade, nonmetastatic *MCT at promising locations* where wide excision is possible. In these cases, surgery alone is mostly curative. A 3-cm *surgical margin* extending at least one fascial plane deep has historically been recommended. Recently, it has been shown that lateral margins of 2 cm and only one fascial plan or even 1 cm lateral and 4 mm deep margins are sufficient to avoid recurrence or metastasis of low- or intermediate-grade MCT. High-grade, aggressive MCT nevertheless should still be resected with at least 3 cm margins due to their infiltrative growth. Preoperative ultrasound or computed tomography is helpful to evaluate the extent of the tumor. Histopathological identification of incomplete resection at the surgical mar-

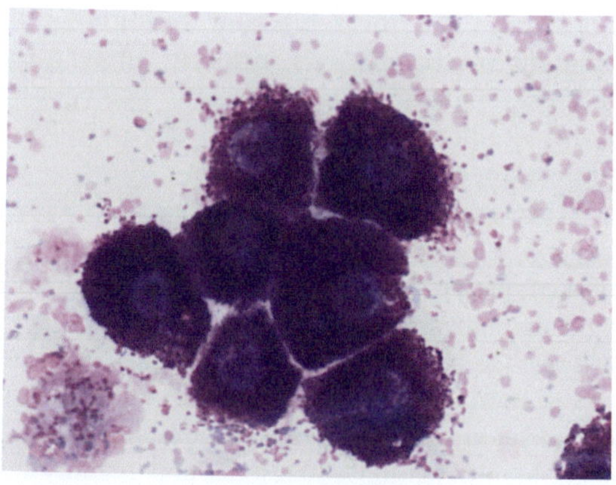

Fig. 4.18 Cytology, cutaneous mast cell tumor grade I/ low grade, dog, May-Grünwald-Giemsa, 1000×. Well-differentiated mast cells with large amounts of fine intracytoplasmic granules (Photo: with permission of Dr. N. Bauer, Faculty of Veterinary Medicine, Justus-Liebig-University, Giessen, Germany)

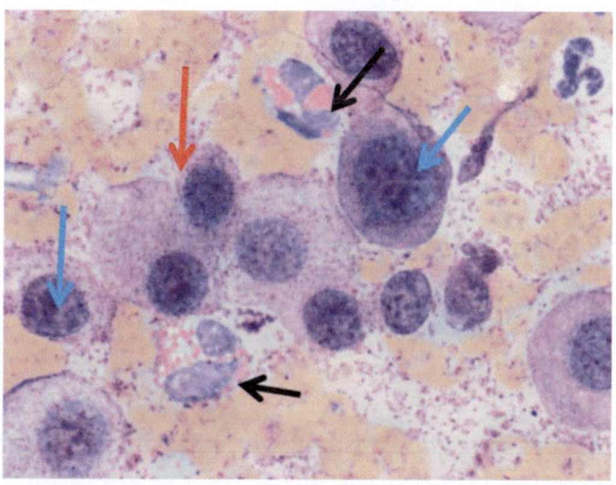

Fig. 4.19 Cytology, cutaneous mast cell tumor grade II/ low grade, dog, May-Grünwald-Giemsa, 1000×. Note the moderately differentiated mast cells (*red arrows*) with moderate amounts of fine dustlike intracytoplasmic granules indicating a moderate grade of differentiation. There is a moderate pleomorphism, anisocytosis, and anisokaryosis and coarse chromatin structure (*blue arrow*) of mast cells. Few scattered eosinophils (*black arrow*) are seen (Photo: with permission of Dr. N. Bauer, Faculty of Veterinary Medicine, Justus-Liebig-University, Giessen, Germany

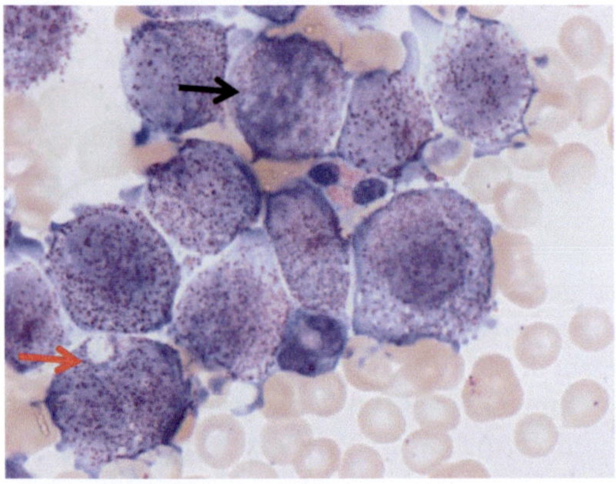

Fig. 4.20 Cytology, cutaneous mast cell tumor grade III/high grade, dog, May-Grünwald-Giemsa, 1000×. Note the presence of moderate to undifferentiated mast cells, mitotic figures (*black arrow*) and erythrophagocytosis (*red arrow*) (Photo: with permission of Dr. N. Bauer, Faculty of Veterinary Medicine, Justus-Liebig-University, Giessen, Germany)

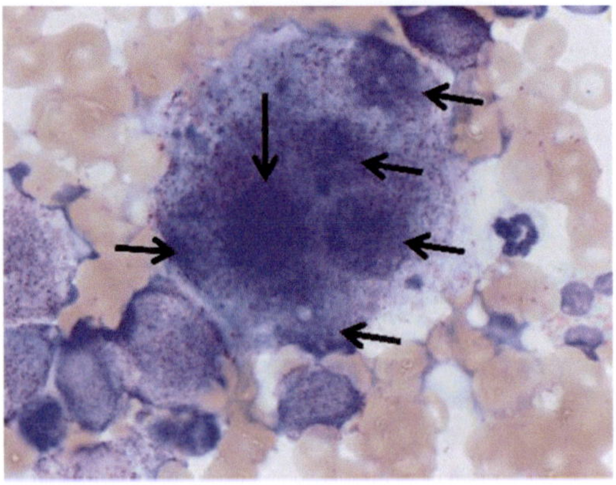

Fig. 4.21 Cytology, cutaneous mast cell tumor grade III/high grade, dog, May-Grünwald-Giemsa, 1000×. Note the presence of bizarre, macrocytic multinucleated undifferentiated mast cells (nuclei marked with *black arrows*) (Photo: with permission of Dr. N. Bauer, Faculty of Veterinary Medicine, Justus-Liebig-University, Giessen, Germany)

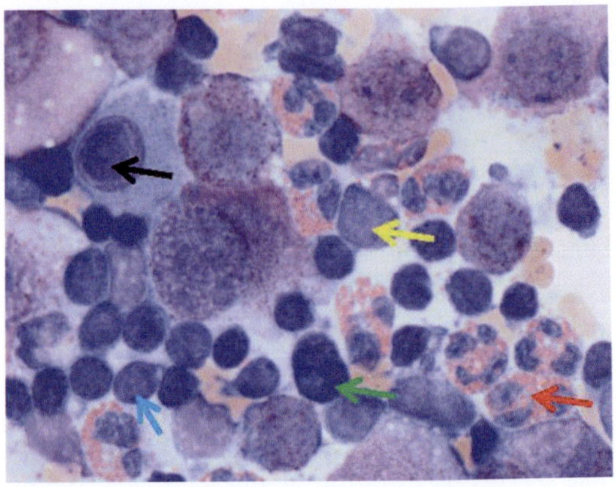

Fig. 4.22 Cytology, lymph node metastasis of a cutaneous mast cell tumor grade III/high grade, dog, May-Grünwald-Giemsa, 1000× (the same dog as in Fig. 4.21). Note the presence of numerous pleomorphic undifferentiated mast cells, some of which with prominent macronucleoli (*black arrow*) and numerous eosinophils (*red arrow*). There are several small mature lymphocytes (*blue arrow*) as well as few plasma cells (*green arrow*) and lymphatic blasts (*yellow arrow*) (Photo: with permission of Dr. N. Bauer, Faculty of Veterinary Medicine, Justus-Liebig-University, Giessen, Germany)

gins is a poor prognostic factor. However, detection of few mast cells at the margin of low-grade tumors does not necessarily lead to tumor recurrence. It has been shown that only 20–30 % of these tumors recur, while 20 % of tumors with free margins also recur. Nevertheless, incomplete margins should be treated with an en bloc resection of the scar with 2 cm margins or additional radiation of the area if possible.

A combination of *surgery and radiotherapy* is the treatment of choice for *MCT in difficult locations* where sufficient margins are not possible. This approach may lead to a long-term control of the disease for low- and intermediate-grade MCT. There is however an ongoing discussion on whether low or intermediate MCT in locations difficult to resect can be successfully excised with margins of less than 0.5 cm without additional radiotherapy or neo-adjunctive chemotherapy. Prednisolone or tyrosine kinase inhibitors (TKI, toceranib, and masitinib) can be used to shrink MCT prior to surgery to increase efficiency of surgery at difficult locations. Radiotherapy certainly increases the probability of disease control.

There are an increasing number of studies showing promising results for *surgery and chemotherapy* of incompletely excised low-to-intermediate MCT when radiotherapy is not possible. *Multidrug protocols* seem to be advantageous over single-drug protocols. *Postoperative administration* of prednisone in combination with vinblastine, a cocktail of prednisone, lomustine, and vinblastine, and prednisone together with vinblastine and cyclophosphamide seem to be efficient even in high-grade tumors or tumors with a high risk of recurrence.

High-grade tumors or tumors with regional or distant metastasis generally have a poor prognosis independent of therapeutic regimen.

Table 4.5 Grading systems for canine mast cell tumors

Grade	Histologic features (percentage of tumors)	Clinical features
Patnaik system		
		Survival rate after 48 months
I	Monomorphic cells, no mitotic figures, only in the dermis (36 %)	83 %
II	Some pleomorphic cells, 0–2 mitotic figures per 400× field, infiltrating the subcutis (43 %)	44 %
III	Dominantly pleomorphic cells, 3–6 mitotic figures, infiltrating the subcutis and deeper (20 %)	6 %
Kiupel system		
Kiupel		Median time to recurrence/ median survival time*
Low grade		14 weeks/23 months
High grade	Per ten 400× fields: >6 mitotic figures or >2 multinucleated cells or >3 bizarre nuclei (at least 10 % of cells vary by at least twofold)	3 weeks/<4 months

HPF = 0.24 mm^2
*Follow-up time at least 28 months

A combination of surgery, radiotherapy of the tumor and the regional lymph node, and chemotherapy is recommended.

Exclusive chemotherapy and *exclusive radiotherapy* without concurrent surgery are usually not efficient for long-term control of bulky MCT and are therefore not recommended.

Treatment with *tyrosine kinase inhibitors (TKIs)* has been established as an alternative treatment option for MCT in recent years. *Toceranib* induces rapid and impressive response rates in almost 50 % of recurrent intermediate- and high-grade MCT, especially in those with activating KIT mutations. Time to tumor progression is restricted under this regimen to 18 weeks. A long-term control of recurrent or unresectable MCT has been achieved in some tumors with the application of the TKI *masitinib*. Inappetence, weight loss, diarrhea, and occasionally vomiting, melena, and myelosuppression are common toxic side effects of both drugs. Unfortunately, resistance to TKI associated *with tumor relapse and disease progression* is a common finding after 6–18 months of treatment for both drugs. Unfortunately, resistance to TKI associated *with tumor relapse and disease progression* is a common finding after 6–18 months of treatment for both drugs.

Presurgical treatment with antihistamine such as diphenhydramine is advised to reduce the systemic effects of mast cell degranulation. In addition, administration of proton pump inhibitors like omeprazole should be considered to prevent gastric lesions.

Prognostic Factors and Markers

The general survival time of dogs with canine MCT is strongly dependent on *tumor grade* (Table 4.5) and to a lesser extent on *clinical staging* (Table 4.4) according to the WHO staging system. In addition, several additional factors are also correlated with prognosis.

Molecular markers are currently *not commonly used* in MCT diagnosis mainly due to the significant and reliable prognostic value of the clinical staging and histologic grading systems. Nevertheless, immunohistochemical analysis of the number of proliferating cells using the *proliferation marker* Ki-67, AgNOR, and PCNA and the pattern and level of *KIT expression* has been shown to be of prognostic value. In addition, the *mutational analysis* of the exon 11 tandem duplication is possible using simple PCR analysis; complete genetic sequence of KIT requires costly genetic sequencing.

■ **Current Trends in Research**

The current research on canine MCT is focusing on the identification of new therapy protocols combining TKI, radiotherapy, and classic chemotherapy agents. In addition, several novel compounds targeting selective inhibitor of nuclear export (SINE), oncolytic retroviruses, pan-bcl-2 blockers, or aurora kinase inhibitors are currently being tested in in vitro assays and clinical trials.

■ **Suggested Further Reading**

(Blackwood et al. 2012; Halsey et al. 2014; Kiupel et al. 2011; London 2013; Meyer et al. 2012, 2013; Patnaik et al. 1984; Stefanello et al. 2015; Thamm and Vail 2007; Welle et al. 2008)

4.1.4.2 Canine Cutaneous Histiocytomas

Box 4.11. Canine Cutaneous Histiocytomas in Three Facts

1. There is ongoing debate whether this monoclonal cell population is a tumor or hyperplasia.
2. Occur in young dogs mainly on the head.
3. Are benign and regress spontaneously.

■ **Epidemiology and Pathogenesis**

Cutaneous histiocytomas are common benign tumors most probably derived from epidermal Langerhans cells. They develop in young dogs under the *age* of 2 years. Their clonal character has been confirmed by genetic analysis. However, there is ongoing debate whether they are real neoplasms or merely reactive hyperplasia, mostly due to the observation of *spontaneous regression*. Tumor regression is associated with an infiltration of lymphocytes and thus is most probably immune mediated.

■ **Clinical Appearance**

Histiocytomas are typically solitary, button-shaped nodules *on the cranial aspect of the body*. They can be rapidly growing and often *regress spontaneously within 1–2 months*. Multiple tumors may be present.

■ **Cytology and Histopathology**

Cytology presents with typical histiocytic cells occasionally admixed with well-differentiated lymphocytes (◘ Figs. 4.23 and 4.24). *Histopathology* is diagnostic due the typical histiocytic cell shape, the wedge-shaped general arrangement of the tumor, and the typical follicular aggregates of lymphocytes at the base of the tumors.

■ **Therapy**

Surgery is curative but not necessary due to the self-limiting nature (spontaneous regression) of the tumors. A successful treatment of multiple histiocytomas with lomustine *chemotherapy* has been described.

■ **Prognostic Factors and Markers**

Immunohistochemical markers are usually not necessary to confirm the diagnosis. Histiocytomas are however typically positive for *CD1a, CD11c, E-cadherin,* and *MHC class II.*

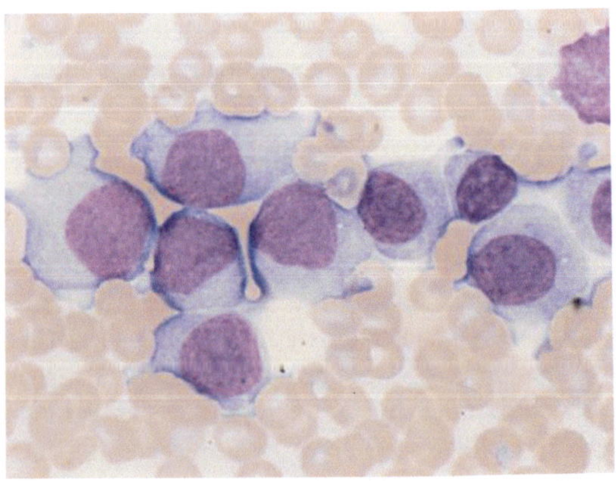

◘ **Fig. 4.23** Cytology, histiocytoma without regression, dog, May-Grünwald-Giemsa, 1000×. Histiocytic cells with eccentrically located nuclei, fine chromatin pattern, and abundant amounts of gray-blue cytoplasm (Photo: with permission of Dr. N. Bauer, Faculty of Veterinary Medicine, Justus-Liebig-University, Giessen, Germany)

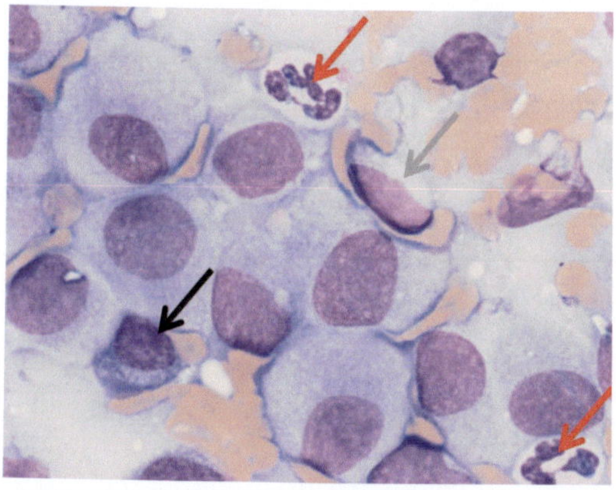

Fig. 4.24 Cytology, histiocytoma with advanced regression, dog, May-Grünwald-Giemsa, 1000×. Note the moderate infiltration with medium-sized lymphocytes (*gray arrow*), plasma cells (*black arrow*) and few neutrophils (*red arrow*) (Photo: with permission of Dr. N. Bauer, Faculty of Veterinary Medicine, Justus-Liebig-University, Giessen, Germany)

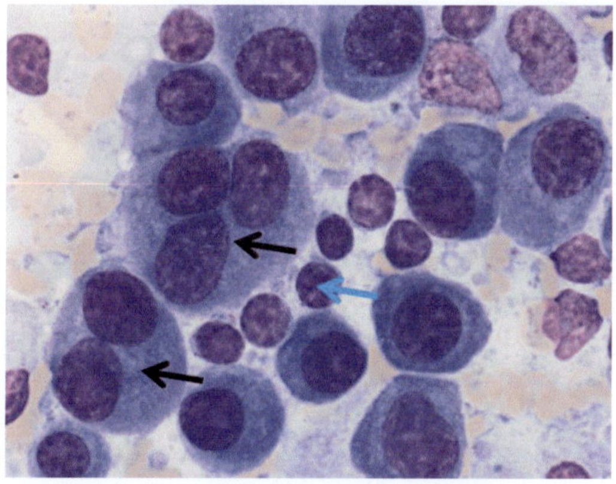

Fig. 4.25 Cytology, cutaneous plasmacytoma, dog, May-Grünwald-Giemsa, 1000×. Note the presence of bi- or multinucleated plasma cells (*black arrow*). Few lymphocytes (*blue arrow*) are also seen (Photo: with permission of Dr. N. Bauer, Faculty of Veterinary Medicine, Justus-Liebig-University, Giessen, Germany)

Suggested Further Reading

(Delcour et al. 2013; Maina et al. 2014; Moore 2014; Pires et al. 2013)

4.1.4.3 Canine Cutaneous Plasmacytomas

Box 4.12. Canine Cutaneous Plasmacytomas in Two Facts

1. Benign tumors.
2. Surgical excision is curative.

Epidemiology and Pathogenesis

Cutaneous plasma cell tumors belong to the group of extramedullary plasmacytomas. They are common *benign* skin tumors of the dog and develop at the *age* of 9–10 years with a predisposition in large *breeds*.

Clinical Appearance

Plasma cell tumors are *solitary, reddish, alopecic, raised nodules* commonly diagnosed at the head and limbs. Hypergammaglobulinemia due to antibody secretion by tumor cells is not observed.

Cytology and Histopathology

Cytologically and histopathologically, plasmacytomas present as an accumulation of *well-differentiated plasma cells* (Fig. 4.25). Bi- or multinucleated cells are common.

Therapy

Complete *surgical excision* is curative. Non-resectable tumors may be treated with prednisone or radiotherapy.

Suggested Further Reading

(Campo 1997; Haga et al. 2013)

4.2 Skin Tumors of the Cat

Squamous cell carcinomas, basal cell tumors, fibrosarcomas, and mast cell tumors are the most common skin tumors of the cat, with each representing 10–20 % of all skin tumors. All other tumors can be considered as rare.

4.2.1 Feline Epithelial Tumors

Squamous cell carcinomas and basal cell tumors are the most common feline epithelial skin tumors. Papillomas, hair follicle tumors, and tumors of the adnexal glands are rare and not described in detail in this chapter.

4.2.1.1 Feline Cutaneous Squamous Cell Carcinoma

Box 4.13. Feline Cutaneous Squamous Cell Carcinomas (SCCs) in Five Facts

1. SCC common on UV-exposed, light-haired areas (pinnae, nasal planum, eyelid)
2. Subtype of potentially *Papillomavirus*-induced Bowenoid in situ carcinoma (BISC)
3. SCC with invasive growth but metastasis rare
4. Surgery with good prognosis at early tumor stages
5. Radiotherapy for difficult location and advanced stages with guarded prognosis

Epidemiology and Pathogenesis

Cutaneous squamous-cell carcinomas (SCC) are a common malignant skin tumor of the cat. In the cat, they are commonly *divided into two tumor types:* UV light-induced invasive SCC and potentially *Papillomavirus*-induced SCC in situ (syn. Bowenoid in situ carcinoma (BISC)).

BISCs are defined as locally invasive (in situ) carcinomas without invasion of the basement membrane of the epidermis. They are thought to be associated with feline *Papillomavirus* infection. Contribution of UV-light exposure in the etiology of BISC in cats is also discussed in the literature, but unlike SCC, these tumors often arise in areas of the body protected from UV light so this is an unlikely cause. BISC occurs in older cats at an *age* > 10 years, without *breed*, *sex*, or hair color predisposition. BISC may progress to invasive SCC.

Invasive SCC usually develop in animals over the *age* of 10 on lightly haired areas of the head that are *exposed to UV light. White pinnae* are the most commonly affected area, while the nasal planum and the eyelids are less frequently affected. There is no sex or breed predisposition for SCC. *Papillomavirus* infection may also be of etiologic relevance for invasive SCC.

Clinical Appearance

BISC present as large, mostly multiple, hairless, pigmented, plaque-like erosions and crusts several cm in diameter. They can occur on any area of the body. Metastasis and invasion are not present by definition (in situ carcinoma). Left untreated the tumors may however progress to invasive SCC. Patients with BISC are at risk of developing new BISC in the future.

Chronic actinic dermatitis is usually the prestage of *SCC*. SCC usually present as plaque-like, erythematous, ulcerated, crust-covered lesions and may be confused with chronic ulcerative dermatitis. They are rarely prominent or papillary. They *grow invasively. Metastasis is rare* but if present is found in the mandibular and retropharyngeal lymph nodes and lungs. In general, survival times of cats with SCC at the pinna are slightly longer (~2.5 years) than that of cats with SCC on the nasal planum. Cats with concurrent lesions on both sites have median survival times of <2 years.

A staging system is available, which is of prognostic relevance for survival and therapy success (◘ Table 4.6)

Cytology and Histopathology

Cytologically, the presence of pleomorphic and anisokaryotic cells is helpful in the diagnosis of SCC (◘ Figs. 4.26 and 4.27).

Histopathologically, *BISC* appear as sharply demarcated supra-basal proliferation of atypical epidermal keratinocytes. Hyperkeratosis and hyperpigmentation may be present. *SCC* consist of invasive groups and cords of moderately to poorly differentiated epithelial cells. Keratinization and keratin pearls are common and help to differentiate SCC from other epithelial tumors.

Therapy

Early *surgery* is the treatment of choice for BISC and SCC at the pinnae; the procedure is associated with a good prognosis if tumor-free margins of at least 1 cm are achieved. Resection of the nasal planum and parts of the eyelid is possible and has a good prognosis if tumor-free surgical margins are achieved.

Radiotherapy is commonly used for treatment of SCC at the nasal planum. Irradiated in situ SCC in this location have a good prognosis of complete remission, while invasive SCC has a guarded prognosis for remission.

Table 4.6 Staging system for feline cutaneous squamous-cell carcinoma (WHO, Owen 1980)

Stage	Description
Tis	Preinvasive carcinoma (carcinoma in situ) not breaching the basement membrane
T1	Tumor <2 cm diameter, superficial or exophytic
T2	Tumor 2–5 cm diameter, or with minimal invasion irrespective of the size
T3	Tumor >5 cm diameter, or with invasion of the subcutis irrespective of the size
T4	Tumor invading other structures such as the fascia, muscle, bone, or cartilage

Photodynamic therapy is a treatment option for SCC on the eyelids and the nasal planum. Treatment often leads to initial complete remission, but in 50 % of cases, recurrences are observed within 1 year.

There are only a few studies on the efficacy of *chemotherapy* for feline cutaneous SCC. These studies have not found significant benefits from doxorubicin, cyclophosphamide, mitoxantrone, and actinomycin. They have found that local application of cisplatin and 5-fluorouracil may be efficient.

Suggested Further Reading

(Bergvall 2013; Munday et al. 2013; Munday et al. 2011; Murphy 2013; Owen 1980)

4.2.1.2 Feline Basal Cell Tumors

Box 4.14. Feline Basal Cell Tumors in Four Facts

1. Benign tumors of the skin at the head
2. May be pigmented
3. Rare basal cell carcinoma with invasion and metastasis
4. Wide surgical excision as treatment of choice

Epidemiology and Pathogenesis

Basal cell tumors (BCT) are a common benign tumor of the cat, which are derived from basal reserve cells of the epidermis. They are common tumors in patients *aged* 8–10 years. *Basal cell carcinomas (BCC)* are a rare malignant version of the

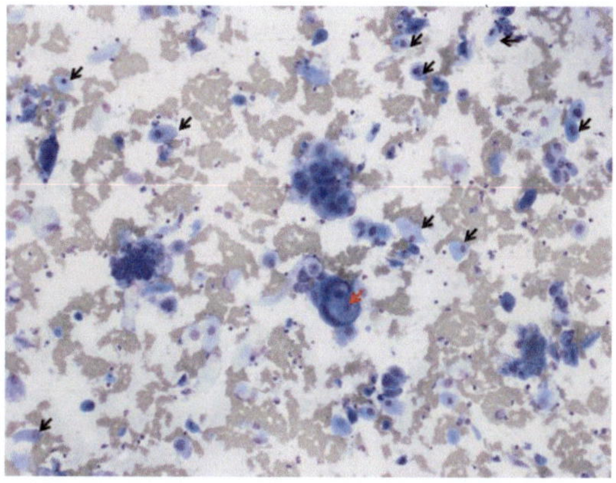

Fig. 4.26 Cytology, cutaneous squamous-cell carcinoma, cat, May-Grünwald-Giemsa, 100×. Note the marked anisocytosis, anisokaryosis, pleomorphism, and variation in nuclear-to-cytoplasm ratio. There are many epithelial cells with asynchronous maturation of nucleus and cytoplasm (*black arrow*), i.e., they possess angular cellular borders and abundant lightly basophilic cytoplasm typical for mature cells but have retained a large, non-pycnotic nucleus typical for immature epithelial cells. Some cells show cell cannibalism (*red arrow*) (Photo: with permission of Dr. N. Bauer, Faculty of Veterinary Medicine, Justus-Liebig-University, Giessen, Germany)

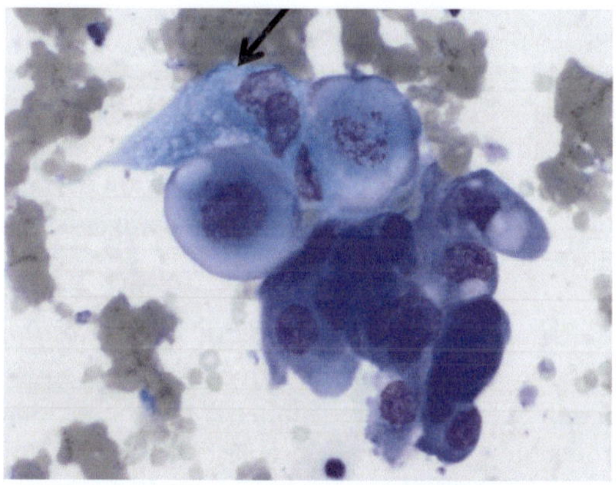

Fig. 4.27 Cytology, cutaneous squamous-cell carcinoma, cat, May-Grünwald-Giemsa, 500×. Note the marked anisocytosis, anisokaryosis, pleomorphism, and variation in nuclear-to-cytoplasm ratio as well as the presence of atypical elongated ("tadpole-like") turquoise epithelial cells with multiple perinuclear vacuoles highly suggestive of squamous-cell carcinoma (*black arrow*) (Photo: with permission of Dr. N. Bauer, Faculty of Veterinary Medicine, Justus-Liebig-University, Giessen, Germany)

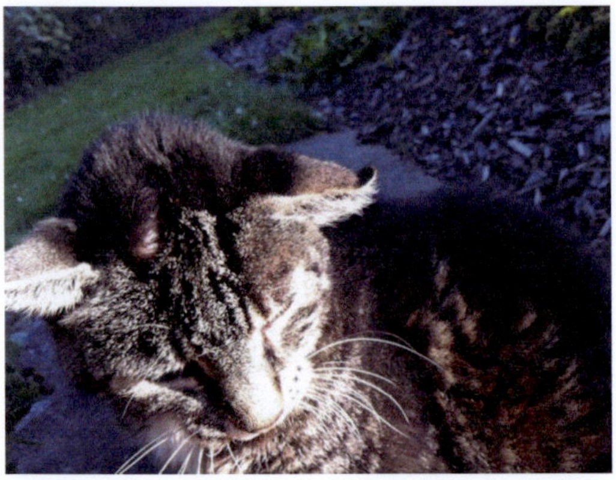

Fig. 4.28 Basal cell tumor, cat presented with a slowly growing, soft, pigmented, cystic mass at the head (Photo: with permission of Dr. N. Bauer, Faculty of Veterinary Medicine, Justus-Liebig-University, Giessen, Germany)

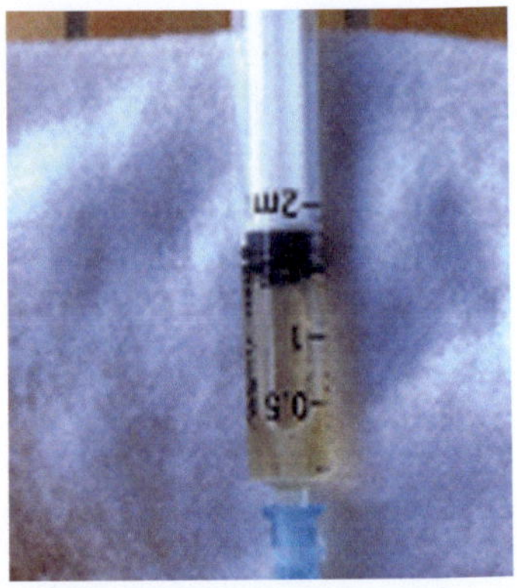

Fig. 4.29 Viscous, yellow fluid aspirated from a basal cell tumor (the same cat as in Fig. 4.28). Note that the fluids aspirated from cystic areas of tumors rarely reveal the etiology, so that also fine-needle aspirates from the margins of the tumor should be taken (Photo: with permission of Dr. N. Bauer, Faculty of Veterinary Medicine, Justus-Liebig-University, Giessen, Germany)

basal cell tumor. BCC grow invasively and can form regional and distant metastases. There is a debate whether basal cell tumors are actually trichoblastomas or apocrine gland adenomas.

Clinical Appearance

Clinically, *BCT* are *well-circumscribed*, button-shaped, hairless nodules commonly located *at the head or neck* (Fig. 4.28). They are often *pigmented* and can be confused with melanomas. They are usually slow growing. *BCC* are faster growing and may *occasionally metastasize* regionally and to distant organs(Fig. 4.29).

Cytology and Histopathology

Cytology of *BCT* presents with a mixture of squamous cells, sebaceous epithelial cells, melanin-containing cells, and fibroblasts (Fig. 4.30). Differentiation of benign BCT from BCC is usually not possible.

On *histopathology, BCT* presents as a well-circumscribed islands of moderately differentiated epithelial cells admixed with a moderately fibrous stroma. *BCC* are differentiated from BCT by their invasive growth at the tumor margins.

Therapy

Wide surgical excision of BCT and most probably of BCC is usually curative. BCT seems to be sensitive to *radiotherapy*, which can be used for the treatment of tumors that are difficult to resect due to their location. The effect of radiotherapy on BCC is unknown.

Suggested Further Reading

(Byam-Cook et al. 2006; Stewart et al. 2006; Stockhaus et al. 2001)

4.2.1.3 Feline Melanomas

Box 4.15. Feline Cutaneous Melanomas in Four Facts

1. Mostly malignant
2. Invasive growth and distant metastasis common
3. May be amelanotic
4. Surgery with wide margins often associated with recurrence

Epidemiology and Pathogenesis

Cutaneous melanomas are rare, *mostly malignant tumors* in the cat. They are tumors of the melanin-producing melanocytes, which are derived from the neural crest and thus neither mesenchymal nor epithelial tumors. There is no *breed* or *sex* predisposition for feline melanomas. The average *age* of cats with the diagnosis of a melanoma is 10–12 years. Melanomas are also found intraocularly or at the eyelids and rarely in the oral cavity (see Chaps. 9 and 16).

Clinical Appearance

Feline cutaneous melanomas are commonly found on the head, the nasal planum, and the

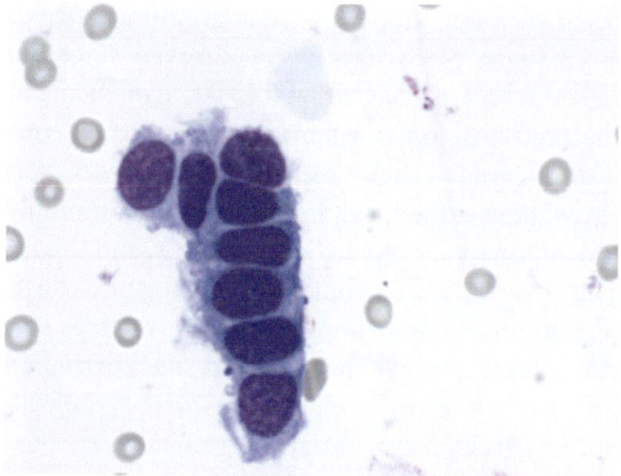

Fig. 4.30 Cytology, basal cell tumor, cat (the same cat as in Fig. 4.28), May-Grünwald-Giemsa, 1000×. Note the cluster of small basaloid cells with centrally located nuclei, fine chromatin pattern, and small amounts of lightly basophilic cytoplasm showing the typical "ribbonlike" growth (Photo: with permission of Dr. N. Bauer, Faculty of Veterinary Medicine, Justus-Liebig-University, Giessen, Germany)

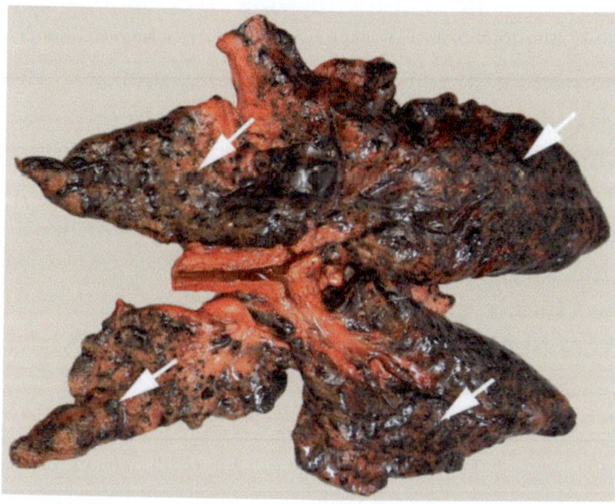

Fig. 4.31 Lung metastases (*white arrows*) of a cutaneous melanoma, cat

digits. They are solitary, sometimes hairless and ulcerated nodules; they are mostly pigmented but can be amelanotic. The *majority of the tumors metastasize* to the regional lymph node, the lung, or other organs (Figs. 4.30 and 4.31). Histologic differentiation of benign and malignant often does not correlate with the actual clinical behavior in the case of cutaneous melanomas.

Cytology and Histopathology

Cytologically, pigmented melanomas present as pigmented epitheloid, spindloid, or even round cell-like tumor cells (Fig. 4.32). The diagnosis of

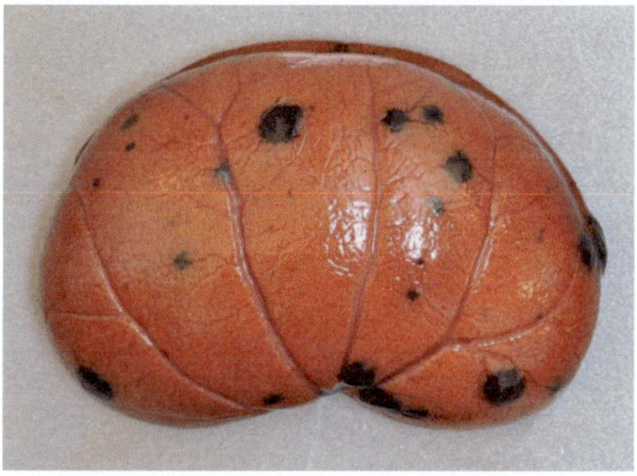

Fig. 4.32 Renal metastases of a cutaneous melanoma, cat

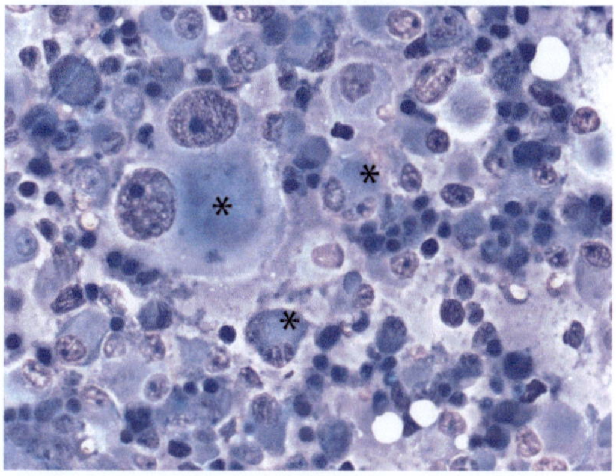

Fig. 4.33 Cytology, cutaneous mostly amelanotic melanoma, May-Grünwald-Giemsa, cat

amelanotic melanoma is challenging cytologically and *histopathologically*. Immunohistochemical detection of S-100 and Melan-A helps to differentiate melanomas from non-neuroectodermal tumors (Fig. 4.33).

Therapy

Surgery with wide tumor margins is the treatment of choice for tumors without detectable metastases. The recurrence rate however is high.

Suggested Further Reading

(Martens et al. 2001; Metcalfe et al. 2013; Stadler et al. 2011)

4.2.2 Mesenchymal Tumors

Malignant mesenchymal tumors in all body areas are commonly designated as *soft tissue sarcomas (STSs)* due to the similarity of their clinical presentation and response to treatment. Commonalities of these tumors are highly invasive growth, high rate of recurrence, and low-to-moderate frequency of local and distant metastases. The term soft tissue sarcomas therefore refers to tumors of different histogenesis such as fibrosarcomas, liposarcomas, and rhabdomyomas.

In cats the term STS is however less often used than in dogs. This may be caused by the smaller variety of mesenchymal tumors in the cat. The most common cutaneous mesenchymal tumor of the cat is the *feline injection-site-associated sarcoma (FISS)*, which is described in detail here. Rhabdomyomas, leiomyosarcomas, and lipomas are very rare in cats.

The *staging and grading systems* initially developed for canine soft tissue sarcomas are occasionally also used for feline soft tissue sarcomas (◻ Table 4.7).

▪ **Suggested Reading**

(Liptak and Forrest 2012)

4.2.2.1 Feline Injection-Site Sarcomas (FISSs)

Box 4.16. Feline Injection-Site-/Vaccine-Associated Sarcomas in Seven Facts

1. Induced by injection-/vaccine-associated inflammation.
2. Repeated injection at the same time as risk factor.
3. Comprehensive vaccination guidelines for risk reduction available.
4. Histopathologic evaluation of tumor margins fails in 20 % of cases.
5. Best results from radical surgery with 5-cm margins or amputation.
6. Post- or preoperative radiotherapy may increase disease-free interval.
7. Chemotherapy of minor relevance.

▪ **Epidemiology and Pathogenesis**

Fibrosarcomas in cats are classified into the more frequent *feline injection-site sarcomas (FISSs)* and the *non-vaccine-/injection-site-associated sarcomas (SAs)* of unknown etiology.

FISS is one of the most common skin tumors of the cat. There is no breed and no sex predisposition. Tumors arise at an average *age* of 8–12 years. FISSs have been observed since the introduction of vaccination into feline medicine in the 1980s. An increased incidence of subcutaneous fibrosarcomas can be seen *months to years after vaccination* at the site of injection, more commonly the interscapular region, lateral thorax, and thighs. This was initially attributed to carcinogenic effects of aluminum-based adjuvants. However, large epidemiologic studies have found *no correlation between any specific adjuvants or vaccine* type with tumor development. Today it is generally accepted that post-vaccination and injection inflammation or most probably any form of chronic inflammation may induce neoplastic transformation of feline subcutaneous myofibroblasts. In particular, the expression of growth factors like TGF and EGF and their receptors in the tumors and mutations of the p53 tumor suppressor gene are thought to be of relevance for the molecular carcinogenesis of FISS.

Two risk factors have been identified for the development of FISS: multiple vaccinations and temperature of the vaccine. The *number of vaccinations* or injections given at a site increases the risk of an FISS developing, i.e., three to four vaccinations (as opposed to one vaccination) in the interscapular region double the risk of sarcoma formation at that site. Furthermore, administration of *cold vaccines* versus room-temperature vaccines is supposed to increase the risk. Several recommendations for the prevention of FISS have been published (► Box 4.17).

Box 4.17. Recommendations for the Prevention of FISS (Hartmann et al. 2015)

1. Vaccination of cats provides essential protection and should not be stopped because of the risk of feline injection-site sarcoma (FISS).
2. Vaccines are not the only injectable medical products associated with FISS.
3. Cats should be vaccinated no more than necessary, in accordance with current guidelines.
4. The interscapular region should generally be avoided. Vaccines should be injected at a site from which a mass can easily be surgically removed, such as distally on a leg or in the skin of the lateral abdomen.

5. Vaccines should be brought to room temperature prior to administration, but should not be kept unrefrigerated for hours.
6. Whenever possible, subcutaneous, rather than intramuscular, injection should be performed.
7. The preference is for non-adjuvanted vaccines over those containing adjuvant, modified live vaccines or recombinant vaccines over inactivated vaccines, and vaccines with a long duration of immunity.
8. Post-vaccination monitoring should be performed. Any lump at the site of injection that is still present 3 months after vaccination, that is larger than 2 cm in diameter, or that is increasing in size 1 month after vaccination should be surgically removed.

In contrast, *non-injection-associated SAs* have an unknown etiology. They are *less common* than FISS and are tumors of *older cats*. They may arise *at any site on the body* but mostly found on the head and distal limbs. *SAs lack the typical FISS inflammation* at all stages of tumor development and size and are thus thought not to be caused by inflammation.

Clinical Appearance

Grossly, *FISS* and *SA* may appear clinically similar, except that SA is found on all body sites and is not more common at vaccination sites. Both are *firm, non-ulcerated, subcutaneous masses* (Fig. 4.34). FISS may appear partially soft or fluctuating due to common cystic spaces. Palpation is a poor indicator of tumor margins; magnetic resonance imaging (*MRI*) and contrast-enhanced computed tomography (*CT*) studies have shown tumor volume to be up to double the size appreciated on palpation. *Metastasis* is observed in up to 25 % of the tumors but usually occurs at later stages of tumor development.

Cytology and Histopathology

Cytology of FISS and SA is characterized by cohesive cluster of spindle cells with marked anisocytosis, anisokaryosis, and pleomorphism. In addition, macrocytic spindle cells with macronuclei and macronucleoli can be seen in highly malignant tumor (Fig. 4.35).

Histopathology of *FISS* is characterized by a poorly circumscribed proliferation of pleomorphic spindle cells around a common necrotic and cystic area within the tumor mass; there is *marked inflammatory infiltration* at the tumor boarders which is not seen with FISA. There is no generally accepted grading system for FISS. 2.1.

Histopathology has a *moderate to poor specificity and sensitivity* to confirm *surgical margins* in the healthy tissue after surgical resection. Even tumors with free margins as diagnosed by a thorough three-dimensional histological approach, which analyzes tumor margins completely in all dimensions, have a recurrence rate of 20 %. This observation has led to the hypothesis that recurrences may actually be new tumors that develop from postsurgical inflammation. The advantage to complete resection is that recurrence after diagnosis of tumor-free margins occurs later than recurrence after incompletely resected tumors.

Therapy

Treatment success of FISS very much depends on early and aggressive therapy to achieve local tumor control.

Aggressive surgery with tumor margins of 5 cm laterally and two fascial planes deep will reduce the recurrence rate to less than 15 %, compared to recurrence after marginal surgery. Aggressive amputation is usually required to achieve sufficient tumor margins for local tumor control; amputation usually requires the complete removal of the limb, dorsal spinous processes, and parts of the scapula and resection of the body wall including several ribs or hemipelvectomy.

Radiotherapy is recommended in addition to aggressive surgery for appropriate treatment of FISS, especially in cases where sufficient tumor margins are not achieved. Both pre- and postoperative radiotherapies are used. The results are however debatable with only 100–300 days of disease-free intervals and 30 % recurrence after *preoperative irradiation* and incomplete resection. Similarly, incomplete resection and *postoperative irradiation* are only associated with a median disease-free interval of approximately 1 year and recurrence of up to 30 %. The time span between

Table 4.7 Staging system for soft tissue sarcomas (Liptak and Forrest 2012)

Stage	Tumor size	Lymph node metastases	Metastasis	Histologic grade
1	T_{any} (any r size)	N0 (none)	M0 (none)	I–II
II	T_{1a} (<5 cm, superficial) T_{1b} (<5 cm, deep) T_{2a} (>5 cm, superficial)	N0 (none)	M0 (none)	III
III	T_{2b} (>5 cm, deep)	N0 (none)	M0 (none)	III
IV	T_{any} (any r size) T_{any} (any r size)	N1 (present) N_{any}	M_{any} M1 (present)	I–III

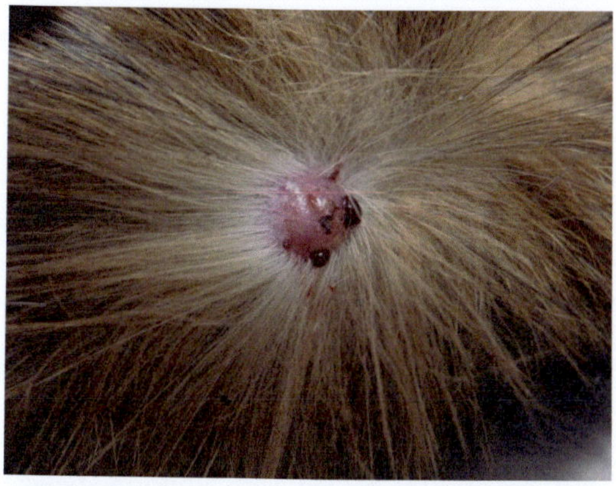

Fig. 4.34 Feline injection-site sarcoma, cat (Photo: with permission of the Faculty of Veterinary Medicine, Justus-Liebig-University, Giessen, Germany)

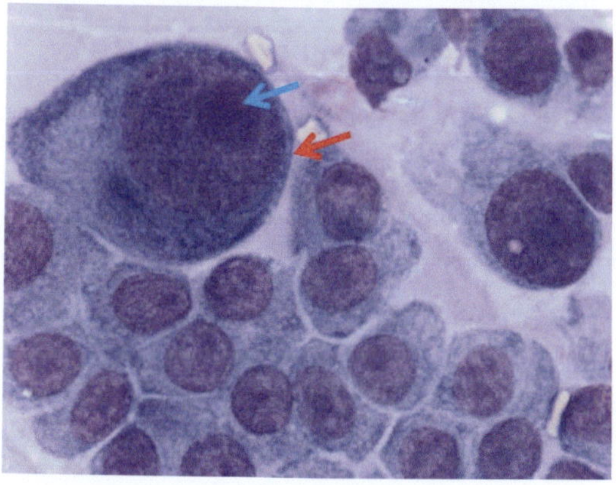

Fig. 4.35 Cytology, feline injection-site-associated sarcoma (FISS), cat (the same cat as in Fig. 4.34), May-Grünwald-Giemsa, 1000×. Note the cohesive cluster of spindle cells with marked anisocytosis, anisokaryosis, and pleomorphism. Several macrocytic spindle cells (*red arrow*) with macronuclei and macronucleoli are seen (*blue arrow*) indicative of a highly malignant tumor (Photo: with permission of Dr. N. Bauer, Faculty of Veterinary Medicine, Justus-Liebig-University, Giessen, Germany)

surgery and radiotherapy should be less than 2 weeks to minimize recurrence rates. *Exclusive radiotherapy* should be restricted to palliative care.

Chemotherapy is of minor relevance in the treatment of FISS but may have some impact on survival times of cats treated with surgery and radiotherapy. An increase in the disease-free interval in cats treated with doxorubicin after surgery has been observed. Exclusive chemotherapy can lead to a short-term (on average 3 months long) response in up to 50 % of treated cats after administration of doxorubicin alone or in combination with cyclophosphamide.

Immunotherapy with intralesional injection of interleukin-2 (IL-2) and surgery may lead to a decrease in the recurrence rate by 50 %.

Prognostic Factors and Markers

Several factors negatively influence the prognosis for FISS (▶ Box 4.18).

Box 4.18. Negative Prognostic for FISS

1. Tumor size >2 cm
2. Incomplete resection
3. Recurrence after excision
4. High-grade tumor
5. Distant metastasis
6. No pre-/postoperative radiotherapy

Suggested Further Reading

(Eckstein et al. 2009; Hendrick and Goldschmidt 1991; Hershey et al. 2000; Kass et al. 2003; Ladlow 2013; Liptak and Forrest 2012; Martano et al. 2011; Richards et al. 2006; Vaccination Guidelines et al. 2010)

4.2.3 Feline Hematopoietic Tumors

Mast cell tumors are the most common cutaneous hematopoietic tumor of the cat. Plasma cell tumors are rare, cutaneous lymphomas (Chap. 6) very rare in the cat.

4.2.3.1 Feline Cutaneous Mast Cell Tumors

Box 4.19. Feline Cutaneous Mast Cell Tumors in Four Facts

1. Often malignant.
2. Show an invasive growth and occasionally distant metastases.
3. Surgery with wide margins is usually curative.

4

Epidemiology and Pathogenesis

Feline mast cell tumors (MCT) are common tumors in the cat; they make up ~10 % of all feline neoplasias. MCT are further classified into three clinically very diverse forms: cutaneous, intestinal, and visceral/systemic MCT (also see Chaps. 6 and 9). *Cutaneous MCTs* are the second most common skin tumor in the cat, making up ~20 % of all cutaneous tumors. Feline cutaneous MCTs are usually diagnosed between the *age* of 2–4 years (atypical form) and 10 years (mastocytic form). Siamese cat *breeds* are predisposed to all forms of MCT.

The *etiology* and *molecular pathogenesis* of feline MCT are mostly unknown. Due to the breed predisposition in Siamese cats, *a genetic basis* is assumed. A contribution of mutations in the *stem cell factor receptor KIT* is hypothesized. Up to two-thirds of cutaneous and splenic/visceral MCT have KIT mutations in the exons 8 and 9, which induce ligand-independent activation of KIT and may thus contribute to proliferation and survival of MCT cells.

Clinical Appearance

Feline cutaneous MCT is usually white to pink, *solitary, firm, well-circumscribed*, or occasionally pruritic, plaque-like, flat, hairless, dermal masses. One-quarter of the tumors are superficially ulcerated on the head and the neck. Cats may present with pruritus and erythema; Darier's sign, which consists in rapid swelling after manipulation due to histamine release, has been reported. *Multiple tumors* are present in 20 % of cats. Metastasis is reported in 0 to 22 % of the tumors. Paraneoplastic, systemic disease is rather uncommon in cats with cutaneous MCT.

A *staging system* for feline tumors exists but its relevance for therapy or prognosis is not confirmed (Table 4.8). Nevertheless, a thorough physical exam and abdominal ultrasound are helpful to identify splenic disease in establishing a general prognosis. A buffy coat analysis for the detection of circulating mast cells is helpful in cats, in contrast to dogs, to identify systemic spread of the tumor. No paraneoplastic syndromes are observed with this tumor type.

Cytology and Histopathology

Cytology of feline MCT is usually diagnostic except for the uncommon atypical form (Fig. 4.36). Unfortunately, cytology is not a reliable method for discriminating benign from malignant tumors or for evaluating tumor grade.

Histopathology is required for unequivocal differentiation of feline cutaneous MCT into their subclasses. Two distinct subclasses of cutaneous MCT in the cat have been reported: the mastocytic MCT (~90 %) and the histiocytic MCT (~10 %). The *mastocytic form* is further subdivided histologically into well-differentiated, compact MCT (up to 90 %) and poorly differentiated, pleomorphic MCT. *Well-differentiated, compact MCT* are mostly benign with uniform, typical

Table 4.8 Staging system for feline mast cell tumors (Henry 2013)

Stage	Description
0	One tumor, completely excised
I	One tumor confined to the skin, no lymph node metastasis
II	One tumor confined to the skin with lymph node metastasis
III	Many/large infiltrating tumors, with/without lymph node metastasis
IV	Any tumor with distant spread of the disease

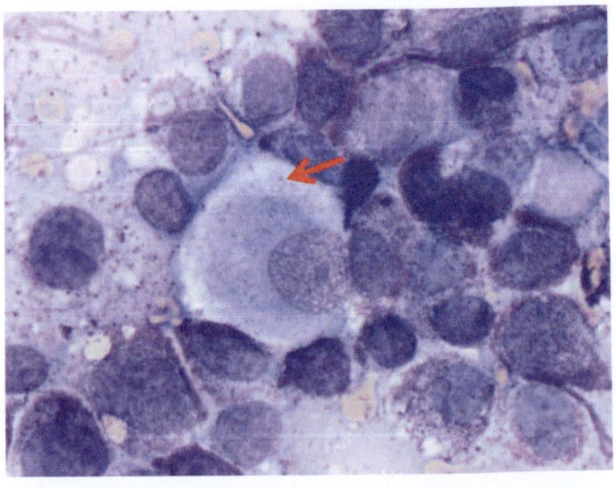

Fig. 4.36 Cytology, mastocytic, poorly differentiated mast cell tumor, cat, May-Grünwald-Giemsa, 1000×. Note the pleomorphic mast cells with moderate to marked anisocytosis, anisokaryosis, and pleomorphism. There are several undifferentiated, large mast cells with rare intracytoplasmic metachromatic granules indicative of a low degree of differentiation (*red arrow*) (Photo: with permission of Dr. N. Bauer, Faculty of Veterinary Medicine, Justus-Liebig-University, Giessen, Germany)

mast cell morphology; they rarely metastasize. *Poorly differentiated, diffuse MCT* have a marked cellular and nuclear pleomorphism, aggressive infiltrative character, and high mitotic index. Metastasis to the lymph nodes and the abdomen may occur but is still the exception even for this malignant subtype. *Histiocytic MCT* possess morphologic features characteristic of histiocytic cells. Similar to the canine cutaneous histiocytoma, they regress spontaneously over a period of several months.

A *grading system* for feline mast cell tumors is not available. The Patnaik system for canine MCT does not have prognostic value for feline MCT.

▪ Therapy

Surgery is the treatment of choice for feline MCT. Simple excision is often curative. Completeness of surgical excision is not significantly correlated with recurrence in well-differentiated feline MCT. Most studies show that tumor recurrence may occur for up to onc-third of cutaneous MCT, regardless of the completeness of surgical excision. Most of these recurring tumors are poorly differentiated MCT.

Chemotherapy is of questionable value as an adjunctive therapy for the treatment of feline MCT. *Lomustine* has been successfully tested and may be helpful for cats with poorly differentiated, locally invasive, or metastatic tumors. Corticosteroids have not been shown to be effective in the treatment of feline MCT. The *tyrosine kinase inhibitor (TKI) imatinib* has effects on feline mast cells in cell culture, and first reports are available on at least partial response in single cases of cats with MCT. The effect of the TKI masitinib or toceranib has not been tested in cats with feline mast cells yet.

Radiotherapy is recommended for incompletely excised tumors but studies proving its efficacy are lacking.

▪ Prognostic Factors and Molecular Marker

As stated previously, the majority of feline MCT carry a *mutation in the KIT* gene exon 8 or 9. Their value as prognostic indicator is however questionable. In contrast, a switch from the normal membrane-bound *KIT protein expression* to cytoplasmic expression in feline MCT cells is associated with poor prognosis. Increased expression of the proliferation marker *Ki67* is also associated with a more aggressive tumor behavior.

▪ Current Trends in Research

There is an ongoing discussion on the relevance of *KIT mutations* and TKI in the treatment of feline cutaneous MCT.

▪ Suggested Reading

(Blackwood et al. 2012; Hoshino et al. 2012; Sabattini et al. 2013)

4.2.3.2 Feline Cutaneous Plasmacytomas

Box 4.20. Feline Cutaneous Plasmacytomas in Three Facts

1. Mostly benign.
2. Present as solitary, raised nodules.
3. Surgery is usually curative.

▪ Epidemiology and Pathogenesis

Cutaneous plasmacytomas are derived from plasma cell tumors. They are rare skin tumors in the cat and develop at an *age* of <10 years.

▪ Clinical Appearance

Cutaneous plasma cell tumors are benign, *solitary, alopecic, raised nodules*, diagnosed on areas of the skin. Metastatic behavior and hypergammaglobulinemia are occasionally described.

▪ Cytology and Histopathology

Plasmacytomas present as an accumulation of *well-differentiated plasmacytoid cells* on cytology and on histopathology. The presence of multinucleated cells is common (◘ Fig. 4.37).

▪ Therapy

Surgical excision is the treatment of choice.

▪ Suggested Further Reading

(Muller et al. 2011; Teixeira et al. 2013; Theon et al. 2007)

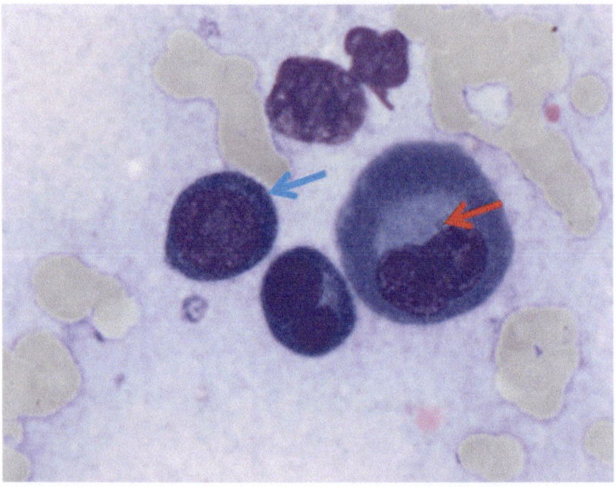

Fig. 4.37 Cytology, plasmacytoma, cat, May-Grünwald-Giemsa, 1000×. Note the atypical, often binucleate plasma cells with moderate to marked anisocytosis, anisokaryosis, and pleomorphism. Occasionally, nuclear fragmentation (*red arrow*) and undifferentiated blastoid (*blue arrow*) cells are seen (Photo: with permission of Dr. N. Bauer, Faculty of Veterinary Medicine, Justus-Liebig-University, Giessen, Germany)

4.3 Equine Skin Tumors

Skin tumors are the most commonly diagnosed neoplasms of the horse. Of these, sarcoids are the most common tumors followed by melanoma. Squamous-cell carcinomas are also observed but mostly occur in the periocular area (see Chap. 16) and the penis (▶ see Chap. 7) and are discussed in their respective chapters.

4.3.1 Equine Sarcoids

Box 4.21. Equine Sarcoids in Four Facts
1. Induced by infection with bovine *papillomaviruses* 1 and 2 (BPV1, BPV2)
2. May grow invasively, often recur, never metastasize
3. Highly variable macroscopic appearance
4. Numerous reported therapy options but none very effective

Epidemiology and Pathogenesis

With a prevalence of up to 10 % of all horses, sarcoids are the *most common tumor of the horse.* Sarcoids have also been reported in other equids like zebras, donkeys, mules, and even giraffes and antelopes. Sarcoids are the result of a multifactorial pathogenesis. However, infection with the *bovine papillomaviruses 1 and 2 (BPV1, BPV2)* is the major factor contributing to their development. Viral DNAs but not infectious virions are consistently detected in the tumors. The amount of viral DNA positively correlates with the aggressiveness of the sarcoid. Due to the nonproductive infection in equine cells, only *direct contact with infected cattle* or *indirect contact via fomites or insect vectors* is infectious. It is unlikely that equine sarcoid material or sarcoid-carrying horses can be infectious to other horses.

The *viral proteins E5, E6,* and *E7* primarily contribute to the neoplastic transformation of equine fibroblasts. Both E5 and E6 upregulate the expression of mitogen-activated protein kinase (MAPK) and thus fibroblast proliferation; E5 also downregulates major histocompatibility complex 1 (MHC-1) and thus contributes to immune evasion of infected fibroblasts.

There is a *breed* predisposition in Appaloosas, Arabians, Quarter horses, and Thoroughbreds. An increased risk has been associated with the *MHC alleles* A3 and W13. Sarcoids are commonly first noticed in young horses at an *age* of 1–7 years but may occur at any age. There is no *gender* or *color* predisposition.

Clinical Appearance

Macroscopically, sarcoids have a *highly variable appearance*, and more than half of the horses may have *multiple tumors*. They usually develop at sites of *previous trauma* or in areas with *thin skin*. Sarcoids are *non-metastatic* but infiltratively growing and thus have a *high recurrence rate* after treatment. Spontaneous regression is rare.

Clinically, sarcoids may be classified in to *six types according to Knottenbelt: occult, verrucous, nodular (types A and B), fibroblastic, malignant, and mixed. Occult sarcoids* are focal areas of alopecia, scaling, hyperkeratosis, and hyperpigmentation; they are located at the neck, face, medial thigh, and shoulder. *Verrucous sarcoids* have a raised, alopecic, irregular surface; they are located at the head, neck, axillae, and groin. *Nodular sarcoids type A* are nodular subcutaneous masses that can be moved freely under the skin while *nodular sarcoids type B* are connected with the subcutis and thus are not movable. Both types are usually haired but may become alopecic and ulcerated. Both are common periocularly, at the groin, and the prepuce. *Fibroblastic sarcoids* are fleshy, ulcerated masses which are pedunculated (type 1) or have a broad invasive base (type 2). They are commonly found at the axillae, groin, legs, and periocularly. *Malignant sarcoids* are particularly aggressive and invasive and may infiltrate lymphatic vessels. Although occult, verrucous and nodular sarcoids may remain static for years; all sarcoids can progress to the more aggressive fibroblastic or malignant type, most commonly after being irritated and traumatized. *Fibroblastic sarcoids* are fleshy, ulcerated masses which are pedunculated (type 1) or have a broad invasive base (type 2). They are commonly found at the axillae, groin, legs, and periocularly. *Malignant sarcoids* are particularly aggressive and invasive and may infiltrate lymphatic vessels. Although occult, verrucous and nodular sarcoids may remain static for years, all sarcoids may progress to the more aggressive fibroblastic or malignant type, most commonly after being irritated and traumatized.

Clinical presentation, *histopathology*, and *PCR* for the detection of BPV DNA are used *for ultimate diagnosis* of equine sarcoids.

▪ Cytology and Histopathology

Cytology of sarcoids usually presents as proliferating fibroblasts and is therefore *not specific enough* to differentiate sarcoids from other nonneoplastic, proliferative lesions like granulation tissue.

Histopathology of sarcoids usually shows a dermal *proliferation of fibroblasts* in a rather mixed-growth pattern usually starting directly at the epidermal basement membrane. Fibroblasts are usually oriented perpendicular to the basement membrane in a so-called "picket fence" pattern. Epidermal proliferation with *rete ridges* extending deep into the dermis may be present.

▪ Therapy

There is no universally effective treatment protocol for equine sarcoids. A *plethora of approaches* has been developed, and any one of these may be applied depending on the specific tumor, location, and clinical equipment.

Surgery can be an effective treatment if resection with wide margins is possible. *Early and radical removal* of small sarcoids has the best prognosis. Nevertheless, a high recurrence rate is seen even with surgical treatment. BPV DNA has been detected up to 2 cm outside the macroscopically perceived tumor. Surgical margins should therefore be generous. A "one-cut, one-blade" policy and a diligent prevention of contact between tumor material and the surgical site may prevent implantation of infected cells into the tumor bed.

Carbon dioxide laser treatment and *cryosurgery* with three cycles of quick freezing and slow thawing of the tumor have been reported as potentially effective in some cases.

Radiotherapy has been reported to be the most effective treatment with very low recurrence rates. However, it is expensive and not easily available. *Interstitial brachytherapy* with implants of a radiation source (iridium, cobalt, radium) injected into the sarcoid is also associated with an efficacy of up to 100 % and very low recurrence rates.

Local chemotherapy with injection or topical application of *cisplatin* or *5-fluorouracil* into the sarcoid has been reported to either induce remission or reduce recurrence rates in the majority of smaller sarcoids. Debulking surgery is often used in combination with local pre- or postoperative chemotherapy.

Antiviral drugs like acyclovir, cidofovir, and xanthates have been used topically and as injections with promising results in a few studies.

Immunomodulatory therapies including intratumoral infection with fragments of *Mycobacterium bovis* (*BCG vaccine*) have been used to stimulate an immune reaction against BPV-infected cells in sarcoids with successful resolution of up to two-thirds of the treated tumors. Finally, treatment attempts using *imiquimod, baypamun*, and *extracts from bloodroot* (*Sanguinaria canadensis*) have been reported.

▪ Prognostic Factors and Marker

Treatment of horses under of 4–6 years old with small tumors at an early stage of development is associated with a good-to-moderate prognosis. Trauma of the sarcoid and recurrence after primary treatment worsen the prognosis significantly.

▪ Suggested Further Reading

(Bergvall 2013; Byam-Cook et al. 2006; Knottenbelt 2006; Martens et al. 2001; Stadler et al. 2011; Stewart et al. 2006)

4.3.2 Equine Melanomas

Box 4.22. Equine Melanomas in Six Facts

1. Common tumor in gray horses.
2. Also present in non-gray horses.
3. Initially benign tumors may become malignant.
4. No evidence for biopsy-induced malignant transformation.
5. Early surgery may be curative.
6. Radiotherapy, local chemo- and immunotherapy, and antitumor vaccination also possible.

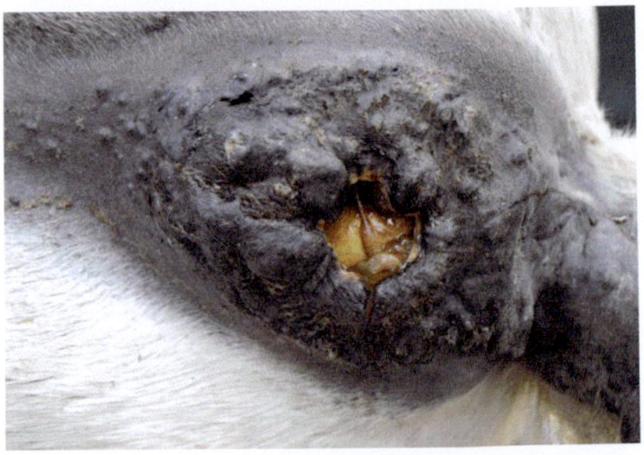

Fig. 4.38 Perianal melanoma, gray horse

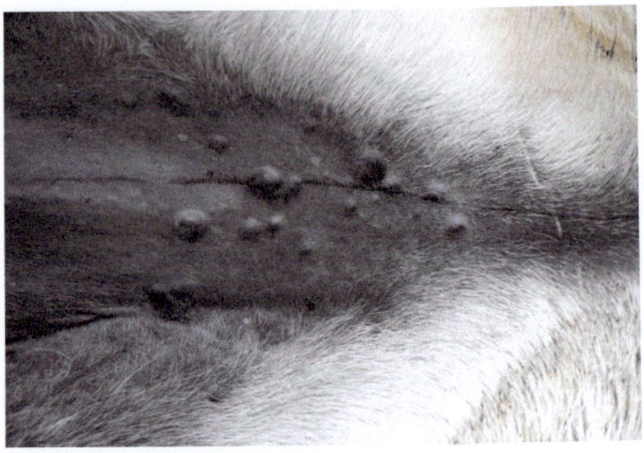

Fig. 4.39 Perineal melanoma, gray horse

Epidemiology and Pathogenesis

Melanomas are a common skin tumor in horses. They develop by neoplastic transformation of cutaneous melanocytes. Melanomas have been reported in horses of all colors. However, *gray horses* are predisposed with a prevalence of up to 80 % at an *age* of 15 years or older. The tumors usually have a long initial benign growth phase but approximately *66 % of them become malignant* with metastasis in distant organs after long periods of dormancy. Although less common, a large fraction of *melanomas in non-gray horses* are *malignant*.

The high incidence of melanomas in gray horses has been associated with the graying process beginning at 5–8 years of age. This graying process and the increased risk of melanoma development are based on a duplication in intron 6 of the *syntaxin 17* (STX17) gene. STX17 activates the extracellular signal-regulated kinase (ERK) pathway and thereby induces melanocyte proliferation. In addition, the role of genetic polymorphisms of the *melanocortin 1 receptor (MC1R)* and its antagonist *agouti signaling protein (ASIP)* has been analyzed for their contribution to the development of equine melanomas but their direct role has not been finally proven.

Clinical Appearance

Cutaneous melanomas of the horse are usually easy to diagnose due to their pigmentation. They are usually *slow growing, pigmented masses* (Figures 4.38 and 4.39). *Amelanotic tumors* are rare but may occur. Melanomas may be deep dermal masses or located more superficially in the dermis and epidermis. The latter may ulcerate at advanced stages. The *most common anatomic sites* for melanomas in the horse are the perianal region, the ventral tail base, the lip, the skin overlying the parotid salivary gland, and the prepuce. Systemic clinical symptoms depend on the site of *distant, lymphogenic metastasis* and include weight loss and colic and neurologic symptoms. There seems to be a slight predisposition of metastasis development for *the serosa overlying the lung, the spleen, and the liver*. Final diagnosis is usually based on the signalment of a gray horse, the coloration of the tumor, and the histopathology. There is no scientific evidence that taking biopsies triggers malignant transformation despite anecdotal rumors. Diagnostic imaging can be used to determine the presence of distant metastasis.

■ **Cytology and Histopathology**

Cytology of pigmented tumors confirms the clinical diagnosis, but is rarely performed by equine practitioners due to the typical clinical picture. *Amelanotic tumors* may be more challenging to diagnose on cytology due to the high variability of the histologic appearance of tumor cells from spindle cell like to an epitheloid.

Histopathology is usually straightforward in pigmented tumors. Amelanotic tumors may resemble sarcoid or epithelial tumors due to the variability of the histologic appearance of pleomorphic tumor cells. Mainly PNL2 and also S100 and PGP9.5 have been used as immunohistochemical markers to support histopathologic diagnosis of amelanotic tumors.

■ **Therapy**

The goal of treatment usually is local disease control and the prevention of metastatic spread. Effective treatment options for internal tumors or metastases are not available.

Surgery is the standard treatment for equine cutaneous melanomas. Due to the observed malignant transformation of equine melanomas over time, it seems reasonable to resect small tumors at an early, benign stage to prevent metastatic disease.

If available and affordable, *radiotherapy* may be an alternative for non-resectable tumors. Both *teletherapy* with an external radiation source and *brachytherapy* with an implantation of the radiation source (iridium, cobalt, radium) directly in or on the tumor have been used with some success.

Local chemotherapy with injection of *cisplatin* and *carboplatin* has been successfully used for treatment of melanomas. Unfortunately, the larger the tumor, the less successful the treatment.

Local immunotherapy using injections of DNA plasmids encoding for *interleukin (IL)-12* and *IL-18* has been tested. Injection of either plasmid led to tumor shrinkage in most horses.

Antitumor DNA vaccination using the human tyrosinase gene, which is almost exclusively expressed in melanocytes, has been tested experimentally in a small cohort of horses and associated with a measurable anti-tyrosinase response and tumor shrinkage.

■ **Suggested Further Reading**

(Jiang et al. 2014; Metcalfe et al. 2013; Muller et al. 2011; Phillips and Lembcke 2013; Rowe and Sullins 2004; Teixeira et al. 2013; Theon et al. 2007)

4.4 Bovine Skin Tumors

Benign virus-induced papillomas are the most common skin tumors in bovines. Squamous-cell carcinomas have also been described and may develop in nonpigmented, mainly periocular ("cancer eye") skin regions in geographic areas with high UV-light intensity, although occurrence is rare.

4.4.1 Bovine Cutaneous Papillomas/Papillomatosis

Box 4.23. Bovine Papillomas in Four Facts

1. Are induced by bovine *Papillomavirus* (BPV) infection.
2. Usually develop early in life, but may be present at any age.
3. Spontaneous regression after several months common.
4. Autogenous vaccines produced with the local BPV strain may help to prevent papillomas.

■ **Epidemiology and Pathogenesis**

Cattle develop papillomas more often than any other domestic animal. The nodules are induced by an infection with one of the currently *13 bovine cutaneous Papillomavirus (BPV) types*. The development of virus-induced papillomas is however not restricted to the skin. Gastrointestinal and urogenital papillomas are also often observed in cattle. There is a *genotype-phenotype relationship* of the BPV type with the anatomic site of papilloma development. BPV-1 and BPV-2 cause fibropapillomas involving both the epithelium and the underlying dermis; BPV-3, BPV-4, BPV-6, BPV-9, BPV-10, BPV-11, and BPV-12 are detected in epithelial papillomas; BPV-5 and BPV-8 are associated with fibropapillomas and epithelial papillomas, and BPV-7 and BPV-13 exclusively are associated with cutaneous papillomas. Nevertheless, most bovine papillomas may contain multiple BPV types. The virus is transmitted via direct contact, fomites, and possibly by insect vectors. Papillomas appear several weeks after exposure and may regress after several months. *Papillomatosis,* concurrent presence of multiple papillomas, is common in young cattle. *Single papillomas* are more common in older animals, which do not always contain BPV DNA.

Clinical Appearance

Papillomas are *single or multiple, prominent or pedunculated, superficially frayed, cauliflower-like tumors*. Fibropapillomas may appear as solid dermal nodules with a papilloma-like surface. Papillomas are most often present on the head, neck, and shoulders and only occasionally on the back and abdomen. Spontaneous regression within months is commonly observed. Although animals develop immunity against the BPV strain, immune suppression and loss of immunity may cause development of new papillomas.

Cytology and Histopathology

Cytology is usually not specific enough for ultimate diagnosis of papillomas.

Histopathologically, papillomas are characterized as plaque-like exophytic neoplasms composed of epithelial cells that form elongated, arborizing papillary projections separated by lamellated keratin. Keratinocytes with basophilic intranuclear inclusion bodies (koilocytes) and numerous intracytoplasmic keratohyalin granules are occasionally present within the superficial layers of the neoplasm. In the superficial dermis, there is often an infiltration by lymphocytes, plasma cells, and some neutrophils.

Therapy

Therapy is usually not necessary due to spontaneous regression of papillomas in cattle. Vaccines are occasionally used to prevent papillomatosis if it is a relevant herd problem but are not therapeutic in cattle that already have lesions. Autogenous vaccines, produced from BPV antigen isolated from papillomas of the herd, are usually more effective than commercially available vaccines. A first vaccination has to be performed in week-old calves to prevent infection and papilloma development since repeated boosting is necessary for protective immunity.

Suggested Further Reading

(Campo 1997; Haga et al. 2013; Nasir and Campo 2008)

Suggested Reading

Abramo F, Pratesi F, Cantile C, Sozzi S, Poli A (1999) Survey of canine and feline follicular tumours and tumour-like lesions in central Italy. J Small Anim Pract 40:479–481

Anderson CL, MacKay CS, Roberts GD, Fidel J (2015) Comparison of abdominal ultrasound and magnetic resonance imaging for detection of abdominal lymphadenopathy in dogs with metastatic apocrine gland adenocarcinoma of the anal sac. Vet Comp Oncol 13:98–105

Bacon NJ, Dernell WS, Ehrhart N, Powers BE, Withrow SJ (2007) Evaluation of primary re-excision after recent inadequate resection of soft tissue sarcomas in dogs: 41 cases (1999–2004). J Am Vet Med Assoc 230: 548–554

Baker-Gabb M, Hunt GB, France MP (2003) Soft tissue sarcomas and mast cell tumours in dogs; clinical behaviour and response to surgery. Aust Vet J 81:732–738

Beckwith-Cohen B, Teixeira LB, Ramos-Vara JA, Dubielzig RR (2014) Squamous papillomas of the conjunctiva in dogs: a condition Not associated with papillomavirus infection. Vet Pathol 52(4):676–680

Belluco S, Brisebard E, Watrelot D, Pillet E, Marchal T, Ponce F (2013) Digital squamous cell carcinoma in dogs: epidemiological, histological, and immunohistochemical study. Vet Pathol 50:1078–1082

Bennett PE, DeNicola DB, Bonney P, Glickman NW, Knapp DW (2002) Canine anal sac adenocarcinomas: clinical presentation and response to therapy. J Vet Intern Med 16:100–104

Bergman PJ (2012) Paraneoplastic hypercalcemia. Top Companion Anim Med 27:156–158

Bergvall KE (2013) Sarcoids. Vet Clin North Am Equine Pract 29:657–671

Blackwood L, Murphy S, Buracco P, De Vos JP, De Fornel-Thibaud P, Hirschberger J, Kessler M, Pastor J, Ponce F, Savary-Bataille K, Argyle DJ (2012) European consensus document on mast cell tumours in dogs and cats. Vet Comp Oncol 10:e1–e29

Bowlt KL, Friend EJ, Delisser P, Murphy S, Polton G (2013) Temporally separated bilateral anal sac gland carcinomas in four dogs. J Small Anim Pract 54:432–436
Brachelente C, Porcellato I, Sforna M, Lepri E, Mechelli L, Bongiovanni L (2013) The contribution of stem cells to epidermal and hair follicle tumours in the dog. Vet Dermatol 24:188–194.e141
Brehm DM, Vite CH, Steinberg HS, Haviland J, van Winkle T (1995) A retrospective evaluation of 51 cases of peripheral nerve sheath tumors in the dog. J Am Anim Hosp Assoc 31:349–359
Brockley LK, Cooper MA, Bennett PF (2013) Malignant melanoma in 63 dogs (2001–2011): the effect of carboplatin chemotherapy on survival. N Z Vet J 61:25–31
Burton JH, Mitchell L, Thamm DH, Dow SW, Biller BJ (2011) Low-dose cyclophosphamide selectively decreases regulatory T cells and inhibits angiogenesis in dogs with soft tissue sarcoma. J Vet Intern Med 25:920–926
Byam-Cook KL, Henson FMD, Slater JD (2006) Treatment of periocular and non-ocular sarcoids in 18 horses by interstitial brachytherapy with iridium-192. Vet Rec 159:337–341
Campo MS (1997) Bovine papillomavirus and cancer. Vet J 154:175–188
Carroll EE, Fossey SL, Mangus LM, Carsillo ME, Rush LJ, McLeod CG, Johnson TO (2010) Malignant pilomatricoma in 3 dogs. Vet Pathol 47:937–943
Chijiwa K, Uchida K, Tateyama S (2004) Immunohistochemical evaluation of canine peripheral nerve sheath tumors and other soft tissue sarcomas. Vet Pathol 41:307–318
de Swarte M, Alexander K, Rannou B, d'Anjou MA, Blond L, Beauchamp G (2011) Comparison of sonographic features of benign and neoplastic deep lymph nodes in dogs. Vet Radiol Ultrasound 52:451–456
Delcour NM, Klopfleisch R, Gruber AD, Weiss AT (2013) Canine cutaneous histiocytomas are clonal lesions as defined by X-linked clonality testing. J Comp Pathol 149:192–198
Demetriou JL, Brearley MJ, Constantino-Casas F, Addington C, Dobson J (2012) Intentional marginal excision of canine limb soft tissue sarcomas followed by radiotherapy. J Small Anim Pract 53:174–181
Dennis MM, McSporran KD, Bacon NJ, Schulman FY, Foster RA, Powers BE (2011) Prognostic factors for cutaneous and subcutaneous soft tissue sarcomas in dogs. Vet Pathol 48:73–84
Dernell WS, Withrow SJ, Kuntz CA, Powers BE (1998) Principles of treatment for soft tissue sarcoma. Clin Tech Small Animal Pract 13:59–64
Eckstein C, Guscetti F, Roos M, Martin de las Mulas J, Kaser-Hotz B, Rohrer Bley C (2009) A retrospective analysis of radiation therapy for the treatment of feline vaccine-associated sarcoma. Vet Comp Oncol 7:54–68
Elmslie RE, Glawe P, Dow SW (2008) Metronomic therapy with cyclophosphamide and piroxicam effectively delays tumor recurrence in dogs with incompletely resected soft tissue sarcomas. J Vet Intern Med 22:1373–1379
Emms SG (2005) Anal sac tumours of the dog and their response to cytoreductive surgery and chemotherapy. Aust Vet J 83:340–343
Haga T, Dong J, Zhu W, Burk RD (2013) The many unknown aspects of bovine papillomavirus diversity, infection and pathogenesis. Vet J 197:122–123
Halsey CH, Gustafson DL, Rose BJ, Wolf-Ringwall A, Burnett RC, Duval DL, Avery AC, Thamm DH (2014) Development of an in vitro model of acquired resistance to toceranib phosphate (Palladia(R)) in canine mast cell tumor. BMC Vet Res 10:105
Hartmann K, Day MJ, Thiry E, Lloret A, Frymus T, Addie D, Boucraut-Baralon C, Egberink H, Gruffydd-Jones T, Horzinek MC and others (2015) Feline injection-site sarcoma: ABCD guidelines on prevention and management. J Feline Med Surg 17(7):606–13
Hendrick MJ, Goldschmidt MH (1991) Do injection site reactions induce fibrosarcomas in cats? J Am Vet Med Assoc 199:968
Henry C, Herrera C (2013) Mast cell tumors in cats: clinical update and possible new treatment avenues. J Feline Med Surg 15(1):41–7
Hershey AE, Sorenmo KU, Hendrick MJ, Shofer FS, Vail DM (2000) Prognosis for presumed feline vaccine-associated sarcoma after excision: 61 cases (1986–1996). J Am Vet Med Assoc 216:58–61
Herzog A, Buchholz J, Ruess-Melzer K, Lang J, Kaser-Hotz B (2013) Combined use of irradiation and DNA tumor vaccine to treat canine oral malignant melanoma: a pilot study. Schweiz Arch Tierheilkd 155:135–142
Hobson HP, Brown MR, Rogers KS (2006) Surgery of metastatic anal sac adenocarcinoma in five dogs. Vet Surg 35:267–270
Hohenhaus AE, Kelsey JL, Haddad J, Barber L, Palmisano M, Farrelly J, Soucy A (2016) Canine cutaneous and subcutaneous soft tissue sarcoma: an evidence-based review of case management. J Am Anim Hosp Assoc 52(2):77–89
Hoshino Y, Mori T, Sakai H, Murakami M, Maruo K (2012) Palliative radiation therapy in a dog with malignant trichoepithelioma. Aust Vet J 90:210–213
Jiang L, Campagne C, Sundstrom E, Sousa P, Imran S, Seltenhammer M, Pielberg G, Olsson MJ, Egidy G, Andersson L, Golovko A (2014) Constitutive activation of the ERK pathway in melanoma and skin melanocytes in Grey horses. BMC Cancer 14:857
Kass PH, Spangler WL, Hendrick MJ, McGill LD, Esplin DG, Lester S, Slater M, Meyer EK, Boucher F, Peters EM, Gobar GG, Htoo T, Decile K (2003) Multicenter case–control study of risk factors associated with development of vaccine-associated sarcomas in cats. J Am Vet Med Assoc 223:1283–1292
Kiupel M, Webster JD, Bailey KL, Best S, DeLay J, Detrisac CJ, Fitzgerald SD, Gamble D, Ginn PE, Goldschmidt MH, Hendrick MJ, Howerth EW, Janovitz EB, Langohr I, Lenz SD, Lipscomb TP, Miller MA, Misdorp W, Moroff S, Mullaney TP, Neyens I, O'Toole D, Ramos-Vara J, Scase TJ, Schulman FY, Sledge D, Smedley RC, Smith K, W Snyder P, Southorn E, Stedman NL, Steficek BA, Stromberg PC, Valli VE, Weisbrode SE, Yager J, Heller J, Miller R (2011) Proposal of a 2-tier histologic grading system for canine cutaneous mast cell tumors to more accurately predict biological behavior. Vet Pathol 48:147–155
Klopfleisch R, Meyer A, Lenze D, Hummel M, Gruber AD (2013) Canine cutaneous peripheral nerve sheath

tumours versus fibrosarcomas can be differentiated by neuroectodermal marker genes in their transcriptome. J Comp Pathol 148:197–205
Knottenbelt DC (2006) A suggested clinical classification for the Equine sarcoid. Pferdeheilkunde 22:479–480
Kung MB, Poirier VJ, Dennis MM, Vail DM, Straw RC (2014) Hypofractionated radiation therapy for the treatment of microscopic canine soft tissue sarcoma. Vet Comp Oncol. doi: 10.1111/vco.12121
Kuntz CA, Dernell WS, Powers BE, Devitt C, Straw RC, Withrow SJ (1997) Prognostic factors for surgical treatment of soft-tissue sarcomas in dogs: 75 cases (1986–1996). J Am Vet Med Assoc 211:1147–1151
Ladlow J (2013) Injection site-associated sarcoma in the cat: treatment recommendations and results to date. J Feline Med Surg 15:409–418
Lange CE, Favrot C (2011) Canine papillomaviruses. Vet Clin North Am Small Anim Pract 41:1183–1195
Langova V, Mutsaers AJ, Phillips B, Straw R (2004) Treatment of eight dogs with nasal tumours with alternating doses of doxorubicin and carboplatin in conjunction with oral piroxicam. Aust Vet J 82:676–680
Lawrence J, Forrest L, Adams W, Vail D, Thamm D (2008) Four-fraction radiation therapy for macroscopic soft tissue sarcomas in 16 dogs. J Am Anim Hosp Assoc 44:100–108
Liptak JM, Forrest LJ (2012) Soft tissue sarcomas. In: Withrow & MacEwen's small animal clinical oncology, 5th edn. Saunders Elsevier, St. Louis, p 357
London CA (2013) Kinase dysfunction and kinase inhibitors. Vet Dermatol 24:181–187.e139–140
Luff JA, Affolter VK, Yeargan B, Moore PF (2012) Detection of six novel papillomavirus sequences within canine pigmented plaques. J Vet Diagn Invest: Off Publ Am Assoc Vet Lab Diagn, Inc 24:576–580
Maina E, Colombo S, Stefanello D (2014) Multiple cutaneous histiocytomas treated with lomustine in a dog. Vet Dermatol 25:559–562, e598–559
Martano M, Morello E, Buracco P (2011) Feline injection-site sarcoma: past, present and future perspectives. Vet J 188:136–141
Martens A, De Moor A, Demeulemeester J, Peelman L (2001) Polymerase chain reaction analysis of the surgical margins of equine sarcoids for bovine papilloma virus DNA. Vet Surg 30:460–467
Masserdotti C, Ubbiali FA (2002) Fine needle aspiration cytology of pilomatricoma in three dogs. Vet Clin Pathol/Am Soc Vet Clin Pathol 31:22–25
Matz BM (2015) Current concepts in oncologic surgery in small animals. Vet Clin North Am Small Anim Pract 45:437–449
McEntee MC, Page RL, Mauldin GN, Thrall DE (2000) Results of irradiation of infiltrative lipoma in 13 dogs. Vet Radiol Ultrasound : Off J Am Coll Vet Radiol Int Vet Radiol Assoc 41:554–556
Metcalfe LV, O'Brien PJ, Papakonstantinou S, Cahalan SD, McAllister H, Duggan VE (2013) Malignant melanoma in a grey horse: case presentation and review of equine melanoma treatment options. Ir Vet J 66:22
Meyer A, Gruber AD, Klopfleisch R (2012) CD25 is expressed by canine cutaneous mast cell tumors but not by cutaneous connective tissue mast cells. Vet Pathol 49:988–997
Meyer A, Gruber AD, Klopfleisch R (2013) All subunits of the interleukin-2 receptor are expressed by canine cutaneous mast cell tumours. J Comp Pathol 149:19–29
Meyer A, Klopfleisch R (2014) Multiple polymerase chain reaction markers for the differentiation of canine cutaneous peripheral nerve sheath tumours versus canine fibrosarcomas. J Comp Pathol 150:198–203
Moore PF (2014) A review of histiocytic diseases of dogs and cats. Vet Pathol 51:167–184
Muller J, Feige K, Wunderlin P, Hodl A, Meli ML, Seltenhammer M, Grest P, Nicolson L, Schelling C, Heinzerling LM (2011) Double-blind placebo-controlled study with interleukin-18 and interleukin-12-encoding plasmid DNA shows antitumor effect in metastatic melanoma in gray horses. J Immunother 34:58–64
Munday JS, Dunowska M, Hills SF, Laurie RE (2013) Genomic characterization of Felis catus papillomavirus-3: a novel papillomavirus detected in a feline Bowenoid in situ carcinoma. Vet Microbiol 165:319–325
Munday JS, O'Connor KI, Smits B (2011) Development of multiple pigmented viral plaques and squamous cell carcinomas in a dog infected by a novel papillomavirus. Vet Dermatol 22:104–110
Munday JS, Tucker RS, Kiupel M, Harvey CJ (2015) Multiple oral carcinomas associated with a novel papillomavirus in a dog. J Vet Diagn Investig : Off Publ Am Assoc Vet Lab Diagn, Inc 27(2):221–225
Murphy S (2013) Cutaneous squamous cell carcinoma in the cat: current understanding and treatment approaches. J Feline Med Surg 15:401–407
Nasir L, Campo MS (2008) Bovine papillomaviruses: their role in the aetiology of cutaneous tumours of bovids and equids. Vet Dermatol 19:243–254
O'Brien MG, Berg J, Engler SJ (1992) Treatment by digital amputation of subungual squamous cell carcinoma in dogs: 21 cases (1987–1988). J Am Vet Med Assoc 201:759–761
Ogilvie GK, Reynolds HA, Richardson RC, Withrow SJ, Norris AM, Henderson RA, Klausner JS, Fowler JD, McCaw D (1989) Phase II evaluation of doxorubicin for treatment of various canine neoplasms. J Am Vet Med Assoc 195:1580–1583
Ottnod JM, Smedley RC, Walshaw R, Hauptman JG, Kiupel M, Obradovich JE (2013) A retrospective analysis of the efficacy of Oncept vaccine for the adjunct treatment of canine oral malignant melanoma. Vet Comp Oncol 11:219–229
Owen LN (1980) Squamous cell carcinoma. In: TNM classification of tumours in domestic, 1st edn. World Health Organization, Geneva, pp 46–47
Patnaik AK, Ehler WJ, MacEwen EG (1984) Canine cutaneous mast cell tumor: morphologic grading and survival time in 83 dogs. Vet Pathol 21:469–474
Phillips JC, Lembcke LM (2013) Equine melanocytic tumors. Vet Clin North Am Equine Pract 29:673–687
Pires I, Alves A, Queiroga FL, Silva F, Lopes C (2013) Regression of canine cutaneous histiocytoma: reduced proliferation or increased apoptosis? Anticancer Res 33:1397–1400
Polton G (2007) Anal sac gland carcinoma in cocker spaniels. Vet Rec 160:244

4

Polton GA, Brearley MJ (2007) Clinical stage, therapy, and prognosis in canine anal sac gland carcinoma. J Vet Intern Med 21:274–280

Prpich CY, Santamaria AC, Simcock JO, Wong HK, Nimmo JS, Kuntz CA (2014) Second intention healing after wide local excision of soft tissue sarcomas in the distal aspects of the limbs in dogs: 31 cases (2005–2012). J Am Vet Med Assoc 244:187–194

Rassnick KM (2003) Medical management of soft tissue sarcomas. Vet Clin N Am-Small 33:517–531

Richards JR, Elston TH, Ford RB, Gaskell RM, Hartmann K, Hurley KF, Lappin MR, Levy JK, Rodan I, Scherk M, Schultz RD, Sparkes AH (2006) The 2006 American association of feline practitioners feline vaccine advisory panel report. J Am Vet Med Assoc 229:1405–1441

Ross JT, Scavelli TD, Matthiesen DT, Patnaik AK (1991) Adenocarcinoma of the apocrine glands of the anal Sac in dogs – a review of 32 cases. J Am Anim Hosp Assoc 27:349–355

Rowe EL, Sullins KE (2004) Excision as treatment of dermal melanomatosis in horses: 11 cases (1994–2000). J Am Vet Med Assoc 225:94–96

Sabattini S, Guadagni Frizzon M, Gentilini F, Turba ME, Capitani O, Bettini G (2013) Prognostic significance of Kit receptor tyrosine kinase dysregulations in feline cutaneous mast cell tumors. Vet Pathol 50:797–805

Smedley RC, Spangler WL, Esplin DG, Kitchell BE, Bergman PJ, Ho HY, Bergin IL, Kiupel M (2011) Prognostic markers for canine melanocytic neoplasms: a comparative review of the literature and goals for future investigation. Vet Pathol 48:54–72

Spangler WL, Kass PH (2006) The histologic and epidemiologic bases for prognostic considerations in canine melanocytic neoplasia. Vet Pathol 43:136–149

Stadler S, Kainzbauer C, Haralambus R, Hainisch E, Brandt S, Brehm W (2011) Successful treatment of equine sarcoids by topical aciclovir application. Vet Rec 168:187–187

Stefanello D, Buracco P, Sabattini S, Finotello R, Giudice C, Grieco V, Iussich S, Tursi M, Scase T, Di Palma S, Bettini G, Ferrari R, Martano M, Gattino F, Marrington M, Mazzola M, Elisabetta Vasconi M, Annoni M, Marconato L (2015) Comparison of 2- and 3-category histologic grading systems for predicting the presence of metastasis at the time of initial evaluation in dogs with cutaneous mast cell tumors: 386 cases (2009–2014). J Am Vet Med Assoc 246:765–769

Stewart AA, Rush B, Davis E (2006) The efficacy of intratumoural 5-fluorouracil for the treatment of equine sarcoids. Aust Vet J 84:101–106

Stockhaus C, Teske E, Rudolph R, Werner HG (2001) Assessment of cytological criteria for diagnosing basal cell tumours in the dog and cat. J Small Anim Pract 42:582–586

Suzuki S, Uchida K, Nakayama H (2014) The effects of tumor location on diagnostic criteria for canine malignant peripheral nerve sheath tumors (MPNSTs) and the markers for distinction between canine MPNSTs and canine perivascular wall tumors. Vet Pathol 51:722–736

Teixeira RB, Rendahl AK, Anderson SM, Mickelson JR, Sigler D, Buchanan BR, Coleman RJ, McCue ME (2013) Coat color genotypes and risk and severity of melanoma in gray quarter horses. J Veterinary Intern Med/Am Coll Vet Intern Med 27:1201–1208

Thamm DH, Vail DM (2007) Mast cell tumors. In: Withrow & MacEwen's small animal clinical oncology, 4th edn. Saunders Elsevier, St. Louis, pp 402–424

Theon AP, Wilson WD, Magdesian KG, Pusterla N, Snyder JR, Galuppo LD (2007) Long-term outcome associated with intratumoral chemotherapy with cisplatin for cutaneous tumors in equidae: 573 cases (1995–2004). J Am Vet Med Assoc 230:1506–1513

Thomson M (2007) Squamous cell carcinoma of the nasal planum in cats and dogs. Clin Tech Small Anim Pract 22:42–45

Vaccination Guidelines G, Day MJ, Horzinek MC, Schultz RD (2010) WSAVA guidelines for the vaccination of dogs and cats. J Small Anim Pract 51:1–32

Vail DM, Withrow SJ, Schwarz PD, Powers BE (1990) Perianal adenocarcinoma in the canine male – a retrospective study of 41 cases. J Am Anim Hosp Assoc 26:329–334

Waropastrakul S, Munday JS, French AF (2012) Infrequent detection of papillomaviral DNA within canine cutaneous squamous cell carcinomas, haemangiosarcomas and healthy skin on the ventrum of dogs. Vet Dermatol 23:197–e41

Webb JL, Burns RE, Brown HM, LeRoy BE, Kosarek CE (2009) Squamous cell carcinoma. Compendium 31:E9

Welle MM, Bley CR, Howard J, Rufenacht S (2008) Canine mast cell tumours: a review of the pathogenesis, clinical features, pathology and treatment. Vet Dermatol 19:321–339

Mammary Tumors

Robert Klopfleisch

R. Klopfleisch (ed.), *Veterinary Oncology*, DOI 10.1007/978-3-319-41124-8_5

Mammary tumors are common tumors in dogs and to a lesser extent in cats, mice, rats, and guinea pigs. They are rarities with no relevance for daily veterinary practice in other animal species.

5.1 Canine Mammary Tumors (CMT)

Box 5.1. Canine Mammary Tumors in Six Facts

1. Most common tumor in the uncastrated female dog.
2. Sex steroid/spaying influences incidence.
3. No known relevant tumor-associated mutations.
4. Staging and histologic grading is of prognostic relevance.
5. Less than 50 % of the tumors are malignant; one quarter or less metastasizes (to the lung).
6. Surgery is the treatment option of choice.

▪ Epidemiology and Pathogenesis

Traditionally, CMT have been considered the *most common tumor of the female dog*. They are still one of the most common tumors of the female dog in Europe, where early spaying practice is uncommon and many dogs are left intact. A potential lifetime risk of greater than 50 % of developing mammary tumors has been reported in Europe. CMT are rare in the United States, where most dogs are spayed during the first year of life. Male dogs are rarely affected by mammary tumors and if so the tumors are histologically and clinically benign.

Age is one of the few undisputed factors with influence on development of CMT. Few tumors are seen before the age of six, and the peak of cases is seen in dogs of 10–14 years.

The general effect of *sex steroids* and spaying on tumor initiation and early carcinogenesis is universally accepted, but the influence of the timing of the procedure is continuously under debate. An early study proposed that *spaying/ovariohysterectomy* before the first estrus reduces the tumor risk 200-fold compared to intact dogs, while spaying after the second estrus has no effect. Several more recent studies and meta-analyses have challenged this simple model and found no effect of age at spaying on tumor risk. Put another way, spaying later in life may also reduce tumor risk. *Estrus suppression* using progesterone derivatives also increases tumor risk and is thus not recommended if spaying is an option. Unlike in humans, where pregnancy and lactation are both thought to reduce breast cancer risk, in dogs the number of *gestations* and *pseudopregnancy* most probably has no influence on tumor development. The effect of sex steroids on tumor progression in CMT is uncertain. All normal mammary gland epithelial cells and most of the epithelial tumor cells in benign mammary tumors express *estrogen* and *progesterone receptor*. In contrast, malignant mammary tumors in dogs (and their metastases) mostly do not express the receptors. This means they are most probably independent of external hormonal stimuli, and spaying at the time of tumor diagnosis is probably not an effective part of treatment.

Breed predisposition may have a minor effect on the development of mammary tumors in dogs; the literature reports contradictory results with several different breeds at potential risk or not, depending on the sources.

The *molecular pathogenesis* of CMT is an area of constant and ongoing research. CMT carcinogenesis is often hypothesized to *have a progressive course to malignancy*, developing from dysplasia to adenoma to malignant tumors. This assumption is mainly based on two observations. The first is that malignant tumors are on average bigger in diameter. The second is that benign and malignant tumor cells are simultaneously present in malignant tumors. However, proving this on a molecular level is difficult. It would require observing tumor growth in situ, which is ethically untenable. *No biologically relevant tumor-inducing mutations* or signaling cascades have been identified so far. One major research focus was the search for spontaneous or hereditary mutations of the *BRCA genes*, DNA repair genes associated with hereditary breast cancer in women. Despite weak hints, no strong correlation has been found between the genetic sequence of BRCA in dogs and clinical outcome or malignant behavior of CMT. Research on more complex malignancy-associated RNA and protein expression patterns is ongoing and generally promising. Unfortunately, so far this research has not been translated in ready-to-use diagnostic assays with prognostic relevance or predictive value for therapy selection.

Clinical Appearance

The incidence of CMT is higher in the *caudal mammary complexes* due to higher amounts of mammary gland tissue (◘ Fig. 5.1). *Primary multiplicity* of tumors is common. This means that several tumors of the same or different histological types develop concurrently and independently within the same complexes. For example, two complexes may independently develop adenocarcinoma, or one complex may develop an adenocarcinoma and the other an adenoma. Evaluation of malignancy is usually not appreciable by palpation of the primary tumor except for the highly malignant *inflammatory mammary carcinomas.* These tumors resemble a severe mastitis, presenting with heat, erythema, and edema in the affected gland. They are also characterized by a marked firmness in the affected mammary complex, surrounding tissues and the hind limbs. This firmness is typical for a neoplastic rather than a solely inflammatory process. Fast growth, a size >5 cm in diameter, ulceration, and associated swelling of the regional lymph node are probable but not definite *signs of malignancy for noninflammatory carcinoma.* The regional lymph node for mammary complexes 1–3 is the axial lymph node; the inguinal lymph node is regional for mammary complexes 3–5. Clinical staging is currently performed according to a modified WHO system (◘ Table 5.1).

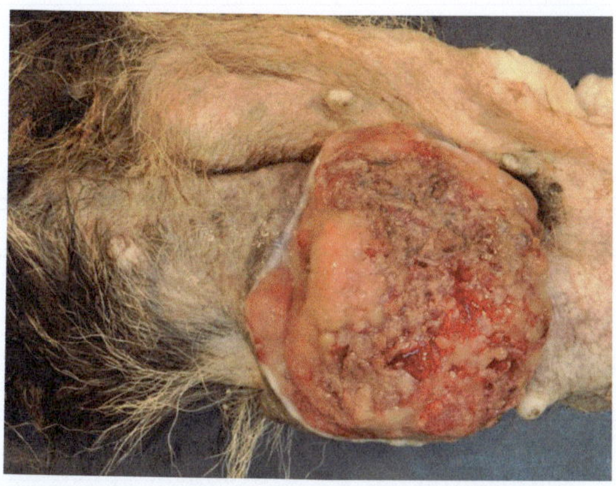

◘ **Fig. 5.1** Ulcerated malignant canine mammary tumor, dog (From the archive of the Institute of Veterinary Pathology, Freie Universität Berlin)

End-stage CMT are characterized by *lymphogenic spread* with involvement of the regional lymph node or a probable direct hematogenic spread with the development of multiple *lung metastases* (◘ Fig. 5.2). Metastasis to other organs is observed in less than 10 % of metastatic tumors. Lateral and dorsoventral *thoracic radiographs* are therefore standard procedure prior to surgery to rule out lung metastasis.

Complete blood count, clinical chemistry, and *urinalysis* are usually normal, but disseminated intravascular coagulation (DIC) may be present in dogs with inflammatory carcinomas. *No paraneoplastic syndrome* is known for this tumor type.

Cytology and Histopathology

Cytology is generally not recommended as it has low specificity and sensitivity for CMT diagnosis. It is also inadequate for tumor grading due to marked intratumoral heterogeneity. In some cases, however, cytology might be helpful to differentiate mammary tumors from other tumors in the mammary region such as mast cell tumors or lymphoma (◘ Figs. 5.3 and 5.4).

Histopathologic analysis using excisional biopsies is the definitive method for diagnosing and grading CMT. Classification of CMT is very complex with more than 40 histologically defined tumor subtypes. Unfortunately, this sophisticated classification is not based on or even correlated with specific clinical behaviors or recommendations for therapy protocols.

CMT in the strict sense are tumors of the epithelial cells of the mammary gland, which are either (malignant) *carcinoma* or (benign) *adenoma. Complex adenoma* and *carcinoma* present with a concurrent proliferation of the perialveolar myoepithelial cells. *Benign mixed tumors*, which are common, contain a neoplastic epithelial component accompanied by nonneoplastic cartilage and bone. Usually *less than 50 % of the tumors are histologically malignant.*

Follow-up studies indicate that less than 50 % of dogs with surgically removed histologically defined adenocarcinomas developed metastases or recurring tumors. A *3-tier grading system* for mammary carcinomas has been developed to improve and standardize the prognostic value of histopathologic diagnosis (◘ Table 5.2). Submission of the respective regional lymph node is recommended as it improves prognostic accuracy for metastatic potential.

Table 5.1 Staging system for CMT (Owen, 1980, WHO classification)

Stage	T (tumor diameter)	N (lymph node metastases)	M (distant metastases)	Survival 1/2 years after mastectomy in %
I	T_1 (<3 cm)	N_0	M_0	97.9/90–98
II	T_2 (3–5 cm)	N_0	M_0	Unknown/90–98
III	T_3 (>5 cm)	N_0	M_0	Unknown/90–98
IV	T_A (any size)	N_1	M_0	(For N_A) 75.8/30–66
V	T_A (any size)	N_A	M_1	14/14–30

N_0 no lymph node metastases, N_1 lymph node metastases, N_A lymph node status irrelevant, M_0 no distant metastases, M_1 distant metastases detected

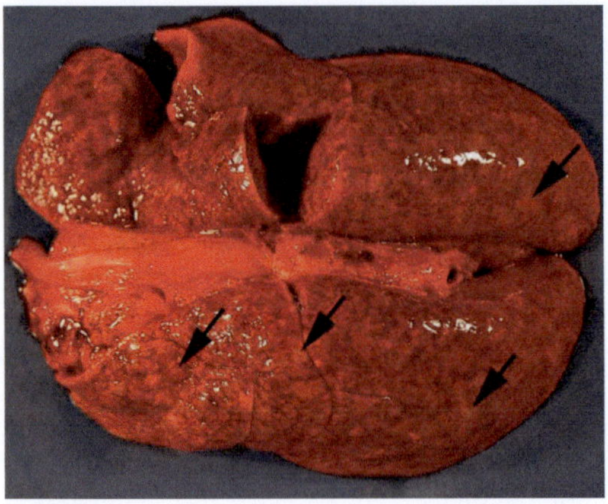

Fig. 5.2 Lung metastases (*black arrow*) of a canine mammary tumor, dog (From the archive of the Institute of Veterinary Pathology, Freie Universität Berlin)

Inflammatory mammary carcinomas are rare, but they are the most aggressive mammary tumor in the dog. They are characterized by macroscopic resemblance to acute mastitis, presenting with edema, firmness, erythema, and pain. Histologically, inflammatory carcinomas lack a discernible tumor mass. They are composed of an accumulation of single or small groups of tumor cells in dermal lymph vessels. Metastasis to distant organs is usually present at the time of tumor diagnosis. Secondary inflammatory carcinomas, which develop from primary solid tumors, are possible.

Therapy

Surgery is still the standard treatment for dogs with mammary tumors. There is an ongoing debate whether nodulectomy, regional mastectomy, or radical mastectomy is the treatment of choice.

Nodulectomy is recommended for small (<1 cm), moveable nodules, which in the majority of the cases are benign. Nodules should be removed with a margin of up to 2 cm to ensure complete resection. If the nodule turns out to be malignant on histopathology, a more extensive secondary excision of the complete gland is recommended.

The idea of *regional mastectomy* is based on the finding that the lymphatic system of mammary glands 1–3 drains to the cranial sternal and axial lymph nodes, while the lymphatic vessels of the mammary glands 4 and 5 drain to the superficial inguinal and the medial iliac lymph nodes. Due to this lymphatic communication, glands 1–3 and/or glands 4 and 5 should be removed en bloc. The regional lymph node should also be removed and submitted for histopathologic analysis of the metastatic potential of the primary tumor.

Unilateral or even bilateral *radical mastectomy* involves the removal of all five mammary glands en bloc. The advantages of radical mastectomy for survival are a matter of debate. The procedure causes a large wound with increased risks for postoperative delayed wound healing. However, due to the primary multiplicity of canine tumors discussed above, radical mastectomy may be indicated. Bilateral mastectomy is only recommended for dogs with pendulous mammary glands, which allow for tension-free wound closure.

Chemotherapy is not a treatment option for CMT. Most of the protocols tested are highly toxic and have had no effect on disease outcome. In

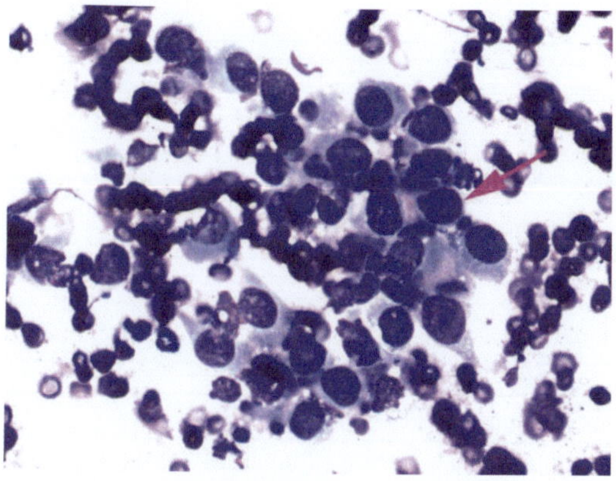

Fig. 5.3 Cytology, low malignant canine mammary tumor, dog, May-Grünwald-Giemsa, 200×. Note the moderately pleomorphic epithelial cells with mild anisocytosis, anisokaryosis, and mild variation in nuclear to cytoplasm ratio (*pink arrow*)

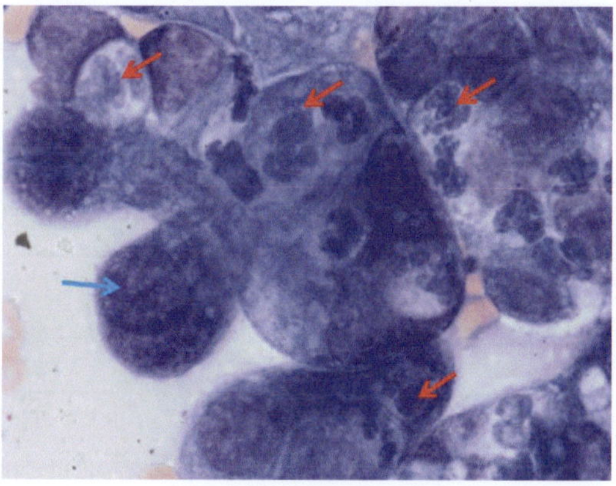

Fig. 5.4 Cytology, anaplastic mammary carcinoma, dog, May-Grünwald-Giemsa, 1000x. Note the highly pleomorphic epithelial cells with marked anisocytosis, anisokaryosis, variation in nuclear to cytoplasm ratio, multiple prominent nucleoli (*blue arrow*), and cell cannibalism of neutrophils (*red arrow*) (Photo: with permission from Dr. N. Bauer, Faculty of Veterinary Medicine, Justus-Liebig-University, Giessen, Germany)

contrast, several in vitro studies on a variety of anticancer drugs have shown an impact on mammary tumor cell proliferation and cell death but lack in vivo confirmation.

The effect of *radiotherapy* or *hormonal therapy* with estrogen modulators like tamoxifen on CMT is unclear. The few available studies cast doubt their effectiveness. Concurrent *ovariohysterectomy* and mastectomy as an adjunct therapy have been discussed repeatedly, but no effect on survival has been shown.

Prognostic Factors and Markers

Tumor staging and grading are important prognostic factors for CMT (Tables 5.1 and 5.2). Tumor size and lymph node metastases can also be used as independent prognostic indicators (Table 5.3). Lack of *estrogen* and *progesterone receptor* expression as shown by immunohistochemistry in CMT indicates a more malignant phenotype and worse prognosis. Due to the lack of expression hormone receptors in most CMT, receptor expression is not routinely analyzed in CMT diagnostics in contrast to human breast cancer. Another receptor commonly analyzed in human breast cancer samples is the *HER2*, the human epithelial growth factor receptor 2. The relevance of immunohistochemical detection of HER2 expression in CMT is unclear. The latest approach to finding biomarkers for CMT has been the detection of mRNA of *circulating tumor cells* (CTC) in the peripheral blood. Strong correlations have been found between CTC and the metastatic behavior of primary tumors.

Current Trends in Research

Current research on CMT focuses on the identification and characterization of cancer stem cells, the identification of effective anticancer drugs, and finding prognostic mRNA and protein expression patterns. Several studies have identified *mammary cancer stem cells* using surface markers like OCT4 and Nanog and confirmed their remarkable chemoresistance and resistance to radiotherapy. Several unrelated *potential chemotherapeutic agents* like the hyaluronan synthesis inhibitor 4-methylumbelliferone; the COX2 inhibitor celecoxib; the nonsteroidal anti-inflammatory drugs tolfenamic acid, piroxicam, and deracoxib; and an oncolytic vaccinia virus have been successfully tested in vivo and are now awaiting clinical approval. Finally, *complex RNA and protein expression* patterns for sensitive and specific discrimination of malignant and benign CMT have been identified using expensive and complex microarray and proteomics technology. But these expression patterns have not been translated into less expensive and easy-to-use diagnostic assays.

Table 5.2 Grading system for CMT (Pena et al. 2013)

Histologic criteria	Points			
A. Tubule formation	1	>75 % tubular morphology		
	2	10–75 % tubular morphology		
	3	<10 % tubular morphology		
B. Nuclear pleomorphism	1	Uniform nuclei, rare nucleoli		
	2	Moderate variation in nuclear size/shape, presence of nucleoli		
	3	Marked variation in nuclear size/shape, often prominent nucleoli		
C. Mitoses per 10 HPF	1	0–9 mitoses/10 HPF		
	2	10–19 mitoses/10 HPF		
	3	≥20 mitoses/10 HPF		
			Rec./Mets.[a]	Cancer death[a]
Total score (A + B + C)	3–5	*Grade 1*	3.4 %	0
Total score (A + B + C)	6–7	*Grade 2*	15.8 %	15.8 %
Total score (A + B + C)	8–9	*Grade 2*	58.8 %	58.8 %

HPF = 0.24 mm^2
[a]Follow-up time at least 28 months

Table 5.3 Prognostic factors for CMT

Factor	Details	Disease-free interval (Beauvais et al. 2012)/ survival time (Chang et al. 2005)
Tumor diameter[a]	<5 cm	112 weeks (Chang et al. 2005)
	>5 cm	40 weeks (Chang et al. 2005)
Lymph node metastases[a]	No	<30 % recurrence after 2 years
	Yes	80 % recurrence after 6 months
	Or	
	No	21 % death rate after 2 years
	Yes	86 % death rate after 2 years

[a]Treated with surgery

5.2 Feline Mammary Tumor (FMT)

Box 5.2. Feline Mammary Tumors in Six Facts

1. Common in the cat but less common than in the dog.
2. Sex steroid/spaying influences incidence.
3. No known relevant tumor-associated mutations.
4. Staging and histologic grading is of prognostic relevance.
5. More than 90 % of the tumors are malignant and metastasize mostly to the lung.
6. Surgery is the treatment option of choice.

Epidemiology and Pathogenesis

The incidence of FMT is half that of CMT. They are nevertheless still a common tumor of the cat, making up approximately 17 % of all feline tumors. FMT are usually diagnosed at the *age* of 10–12 years. A *breed* predilection has been observed for Siamese cats. In rare cases male cats may also develop mammary tumors, similar to dogs.

Sex steroids and early spaying have an effect on tumor initiation and early carcinogenesis. *Spaying* before the age of 1 year reduces the risk of mammary tumor development by up to 90 %. In contrast, *estrus suppression* using progesterone derivatives increases tumor risk by threefold in females and is thus not recommended if spaying is an option. The effect of sex steroids on tumor progression and malignant behavior is questionable. As mentioned in the discussion of canine mammary tumors, normal mammary gland epithelial cells and benign mammary tumor cells express *estrogen* and *progesterone receptors*. Very few malignant tumors express these receptors in felines, and in those that do, only a few tumor cells are affected. Thus, unlike human breast cancer, both canine and FMT are most probably not responsive to external hormonal stimuli.

Other than the influence of sex steroids in early carcinogenesis, the *molecular pathogenesis* of FMT is unclear. Much effort has been invested in analyzing the malignancy potential of overexpression of *HER2,* but nothing significant has been identified. Cyclooxygenase-2 (COX2) and vascular endothelial growth factor receptor 2 (VEGFR2) expression has however been associated with slightly shorter survival in felines. *No biologically relevant tumor-inducing mutations* or signaling cascades have been identified so far.

▪ Clinical Appearance

All four mammary glands of felines, two thoracic and two abdominal, can be affected by mammary tumors. There may however be a slight predisposition of the caudal glands, as in dogs. FMT are usually single subcutaneous, sometimes ulcerated or cystic masses. Macroscopic distinction between benign and malignant tumors is difficult to impossible. Since up to 90 % of the tumors are histologically malignant, all masses in the feline mammary glands should be treated as such until proven otherwise. Multiple mammary masses are possible but less common than in the dog. Signs of inflammation, edema, swelling, firmness, erythema, pain, and regional and distant metastases have been seen in the few cases of highly aggressive inflammatory carcinomas. They are difficult to differentiate from acute mastitis or nonneoplastic fibroadenomatous hyperplasia.

The *tumor diameter* is part of the *WHO staging system* and strongly influences the prognosis (◘ Table 5.4). *Lymph node metastasis* is present in up to 90 % of cats with mammary tumors at the time of surgery. Axillary lymph nodes, inguinal and to a lesser extent sternal lymph nodes, are most commonly affected. *Pulmonary metastases* are common in cats with mammary tumors, and, similar to the dog, they are the most common cause of death and euthanasia in patients with mammary tumors. Lateral and dorsoventral *thoracic radiographs* are therefore standard procedure prior to surgery to rule out lung metastasis.

Complete blood count, blood chemistry, and *urinalysis* are usually normal. *No paraneoplastic syndromes* are known for this tumor type.

◘ Table 5.4 Staging system for FMT (Owen, 1980, WHO classification)

Stage	T (tumor diameter)	N (lymph node metastases)	M (distant metastases)	Average survival time
I	T_1 (<2 cm)	N_0	M_0	29 months
II	T_2 (2–3 cm)	N_0	M_0	12.5 months
III	T_3 (>3 cm) $T_{1,2}$ (<3 cm)	N_0 N_1	M_0 M_0	9 months
IV	T_A (any size)	N_1	M_1	1 months

N_0 no lymph node metastases, N_1 lymph node metastases, M_0 no distant metastases, M_1 distant metastases detected

5.2.1 Cytology and Histopathology

Fine-needle aspiration of FMT is more helpful than in dogs since most of the tumors are malignant. Cytology is nevertheless not a reliable method for discriminating benign from malignant tumors or for evaluating tumor grade.

Histopathologic analysis using tissue biopsies is the definitive technique to diagnose and grade FMT. Up to 90% of FMT are classified as malignant carcinomas. These may be further subclassified into histologic subtypes according to their growth pattern, but the prognostic relevance of these subtypes is questionable. A *3-tier grading system* for mammary carcinomas to improve and standardize the prognostic value of the histopathologic diagnosis has been developed and is increasingly used (◘ Table 5.5). In addition to the features involved in the grading system, tumor size and lymph node involvements are considered prognostic features strongly correlated with malignancy. Tumors with a maximum diameter of >3 cm are associated with a survival of 5 months or less, while cats with tumors <2 cm in diameter may survive for 12 months or more.

Inflammatory mammary carcinomas seem to be rare in cats, and only four cases, all with survival times of only a few days until euthanasia, have been described so far. Histologically, embolism of tumor cells can be seen in superficial dermal lymphatic vessels, with severe secondary inflammation.

Benign tumors represent around 10% of all FMT. They are further classified as simple or complex adenomas or fibroadenomas although this subclassification is irrelevant for prognosis. Complex tumors with concurrent proliferation of myoepithelial cells or mixed tumors with cartilage and bone are extremely rare in cats, in contrast to dogs where they are common.

Fibroadenomatous hyperplasia is a nonneoplastic, primarily noninflammatory, progesterone-induced massive proliferation of the mammary glands. Usually multiple glands are affected, but on occasion lesions are found in only one gland. It occurs in young cats <2 years of age after estrus or during pregnancy. Removal of the hormonal stimulus by ovariohysterectomy leads to regression of the swelling in most cases.

▪ Therapy

Surgery is still the standard treatment for FMT. The *lymphatic drainage* of the feline mammary glands is most probably *highly connected*. It is assumed that the first and second (thoracic) glands drain mostly to the axillary lymph node, the third and maybe the second gland to the axillary and the inguinal lymph nodes, and the fourth (inguinal) gland only to the inguinal lymph node. In addition, left and right mammary glands also

◘ **Table 5.5** Grading system for FMT (Mills et al. 2013)

Histologic criteria	Points			
A. Lymphovascular invasion	0	Absent		
	1	Present		
B. Nuclear form	0	<5% abnormal		
	1	>5% abnormal		
C. Mitoses per 10 HPF	0	<62		
	1	>62		
			Median survival, months	Survival at 18 months, %
Total score (A+B+C)	0	*Grade 1*	31	82
Total score (A+B+C)	1	*Grade 2*	14	37
Total score (A+B+C)	2–3	*Grade 2*	8	18

HPF = 0.22 mm^2

seem to communicate. Unilateral or even bilateral *complete mastectomy* is recommended as the treatment of choice due to the aggressive character of these tumors and the close communication between structures. Radical mastectomy significantly reduces the probability of recurrence. A 2-week interval is recommended between procedures in bilateral mastectomy. The inguinal lymph node is located adjacent and caudal to the fourth gland and should always be removed and submitted for biopsy. Due to the distant location of the axillary lymph node, it should be removed only if enlarged or positive in fine-needle aspirates; removal does increase survival time. *Ovariohysterectomy* at the time of mastectomy has no benefit on survival or tumor recurrence. It should be considered if a fibroadenomatous hyperplasia is confirmed or suspected.

Chemotherapy with doxorubicin alone or with cyclophosphamide may have some beneficial effects on non-resectable tumors. A metronomic approach with long application of low doses of vincristine, cyclophosphamide, and methotrexate has been shown to prolong survival and disease-free interval. The effect of chemotherapy treatment as an adjunct to surgery is not confirmed but may increase survival time by up to 600 days.

Radiotherapy and *anti-hormonal therapy* have no proven effect in the treatment of FMT.

Prognostic Factors and Markers

Studies on the correlation between overexpression of *HER2* and overall survival are contradictory. In addition, there is only insufficient information on whether FMT also loose estrogen and progesterone expression with increasing malignancy as it is common in canine mammary tumors. However, cyclooxygenase-2 (*COX2*) and vascular endothelial growth factor receptor 2 (*VEGFR2*) expression in FMT has been associated with slightly shorter survival times. COX2 and VEGFR2 could thus act as potential therapeutic targets for mammary tumors in this species. More prognostic factors for FMT are presented in Table 5.6.

Current Trends in Research

The majority of recent studies on FMT focuses on the analysis of protein and mRNA and protein expression patterns of several genes involved in apoptosis, cell adhesion, or growth factor signaling. In addition, evidence of FMT stem cells has been found and coupled with insights into radiotherapy and chemotherapy resistance and may open the way for understandings of FMT biology. Several research groups are also trying to apply the molecular classification scheme of human breast cancer based on estrogen, progesterone, and HER2 protein expression to FMT, to evaluate the applicability of felines as a model for human disease.

Table 5.6 Prognostic factors for FMT

Factor	Details	Disease-free interval (Beauvais et al. 2012)/ survival time (Chang et al. 2005)
Tumor diameter[a]	<3 cm	21–24 months (Beauvais et al. 2012)
	>3 cm	4–12 months (Beauvais et al. 2012)
	Or	Or
	<2 cm[b]	450 days (Chang et al. 2005)
	2–3 cm[b]	448 days (Chang et al. 2005)
	>3 cm[b]	200 days (Chang et al. 2005)
Metastatic disease[b]	No	>2100 days (Chang et al. 2005)
	Yes	331 days (Chang et al. 2005)
Location of metastasis[b]	Lymph node	>1543 days (Chang et al. 2005)
	Lung	331 days (Chang et al. 2005)
	Pleura	188 days (Chang et al. 2005)
Type of mastectomy[b]	Regional	428 days
	Unilateral radical	348 days
	Bilateral radical	917 days

[a]Treated with surgery
[b]Treated with mastectomy and doxorubicin

▪ Suggested Reading

(Hughes and Dobson 2012; Mills et al. 2015; Morris 2013; Novosad et al. 2006; Pang et al. 2013; Perez-Alenza et al. 2004; Viste et al. 2002)

Suggested Reading

Beauvais W, Cardwell JM, Brodbelt DC (2012) The effect of neutering on the risk of mammary tumours in dogs--a systematic review. J Small Anim Pract 53:314–322

Chang SC, Chang CC, Chang TJ, Wong ML (2005) Prognostic factors associated with survival two years after surgery in dogs with malignant mammary tumors: 79 cases (1998–2002). J Am Vet Med Assoc 227:1625–1629

da Costa A, Kohn B, Gruber AD, Klopfleisch R (2013) Multiple RT-PCR markers for the detection of circulating tumour cells of metastatic canine mammary tumours. Vet J 196:34–39

Hughes K, Dobson JM (2012) Prognostic histopathological and molecular markers in feline mammary neoplasia. Vet J 194:19–26

Klopfleisch R, Lenze D, Hummel M, Gruber AD (2010) Metastatic canine mammary carcinomas can be identified by a gene expression profile that partly overlaps with human breast cancer profiles. BMC Cancer 10:618

Klopfleisch R, von Euler H, Sarli G, Pinho SS, Gartner F, Gruber AD (2011) Molecular carcinogenesis of CMT: news from an old disease. Vet Pathol 48:98–116

Mills SW, Musil KM, Davies JL, Hendrick S, Duncan C, Jackson ML, Kidney B, Philibert H, Wobeser BK, Simko E (2015) Prognostic value of histologic grading for feline mammary carcinoma: a retrospective survival analysis. Vet Pathol 52:238–249

Morris J (2013) Mammary tumours in the cat: size matters, so early intervention saves lives. J Feline Med Surg 15:391–400

Novosad CA, Bergman PJ, O'Brien MG, McKnight JA, Charney SC, Selting KA, Graham JC, Correa SS, Rosenberg MP, Gieger TL (2006) Retrospective evaluation of adjunctive doxorubicin for the treatment of feline mammary gland adenocarcinoma: 67 cases. J Am Anim Hosp Assoc 42:110–120

Pang LY, Cervantes-Arias A, Else RW, Argyle DJ (2011) Canine mammary cancer stem cells are radio- and chemoresistant and exhibit an epithelial-mesenchymal transition phenotype. Cancers (Basel) 3:1744–1762

Pang LY, Blacking TM, Else RW, Sherman A, Sang HM, Whitelaw BA, Hupp TR, Argyle DJ (2013) Feline mammary carcinoma stem cells are tumorigenic, radioresistant, chemoresistant and defective in activation of the ATM/p53 DNA damage pathway. Vet J 196:414–423

Pena L, De Andres PJ, Clemente M, Cuesta P, Perez-Alenza MD (2013) Prognostic value of histological grading in noninflammatory canine mammary carcinomas in a prospective study with two-year follow-up: relationship with clinical and histological characteristics. Vet Pathol 50:94–105

Perez-Alenza MD, Jimenez A, Nieto AI, Pena L (2004) First description of feline inflammatory mammary carcinoma: clinicopathological and immunohistochemical characteristics of three cases. Breast Cancer Res 6:R300–R307

Rivera P, von Euler H (2011) Molecular biological aspects on canine and human mammary tumors. Vet Pathol 48:132–146

Sleeckx N, de Rooster H, Veldhuis Kroeze EJ, Van Ginneken C, Van Brantegem L (2011) Canine mammary tumours, an overview. Reprod Domest Anim 46:1112–1131

Viste JR, Myers SL, Singh B, Simko E (2002) Feline mammary adenocarcinoma: tumor size as a prognostic indicator. Can Vet J 43:33–37

Yamagami T, Kobayashi T, Takahashi K, Sugiyama M (1996) Prognosis for canine malignant mammary tumors based on TNM and histologic classification. J Vet Med Sci 58:1079–1083

Hematopoietic Tumors

Manfred Henrich

R. Klopfleisch (ed.), *Veterinary Oncology*, DOI 10.1007/978-3-319-41124-8_6

6.1 Lymphatic Tumors

Lymphatic tumors in veterinary patients resemble non-Hodgkin's lymphomas in humans. They are a systemic neoplastic disease of lymphocytes or their precursors. They are a highly heterogeneous group of malignant tumors with varied biologic behavior due to their origin from different types of lymphocytes, despite the common terminology, which designates them all as lymphomas.

6

6.1.1 Canine Lymphomas

Box 6.1. Canine Lymphomas in Four Facts

1. Common tumors in dogs.
2. Many different types with different biologic behavior exist.
3. Clinical symptoms related to location and extend of tumor infiltration.
4. Chemotherapy is the treatment of choice.

Epidemiology and Pathogenesis

Lymphomas are one of the most common neoplasms in dogs. Middle-*aged* to older dogs are at a higher risk; intact females are at a lower risk. Boxers, bullmastiffs, bulldogs, basset hounds, St. Bernards, Scottish terriers, Airedale terriers, Bouvier des Flandres, Labrador retrievers, and Rottweilers are predisposed. There is also a predisposition for some *breeds* to develop distinct types of lymphomas, e.g., T-cell lymphomas in boxers, spitz, and Asian dog breeds and B-cell lymphomas in cocker spaniels and basset hounds. This breed predisposition implies that there are genetic factors for the development of lymphomas. An *infectious etiology* has not been confirmed in dogs so far. Exposure to herbicides, particularly 2,4-dichlorophenoxyacetic acid (a common weed killer and one of the ingredients in agent orange), is reported to increase the risk of lymphomas in dogs.

Molecular abnormalities found in canine lymphomas include chromosomal aberrations (trisomy 13 and 31, monosomy 14), aberrations in the expression of certain tumor suppressor genes and oncogenes (p53, Rb, N-ras, and p16), and telomerase activity.

Clinical Appearance

Clinical symptoms are variable and depend on location and size of the tumor or neoplastic infiltration of other organs. *Aggressive multicentric lymphoma* is the most common form followed by *gastrointestinal* (*alimentary*), *mediastinal*, *cutaneous, and extra-nodal.*

Lymphomas can arise anywhere outside the lymphatic system (primary extra-nodal forms), but the skin, central nervous system, eyes, heart, bladder, and nasal mucosa are the most frequently affected extra-nodal locations.

The first clinical sign of *multicentric lymphoma* is generalized, non-painful swelling of lymph nodes, often accompanied by enlargement of the liver and spleen (Fig. 6.1). Involvement of the bone marrow is common and is associated with leukopenia and/or anemia. Nonspecific symptoms like anorexia, diarrhea, vomiting, weight loss, and fever are observed in some patients.

Animals with *gastrointestinal lymphoma* may present with vomiting, anorexia, diarrhea, weight loss, icterus, and tenesmus. On physical examination, hepatosplenomegaly and mid-abdominal or cranial abdominal masses may be noted.

Dogs with *mediastinal lymphoma* have masses within the cranial mediastinum due to enlargement of either mediastinal lymph nodes or the

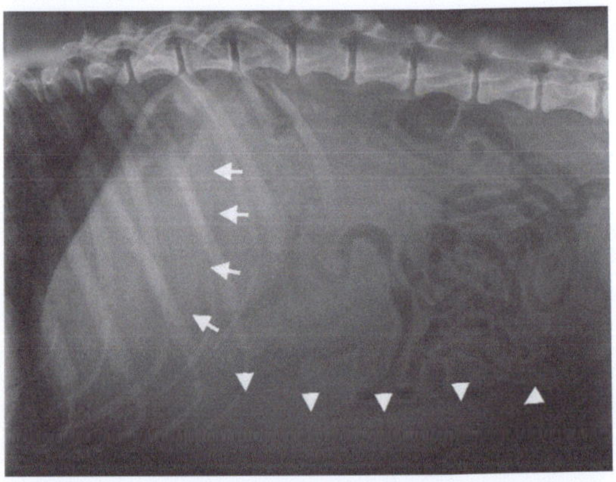

Fig. 6.1 Lateral abdominal radiograph of a dog with multicentric lymphoma. The spleen (*arrowheads*) is markedly enlarged, and there is a space-occupying mass (enlarged mesenteric lymph nodes) between the caudal margin of the stomach (*arrows*) and replacing the intestine caudally (Photo: with permission of Dr. Antje Hartmann, Vetsuisse Faculty University of Bern, Bern, Switzerland, and the Department of Veterinary Clinical Sciences, Clinic for Small Animals, Surgery, Justus-Liebig-University Giessen, Giessen, Germany)

thymus. Clinical signs are associated with the mass effect of the tumor compressing adjacent organs, most notably the lung, resulting in dyspnea. Tumor-associated pleural effusion may contribute to the compression of the lung. Compression/invasion of the cranial vena cava can cause head and forelimb edema. Stenosis of the esophagus due to the mass effect can result in regurgitation.

Cutaneous lymphoma represents 1 % of canine skin tumors and appears in two forms: epitheliotropic and non-epitheliotropic lymphoma. *Epitheliotropic lymphoma* (syn. mycosis fungoides) is a multifocal to widespread tumor that can be highly variable and mimic any inflammatory skin disease. Clinical forms can be principally subdivided into *exfoliative erythroderma* (generalized erythema, scaling, depigmentation, alopecia, and variable pruritus), *solitary or multiple nodules or plaques* (scaly, erythematous, and crusted swellings that may coalesce, erode, or ulcerate, but seldom regress), *ulcerative oral forms*, and *lymphomas with mucocutaneous localization*. *Non-epitheliotropic lymphoma* appears as single or multiple nodules in the dermis or subcutis. Any site of the body can be involved; however, oral forms are less common. The nodules may ulcerate. Swelling of the regional lymph nodes is common.

Paraneoplastic syndromes (i.e., signs caused by the neoplasia but unrelated to the mass effect of the tumor or its metastases) can occur with lymphoma. Anemia and hypercalcemia of malignancy are two of the most common paraneoplastic syndromes of lymphoma. The latter is due to the production of parathyroid hormone-related peptide (PTHrP) by the tumor cells. Clinically animals show polyuria and polydipsia, vomiting, and dehydration. In severe cases constipation, hypertension, twitching, weakness, shaking, depression, vomiting, bradycardia, stupor, and possibly coma and death can occur.

Staging

The WHO *clinical staging system* discussed in previous chapters can be used to stage lymphomas in veterinary medicine (Table 6.1).

Table 6.1 System for the staging of lymphomas in domestic animals according to the WHO, (Owen 1980)

Stage
1 Involvement limited to a single node or lymphoid tissue in a single organ
2 Involvement of many lymph nodes in a regional area (± tonsils)
3 Generalized lymph node involvement
4 Liver and/or spleen involvement (± stage 3)
5 Manifestation in the blood and involvement of the bone marrow and/or other organ systems (± stage 1–4)
Each stage is subclassified into:
(a) Without systemic signs
(b) With systemic signs

Classification

The classification of lymphomas is very complex and different classification schemes exist. Clinically lymphomas are classified by anatomical site (multicentric, gastrointestinal (alimentary), mediastinal, cutaneous, and extra-nodal). Other classification schemes include histological and immunohistologic features.

The WHO histological classification of hematopoietic tumors of domestic animals is widely used by veterinary pathologists and includes anatomic, histologic, and immunohistologic (B-cell or T-cell phenotype) criteria. However, some studies also use criteria of other classification schemes (e.g., Working Formulation (WF), updated Kiel classification); it is especially common to grade lymphomas as high, intermediate, and low grade. The accuracy of the WHO classification was confirmed in one study with 300 cases; another subsequent study associated WHO classification with survival, thereby combining the WHO criteria with a grading scheme (Table 6.2).

Cytology and Histopathology

Cytology of lymphomas (Figs. 6.2 and 6.3) is an appropriate and minimally invasive diagnostic procedure. It is diagnostically reliable in cases of high numbers of immature cells (>50 % of the cell population). However, accurate diagnosis by cytology may be impaired by the presence of low numbers of recognizable neoplastic cells (Fig. 6.4) and/or a high background of reactive lymphocytes (Fig. 6.5). The same is true for well-differentiated (small type) lymphomas, in which neoplastic cells do not differ morphologically from nonneoplastic lymphocytes.

Table 6.2 Grading of lymphomas classified according to the WHO (Valli et al. 2013)

B-cell lymphomas	T-cell lymphomas
Indolent B-cell lymphomas	*Indolent T-cell lymphomas*
Marginal zone lymphomas	T-zone lymphomas
Mantle cell lymphomas	*Low-grade T-cell lymphomas*
Follicular lymphomas	T-cell anaplastic large cell lymphomas
Low-grade B-cell lymphomas	Enteric T-cell lymphomas
Diffuse large B-cell lymphomas LO IB	Cutaneous T-cell lymphomas
Diffuse large B-cell lymphomas LO CB	*High-grade T-cell lymphomas*
T-cell-rich large B-cell lymphomas	Peripheral T-cell lymphomas
B-cell small lymphocytic lymphomas	T-cell lymphoblastic lymphomas
B-cell chronic lymphocytic leukemia	T-cell lymphoblastic lymphomas cleft
Diffuse intermediate B-cell lymphomas	
Intermediate-grade B-cell lymphomas	
Diffuse large B-cell lymphomas mid CB	
Diffuse large B-cell mid IB	
Plasmacytomas	
Lymphoid lymphomas	
High-grade B-cell lymphomas	
Diffuse large B-cell lymphomas HI CB	
Diffuse large B-cell lymphomas HI IB	
Burkitt-like lymphomas	
B-anaplastic large cell lymphomas	
B-cell lymphoblastic lymphomas	
B-cell lymphoblastic lymphomas cleft	
Plasmablastic lymphomas	

LO low mitotic rate, *mid* moderate mitotic rate, *HI* high mitotic rate, *IB* immunoblastic, *CB* centroblastic

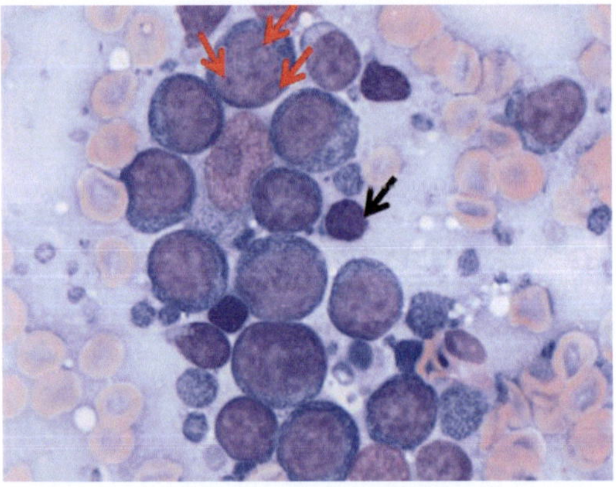

Fig. 6.2 Cytology, lymphoma, lymph node, dog, May-Grünwald-Giemsa 1000×. In cytological specimens, the diagnosis of lymphoma is based on the presence of >50 % lymphatic blasts. In this dog, approximately 80 % lymphatic blasts and only rare small mature lymphocytes (*black arrow*) are seen. The lymphatic blasts are medium sized (approximately 2× the diameter of an erythrocyte) and possess eccentrically located nuclei, a finely stippled chromatin with several marginal, prominent nucleoli (*red arrow*) and moderate amounts of basophilic cytoplasm. The cellular morphology is typical for a polymorphic centroblastic B-cell lymphoma (Photo: with permission of Dr. N. Bauer, Faculty of Veterinary Medicine, Justus-Liebig-University Giessen, Giessen, Germany)

Growth patterns and associated architectural alterations can be assessed with *histological examination* of affected tissues. The abovementioned classification requires histologic examination in conjunction with immunohistochemistry (for the assessment of the lineage, i.e., B- or T-cell).

The morphology of neoplastic lymphocytes differs according to the type of lymphoma. Cells of undifferentiated lymphomas resemble lymphoblasts. Cells of well-differentiated (small cell) lymphomas may be undistinguishable from non-neoplastic lymphocytes. Lymphomas often show a diffuse, sheetlike infiltration of the tissue with effacement of the original architecture. However, exceptions with specific growth patterns exist, e.g., follicular lymphomas.

Assessment of Clonality

In some cases, neoplastic lymphocytic proliferation cannot be distinguished from reactive proliferation by cytology or histology alone. In these cases, assessing the clonality of the lymphocytes by *clonality assays* can aid in establishing a final diagnosis. Neoplastic lymphocytes in lymphomas originate from a single transformed cell. The neoplastic

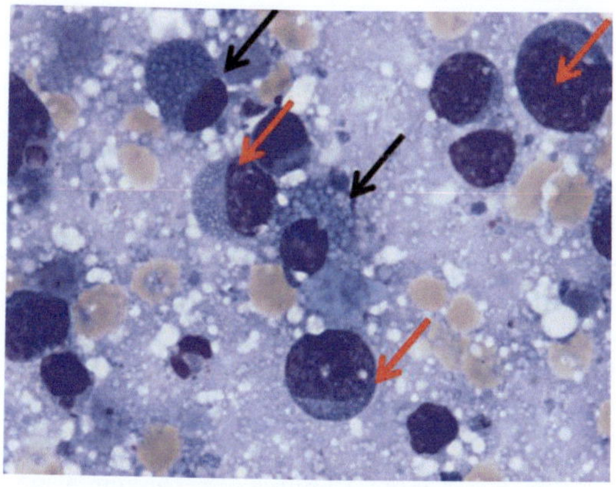

Fig. 6.3 Cytology, B-cell lymphoma with Mott cell differentiation, lymph node, dog, May-Grünwald-Giemsa 1000×. There are many medium-sized to large lymphatic blasts (of a diameter ranging between 2 and 3 red blood cells, *red arrow*) with eccentrically located slightly indented nuclei, reticular chromatin pattern, and small to moderate amounts of basophilic cytoplasm containing rare to many small clear vacuoles. The presence of several mature plasma cells with multiple intracytoplasmic vacuoles (Mott cells, *black arrow*) is indicative of a B-cell lymphoma with Mott cell differentiation as rarely described in dogs and cats. Histopathology confirmed the presence of immunoglobulin G (IgG)-positive cells (Photo: with permission of Dr. N. Bauer, Faculty of Veterinary Medicine, Justus-Liebig-University Giessen, Giessen, Germany)

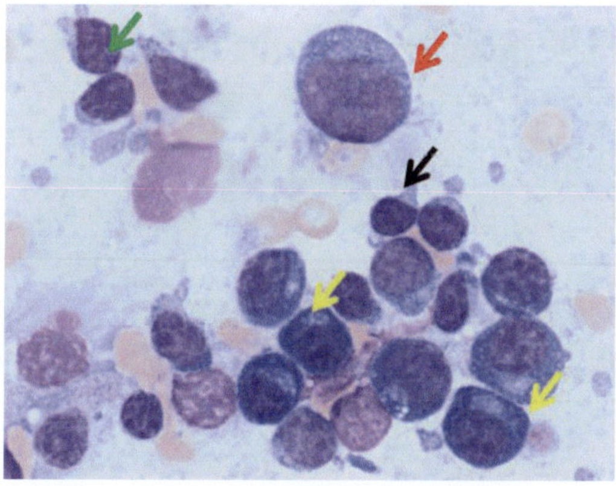

Fig. 6.4 Cytology, reactive hyperplasia, lymph node in a dog with leishmaniasis, May-Grünwald-Giemsa 1000×. There is a mixed cellular population consisting of many plasma cells (*yellow arrow*) as well as several small mature (*black arrow*) and medium-sized (*green arrow*) lymphocytes. Few lymphatic blasts (*red arrow*) are also present. In this case, underlying high-grade lymphoma characterized by a percentage of lymphatic blasts exceeding 50 % is very unlikely, although very early stages cannot be entirely ruled out. However, such early cases would also be difficult to detect with histopathology (Photo: with permission of Dr. N. Bauer, Faculty of Veterinary Medicine, Justus-Liebig-University Giessen, Giessen, Germany)

progeny is therefore genetically monoclonal. In contrast, reactive lymphocytes are a heterogeneous population of cells recruited to the focus of inflammation and are consequently polyclonal in nature.

Lymphocytes rearrange their antigen receptor genes during their development. Subsequently each cell carries a unique gene sequence coding for an unique antigen receptor. A *PCR for antigen receptor rearrangement* (*PARR*) utilizes this variation in the genome to differentiate a monoclonal population (identical sequence in each neoplastic cell) from a polyclonal population (mixture of difference sequences in nonneoplastic cells). The PARR is not sensitive or specific enough to be suitable as a stand-alone diagnosis of lymphomas. Results must be interpreted in the context of histology, immunohistochemistry, and clinical data. Furthermore, clonality assays cannot replace immunohistochemistry/-cytology for the determination of the lineage (B- or T-cell).

Therapy

Chemotherapy using variations of "CHOP" combination protocols (cyclophosphamide, doxorubicin [=*h*ydroxydaunorubicin], vincristine [=Oncovin], prednisone) is the preferred therapy for canine lymphoma. A modified *Madison Wisconsin* protocol, a CHOP-based protocol, is widely used by veterinary oncologists. The median overall survival times (OST) of dogs with multicentric lymphomas treated with CHOP-based protocols are about 8–12 months; unfortunately less than 25 % of these dogs survive longer than 2 years.

Surgery may be beneficial in solitary forms of lymphomas if multicentric involvement can be ruled out.

Radiation therapy may also be feasible for solitary forms of lymphoma or as palliative therapy and/or to deplete the bone marrow for bone marrow or stem cell transplantation.

Prognostic Factors and Markers

Per definition, lymphomas are malignant. However, due to the variety of lymphoma types, prognosis of the disease is highly variable with very aggressive forms on one side of the spectrum and very slow progressive (indolent) forms on the other side.

Overall, *T-cell lymphomas* are reported to have shorter survival times and remissions. Furthermore, *WHO substage b* (with clinical signs) is also associated with poorer outcomes. *Grading* the WHO stages and associating them with survival time allow us to associate histology with prognosis.

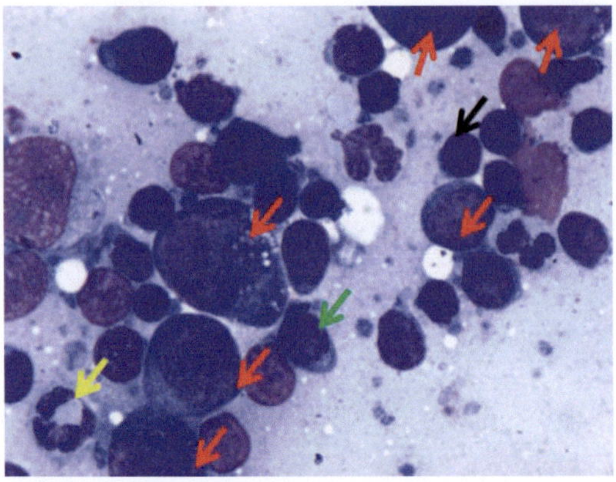

Fig. 6.5 Cytology, follicular hyperplasia, abdominal lymph node, 8-month-old Maine Coon cat, May-Grünwald-Giemsa 1000×. There are approximately 40 % pleomorphic, medium-sized to large lymphatic blasts (*red arrow*) interspersed with several small mature (*black arrow*) and medium-sized (*green arrow*) lymphocytes. Few nondegenerate neutrophils (*yellow arrow*) are also present. In this case, reactive hyperplasia with a markedly increased amount of lymphatic blasts cannot be differentiated from high-grade lymphoma in an early stage as the percentage of lymphatic blasts is close to 50 %, the threshold to diagnose lymphoma. Histopathology is required to differentiate between both diagnoses. In this case, it revealed follicular hyperplasia (Photo: with permission of Dr. N. Bauer, Faculty of Veterinary Medicine, Justus-Liebig-University Giessen, Giessen, Germany)

High-grade lymphomas are associated with higher mortality rates than intermediate- or low-grade lymphomas. Another factor with influence on prognosis is *anatomical site* (diffuse lymphomas of the skin or gastrointestinal tract, hepatosplenic lymphomas, and lymphomas of the central nervous system are associated with poorer prognosis). Furthermore, the *frequency of AgNORs* (argyrophilic nucleolar organizer regions) on immunohistochemistry as well as the *potential doubling time* (*Tpot*) can be used as predictors of outcome in dogs.

▪ Current Trends in Research

The aim of many studies is to improve the diagnosis, prognosis, and therapy of canine lymphomas. Identification of factors associated with survival and response to therapy can result in a more accurate prognosis. New therapeutic approaches and agents are tested in lymphoma cell lines and in clinical trials.

▪ Suggested Reading

(Mortier et al. 2012; Richards and Suter 2015; Marconato et al. 2013; Valli et al. 2013; Valli et al. 2011; Gross et al. 2008)

6.1.2 Canine Lymphocytic Leukemia

Lymphocytic leukemia is defined as a lymphoid neoplasm with extensive involvement of the bone marrow that usually (though it does not have to) goes along with large numbers of *neoplastic cells in the peripheral blood*. Leukemias without detectable tumor cells in the peripheral blood are termed "aleukemic leukemias." The distinction between leukemia and stage 5 lymphomas is subjective.

Box 6.2. Canine Lymphocytic Leukemia in Six Facts

1. A lymphoid neoplasm with extensive bone marrow involvement.
2. Neoplastic lymphocytes often numerous in peripheral blood.
3. Aleukemic leukemias (without neoplastic cells in peripheral blood) exist.
4. Acute forms are very aggressive with poor prognosis.
5. Chronic forms are very slow progressive.
6. Chemotherapy is the treatment of choice.

▪ Epidemiology and Pathogenesis

Lymphocytic leukemia affects many different *breeds*, although a prevalence of large and giant breeds (e.g., German shepherds and retrievers) is reported. Mean *age* at diagnosis is usually around 7–10 years. There is no *sex predisposition* to the disease or certain subtypes. The etiology and exact pathogenesis, as with canine lymphomas, remain unclear. Genetic factors likely contribute to the development of the disease.

▪ Clinical Appearance

Overt clinical signs are dependent on the type of leukemia.

Animals with *chronic lymphocytic leukemia* (*CLL*) usually present with mild symptoms (lethargy, loss of appetite, vomitus, diarrhea, lameness, and slightly enlarged lymph nodes and spleen) or no symptoms. White blood count usually reveals a marked lymphocytosis of mature lymphocytes that may appear morphologically normal but can be functionally abnormal. Concurrent abnormalities include mild anemia, thrombocytopenia, and neutropenia. Severity of symptoms and hematological abnormalities may increase over the course of the disease. Monoclonal gammopathy, hemolytic anemia, pure red cell aplasia, and in some cases hypercalcemia are the paraneoplastic syndromes associated with CLL.

Animals with *acute lymphoblastic leukemia* (*ALL*) usually have more pronounced clinical signs with lymphadenopathy, hepato- and splenomegaly, anorexia, weight loss, and lethargy. Massive infiltration and destruction of the bone marrow lead to myelosuppression and eventually myelophthisis, resulting in severe anemia, thrombocytopenia, and neutropenia. Infiltration of extramedullary sites can cause symptoms related to the affected organ or tissue.

Cytology and Histopathology

Cytological examination of the bone marrow (Fig. 6.6) and peripheral blood (Fig. 6.7) can be helpful in diagnosing lymphocytic leukemia. Bone marrow aspirates may be redundant and thus avoided if cytology of peripheral blood shows marked lymphocytosis and differential diagnoses of nonneoplastic lymphocytosis (e.g., chronic ehrlichiosis, IL-2 administration, post-vaccine lymphocytosis) can be ruled out (e.g., by PARR analysis, predominance of one phenotype, or atypical lymphocytes). However, the characteristic feature of lymphocytic leukemia is the infiltration of the bone marrow by neoplastic cells. In *ALL* lymphoblasts are detectable in aspirates in high numbers, whereas in *CLL* mature cells predominate.

Histopathology of bone marrow core biopsies is especially useful if aspiration of the bone marrow is not diagnostic. Immunohistochemistry is useful for differentiating ALL from acute myeloid leukemia in cases of premature cells on histopathology.

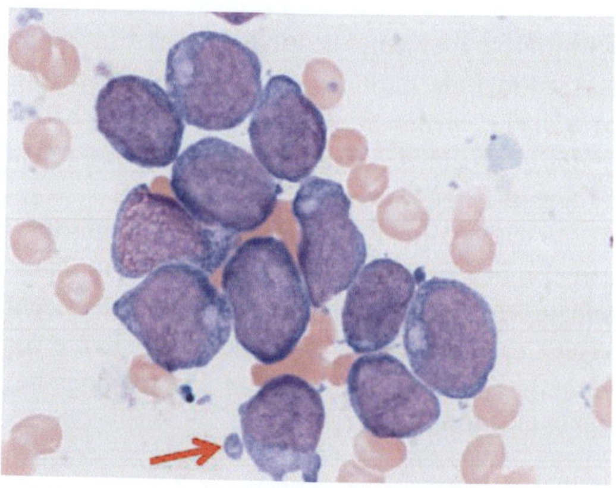

Fig. 6.6 Cytology, acute lymphocytic leukemia, subleukemic stage, bone marrow aspirate, dog, May-Grünwald-Giemsa 1000×. The dog was presented with a pancytopenia and rare lymphatic blasts in the peripheral blood. The bone marrow aspirate was highly cellular, and normal hematopoietic precursor cells are replaced by large lymphoblasts with a diameter of >2.5 erythrocytes. They possess eccentrically located slightly indented nuclei, a finely stippled chromatin pattern, and moderate amounts of a lightly basophilic cytoplasm with clear perinuclear halo. Typical for lymphatic cells is the presence of cytoplasmic fragments (*red arrow*) (Photo: with permission of Dr. N. Bauer, Faculty of Veterinary Medicine, Justus-Liebig-University Giessen, Giessen, Germany)

Therapy

Chlorambucil is the *chemotherapy* agent of choice for the treatment of *CLL*. Whether or not therapy is indicated depends on the clinical signs and hematologic changes. Surveillance (clinical examination, complete blood count) is recommended during the indolent phase instead of medication. Due to the aggressive nature of *ALL*, the disease requires aggressive chemotherapy (CHOP-based protocols) and/or bone marrow or stem cell transplantation (currently rarely applied in veterinary medicine).

Prognostic Factors and Markers

The most important prognostic factor is the type of leukemia. *CLL* usually progresses slowly, and on average veterinary patients survive 1–3 years

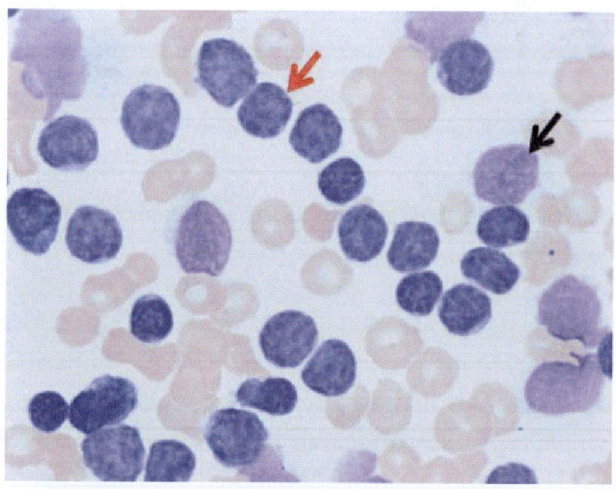

Fig. 6.7 Cytology, chronic lymphocytic leukemia, blood smear, dog, May-Grünwald-Giemsa 1000×. There is a severe leukocytosis based on a severe lymphocytosis. The lymphocytes are mainly small and mature (*red arrow*). The presence of several large lymphocytes, however, indicates the progression into a more accelerated phase of proliferation. Several naked nuclei (*black arrow*) are also present mainly due to the relatively high fragility of lymphatic cells (Photo: with permission of Dr. N. Bauer, Faculty of Veterinary Medicine, Justus-Liebig-University Giessen, Giessen, Germany)

with a good quality of life. Factors associated with longer survival times are T-cell phenotype, low lymphocyte numbers in the peripheral blood, older age, and absence of anemia. Veterinary patients with *ALL* have a very poor prognosis even with therapy; survival times range from days to about 8 months.

- **Suggested Reading**

(Adam et al. 2009; Hodgkins et al. 1980; Leifer and Matus 1986; Couto 1985; Matus et al. 1983; Morris et al. 1993)

6.1.3 Feline Lymphomas

Box 6.3. Feline Lymphomas in Six Facts

1. Common tumors in cats.
2. Can be caused by the feline leukemia virus (FeLV).
3. After the 1980s (FeLV eradication), the number of FeLV-positive lymphomas decreased.
4. Many different types with different biologic behavior exist.
5. Clinical symptoms related to location and extent of tumor infiltration.
6. Chemotherapy is the treatment of choice.

- **Epidemiology and Pathogenesis**

Hematopoietic tumors represent up to 50 % of cancers diagnosed in cats. Of these 50–90 % are lymphomas.

The signalment and characteristics of feline lymphomas have changed with the eradication and vaccination programs for feline leukemia virus (FeLV) in the early 1980s. *FeLV-associated lymphomas* often appeared in young cats (median *age* 4–6 years). These patients often showed mediastinal forms of the disease. The frequency of lymphomas has increased over the years despite the fact that the number of FeLV-associated lymphomas decreased with the eradication of FeLV infections. A change in the age of affected patients and the anatomical location of lesions are notable. Veterinary patients with *non-FeLV-associated lymphomas* are now older (median age 9.5 years), and gastrointestinal (primarily intestinal) lymphomas now dominate. There is a *breed* predisposition for Siamese and Oriental cats; a sex predisposition is not confirmed.

FeLV infection is a high risk factor for the development of lymphomas. About 55–70 % of lymphomas were positive for FeLV before the introduction of FeLV vaccines. The integration of FeLV provirus into the lymphocyte's DNA can trigger the development of the neoplasia. *FeLV-associated lymphomas* are more often T-cell origin neoplasias with mediastinal (thymic) or multicentric lesions and involvement of peripheral lymph nodes.

Feline immunodeficiency virus (FIV) infection also increases the risk of developing lymphoma. As the virus was not frequently found within tumor tissues, an indirect effect (immunosuppression) is assumed.

Chronic inflammation is another proposed risk factor for the development of lymphoma in cats. Some studies have found an association between inflammatory bowel disease and the development of lymphomas, but this finding is not supported in all studies.

- **Classification**

Clinically feline lymphoma can be *classified by anatomical site*. The anatomical classification within the literature is inconsistent, but many studies include *multicentric, gastrointestinal (alimentary), mediastinal (thymic), and extranodal/unclassified forms* (e.g., nasal, renal, cutaneous, CNS lymphomas).

As with canine lymphomas, feline lymphomas can also be *classified by histology and immunohistology*. However, a combination of the recent WHO classification with a grading scheme for feline lymphoma similar to the one for dogs has not yet been published.

- **Clinical Appearance**

The clinical signs are associated with the type of lymphoma and affected anatomic sites.

Cats with *multicentric lymphomas* may present with single enlarged peripheral lymph nodes or nodes of a lymph region. Further clinical signs are associated with the involved lymph centers and organs.

Patients with *gastrointestinal forms* present with corresponding signs (e.g., weight loss, vomiting, diarrhea, and anorexia). Abdominal masses or thickened intestinal walls (◻ Fig. 6.8) can

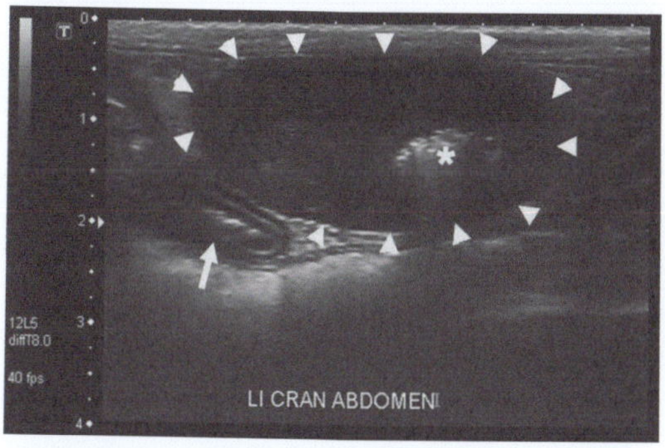

Fig. 6.8 Sonographic picture of a cat with intestinal lymphoma. Note the enlarged intestinal loop (*arrowheads*) with loss of the typical intestinal wall layers (as seen in the adjacent loop (*arrow*)). The mural striation of the intestinal wall is replaced by a hypoechoic circumferential wall thickening. The lumen (*) contains gas, which results in a hyperechoic signal (Photo: with permission of Dr. Antje Hartmann, Vetsuisse Faculty University of Bern, Bern, Switzerland, and the Department of Veterinary Clinical Sciences, Clinic for Small Animals, Surgery, Justus-Liebig-University Giessen, Giessen, Germany)

often be palpated. Progression depends on the type of lymphoma. Lymphocytic forms progress more slowly (months) than lymphoblastic forms (days or weeks).

Mediastinal forms are associated with respiratory signs (tachypnea, dyspnea), non-compressible cranial thorax, and often pleural effusion containing neoplastic cells.

Cats with *nasal lymphomas* present with symptoms related to the upper respiratory tract (e.g., nasal discharge, upper respiratory noise, ocular discharge, epistaxis). In extreme cases they can present with facial deformation.

Renal lymphoma is associated with signs of renal failure (polyuria/polydipsia, loss of appetite, weight loss). Irregular, often bilateral, enlargement of the kidneys is palpable (Fig. 6.9).

Cutaneous lymphomas represent ~3 % of feline skin tumors and appear in two forms: epitheliotropic and non-epitheliotropic lymphomas. *Non-epitheliotropic lymphoma* is the most common form of cutaneous lymphoma in cats. It appears as single or multiple nodules in the dermis or subcutis. Any site of the body can be involved. The oral mucosa is less commonly affected. The nodules may ulcerate, and swelling of the regional lymph nodes is common. *Epitheliotropic lymphomas* are similar to those described above for the dog.

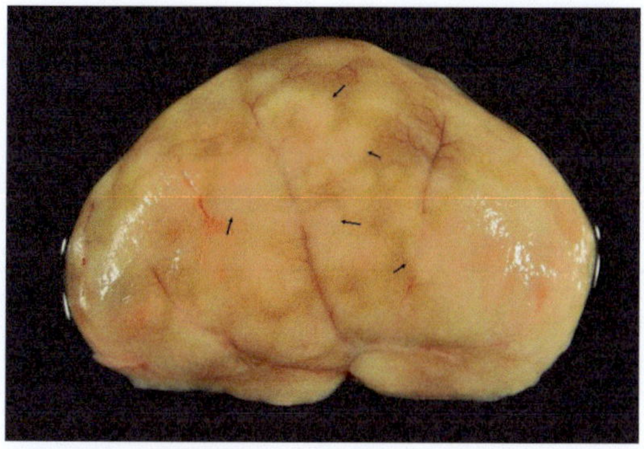

Fig. 6.9 The kidney of a cat with renal lymphoma. The tumor shows a multifocal to coalescing infiltration (*arrows*) of the renal parenchyma

Cats with *lymphomas of the CNS* show signs associated with the location within the CNS (intracranial, spinal) including seizures, behavioral changes, ataxia, paresis or paralysis, blindness, and many more, often combined with systemic signs like anorexia and lethargy.

Paraneoplastic syndromes (i.e., signs caused by the neoplasia but unrelated to the mass effect of the tumor or its metastases) can occur in cats with lymphomas, but they are less frequent than in dogs. Hypercalcemia of malignancy due to the production of parathyroid hormone-related peptide (PTHrP) can lead to anorexia, polyuria and polydipsia, weight loss, lethargy, and weakness.

Staging

The WHO clinical staging system can be used for staging feline lymphoma (see Table 6.1), but a staging system proposed by (Mooney and Hayes 1986) is used as well (see Table 6.3).

Cytology and Histopathology

Cytology is a minimally invasive procedure that can be diagnostic for lymphoma if an adequate number (>50 % of the cell population) of clearly neoplastic cells can be identified (Fig. 6.10). However, accurate diagnosis by cytology may be impaired by the presence of low numbers of recognizable neoplastic cells and/or a high background of reactive lymphocytes. The same is true for well-differentiated (small cell) lymphomas, in which neoplastic cells do not differ morphologically from nonneoplastic lymphocytes.

Histopathology may face the same problems, but it has the advantage of showing growth patterns and architectural alterations caused by the growth and

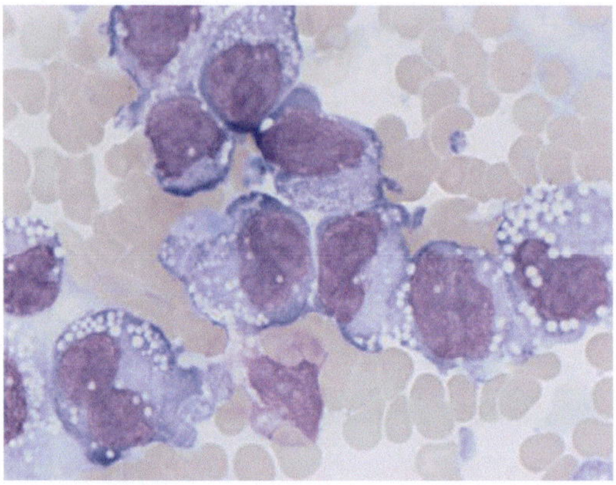

Fig. 6.10 Cytology, lymphoma, lymph node, cat, May-Grünwald-Giemsa 1000×. In cytological specimens, the diagnosis of lymphoma is based on the presence of >50 % lymphatic blasts. In this cat, almost 100 % lymphatic blasts are seen. The lymphatic blasts are large (approximately >2.5× the diameter of an erythrocyte) and possess eccentrically located irregular to indented nuclei, a reticular to clumped chromatin, indistinct nucleoli, and large amounts of lightly basophilic cytoplasm containing several clear vacuoles. Rarely, binuclear cells (*bottom left*) are seen. The cellular morphology is typical for an anaplastic T-cell lymphoma (Photo: with permission of Dr. N. Bauer, Faculty of Veterinary Medicine, Justus-Liebig-University Giessen, Giessen, Germany)

infiltration of the tumor cells. Due to the high variability of the different types of lymphomas, neoplastic lymphocytes differ considerably, and morphological identification can be difficult. Cells of well-differentiated (small cell) lymphomas show high similarity with nonneoplastic lymphocytes, but less differentiated lymphomas exist as well. Cells of these tumors resemble lymphoblasts. The histologic growth pattern is often a diffuse, sheetlike infiltration with effacement of the original architecture. However, some lymphomas, e.g., follicular lymphomas, show a different growth pattern.

Assessment of Clonality

▶ See Sect. 6.1.1.

Therapy

Chemotherapy is the treatment of choice for feline lymphoma due to their systemic character. As with canine lymphomas, modifications of the CHOP protocol (*c*yclophosphamide, doxorubicin [= *h*ydroxydaunorubicin], vincristine [= Oncovin], *p*rednisone) are used. These protocols are suitable to treat all lymphomas except the well-differentiated types. Cats do not respond to treatment as well as dogs (response rates of 50–80 % with median remission and survival durations of 4–6 months), but they often suffer fewer side effects of the therapy.

Radiation therapy is useful for solitary forms. A high rate of complete remissions can be achieved with radiation therapy in feline nasal lymphoma.

Table 6.3 System for the staging of feline lymphomas according to (Mooney and Hayes 1986)

Stage 1
Single tumor (extra-nodal) or single anatomic site (nodal)
Includes primary intrathoracic tumors
Stage 2
Single tumor (extra-nodal) with regional lymph node involvement
Two or more nodes on same side of the diaphragm
Two extra-nodal tumors ± regional lymph node involvement on same side of the diaphragm
Resectable primary gastrointestinal tumor ± involvement of associated mesenteric lymph node
Stage 3
Two extra-nodal tumors on opposite sides of the diaphragm
Two or more nodes on opposite sides of the diaphragm
All extensive primary non-resectable intra-abdominal disease All paraspinal and epidural tumors, regardless of other tumor sites
Stage 4
Stages 1, 2, or 3 with involvement of the spleen and/or liver
Stage 5
Stages 1, 2, 3, or 4 with initial involvement of the CNS or bone marrow or both

Prognostic Factors and Markers

Prognosis depends on the *type and anatomical location* of the lymphomas in cats. Gastrointestinal lymphoma has a significantly shorter survival time than mediastinal and nasal lymphoma. As a grading scheme correlated with the WHO classification scheme is lacking, prognosis regarding the *cell type* is based on the cellular assessment of the Kiel classification. High-grade lymphomas have significantly shorter survival times than low-grade lymphomas. Unlike in the dog, a prognostic value of the *immunophenotype* (i.e., B- or T-cell lymphomas) has *not been confirmed.*

Current Trends in Research

Many of the recently published studies aim to improve diagnosis, therapy, and prognosis of feline lymphoma. Evaluating different approaches or therapeutic agents may help to improve therapeutic strategies and increase the success of lymphoma treatment.

Suggested Reading

(Hardy 1981; Vail et al. 1998; Louwerens et al. 2005; Carreras et al. 2003; Ragaini et al. 2003; Hart et al. 1994)

6.1.4 Feline Lymphocytic Leukemia

Lymphocytic leukemias are neoplastic lymphoid proliferations with extensive involvement of the bone marrow. Usually, large numbers of neoplastic cells can be found in the peripheral blood; these are absent in aleukemic leukemia. It can be difficult in some cases and virtually impossible in others to differentiate between leukemia and stage 5 lymphoma.

Box 6.4. Feline Lymphocytic Leukemia in Seven Facts

1. A lymphoid neoplasm with extensive bone marrow involvement.
2. Neoplastic lymphocytes often numerous in peripheral blood.
3. Aleukemic leukemias (without neoplastic cells in peripheral blood) exist.
4. Acute forms are very aggressive with poor prognosis and often associated with feline leukemia virus (FeLV) infections.
5. With the declining incidence of FeLV infections, the incidence of feline leukemia is also declining.
6. Chronic forms are very slow progressive.
7. Chemotherapy is the treatment of choice.

Epidemiology and Pathogenesis

During the FeLV era, *acute lymphocytic leukemia (ALL)* was the most common type of leukemia seen in cats. However, after the FeLV eradication and vaccination programs in the 1980s, this tumor type is seldom encountered, and the recent literature regarding the disease is sparse. The majority of cats with ALL are *FeLV positive*, and the disease affects young cats (*age* less than 4 years).

Chronic lymphocytic leukemia (CLL) is only rarely diagnosed in cats. The current incidence of the disease in cats is unknown. Cats with CLL are older (median *age* 12.5 years) and these tumors are usually *FeLV negative*. There is no *sex* predisposition for lymphocytic leukemia.

Clinical Appearance

Cats with *ALL* usually present in good condition with an acute onset of nonspecific signs like lethargy, anorexia, vomitus, diarrhea, weight loss, and polyuria/polydipsia.

CLL is a neoplasia with indolent (slow progressive) behavior. If symptomatic at all, cats with CLL present with lethargy, reduced appetite, and weight loss. In many cases, an enlarged spleen can be palpated.

Cytology and Histopathology

Cytological examination of the bone marrow and peripheral blood (Fig. 6.11) can be helpful in diagnosing lymphocytic leukemia. Bone marrow aspirates may be redundant and thus avoided if cytology of peripheral blood shows marked lymphocytosis and differential diagnoses of nonneoplastic lymphocytosis (e.g., chronic ehrlichiosis, IL-2 administration, postvaccine lymphocytosis) can be ruled out (e.g., by PARR analysis, predominance of one phenotype, or atypical lymphocytes). However, the characteristic feature of lymphocytic leukemia is the infiltration of the bone marrow by neoplastic cells. In *ALL* lymphoblasts are detectable in aspirates in high numbers, whereas in *CLL* mature cells predominate.

Histopathology of bone marrow core biopsies is especially useful if aspiration of the bone marrow is not diagnostic. Immunohistochemistry is useful for differentiating ALL from acute myeloid leukemia in cases of premature cells on histopathology.

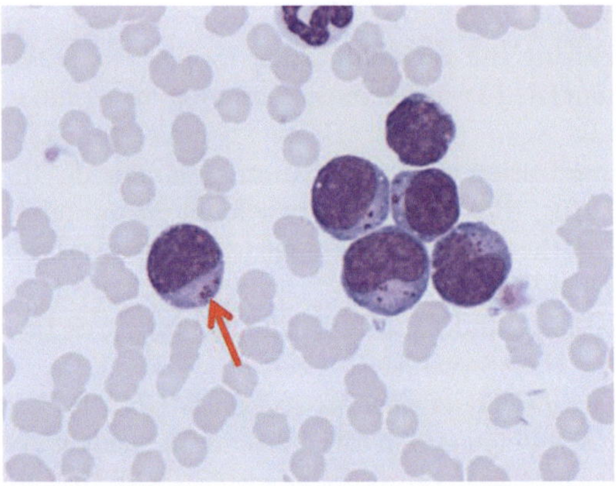

Fig. 6.11 Cytology, acute lymphoblastic leukemia involving large granular lymphocytes (LGL), blood smear, cat, May-Grünwald-Giemsa 1000×. There are many large lymphocytes with round to indented nuclei, finely stippled chromatin pattern, mainly indistinct nucleoli, and several perinuclear azurophilic granules (*red arrow*). Differential diagnosis is LGL lymphoma, which is in the cat mainly arising from the gastrointestinal tract. Involvement of the spleen leads to a leukemic stage (Photo: with permission of Dr. N. Bauer, Faculty of Veterinary Medicine, Justus-Liebig-University Giessen, Giessen, Germany)

■ Therapy

Response to *chemotherapy* is poor in cats with *ALL*. A combination of vincristine and prednisone has been shown to result in complete remission in 27 % of treated cats. Therapy of *CLL* with chlorambucil and prednisone results in a median survival of about 14 months with 88 % percent of the cats achieving complete or partial remission.

■ Prognostic Factors and Markers

As in dogs, the type of leukemia strongly influences the prognosis. Patients with *ALL* have a very poor prognosis with short survival times. Patients with *CLL* have a better prognosis and longer survival time due to the indolent nature of CLL.

■ Suggested Reading

Campbell et al. (2013), Cotter (1983)

6.2 Plasma Cell Tumors of Cats and Dogs

The following plasma cells tumors are listed in the WHO classification of hematopoietic tumors of domestic animals:

- Indolent plasmacytomas
- Anaplastic plasmacytomas
- Plasma cell myelomas (multiple myelomas)

The term *myeloma-related disorders* (*MRD*) can be used to describe all neoplasias of plasma cells or immunoglobulin-secreting B-lymphocyte precursors. Besides the tumors described in the WHO classification, MRD also includes:

- Solitary plasmacytomas of the bone
- Macroglobulinemia
- Immunoglobulin-secreting lymphomas
- Myeloma cell leukemia

The following chapter will concentrate on plasma cell myelomas and plasmacytomas as they are the most common forms of plasma cell tumors.

6.2.1 Plasma Cell Myelomas (Multiple Myelomas) of Cats and Dogs

Plasma cell myelomas are characterized by a systemic proliferation of neoplastic plasma cells. Multiple bone marrow sites, often within the axial skeleton, are usually affected (hence the name "multiple myelomas").

Box 6.5. Plasma Cell Myelomas in Five Facts

1. Systemic proliferation of neoplastic plasma cells often in multiple bone marrow sites.
2. Infiltration of the bone marrow leads to osteolytic lesions.
3. Primarily found in older dogs, less in other species.
4. Clinical signs attributed to bone involvement and circulating (components of) immunoglobulin.
5. Chemotherapy is the treatment of choice.

■ Epidemiology and Pathogenesis

Plasma cell myeloma is a malignant disease of older dogs (*age* 8–9 years). Cats and other domestic animals are rarely affected; if the disease appears in other species, they are also usually older patients. A *sex* predisposition has not been confirmed. The etiology of the disease is unknown. Chronic immune stimulation (*chronic inflammation*), exposure to carcinogens, and *breed* predispositions (German shepherd dogs are overrepresented in one study) have been suggested to contribute to the development of the disease.

▪ Clinical Appearance

Dogs with plasma cell myelomas often present with *lameness*. Multifocal osteolytic lesions can be identified radiographically (◘ Fig. 6.12).

In *cats*, lameness is reported in variable percentages, and this species often shows *nonspecific signs* like weight loss, reduced appetite, vomiting, and diarrhea. Multiple extramedullary manifestations (particular in the spleen, liver, and lymph nodes) have been found in a considerable number of cases. Sometimes, these cases lack bone marrow involvement and are considered as *aggressive, multicentric, non-cutaneous, extramedullary plasmacytomas*. However, the distinction from plasma cell myelomas is blurred, and this tumor is often subsumed under the plasma cell myelomas.

The malignant plasma cells often produce large quantities of a single type or part of immunoglobulin (*M component*). Therefore, beside clinical signs due to infiltration of neoplastic cells into the bone and organs, clinical signs are also due to high amounts of circulating M component and its excretion or storage. Frequent clinical signs include bleeding diathesis (e.g., as epistaxis, retinal bleeding), hyperviscosity syndrome, renal failure, immunodeficiencies, cardiac failure, and CNS signs.

Additional *clinical pathology findings* include anemia, hypoalbuminemia, proteinuria (including excretion of immunoglobulin light chain proteins, so-called Bence Jones proteins), hypercalcemia, and azotemia.

▪ Cytology and Histopathology

Bone marrow aspiration (◘ Fig. 6.13) or *bone marrow core biopsies* are required for definitive diagnosis. In plasma cell myelomas the number of plasma cells in the marrow exceeds the normal *number of plasma cells* (<5 %). A cutoff level of 20 % plasma cells in the sample is recommended (>10 % in the cat, if cells are atypical). Due to the uneven distribution of the neoplastic foci, multiple aspirates or biopsies might be necessary. In most cases, neoplastic cells are uniformly shaped with regular nuclei, occasional binucleated cells, and abundant cytoplasm. Mitotic rate is below the mitotic rate of the surrounding bone marrow. In forms that are more aggressive, the cells show increasing anisocytosis and anisokaryosis with high mitotic rates.

Benign bone marrow plasmacytosis is the main *differential diagnosis* for plasma cell myelomas; benign plasmacytosis tends to have less cytoplasmic volume, but definitive diagnosis should be based on two or more of the typical findings, including osteolysis, atypical plasmacytosis, monoclonal gammopathy, and/or proteinuria (Bence Jones proteins).

▪ Therapy

The aim of treatment for myeloma is to reduce the tumor cell mass and to treat secondary effects of the tumor and its secreted proteins.

Chemotherapy (melphalan in combination with prednisone) is effective in dogs to reduce the number of tumor cells and the amount of circulating M component. Nevertheless, complete elimination is rare and relapses are common. *Mean survival time* of dogs is 1.5 years. Cats respond less

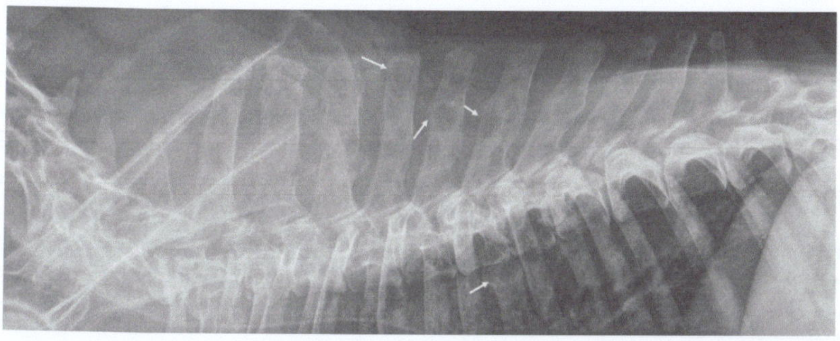

◘ **Fig. 6.12** Lateral radiograph of the thoracic spine of a dog with plasma cell myeloma. Within the vertebral bodies, dorsal spinous processes and the ribs are multiple foci of osteolysis (*arrows*). The "punched out" appearance of the lesions are typical for plasma cell myelomas (Photo: with permission of Dr. Antje Hartmann, Vetsuisse Faculty University of Bern, Bern, Switzerland, and the Department of Veterinary Clinical Sciences, Clinic for Small Animals, Surgery, Justus-Liebig-University Giessen, Giessen, Germany)

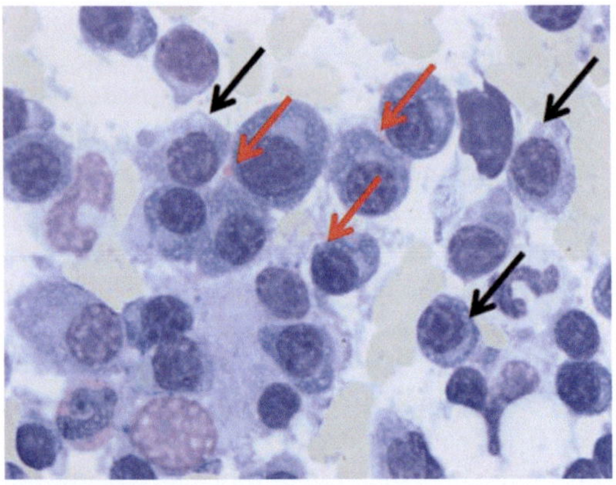

Fig. 6.13 Cytology, plasma cell myeloma, bone marrow aspirate, dog, May-Grünwald-Giemsa 1000x. Note the dominance of plasma cells with atypical lightly basophilic vacuolar cytoplasm (*black arrow*). Some plasma cells show eosinophilic material associated with the cellular border (so-called flame cells or flaming plasma cell, *red arrow*) indicative of an IgA-producing multiple myeloma (Photo: with permission of Dr. N. Bauer, Faculty of Veterinary Medicine, Justus-Liebig-University Giessen, Giessen, Germany)

favorable to chemotherapy with common relapses and survival times of less than 6 months. However, long-term survival (>1 year) has been reported.

After chemotherapy has been initiated, *tumor sequela may be treated*; this includes plasmapheresis for the treatment of the hyperviscosity syndrome, treatment of hypercalcemia, fluid therapy for the renal involvement, and orthopedic treatment of pathologic fractures.

Prognostic Factors and Markers

The presence of widespread osteolysis, hypercalcemia, or excretion of Bence Jones proteins is negatively correlated with survival in dogs.

Suggested Reading

(Osborne et al. 1968; Matus et al. 1986; MacEwen and Hurvitz 1977; Mellor et al. 2006; Mellor et al. 2008)

6.2.2 Plasmacytomas in Dogs and Cats

Solitary plasmacytomas develop either in the bone (solitary osseous plasmacytomas) or in the soft tissue (extramedullary plasmacytomas). These tumors are focal proliferations of atypical plasma cells.

Box 6.6. Plasmacytomas in Five Facts

1. Tumor of mature dogs and rarely cats.
2. Plasmacytomas in the skin and oral cavity are benign.
3. Solitary osseous plasmacytomas can evolve to plasma cell myelomas.
4. Surgical excision is curative for skin tumors.
5. Chemotherapy and radiation therapy additionally applied in some tumors.

Epidemiology and Pathogenesis

Plasmacytomas are infrequently seen in dogs and only rarely in cats. Patients are usually older (median *age*, 9–10 years in dogs) with no *sex* predisposition. Dog *breeds* with a higher risk of developing plasmacytomas are American and English cocker spaniels and West Highland white terriers. A higher risk is presumed in Yorkshire terriers, boxers, German shepherds, and Airedale terriers.

Clinical Appearance

Extramedullary plasmacytomas in dogs are usually found in the *skin* and less often in *oral mucous membranes* or mucosa of the rectum and colon. Other sites of the body (e.g., the stomach, small intestine, spleen, liver, genitalia, eyes, uterus, and lung) are occasionally affected as well. Tumors in the skin are single, soft, slightly raised nodules with no associated clinical signs. Tumors in the gastrointestinal tract can be associated with nonspecific gastrointestinal signs. Colorectal involvement can lead to tenesmus, hemorrhage (rectal bleeding, hematochezia), or rectal prolapse. The clinical course of disease depends on the type of plasmacytomas.

Indolent plasmacytomas are considered to be benign tumors, whereas *anaplastic plasmacytomas* are considered to be malignant but with slow progression and rare metastases.

Solitary osseous plasmacytomas appear within the bones as single lesions but often evolve to multiple myelomas in the course of the disease. Clinical presentation depends on the bone involved; lameness and pain present with long bone involvement and neurologic signs with vertebral involvement.

Cytology and Histopathology

Cytology of plasmacytomas is often diagnostic. In some tumors, cells resemble well-differentiated plasma cells (Fig. 6.14), but in others, they are

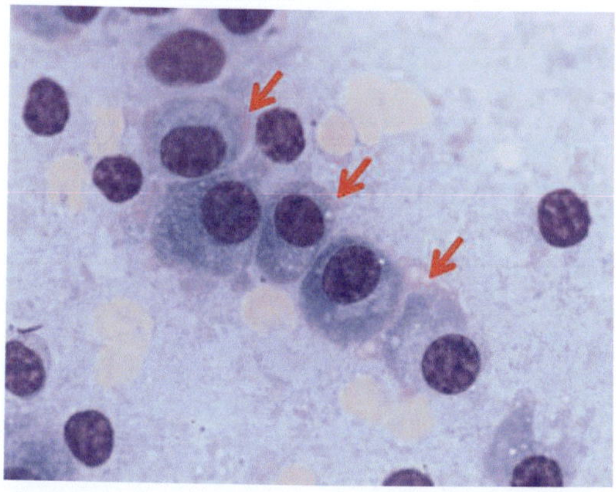

■ **Fig. 6.14** Cytology, plasmacytoma lymph node, dog, May-Grünwald-Giemsa 1000x. In the lymph node, infiltration with neoplastic plasma cells cannot be differentiated from reactive plasma cells, unless the tumor cells are of atypical morphology. In this case, plasmacytoma can be easily detected due to the dominance of so-called flame cells (or flaming plasma cells, *red arrows*) consistent with a clonal proliferation of IgA-producing plasma cells characterized by ruffled magenta-staining cellular margins (Photo: with permission of Dr. N. Bauer, Faculty of Veterinary Medicine, Justus-Liebig-University Giessen, Giessen, Germany)

less differentiated. *Indolent plasmacytomas* present *histologically* as tumors composed of sheets of uniform large cells with eccentrically placed round to oval nuclei and deeply stained cytoplasm (■ Fig. 6.15). Binucleation occurs infrequently and mitoses are rare. *Anaplastic plasmacytomas* show marked anisokaryosis, hyperchromicity, frequent binucleation, and mitoses.

■ Therapy

Surgical excision is the therapy of choice for *extramedullary plasmacytomas*. Adjuvant *chemotherapy* (melphalan and prednisone) or *radiation* can be supportive for recurrent or incompletely removed tumors.

Treatment of *solitary osseous plasmacytomas* depends on the bone involved and associated complications. *Surgical excision* is recommended in cases of instable fractures and/or neurologic signs due to spinal cord compression. *Radiation* therapy alone is suitable for patients with stable fractures or as palliative therapy. Tumors in the axial bones can be treated with either surgical excision or radiation therapy.

■ Prognostic Factors and Markers

Anatomic location is an important prognostic factor. Extramedullary plasmacytomas in the skin and oral cavity are considered benign, whereas tumors in other locations show a higher risk of metastasis to local lymph nodes. Plasmacytomas of the rectal mucosa are less biologic aggressive and surgical excision is usually curative. Solitary osseous plasmacytomas have a less favorable diagnosis since most progress to multiple myelomas. However, the time from local disease to systemic disease may be in the range of months to years. The *microscopic appearance* is useful in differentiating benign indolent plasmacytomas from the (low) malignant anaplastic plasmacytomas.

■ Suggested Reading

(Platz et al. 1999; Meis et al. 1987; Baer et al. 1989)

6.3 Histiocytic Tumors

Proliferations of histiocytic cells are common in dogs and less common in cats. Histiocytes are a heterogeneous group of cells derived from the dendritic or macrophage cell line. Several entities of histiocytic proliferative disorders exist.

6.3.1 Canine Histiocytic Tumors

6.3.1.1 Cutaneous Histiocytomas

Cutaneous histiocytomas are common benign skin tumors mostly of young dogs (► see Chap. 4).

6.3.1.2 Histiocytic Sarcomas

Histiocytic sarcomas (*HS*) derive from interstitial dendritic cells. These can be found in the perivascular region of many organs, with the exception of the brain (here they are only found in the meninges and choroid plexus). A related but distinct form of HS is called *hemophagocytic histiocytic sarcomas*. This variant originates from macrophages.

Box 6.7. Histiocytic Sarcomas in Six Facts

1. Malignant tumor of dendritic cells.
2. Bernese Mountain Dogs are predisposed.
3. Localized or disseminated ("malignant histiocytosis").
4. Disseminated HS has a poor prognosis.
5. Localized HS has a more favorable prognosis.
6. Therapy of choice: surgical excision (localized) or chemotherapy (disseminated).

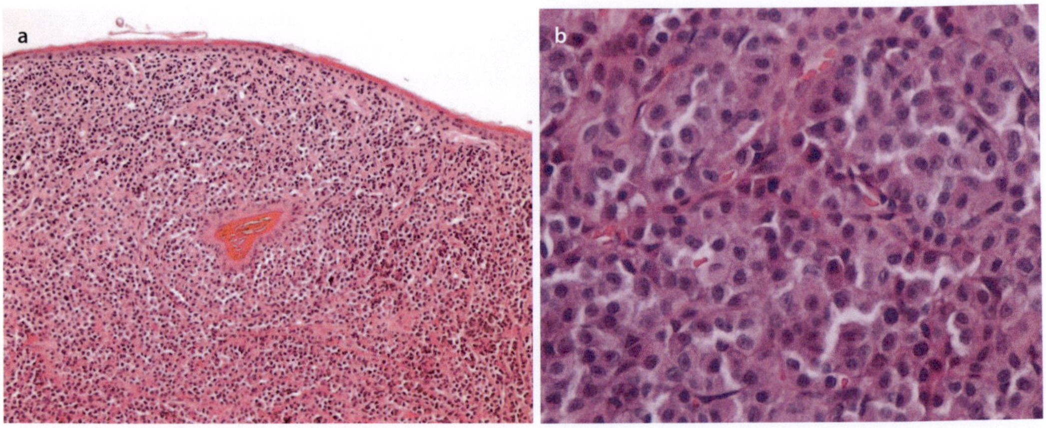

◘ **Fig. 6.15** Histology of the skin of a dog with solitary cutaneous plasmacytoma. (**a**) The dermis shows a sheetlike infiltration with neoplastic cells (hematoxylin and eosin, 100×). (**b**) Higher magnification of A. Neoplastic cells are large, relatively uniform with eccentrically placed round to oval nuclei and deeply stained cytoplasm (hematoxylin and eosin, 400×)

Epidemiology and Pathogenesis

Histiocytic sarcomas are a disease mainly seen in dogs and only rarely in other species, including cats (see below), horses, and cattle. *Bernese Mountain Dogs* are predisposed to histiocytic sarcomas, but Rottweilers, golden retrievers, and flat-coated retrievers have an increased incidence as well. In other breeds, the disease occurs sporadically. The mode of inheritance in Bernese Mountain Dogs is reported to be polygenetic. There is a similarity to histiocytic sarcomas in humans; similar genetic loci are affected (tumor suppressor genes: CDKN2A, RB1, and PTEN). Age of initial diagnosis is between 6 and 8.5 years. A sex predisposition has not been found.

The *hemophagocytic histiocytic sarcoma* also shows a predisposition for Bernese Mountain Dogs, as well as Rottweilers and retrievers. The range of age at diagnosis, 2.5–13 years, is slightly broader than in the non-hemophagocytic variant.

Clinical Appearance

Histiocytic sarcomas can be *focal* (*localized HS*) within a single organ or site of the body or systemic. If the disease spreads beyond the local lymph node, it is called *disseminated histiocytic sarcoma* (previously *malignant histiocytosis*). It is commonly detected in the lung, spleen, and lymph nodes.

Localized HS often occurs initially in the subcutis of the limbs, but other sites like the spleen, liver, lung, brain, nasal or oral cavity, and joints are primary sites as well. Spreading occurs first to the draining lymph node and subsequently to distant sites (often the liver and lung, if not primarily involved).

Affected organs of the *hemophagocytic HS* are the spleen, liver, bone marrow, and lung.

Clinical signs depend on the organ involved but include nonspecific systemic signs (like anorexia, weight loss, and lethargy). The mass effect of thoracic tumors (especially within the lung, ◘ Fig. 6.16) leads to coughing and other respiratory signs. Involvement of the CNS can result in neurologic signs (e.g., seizures, ataxia, and paralysis). Articular HS is associated with lameness.

Clinical pathology findings include mild anemia, which can be profound in cases of hemophagocytic HS, thrombocytopenia, and rare hypercalcemia.

Localized and disseminated HS present as solitary or multiple white masses with a smooth cut surface, whereas the *hemophagocytic variant* infiltrates the affected organs diffusely without formation of nodular tumor masses.

Cytology and Histopathology

Cytology shows pleomorphic histiocytic cells with marked anisocytosis and anisokaryosis (◘ Figs. 6.17 and 6.18). The cells are often bi- or multinucleated with a variable number of mitoses. Differentiation of benign histiocytic proliferations from histiocytic sarcomas can be difficult

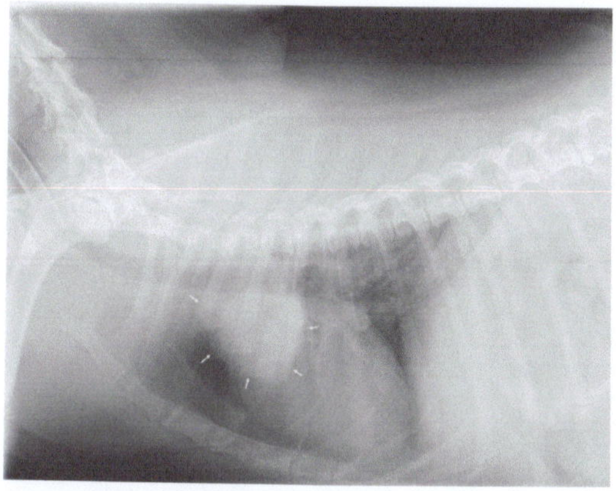

Fig. 6.16 Lateral thoracic radiograph a Bernese Mountain Dog with histiocytic sarcoma. Note the solitary space-occupying lesion (*arrows*) within the caudal part of the left cranial lobe of the lung (Photo: with permission of Dr. Antje Hartmann, Vetsuisse Faculty University of Bern, Bern, Switzerland, and the Department of Veterinary Clinical Sciences, Clinic for Small Animals, Surgery, Justus-Liebig-University Giessen, Giessen, Germany)

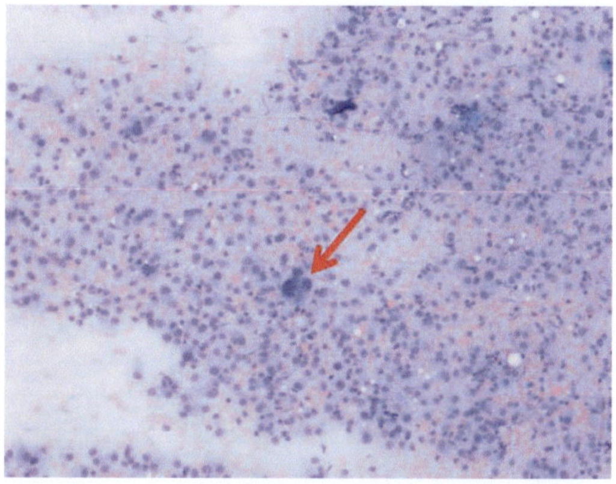

Fig. 6.17 Cytology, histiocytic sarcoma, thoracic mass, mixed-breed dog, May-Grünwald-Giemsa 100×. Note the presence of histiocytic giant cells diagnostic for histiocytic sarcoma (*red arrow*) (Photo: with permission of Dr. N. Bauer, Faculty of Veterinary Medicine, Justus-Liebig-University, Giessen, Germany)

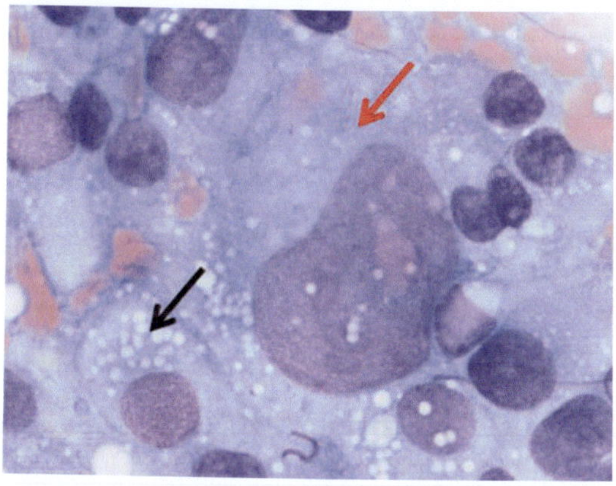

Fig. 6.18 Cytology, histiocytic sarcoma, thoracic mass, mixed breed dog (same dog as in Fig. 6.17), May-Grünwald-Giemsa 1000x. Note the presence of smaller (*black arrow*) histiocytic cells without phagocytic activity as well as larger atypical histiocytes with macronuklei (*red arrow*). (Photo: with permission of Dr. N. Bauer, Faculty of Veterinary Medicine, Justus-Liebig-University Giessen, Giessen, Germany)

with cytology alone. Sheets of large, pleomorphic cells, often multinucleated with numerous bizarre mitoses (Fig. 6.19), are seen on *histopathology* of HS. Sometimes a spindle cell component can be observed as well. Due to the pleomorphism, anaplastic tumors of different origin need to be ruled out by immunohistology. The hemophagocytic subtype shows marked erythrophagocytosis in cytology and histology.

Therapy

Wide *surgical excision* of localized HS can be curative if the tumor has not spread.

Treatment of disseminated HS with *lomustine* showed about a 50 % response rate, with prolonged survival times (median 172 days) compared to nonresponding dogs (median 60 days).

Prognostic Factors and Markers

The main prognostic factor is the type of histiocytic sarcoma involved. The median survival time of dogs with *localized HS* in a study with 11 dogs was 5.3 years. The aggressive behavior of the *disseminated HS* causes a very fast progressive disease, which results in a poor prognosis. Data of survival times is scarce; patients were euthanized shortly after diagnosis in many reported cases. Dogs with *hemophagocytic HS* are reported to have a survival time of 2–32 weeks (median about 7 weeks).

Suggested Reading

(Moore 2014; Fulmer and Mauldin 2007; Affolter; Moore 2002 and , Moore 2006)

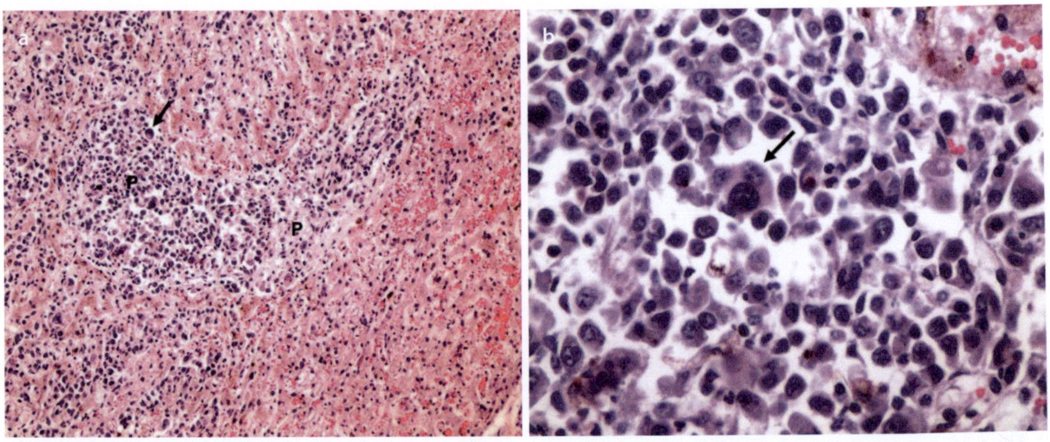

Fig. 6.19 Histology of the liver of a Bernese Mountain Dog with histiocytic sarcoma. (**a**) There is extensive infiltration of the liver sinusoids and the portal areas (P) with neoplastic cells, including multiple tumor giant cells (*arrow*) (hematoxylin and eosin, 100×). (**b**) Higher magnification of A. Note the high level of pleomorphism of the neoplastic cells including the tumor giant cells (*arrow*) (hematoxylin and eosin, 400×)

6.3.2 Feline Progressive Histiocytosis

Feline progressive histiocytosis originates from interstitial dendritic cells of the skin and represents a low-grade histiocytic sarcoma.

Box 6.8. Feline Progressive Histiocytosis in Four Facts

1. A slowly progressive tumor of interstitial dendritic cells of the skin.
2. Begins with solitary cutaneous nodules.
3. Often becomes systemic in the course of the disease
4. There is no effective therapy and the long-term prognosis is poor.

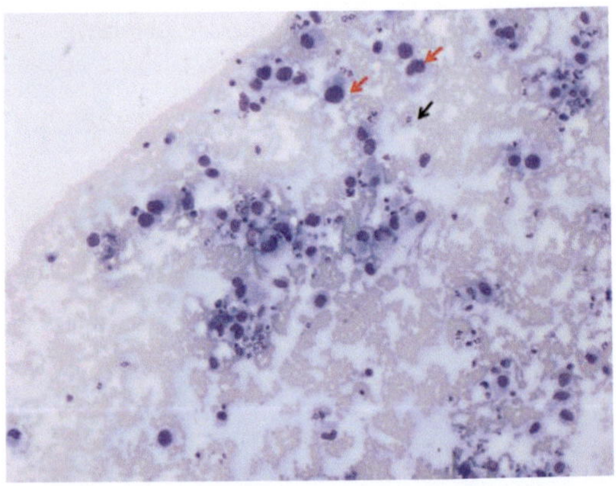

Fig. 6.20 Cytology, feline progressive histiocytosis, skin tumor, mandibular area, cat, May-Grünwald-Giemsa 100×. There are numerous pleomorphic large histiocytic giant cells with round to kidney-shaped nuclei diagnostic for progressive histiocytosis (*red arrow*). Their atypically large size can be easily seen in comparison with a neutrophil (*black arrow*): a benign histiocytic cell would possess nuclei that are much smaller than a neutrophil

▪ Epidemiology and Pathogenesis

Feline progressive histiocytosis is a disease of middle-aged to older cats (7–17 years).

▪ Clinical Appearance

The disease presents *initially as a solitary cutaneous nodule*, which usually progresses to multiple non-painful, non-pruritic nodules, papules, or plaques. Lesions can be alopecic and ulcerated. Affected sites are the head, trunk, and distal limbs. The lesions may wax and wane; regression does not occur. Instead, many cats develop *metastases* to regional lymph nodes and internal organs *during the course of the disease* including the lungs, liver, spleen, and kidneys.

▪ Cytology and Histopathology

Early lesions are composed of well-differentiated histiocytes (Fig. 6.22). Reactive lesions due to infectious agents have to be ruled out. In the

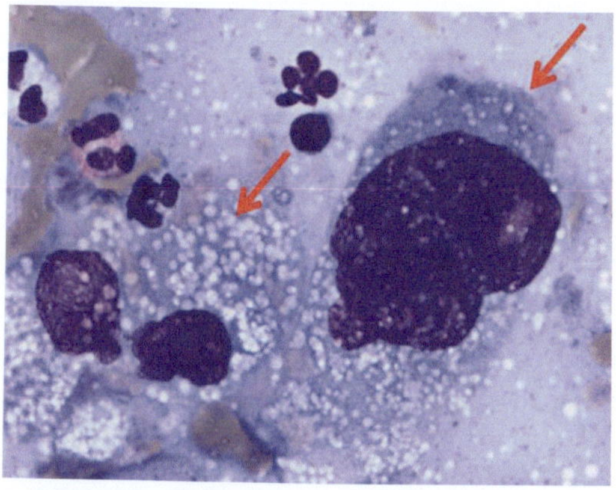

■ **Fig. 6.21** Cytology, feline progressive histiocytosis, skin tumor, mandibular area, cat (the same cat as in Fig. 6.20), May-Grünwald-Giemsa 1000×. There are highly pleomorphic large histiocytic giant cells (*red arrow*) with marked anisocytosis, anisokaryosis, pleomorphism, and indented nuclei with rough chromatin structure (Photo: with permission of Dr. N. Bauer, Faculty of Veterinary Medicine, Justus-Liebig-University Giessen, Giessen, Germany)

course of the disease, criteria of malignancy (atypical cells, bizarre mitoses, and multinucleated cells) are frequently seen (■ Figs. 6.20 and 6.21).

Therapy

No treatment has been reported.

Prognostic Factors and Markers

The disease shows a slow progression. However, due to the lack of an efficient therapy, the prognosis is poor.

Suggested Reading

(Moore 2014; Affolter and Moore 2006)

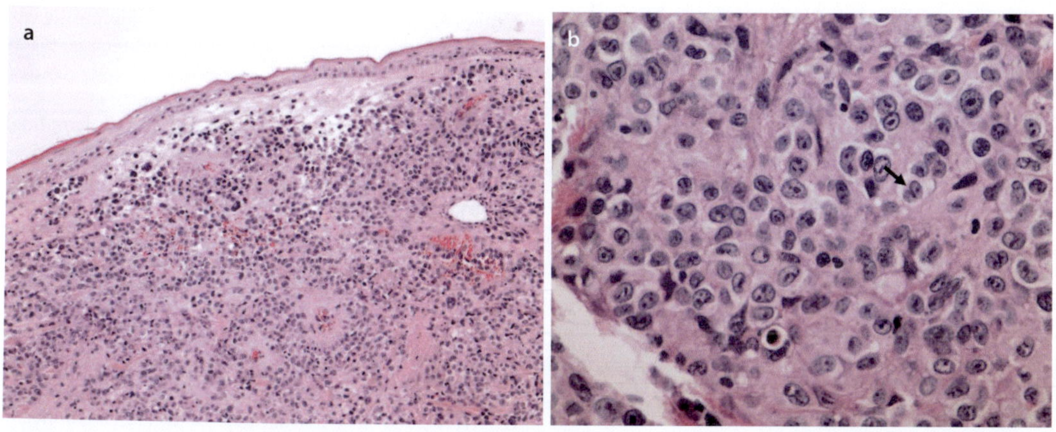

■ **Fig. 6.22** Histology of the skin of a cat with progressive histiocytosis. (**a**) There is a sheetlike infiltration of the dermis with neoplastic cells (hematoxylin and eosin, 100×). (**b**) Higher magnification of A. Neoplastic cells have large amounts of cytoplasm and large round to oval, sometimes indented (*arrow*) nuclei (hematoxylin and eosin, 400×)

Suggested Reading

Adam F, Villiers E, Watson S, Coyne K, Blackwood L (2009) Clinical pathological and epidemiological assessment of morphologically and immunologically confirmed canine leukaemia. Vet Comp Oncol 7(3):181–195. doi:10.1111/j.1476-5829.2009.00189.x

Affolter VK, Moore PF (2002) Localized and disseminated histiocytic sarcomas of dendritic cell origin in dogs. Vet Pathol 39(1):74–83

Affolter VK, Moore PF (2006) Feline progressive histiocytosis. Vet Pathol 43(5):646–655. doi:10.1354/vp.43-5-646

Baer K, Patnaik A, Gilbertson S, Hurvitz A (1989) Cutaneous plasmacytomas in dogs: a morphologic and immunohistochemical study. Vet Pathol Online 26(3):216–221

Campbell MW, Hess PR, Williams LE (2013) Chronic lymphocytic leukaemia in the cat: 18 cases (2000–2010). Vet Comp Oncol 11(4):256–264. doi:10.1111/j.1476-5829.2011.00315.x

Carreras JK, Goldschmidt M, Lamb M, McLear RC, Drobatz KJ, Sorenmo KU (2003) Feline epitheliotropic intestinal malignant lymphomas: 10 cases (1997–2000). J Vet Intern Med 17(3):326–331

Cotter S (1983) Treatment of lymphomas and leukemia with cyclophosphamide, vincristine, and prednisone. II. Treatment of cats. J Am Anim Hosp Assoc 19(2):166–172

Couto CG (1985) Clinicopathologic aspects of acute leukemias in the dog. J Am Vet Med Assoc 186(7):681–685

Couto CG, Rutgers HC, Sherding RG, Rojko J (1989) Gastrointestinal lymphomas in 20 dogs. A retrospective study. J Vet Intern Med 3(2):73–78

Fulmer AK, Mauldin GE (2007) Canine histiocytic neoplasia: an overview. Can Vet J 48(10):1041

Gross TL, Ihrke PJ, Walder EJ, Affolter VK, (eds) (2008) Lymphocytic tumors. In: Skin diseases of the dog and cat. Blackwell Science Ltd, Oxford pp 866–893. doi:10.1002/9780470752487.ch37

Hardy WD Jr (1981) Haematopoietic tumors of cats. J Am Anim Hosp Assoc 17:921–940

Hart JR, Shaker E, Patnaik AK, Garvey MS (1994) Lymphocytic-plasmacytic enterocololitis in cats: 60 cases (1988–1990). J Am Anim Hosp Assoc 30(5):505–514

Hodgkins EM, Zinkl JG, Madewell BR (1980) Chronic lymphocytic leukemia in the dog. J Am Vet Med Assoc 177(8):704–707

Leifer CE, Matus RE (1986) Chronic lymphocytic leukemia in the dog: 22 cases (1974–1984). J Am Vet Med Assoc 189(2):214–217

Louwerens M, London CA, Pedersen NC, Lyons LA (2005) Feline lymphomas in the post-feline leukemia virus era. J Vet Intern Med 19(3):329–335

MacEwen EG, Hurvitz AI (1977) Diagnosis and management of monoclonal gammopathies. Vet Clin North Am 7(1):119–132

Marconato L, Gelain ME, Comazzi S (2013) The dog as a possible animal model for human non-Hodgkin lymphomas: a review. Hematol Oncol 31(1):1–9. doi:10.1002/hon.2017

Matus RE, Leifer CE, MacEwen EG (1983) Acute lymphoblastic leukemia in the dog: a review of 30 cases. J Am Vet Med Assoc 183(8):859–862

Matus RE, Leifer CE, MacEwen EG, Hurvitz AI (1986) Prognostic factors for multiple myelomas in the dog. J Am Vet Med Assoc 188(11):1288–1292

Meis JM, Butler JJ, Osborne BM, Ordonez NG (1987) Solitary plasmacytomas of bone and extramedullary plasmacytomas. A clinicopathologic and immunohistochemical study. Cancer 59(8):1475–1485

Mellor PJ, Haugland S, Murphy S, Smith KC, Holloway A, Archer J, Powell RM, Polton GA, Tasker S, McCormick D, Tempest ME, McNeil PE, Scase TJ, Knott CD, Bonfanti U, Villiers EJ, Argyle DJ, Herrtage ME, Day MJ (2006) Myelomas-related disorders in cats commonly present as extramedullary neoplasms in contrast to myelomas in human patients: 24 cases with clinical follow-up. J Vet Intern Med 20(6):1376–1383

Mellor PJ, Haugland S, Smith KC, Powell RM, Archer J, Scase TJ, Villiers EJ, McNeil PE, Nixon C, Knott C, Fournier D, Murphy S, Polton GA, Belford C, Philbey AW, Argyle DJ, Herrtage ME, Day MJ (2008) Histopathologic, immunohistochemical, and cytologic analysis of feline myelomas-related disorders: further evidence for primary extramedullary development in the cat. Vet Pathol Online 45(2):159–173. doi:10.1354/vp.45-2-159

Mooney SC, Hayes AA (1986) Lymphomas in the cat: an approach to diagnosis and management. Semin Vet Med Surg (Small Anim) 1(1):51–57

Moore PF (2014) A review of histiocytic diseases of dogs and cats. Vet Pathol 51(1):167–184. doi:10.1177/0300985813510413

Moore PF, Affolter VK, Vernau W (2006) Canine hemophagocytic histiocytic sarcomas: a proliferative disorder of CD11d + macrophages. Vet Pathol 43(5):632–645. doi:10.1354/vp.43-5-632

Morris JS, Dunn JK, Dobson JM (1993) Canine lymphoid leukaemia and lymphomas with bone marrow involvement: a review of 24 cases. J Small Anim Pract 34(2):72–79. doi:10.1111/j.1748-5827.1993.tb02613.x

Mortier F, Daminet S, Vandenabeele S, Van de Maele I (2012) Canine lymphomas: a retrospective study (2009–2010). Vlaams Diergeneeskundig Tijdschrift 81(6):341–351

Osborne CA, Perman V, Sautter JH, Stevens JB, Hanlon GF (1968) Multiple myelomas in the dog. J Am Vet Med Assoc 153(10):1300–1319

Owen LN (1980) TNM classification of tumours in domestic animals. World Health Organization, Geneva

Platz SJ, Breuer W, Pfleghaar S, Minkus G, Hermanns W (1999) Prognostic value of histopathological grading in canine extramedullary plasmacytomas. Vet Pathol 36(1):23–27

Ragaini L, Aste G, Cavicchioli L, Boari A (2003) Inflammatory bowel disease mimicking alimentary lymphosarcomas in a cat. Vet Res Commun 27(Suppl 1):791–793

Richards KL, Suter SE (2015) Man's best friend: what can pet dogs teach us about non-Hodgkin's lymphomas? Immunol Rev 263(1):173–191. doi:10.1111/Imr.12238

Vail DM, Moore AS, Ogilvie GK, Volk LM (1998) Feline lymphomas (145 cases): proliferation indices, cluster of differentiation 3 immunoreactivity, and their association with prognosis in 90 cats. J Vet Intern Med 12(5):349–354

Valli VE, San Myint M, Barthel A, Bienzle D, Caswell J, Colbatzky F, Durham A, Ehrhart EJ, Johnson Y, Jones C, Kiupel M, Labelle P, Lester S, Miller M, Moore P, Moroff S, Roccabianca P, Ramos-Vara J, Ross A, Scase T, Tvedten H, Vernau W (2011) Classification of canine malignant lymphomas according to the World Health Organization criteria. Vet Pathol 48(1):198–211. doi:10.1177/0300985810379428

Valli VE, Kass PH, San Myint M, Scott F (2013) Canine lymphomas: association of classification type, disease stage, tumor subtype, mitotic rate, and treatment with survival. VetPathol50(5):738–748.doi:10.1177/0300985813478210

Urogenital Tract Tumors

Stephanie Plog

R. Klopfleisch (ed.), *Veterinary Oncology*, DOI 10.1007/978-3-319-41124-8_7

7.1 Urinary Tract Tumors

7.1.1 Canine Renal Tumors

In general, renal tumors are rare in dogs, but if they occur, they are *mostly malignant*. Adenomas constitute only 15 % of primary neoplasms. Malignant tumors can occur uni- or bilaterally, and *carcinomas* are the most common canine renal neoplasms.

7.1.1.1 Epithelial and Mesenchymal Tumors

Box 7.1. Canine Renal Epithelial and Mesenchymal Neoplasms in Five Facts

1. Mostly malignant
2. Tumors of old dogs, exception: cystadenocarcinomas
3. Clinical signs often unspecific
4. Therapy of choice in cases with unilateral tumors is nephrectomy
5. Commonly metastasize to the lymph nodes, lung, and liver

Epidemiology and Pathogenesis

Epithelial kidney tumors in the dog are divided mainly into *renal cell carcinomas* (*RCC*) and *transitional cell carcinomas*. Primary tumors of the kidneys are mostly *malignant*. Metastases to the kidneys have been described.

Renal cell carcinomas (*RCC*) arise from epithelium of renal tubules and are the *most common* epithelial tumors in the canine kidney. They often occur *bilaterally* and can be highly invasive. The mean age is 8 years, with predisposition of male dogs.

Cystadenocarcinomas are a variant of epithelial tumors in the kidney that occur simultaneously with *nodular dermatofibrosis* mainly in German Shepherd dogs, similar to uterine tumors. This disease is caused by a mutation in the *folliculin* gene, and affected dogs usually present with skin tumors at the age of 6 years. Concomitantly occurring renal cystadenocarcinomas are usually bilateral. Occurrence of *cystadenomas* has been described as well.

Transitional cell carcinomas arise from the lining of the *renal pelvis* and are rare tumors in the canine kidney. In comparison to renal cell carcinomas, metastasis to the lung is seen less often.

Mesenchymal tumors of the kidney include *hemangiosarcomas* and *fibrosarcomas* and various *metastases* from distinct primary focuses that have to be excluded before the diagnosis of a primary renal mesenchymal tumor can be made. *Hemangiomas* are reported to be *the most common benign tumors* in the canine kidney.

Clinical Appearance

Clinical findings in dogs affected by renal tumors are usually *unspecific*, including weight loss, polyuria, lethargy, and hematuria. Some authors say that *hematuria* is seen more often in transitional cell tumors. Clinical signs are mainly attributed to the *destruction of the renal parenchyma* and can mirror those caused by nonneoplastic lesions. Sometimes a painful abdominal mass can be palpated. *Blood chemistry* might reveal polycythemia, anemia, azotemia, neutrophilia, or hypercalcemia. Additional findings like bone metastasis and hypertrophic osteopathy due to pulmonary metastases are rarely described. Since most of the renal neoplasms have already metastasized to the lung, lymph nodes, liver, or heart at the time of diagnosis, *radiography of the thorax* and *abdominal ultrasonography* should be included in every case of suspected renal neoplasia. Metastasis to the skin has also been reported.

Cytology and Histopathology

Renal *clear cells* with vacuolated cytoplasm might be visible in smears of renal carcinomas, but this finding is not pathognomonic, and histopathology is needed for definitive diagnosis and identifying invasion and complete excision. Histologically, a variety of *different subtypes* and *cell types* can be found in renal cell carcinomas, and the clear cell variant is associated with a significantly decreased survival time. Mitotic index (<10 mitoses, 10–30 mitoses, >30 mitoses in 10 high power fields) in RCC is assumed to be an important prognostic variable for the survival time.

Therapy

The therapy of choice in unilateral renal tumors is *nephrectomy*, independent of the type of tumor. Removal of the ureter and adjacent tissue might be necessary and is generally recommended. Particular care should be taken to avoid *spread* of neoplastic cells into the abdominal cavity during surgery. Chemotherapeutic approaches are not useful in primary renal tumors in the dog, and survival times did not differ between treated and nontreated animals in a recent study. Successful treatment with surgical excision of the neoplastic kidney is largely dependent on the functionality of the contralateral kidney.

▪ Prognosis

Although *pulmonary metastases* are present at the time of diagnosis in most cases, survival times of up to 5 years after nephrectomy have been reported. Epithelial tumors are associated with longer survival times than mesenchymal tumors. Renal hemangiosarcomas have a better prognosis than hemangiosarcomas in other organs. *Hemoabdomen* due to rupture of the neoplasm, hematuria, and cachexia are *negatively correlated* with survival.

7.1.1.2 Canine Nephroblastomas

Box 7.2. Canine Nephroblastomas of the Kidney in Five Facts

1. Occur in young adult dogs
2. Can become huge palpable abdominal masses
3. Usually unilateral
4. Nephrectomy as the therapy of choice
5. Prognosis depends on the degree of differentiation

▪ Epidemiology and Pathogenesis

Nephroblastomas originate from *primitive nephrogenic blastema* and can also contain cartilage or muscle, suggesting pluripotent mesenchymal origin. In contrast to other tumors of the kidney, nephroblastomas commonly occur at a *younger age*. Malignancy of the tumor is dependent on its degree of *differentiation*. Nephroblastomas can become huge, causing severe abdominal distension, but are usually *unilateral*. In over 50 % of cases, *metastases* to the lung and liver are seen. Nephroblastomas can also occur as intradural neoplasms of the spinal canal.

▪ Clinical Appearance

The clinical appearance in dogs with nephroblastomas is mainly unspecific, similar to the other renal tumors (▶ see Sect. 7.1.1.1). As 75 % of dogs with nephroblastomas develop *pulmonary metastasis*, radiographic examination of the thorax should be included. Palpable abdominal masses might be detected in some cases.

▪ Cytology and Histopathology

Nephroblastomas are usually composed of blastemal, epithelial, and stromal components and can have a *variable appearance*. Thus, cytology is usually not sufficient and histopathology is needed for the definitive diagnosis. Histologically, *primitive glomeruli* can be seen along with loose *mesenchymal* cells and underdeveloped *tubules*. Diagnosis may be confirmed by *anti-C-19* immunohistochemical staining.

▪ Therapy and Prognosis

Nephrectomy is the method of choice, and there is no reliable information about the usefulness of chemotherapeutics. *Prognosis* is dependent on the *histological appearance* of the tumor, and well-differentiated tumors composed of clearly identifiable tubules and glomeruli have a better prognosis than nephroblastomas with anaplastic or sarcomatoid growth.

7.1.1.3 Malignant Lymphomas

Details on canine lymphomas are given in Chap. 6 (Hematopoietic Tumors). In general, renal lymphomas can occur uni- or bilaterally and are considered *rare* in dogs. *Polycythemia* occurs commonly in association with renal lymphomas. *Pyelectasis* is a common finding in ultrasonography, as are the loss of corticomedullary distinction and renomegaly. Nephrectomy is usually *not* the therapy of choice, but *chemotherapeutic* approaches using COP or CHOP protocols do yield good results, with median survival rates of up to 295 and 309 days, respectively. In most cases, *blastoid cells* can be identified as the main cell population in *cytology* and point toward the presence of a renal lymphoma.

▪ Suggested Reading

(Batchelor et al. 2006; Battaglia et al. 2005; Bryan et al. 2006; Chiang et al. 2007; Crow et al. 1995; Durno et al. 2011; Edmondson et al. 2015; Hayes and Fraumeni 1977; Locke and Barber 2006; Moc and Lium 1997; Militerno et al. 2003; Taylor et al. 2014)

7.1.2 Canine Urinary Bladder Tumors

Tumors of the urinary bladder are the *most common* neoplasms of the canine urinary tract. Most of them are *transitional cell carcinomas*. Clinical diagnosis can be difficult because the clinical signs are unspecific, and the prognosis is dependent on *staging*, degree of urinary tract *obstruction*, and histological *subclassification*.

7.1.2.1 Transitional Cell Carcinomas/TCC

Box 7.3. Transitional Cell Carcinomas of the Urinary Bladder in Six Facts

1. Most common urinary bladder tumor in dogs, especially neutered dogs
2. Associated with contact between urothelium and carcinogens
3. Often invasive, metastasizing, and obstructing
4. Commonly located at the trigone
5. Clinical staging: TNM system
6. Effective therapeutic approaches: combination of surgery and medical treatment

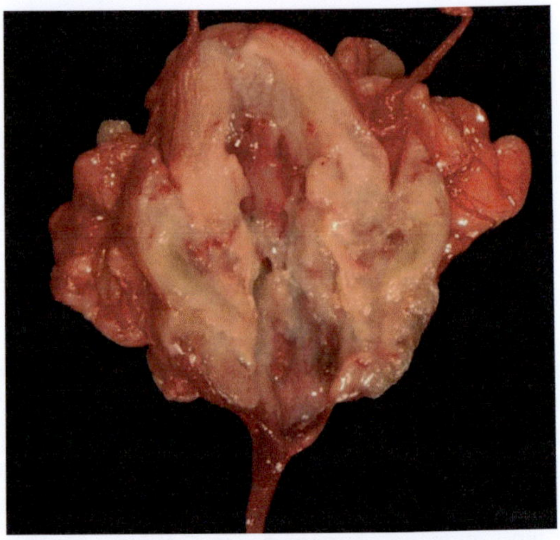

Fig. 7.1 Invasive transitional cell tumor of the urinary bladder of the dog (with permission of P. Schlieben, Landeslabor Frankfurt/Oder and the Archive of the Institute for Veterinary Pathology and R. Klopfleisch, Freie Universität Berlin, Germany)

Epidemiology and Pathogenesis

Transitional cell carcinomas of the urinary bladder are the most common urogenital neoplasms in the dog and arise from the epithelial lining of the urinary bladder. They are often *invasive* and located in the *trigone* region (Fig. 7.1). Primary neoplasms of the urethra are rare, but transitional cell carcinomas of the urinary bladder often infiltrate the urethra. *Neutered* dogs are more likely to develop TCC than intact dogs, and female sex is considered a risk factor, as is prolonged *exposure* of the urinary bladder to various *carcinogens* like cyclophosphamide or older insecticides, herbicides, or pesticides. There seems to be a *breed predisposition* for Scottish Terriers, West Highland White Terriers, Fox Terriers, Shetland Sheepdogs, Beagles, and Collies, and obesity is another risk factor. Affected dogs are usually approximately *10 years* old. Urinary tract obstruction is common.

Clinical Appearance

Main symptoms are pollakiuria, hematuria, dysuria, and – later in the disease – anuria due to urinary tract obstruction. These *unspecific* symptoms are comparable to those of nonneoplastic diseases, and they can even resolve temporarily with antibiotics. Concurrent urinary tract infections are common. *Sonography* is the standard procedure for detecting a urinary bladder neoplasm, and loss of the typical layered arrangement of the urinary bladder wall can hint toward malignant infiltrative growth. TCC can be *polypoid, sessile,* or *papillary*. Differentials include polyps which are often stalked and located in the apex region as well as polypoid cystitis. Endoscopic examination allows for a closer investigation of location, morphology, and dimensions of the neoplasm. *Metastasis* is common, but often late, and usually occurs to the lymph nodes, liver, and lung, and some say that care has to be taken during *cystocentesis* to *avoid seeding of tumor cells*. Catheterization might be the method of choice to collect urine. Metastases to the skin adjacent to the vulva or prepuce as well as metastasis to the bone have also been described.

Clinical *staging* of TCC of the urinary bladder is performed using a World Health Organization (WHO) system (Table 7.1).

Cytology and Histopathology

Cytology can be useful when *dysplastic tumor cells* are visible in the urine, but sensitivity is low. Histology is the method of choice to reach a definitive diagnosis. Histologically, the tumor can be classified according to invasive *growth*, *pattern*

Table 7.1 Clinical staging system for transitional cell carcinomas (Owen 1980)

TNM stage	Category
T	*Primary tumor*
T0	Neoplastic growth not evident
T1	Superficial papillary tumor
T2	Invasion into urinary bladder wall, induration
T3	Invasion into adjacent tissues (prostate, uterus, vagina, intestine)
N	Regional lymph nodes (*Lnn. iliacimediales*)
N0	No involvement
N1	Involvement of regional lymph nodes
N2	Additional involvement of further lymph nodes (*Lnn. lumbales aortici, Lnn. hypogastrici, Lnn. sacrales*)
M	Distant metastases
M0	No distant metastasis
M1	Distant metastasis (lung, bone, brain, etc.)

(papillary, non-papillary), and tumor *grade*. Multiple layers of neoplastic urothelium covering a tumor stalk are common, and *invasion* into the stalk and surrounding stroma as well as desmoplasia are often associated with *metastasis*. Non-papillary and infiltrating variants are most likely to metastasize. There may be areas of glandular or squamous metaplasia. Immunohistochemical staining for *uroplakin III* can be useful in cases of undifferentiated tumors. Another marker for neoplastic transformation is *COX-2* which was assumed to be expressed in neoplastic cells only. However, a recent study revealed COX-2 to be expressed in proliferative epithelium as well, and this marker has to be interpreted with caution.

▪ Therapy

Surgery is useful for obtaining specimens for histopathology, restoration of urine flow, and removal of the neoplasm. During surgical removal special care has to be taken to avoid metastasis seeding. Unfortunately, complete resection is often impossible, and recurrence is common. Stents can help to reduce obstruction and may thus prolong survival time. *Chemotherapy*, often given as a combination therapy with COX inhibitors, can be a promising alternative to surgery and often leads to partial remission or stable disease. Especially multiple different treatment protocols used subsequently can result in control of the disease. Piroxicam or deracoxib, *COX inhibitors*, can result in good quality of life and stable disease when used as single agent, and survival times of up to 2 years have been reported. Localized application of mitomycin C and photodynamic agents yielded inconsistent results, and severe side effects were seen. Immunotherapy is not promising in dogs. *Radiation* therapy in combination with surgery is also possible, but an impairment of life quality due to extensive fibrosis often accompanies the therapy. However, a recent study reported good results with 10 once-daily fractions of 2.7 Gy without significant late side radiation effects and with a survival time of up to 767 days. All patients clinically benefited from this therapy. *Regular urine analysis* to check for secondary bacterial infections is crucial.

▪ Prognostic Factors

Survival is strongly associated with the *TNM clinical staging* (Table 7.1). More advanced TNM stage is associated with younger age, prostate involvement, and higher T stage, with the longest median survival being 234 days. *Prognosis* is also dependent on the *location* of the tumor, *invasion* of the urethra and surrounding tissue, *obstruction* of the urinary tract, and histological *subclassification*. *Ultrasonographically*, involvement of the urinary bladder wall, trigone location, and the presence of a heterogeneous mass are associated with poorer prognosis.

7.1.2.2 Other Epithelial Neoplasms of the Urinary Bladder

Squamous cell carcinomas (SCC), *undifferentiated carcinomas*, and *adenocarcinomas* of the urinary bladder are far less common than TCC. Adenocarcinomas and SCC show non-papillary growth and are often ulcerated. They do not metastasize as often as transitional cell carcinomas. *SCC* can also occur in the *urethra* of female dogs. Since all of them are rare, no information regarding predispositions can be given. *Papillomas* can be multiple and either pedunculated or sessile. The transitional epithelium covering papillomas is well differentiated, but squamous metaplasia might be seen. Hematuria due to ulcerations is a common clinical finding. Notably, urinary bladder papillomas in dogs can undergo *malignant transformation*.

7.1.2.3 Mesenchymal Tumors

All mesenchymal tumors of the urinary bladder are *rare* in the dog, and most of these are benign fibromas and leiomyomas. Leiomyosarcomas can show local invasion, but metastasis is rare.

A special type of mesenchymal tumours is the *botryoid rhabdomyosarcoma* which occurs in the lower urinary tract in *young* dogs of *large* breeds, especially St. Bernard dogs, and is assumed to arise from embryonal rests of myoblasts. *Female* dogs are overrepresented. These tumors are often located at the *trigone* and are thus difficult to resect, similar to TCC, and they also show *infiltrative* growth and a tendency to *metastasize*. Histopathology is necessary for definitive diagnosis, and strap cells, multinucleated cells, and sometimes cross striation are the hallmarks of the tumor.

▪ Suggested Reading

(Budreckis et al. 2015; Cannon and Allstadt 2015; Choy and Fidel 2016; Fulkerson and Knapp 2015; Gerber and Rees 2009; Glickman et al. 2004; Glickman et al. 1989; Hanazono et al. 2014; Hosoya et al. 2013; Kobayashi et al. 2004; Love and Walshaw 1989; McMillan et al. 2011; Mutsaers et al. 2003; Nolan et al. 2015; Patrick et al. 2006; Ramos-Vara et al. 2003; Reed et al. 2012; Rocha et al. 2000; Sledge et al. 2015; Valli et al. 1995; Vignoli et al. 2007)

7.1.3 Feline Renal Tumors

With the exception of renal lymphomas, neoplasms of the feline kidney are rare. It is nonetheless pivotal to distinguish between renal lymphomas and other tumors since therapeutic approaches differ.

7.1.3.1 Feline Renal Lymphomas

Box 7.4. Feline Renal Lymphomas in Six Facts

1. Most common renal neoplasm in cats
2. Diffuse or nodular
3. Usually bilateral, even with unilateral appearance
4. Typical ultrasonographic features: enlargement, loss of corticomedullary distinction, and characteristic hypoechoic rim
5. Therapy of choice: chemotherapy
6. Definitive diagnosis often obtained via cytology

▪ Epidemiology and Pathogenesis

Renal lymphoma is the *most common* renal neoplasm of the cat, often being part of a multicentric lymphoma (▶ see Chap. 6). The kidney is either the *primary* site of neoplastic growth or involved in *metastatic* distribution. *Involvement of other organs* besides the kidneys at the time of diagnosis is nearly always present, and in virtually all cases both kidneys are affected even if only unilateral enlargement is encountered. Mean age is *8 years*, and the majority of cases are *FeLV negative*. Renal lymphomas are mainly *B cell* lymphomas.

▪ Clinical Appearance

Signs of renal lymphomas include *anorexia, weight loss, polyuria, and polydipsia*, but since renal lymphomas can also metastasize to the CNS, first signs can also include *central nervous symptoms*. Palpable unilaterally or bilaterally enlarged kidney(s) may be detected, and radiography is useful to confirm the regular or irregular enlargement. The most distinctive feature in *ultrasonography* is a *hypoechoic rim* surrounding the renal cortex which is thought to arise from the commonly seen *invasion of lymphoblasts* into the renal capsule and is *highly suspicious* for renal lymphomas. An additional change seen in ultrasonography is *loss of the corticomedullary distinction*. Diagnosis should be confirmed by cytology or histology of tru-cut biopsies.

▪ Cytology and Histopathology

In most cases of renal lymphomas, *cytology* after fine needle aspiration under ultrasonographic control is diagnostic, showing *uniform lymphoblastic cells* with a high mitotic rate and only few mature lymphocytes. Histopathology is useful in cases with a more mixed cell population to distinguish between renal lymphomas and *chronic interstitial nephritis*. *Liquor* examination in cases of CNS involvement might reveal lymphoblasts, but the absence of neoplastic cells does not rule out a lymphoma.

▪ Therapy and Prognosis

The therapy of choice for renal lymphomas is *chemotherapy*. Nephrectomy is neither necessary nor curative since at time of diagnosis the involvement of other organs is likely. The most commonly used chemotherapeutic approach is the *COP combination* with cyclophosphamide, vincristine, and prednisolone. If *CNS involvement* is suspected, an additional treatment with lomustine or cytosine arabinoside is useful. The use of doxorubicin should be avoided since this drug is nephrotoxic in cats, and special care should be taken regarding myelosuppressive effects and worsening of the general condition.

Renal lymphomas can respond well to chemotherapy, and survival times of up to 5 years have been reported. Nonetheless, the prognosis for renal lymphomas is worse than for other lymphomas in the cat and worsens with involvement of the CNS. *Prednisolone administration* before chemotherapy is thought to be a negative prognostic factor. In contrast, the *degree of azotemia* and/or *renal enlargement* should *not* be noncritically assessed as prognostic factors and should not be the only reason to decide against chemotherapy, as long as the cat's general condition is good.

7.1.3.2 Other Renal Tumors in the Cat

Compared with renal lymphomas, other renal tumors in cats are rare. The median age is *10 years* and usually only one kidney is affected, so that – in contrast to renal lymphomas – *nephrectomy* is often reasonable, but should be combined with chemotherapy. The most commonly encountered renal tumors in the cat besides renal lymphomas are *renal carcinomas* and *transitional cell tumors.* The clinical and histopathological features are similar to those of the respective tumors in the dog. Benign tumors in the feline kidney are extremely rare.

▪ Suggested Reading

(Gabor et al. 1998; Henry et al. 1999; Mooney et al. 1987; Taylor et al. 2009; Vail et al. 1998; Valdes-Martinez et al. 2007)

7.1.4 Feline Urinary Bladder Tumors

There is very *low prevalence* of urinary bladder tumors in cats, and they account for less than 1 % of all feline neoplasms. If they occur, affected cats are usually older (12–15 years), and *transitional cell carcinomas* are most common, *but lymphomas are also described.* Clinical signs are as unspecific as they are in the dog, and concurrent urinary tract infections are frequent. In contrast to dogs, TCC are most commonly seen in non-trigonal areas. Histopathological features and treatment options are similar to those in dogs, although a *combination* of *surgery* and *chemotherapy* is the most promising approach. There is no detailed staging system for cats. Survival times of up to 261 days have been reported. Other urinary bladder tumors are exceptional.

▪ Suggested Reading

(Brearley et al. 1986; Osborne et al. 1968; Patnaik et al. 2008; Walker et al. 1993; Wilson et al. 2007; Wimberly and Lewis 1979)

7.1.5 Equine Renal Tumors

In general, renal tumors are uncommon in the horse, but the most common primary renal tumor is the *renal carcinoma* (TCC or adenocarcinoma). Carcinomas are usually found in *older* horses and have been reported to *metastasize.* Interestingly, *renal adenomas* are not as rare as in other species, but are frequently incidental findings, solitary, and well differentiated.

▪ Suggested Reading

(Haschek et al. 1981; Rhind et al. 1999; van Mol and Fransen 1986; Wise et al. 2009)

7.1.6 Equine Urinary Bladder Tumors

Primary urinary bladder tumors are uncommon in the horse. *Squamous cell carcinomas* (*SCC*) are most frequently described, followed by transitional cell carcinomas (TCC), polyps, rhabdomyosarcomas, and lymphomas. They are often *ulcerated* and can cause hematuria. SCC are histologically characterized by the lack of transitional cell areas, and they are less likely to metastasize than TCC. Similarly to dogs, the prognosis is dependent on invasiveness and occurrence of metastasis.

▪ Suggested Reading

(Fischer et al. 1985; Hurcombe et al. 2008; Patterson-Kane et al. 2000; Turnquist et al. 1993; Zantingh et al. 2012)

7.1.7 Bovine Renal Tumors

Renal tumors are rare neoplasms in cattle, and the most frequent neoplasms are *renal carcinomas. Cows* are more frequently affected than males which might be rather attributable to the fact that cows predominate in the population than being a true gender predisposition. In contrast to dogs and cats, the *metastatic rate* is *low* in cattle, but renal carcinomas are frequently *bilateral*. Distinctive features in cows are *proteinaceous secretions*, deposition of *hemosiderin*, and occurrence of *corpora amylacea*. Renal adenomas are more common in cattle than in dogs and cats and are usual incidental findings.

■ **Suggested Reading**

(Kelley et al. 1996; Nielsen et al. 1976b)

7.1.8 Bovine Urinary Bladder Tumors

There is a wide variety of neoplastic disease in the urinary bladder of cattle, accounting for economic losses in some areas of the world. Although they can be classified according to the WHO classification scheme of urinary bladder tumors in humans, from an economic point of view, their *pathogenesis* and *outcome* are more important than their subclassification. The most frequently observed symptom is *hematuria*, and the complex of various urinary bladder neoplasms in cattle is well known as *enzootic hematuria*.

7.1.8.1 Enzootic Hematuria

Box 7.5. Enzootic Hematuria in Six Facts

1. Commonly seen in areas in which bracken fern is common
2. Economically important disease in cattle in certain areas of the world
3. Development of a variety of urinary bladder tumors
4. Ptaquiloside of bracken fern as carcinogenic substance; BPV infection is cocarcinogenic
5. Hematuria often the only clinical sign
6. Ptaquiloside ingestion as possible threat for people

■ **Epidemiology and Pathogenesis**

Although this syndrome is seen *worldwide*, the incidence is varying and there are areas of the world in which up to 90 % of cattle can be affected. The *ingestion of ferns*, especially *bracken fern*, plays a major role in the development of urinary bladder tumors in cattle. Bracken fern is so far the only plant known to cause neoplastic disease in animals, and it contains several *carcinogenic substances*, *ptaquiloside* being the most important. Acute intoxication leads to severe hemorrhages in the urinary bladder, but in most cases ongoing *hematuria* is caused by the development of *ulcerated tumors* which are often located in ventral and lateral areas of the urinary bladder, the main sites of contact with urine.

A *variety of tumors* occur in the urinary bladder under the influence of bracken fern, and the most common are papillomas, fibromas, hemangiomas, hemangiosarcomas, and carcinomas. *More than one type* of neoplasm or mixed tumors can occur together. Local *invasion* is often seen in malignant tumors, and *metastasis* can be observed in *up to 10 %*. Bracken fern also drives the progression from benign urinary bladder tumors like papillomas to invasive squamous cell carcinomas. Furthermore, chronic bracken fern intoxication causes *immunosuppression* and promotes chronic *papillomatosis*, which is an important *cofactor* in neoplastic transformation. There are several different bovine papillomavirus (BPV) types known worldwide, but their importance as cocarcinogens varies, dependent on the tissue. Concerning neoplasms in the urinary bladder, *BPV-1*, *BPV-2*, and *BPV-13* are known to play an important role, and BPV-2 has also been found in the urothelium of healthy cattle. Many urinary bladder tumors express DNA encoding the *BPV-2 E5 oncoprotein* which causes neoplastic transformation by several molecular ways.

The occurrence of neoplastic disease due to bracken fern ingestion in cattle has also been linked to a high incidence of gastrointestinal tumors in humans, occurring mainly in areas in which bracken fern is common. Worldwide research is currently focusing on possible routes of intoxication (including consumption of contaminated milk) and possible consequences for people.

■ **Clinical Appearance**

Hematuria is the most common – but very unspecific – clinical sign of chronic bracken fern toxicity. This can also be caused by *acute* bracken fern *intoxication* or *urocystitis* which is seen commonly in concurrence with neoplastic growth.

Histopathology and Special Stains

On the basis of their growth pattern, tumors can be grouped into *four* distinct *categories*: *flat*, *exophytic* or papillary, *endophytic*, and *invasive*. It is important to note that hyperplastic and metaplastic changes often develop into malignant tumors. Immunohistochemical *uroplakin* intensity has been reported to decrease with growing malignancy of the urinary bladder tumors.

Therapy

Since enzootic hematuria is *incurable*, strong efforts are made to prevent the occurrence of enzootic hematuria rather than to treat already existing neoplasms in cattle. One approach is the development of inactivated and saponized *BPV-2 vaccines*.

Suggested Reading

(Ambrosio et al. 2001; Castillo et al. 1998; Cota et al. 2014; Hopkins 1986; Pires et al. 2010; Pathania et al. 2011; Pathania et al. 2012; Roperto et al. 2010; Sharma et al. 2013; Xu 1992)

7.2 Tumors of the Female Genital Tract

7.2.1 Ovarian Tumors

7.2.1.1 Canine Ovarian Tumors of the Dog

Ovarian tumors are *rare* in dogs with a prevalence of 0.5–1.2 % worldwide, most likely due to the practice of ovariohysterectomy in most areas of the world. The most common ovarian tumors in the dog are *epithelial* tumors. The *prognosis* is not dependent on histological type but on complete *excision* and *metastatic growth*.

Canine Epithelial Ovarian Tumors

Box 7.6. Epithelial Tumors of the Canine Ovary in Four Facts

1. Most common ovarian tumor in the bitch
2. Benign and malignant tumors, the latter being prone to intra-abdominal metastasis
3. Clinical signs often unspecific
4. Ovariohysterectomy is the therapy of choice

Epidemiology and Pathogenesis

Epithelial ovarian tumors arise from the *outer surface* of the ovary, and the majority is *malignant*. They can be divided into several histological subtypes. *Metastases*, especially seeding metastasis into the *abdominal cavity* and metastasis to the lymph nodes, liver, or omentum, are frequent. Epithelial ovarian tumors are more commonly *bilateral* than other ovarian tumors. Benign variants include rete adenomas, papillary adenomas, and cystadenomas. Epithelial ovarian tumors mainly develop in *older dogs* (mean age 10 years). *Pointers* seem to be predisposed.

Clinical Appearance

The main clinical signs result from the large palpable *abdominal mass* that causes displacement of the abdominal organs. Hormonal dysfunction is not to be expected with epithelial tumors, but *hypercalcemia* due to the production of PTH-rp (parathyroid hormone-related peptide) has been observed with ovarian adenocarcinomas. Ultrasonography is of use for the definitive diagnosis as well as for detection of metastases and uterine abnormalities. *Malignant* tumors appear mainly *solid* whereas *benign* tumors are often *cystic*. Thoracic radiographs may also be useful for excluding metastatic spread.

Cytology and Histopathology

Because of the high *risk of tumor seeding*, transabdominal aspiration is not indicated. *Abdominal fluid* may contain malignant epithelial tumor cells and can be useful for diagnosis. Histopathologically, the tumors can be classified into *subtypes*, but these are *without* any *prognostic consequences*. Differentiation between adenomas and adenocarcinomas is based on extension and invasion, mitotic index, and size. Immunohistochemically, epithelial ovarian tumors express *cytokeratin*, *vimentin*, *HBME-1*, and *desmin*, but not inhibin-α which is a specific marker for granulosa-theca cell tumors and can be used to distinguish these two tumors.

Therapy and Prognosis

The therapy of choice for epithelial ovarian tumors – as for any other ovarian tumor – is complete *ovariohysterectomy*. Bloodwork, especially the control of *thrombocytopenia*, is necessary prior to surgery because of possible *myelosuppressive effects* due to estrogen production. Exclusion of abdominal seeding metastases should follow ovariohysterectomy. The prognosis is generally good in the absence of metastases.

Canine Granulosa-Theca Cell Tumors

The *second most common* tumor of the canine ovary is the granulosa-theca cell tumor (or granulosa cell tumor), belonging to the group of sex cord-stromal tumors. They arise from the gonadal stroma and can produce a *variety of hormones* which are often responsible for *clinical signs* like vulvar enlargement, discharge, persistent estrus or pancytopenia (due to estrogen production), or cystic endometrial hyperplasia and pyometra (due to progesterone production). About *20%* of granulosa-theca cell tumors in the dog are *malignant*. When *metastases* occur, they are frequently to the *lymph nodes*, *pancreas*, or *lungs*. Abdominal seeding is not as common as with epithelial tumors, but does occur. *English Bulldogs*, *Boston Terriers*, and *German Shepherds* are described to be predisposed. An enhanced risk is reported when *residual ovarian tissue* is present after insufficient ovariohysterectomy. Immunohistochemistry with *inhibin-α* can be used to confirm the diagnosis. Besides specific hormonal effects, clinical signs are unspecific, and ovariohysterectomy is the therapy of choice.

Canine Teratomas and Dysgerminomas

Teratomas and dysgerminomas arise from primordial germ cells of the ovary and are often accompanied by uterine changes like *pyometra* or *endometrial hyperplasia* as well as *cystic* changes in the contralateral *ovary*. *Dysgerminomas* are usually unilateral, and metastatic rate is low (approximately 30%). They are comprised of a uniform cell population with germ cell appearance, and they usually do not form cysts. *Teratomas* are composed of cell populations of at least *two germ cell layers*, often including a variety of tissues like muscle, hair, adipose tissue, nervous tissue, etc. *Malignant* variants are not uncommon, and *metastasis*, mainly within the abdominal cavity, is reported in up to *50%* of cases. Teratomas may also be seen in younger bitches. *Ovariohysterectomy* is the therapeutic method of choice.

Other Tumors of the Canine Ovary

Other less common tumors of the ovary in the bitch include *thecomas* and *luteomas* which are benign sex cord-stromal tumors as well as rare mesenchymal tumors like *hemangiosarcomas*. Although rarely seen, the ovaries can also be the site of metastasis.

▪ Suggested Reading

(Akihara et al. 2007; Banco et al. 2011; Buijtels et al. 2010; Diez-Bru et al. 1998; Hori et al. 2006; McCandlish et al. 1979; Nielsen et al. 1976a; Patnaik and Greenlee 1987; Riccardi et al. 2007; Rota et al. 2013)

7.2.1.2 Feline Ovarian Tumors

The most common tumors in the feline ovary are *sex cord-stromal tumors*, and the most frequently observed is the granulosa-theca cell tumor.

7.2.1.3 Feline Granulosa-Theca Cell Tumor

Box 7.7. Feline Granulosa-Theca Cell Tumors in Five Facts

1. Most common ovarian tumor in cats, 50% malignant
2. Clinical signs often associated with hormone production
3. Some metastasize widely
4. Transabdominal aspiration or biopsy not indicated, but abdominal effusion can be useful for diagnosis
5. Therapy of choice: ovariohysterectomy

▪ Epidemiology and Pathogenesis

The *granulosa-theca cell tumor* is the *most frequent* ovarian tumor in the cat. 50 % of them exhibit *malignant* behavior. Similar to dogs, they are able to produce a variety of *hormones* which are often responsible for *clinical signs*. They are often *unilateral. Metastases* can be *widespread* including the peritoneum and omentum, lumbar lymph nodes, diaphragm, liver, kidney, spleen, and lung.

▪ Clinical Appearance

Similar to the dog, clinical signs are rather *unspecific* but can be dominated by the hormones produced by the tumor (▶ see section “Canine Granulosa-Theca Cell Tumors”). The space-occupying mass in the abdomen can also lead to lethargy, vomiting, and ascites.

▪ Cytology and Histopathology

Because of the high risk of tumor seeding, transabdominal aspiration is not indicated. *Abdominal fluid* can contain malignant epithelial tumor cells and can be used for diagnostic purposes. Histologically, cells in these tumors may resemble normal follicles, but the histologic arrangement is usually varied, and they often include *gland-like* or *rosette* patterns. In some well-differentiated tumors, *Call-Exner bodies* composed of protein globules surrounded by tumor cells can be detected histologically, but in most cases the arrangement of cells is more diffuse.

▪ Therapy and Prognosis

The therapy of choice is complete *ovariohysterectomy*, and careful exploration of the abdominal cavity for metastasis is crucial. *Prognosis* is dependent on *complete removal* and presence or absence of *metastases*.

Other Feline Ovarian Tumors

The *second* most common ovarian tumor in cats is the *dysgerminoma*, accounting for approximately 15 % of ovarian tumors. They are characterized by their often *large* size, *bilateral* growth, and *metastatic* spread in up to 33 % of cases. They usually do not show cyst formation. *Teratomas* and *epithelial* ovarian tumors are *rare*, and mesenchymal tumors are obviously not of importance in the feline ovary. The ovary can be the site of *metastasis of malignant lymphomas* (▶ see Chap. 6) in cats that are affected by multicentric lymphomas.

▪ Suggested Reading

(Cellio and Degner 2000; Gelberg and McEntee 1985)

Equine Ovarian Tumors

Granulosa-theca cell tumors are the most common ovarian tumors in the mare. Similar to other species, they can produce *estrogen* and *progesterone*, accounting for some of the clinical signs. In addition, the granulosa-theca cell tumors in horses frequently produce *testosterone*, and *male behavior* can be observed in mares with high blood testosterone levels. The tumor is often *unilateral*, and *atrophy* of the *contralateral ovary* is usually seen, which might be due to *inhibin-α* production. Function of the contralateral ovary can be restored after removal of the neoplastic ovary. Cyst formation and hemorrhage are common. *Surgery* of the ovary is the therapy of choice. Other tumors, including epithelial tumors, tumors of germ cells, and mesenchymal tumors, are rarely found in the equine ovary.

▪ Suggested Reading

(Bailey et al. 2002; McCue 1992; McCue et al. 2006; Norris et al. 1968; Stabenfeldt et al. 1979)

7.2.1.4 Bovine Ovarian Tumors

The most important ovarian tumor of cows is the *granulosa-theca cell tumor*. These tumors in cattle are mostly *benign* and *unilateral*, but metastases can occur. A predisposition is known for *daughters* of affected cows. After the unilateral tumor has been removed, a similar tumor develops in the *contralateral* ovary is seen in some cases. In early stages, a well-differentiated form with the presence of *Call-Exner bodies* composed of protein globules surrounded by tumor cells may be present. Due to the hormonal activity of the tumor, some affected cows show *nymphomania*. Tumors of the germ cells occur in cattle but are rare. *Surgery* is the treatment of choice. Only a few cases of epithelial ovarian tumors in cattle have been reported. *Vascular hamartomas* might be present in the ovaries of cattle and should not be confused with true neoplasms. A distinctive feature of this species is the occurrence of neoplastic cells of *malignant lymphomas in the corpora lutea*.

▪ Suggested Reading

(Dobson et al. 2013; El-Sheikh Ali et al. 2013; Garcia Iglesias et al. 1991; MacLachlan 1987; Meganck et al. 2011)

7.2.2 Uterine and Vaginal Tumors

7.2.2.1 Canine Uterine and Vaginal Tumors

In the dog, the most common tumors in the uterus and vagina are *leiomyomas*. Uterine tumors in dogs are not as common as vaginal tumors. *Middle-aged to older* dogs are often affected. Tumors can also be found at *uterus stumps* after incomplete ovariohysterectomy. Pregnancies do not protect from the development of uterine tumors.

Leiomyomas/Leiomyosarcomas

Box 7.8. Canine Leiomyomas/Leiomyosarcomas in Four Facts

1. Arise from smooth muscle of the uterus or vagina
2. Vaginal tumors more common than uterine
3. Most often benign
4. Ovariohysterectomy is usually curative, but leiomyosarcomas can metastasize widely

▪ Epidemiology and Pathogenesis

Leiomyomas arise from smooth muscle cells of the uterus or vagina, and although the malignant variant (leiomyosarcoma) occurs, the benign form is far more common. They occur focally or at multiple sites. They usually occur in *middle-aged to older* dogs without breed predisposition. *Leiomyomas* are nonrecurring after surgery, nonmetastatic, noninvasive, and slowly growing. They cannot be distinguished macroscopically from their malignant counterpart. For *vaginal leiomyosarcomas*, wide *metastasis* has been reported. Vaginal *leiomyomas* are often *hormone dependent*, and they commonly occur together with ovarian cysts or granulosa-theca cell tumors, endometrial or mammary hyperplasia, or mammary neoplasm.

Multifocal leiomyomas can occasionally occur together with renal cystadenomas and *nodular dermatofibrosis* in German Shepherd dogs.

▪ Clinical Appearance

Uterine leiomyomas are often *incidental* findings because they grow slowly and do not invade or metastasize. However, they can reach considerable size and cause symptoms due to *abdominal distension. Unspecific* clinical signs like polydipsia/polyuria, vomiting, and weight loss may occur, as well as abnormal estrus cycles and vaginal discharge. Leiomyosarcomas can appear as glandular cystic hyperplasia in ultrasonography. They have a glassy, white, or fleshy appearance. *Vaginal leiomyomas* often *protrude* from the *vulva*, and *vaginal bleeding, discharge,* or *dysuria/hematuria* can accompany this finding. Distinction is made between intra- and extraluminal vaginal leiomyomas, the latter often growing within the vaginal wall, causing coprostasis and swelling of the perineal region. Vaginal and rectal palpation, vaginoscopic examination, and cytology might be useful. Since the presence of the malignant variant cannot be ruled out grossly, *ultrasonographic examination* and *thoracic radiography* are useful to exclude metastatic spread. Ultrasonography of the uterine neoplasm is often variable. In *vaginal leiomyoma*, degenerative changes can lead to *liquefaction* and *cyst* formation. In contrast to vaginal prolapse, which is an important differential, tumors may be poorly circumscribed, are often located in the cranial portion of the vagina, and might be ulcerated and cause bloody discharge.

▪ Cytology and Histopathology

Although smooth muscle cells with elongated cytoplasm and blunt-ended (*cigar-shaped*) nuclei might be detectable in cytology, *histopathology* is inevitable for assessing complete excision and dignity. Leiomyomas are composed of spindle-shaped cells arranged in streams, bundles, or whorls with blunt-ended nuclei, indistinct cell borders, and eosinophilic fibrillary cytoplasm, with abundant stroma. The distinction between *leiomyomas* and *leiomyosarcomas* is basically made on *infiltrative* growth and *polymorphism* of the cells – even in the malignant variant, the *mitotic rate* may be *low*. Immunohistochemistry for smooth muscle actin (*SMA*) can be useful for the definitive diagnosis.

▪ Therapy and Prognosis

Complete *excision* of the neoplastic mass is recommended for vaginal and uterine leiomyomas, and *ovariohysterectomy* is the therapy of choice for the latter. Subtotal vaginectomy might be a possibility in some cases. Surgery is curative for benign tumors and usually – if complete – also for leiomyosarcomas. The presence of *metastasis* worsens the prognosis, and the patient has to be checked for local recurrence on a regular base.

Other Uterine and Vaginal Tumors

Fibrosarcomas, hemangiosarcomas, and lymphomas have been reported in the uterus of dogs, although they are rare, similar to *benign mesenchymal tumors. Epithelial* tumors are equally rare, but if they occur they are mostly *malignant*. A variety of mesenchymal tumors can be seen in the vagina and vulva of dogs, including lipoma in young dogs. Besides leiomyoma and leiomyosarcomas, the most common tumors in the vagina and vulva of dogs are *fibromas, fibroleiomyomas,* and *polyps.* Epithelial tumors occur rarely. Complete *excision* and *histopathology* are needed for the definitive diagnosis, and metastasis should be ruled out in case of suspected malignancy. Complete surgical excision/ovariohysterectomy is the therapy of choice. In case of extraluminal masses, a dorsal episiotomy can be useful.

▪ Suggested Reading

(Cave et al. 2002; Manothaiudom and Johnston 1991; Murphy et al. 1994; Nelissen and White 2012; Patsikas et al. 2014; Thacher and Bradley 1983; Tsioli et al. 2011; Weissman et al. 2013)

7.2.2.2 Feline Uterine and Vaginal Tumors

Feline Uterine Adenocarcinomas

Box 7.9. Feline Uterine Adenocarcinomas in Four Facts

1. Most common tumor in the feline uterus
2. Can metastasize widely, including the CNS, abdominal organs, and lung
3. Immunohistochemical markers include COX-2 and cytokeratin
4. Ovariohysterectomy is the therapy of choice; prognosis depends on metastatic spread

▪ Epidemiology and Pathogenesis

The most common tumor in the feline uterus is the *adenocarcinoma* arising from the uterine gland epithelium, which can also arise in the uterine stump. *Widespread metastases* into nearly every organ have been reported.

▪ Clinical Appearance

Similar to uterine tumors in dogs, clinical signs are often nonspecific, including *inappetence, polydipsia, polyuria,* or *vomiting.* Abdominal distension and other signs associated with space occupation can be observed as well. Complete *staging* including radiography of the thorax and abdominal ultrasonography is recommended because of a high *metastatic risk.* Since metastatic spread can also involve the *brain, central nervous signs* may accompany other clinical symptoms.

▪ Cytology and Histopathology

Although cytology can be helpful in confirming the suspected diagnosis, *histopathological* examination of the excised neoplasm is needed for definitive diagnosis and assessing *invasiveness* and *surgical margins.* Immunohistochemically, these tumors routinely express *cytokeratin, COX-2, E-cadherin,* and *β-catenin.*

▪ Therapy and Prognosis

Ovariohysterectomy is recommended for the therapy of uterine carcinomas. The prognosis largely depends on the presence of *metastasis.* Most uterine adenocarcinomas have already metastasized at the time of diagnosis. Chemotherapeutic approaches are not well established yet.

Mesenchymal and Metastatic Tumors

In the feline uterus, *mesenchymal* tumors, including leiomyosarcomas, rhabdomyosarcomas, fibrosarcomas, and muellerian tumors, have been reported, as well as their benign counterparts (leiomyoma, fibroma). Lipomas and hemangiomas also occur. The uterus of cats can be involved in multicentric tumor spread of *malignant lymphoma* (▶ see Chap. 6). All of these primary tumors are rare compared to uterine adenocarcinomas, and the treatment of choice is always complete *ovariohysterectomy.*

In contrast, the *most common vaginal tumor* in cats is the *leiomyoma,* similar to the situation in dogs, although vaginal tumors in the cat are generally rare. They occur most commonly in older queens. Diagnostic approaches, therapy, and prognosis are similar to vaginal leiomyomas in dogs (▶ see Sect. 7.2.2.1).

▪ Suggested Reading

(Anderson and Pratschke 2011; Cooper et al. 2006; Gil da Costa et al. 2009; Miller et al. 2003; Sato et al. 2007)

7.2.2.3 Equine Uterine and Vaginal Tumors

Uterine tumors are *very rare* in horses. Of these, *leiomyomas* appear to be the most common. Case reports also describe a variety of other mesenchymal tumors. Uterine leiomyomas in the mare are either *pedunculated* or *intramural.* Clinical signs and diagnostic features are comparable to those of the bitch and the queen. Leiomyomas usually have *a good prognosis* after complete removal, but the prognosis for *leiomyosarcomas* is *guarded*. Epithelial tumors are exceptional.

- **Suggested Reading**

(Broome et al. 1992; Govaere et al. 2011; Hurcombe et al. 2008)

7.2.2.4 Bovine Uterine and Vaginal Tumors

Carcinomas are the most frequent tumors of the bovine uterus, and conversely, cows seem to be affected by uterine carcinomas more frequently than other species. The tumors can be *single* or *multiple* and often show a strong *desmoplastic reaction* which results in a firm and contracted appearance. *Metastasis* is not uncommon, and the regional *lymph nodes* and the *lung* are usually involved. *Leiomyomas* also occur and resemble their counterparts in the bitch and queen with regard to appearance and prognosis. The uterus can be a site of metastatic spread of malignant *lymphomas* as well.

Vaginal tumors are not common in cows, but *fibropapillomas* in the *vulva* have been described and are thought to be caused by *bovine papillomavirus* (*BPV*)*-1* infection. Large nuclei, prominent bizarre nucleoli, and *high mitotic rate* are common and should not be interpreted as signs of malignancy. *Desmoplasia* and surface *ulceration* can occur. Vulvar fibropapillomas usually *spontaneously regress* within 6 months.

- **Suggested Reading**

(Elsinghorst et al. 1984; Elzein et al. 1991; Garcia-Iglesias et al. 1995)

7.3 Tumors of the Male Genital Tract

7.3.1 Testicular Tumors

7.3.1.1 Canine Testicular Tumors

Testicular tumors are common in dogs, and the *cryptorchid* testis is especially predisposed for developing neoplasms. More than one type of tumor can occur together in one testis. Metastatic risk depends on the type of tumor. Dogs often present clinically with symptoms ascribed to *hormonal activity* of the tumor, especially in the case of interstitial cell tumors and Sertoli cell tumors.

Box 7.10. Canine Testicular Tumors in Five Facts

1. Most common testicular tumors in the dog are seminomas, Sertoli cell tumors, and interstitial cell tumors
2. Adult to old dogs most commonly affected, cryptorchidism as an important predisposition
3. Sertoli cell tumors and interstitial cell tumors cause feminization and myelosuppression
4. Metastatic spread reported for up to 15 % of Sertoli cell tumors, also seen in seminomas
5. Castration is always the therapy of choice, regardless of the type of tumor

- **Epidemiology and Pathogenesis**

Testicular tumors are *common* in the dog, with *up to 17%* of a population affected. The main important types are *seminomas, Sertoli cell tumors,* and *interstitial cell tumors* (syn. Leydig cell tumors), but mixed germ cell sex cord-stromal tumors (neoplastic Sertoli and germ cells) also occur. Most testicular tumors in the dog are *benign*, although malignant Sertoli cell tumors and seminomas have been reported. The only way to confirm malignancy is *detection of metastasis. Mature* and *old* animals are usually affected, and the *right testicle* is more often affected than the left. Seminomas are derived from cells of the spermatogenic population, thus resembling dysgerminomas in the ovary. Sertoli cell tumors are of gonadostromal origin and are comparable with granulosa-theca cell tumors in bitches. Interstitial cell tumors are derived from the endocrine gonadostromal cell population. Mixed tumors also occur. Teratomas are very rare in the dog. *Cryptorchidism* is a *risk factor* especially for the development of Sertoli cell tumors and seminomas. Interstitial tumors are often bilateral and/or multiple. Adenomas/adenocarcinomas arising from the rete testis are rare.

- **Clinical Appearance**

The main clinical finding in non-cryptorchid dogs is unilateral *enlargement* of the testis, often accompanied by *atrophy* of the *contralateral* testis. Clinical signs suspicious for testicular tumors include symptoms that are caused by *hormonal imbalances* in both cryptorchid and non-cryptorchid dogs. *Feminization* including vulvar swelling, gynecomastia and galactorrhea, bilateral alopecia (◘ Fig. 7.2), and testicular atrophy are often seen, and high *estradiol concentration* in the blood can lead to *bone marrow depletion*, which is a serious consequence. Feminization, particularly common in Sertoli cell tumors of cryptorchid testes, tends to be reversible after removal of the testis, but the bone marrow depletion may be permanent. *Squamous metaplasia* of the *prostate* can lead to symptoms of prostatic lesions, thus thorough examination of the testis is necessary in all cases with prostatic symptoms. Inhibin production with inhibiting effects on LH and FSH production has also been described in Sertoli cell tumors, leading to reduced testosterone production. *Interstitial cell tumors* are capable of producing *testosterone*, and *hyperandrogenism* with dominant behavior in affected dogs has been described, but elevated *estrogen* levels are observed more often. *Perianal gland* and *tail gland hyperplasia* as well as *prostatic enlargement* can accompany *interstitial cell tumors*. There is only one description of hormonal imbalance in a patient with seminoma. They usually do not produce hormones. *Hypertrophic osteopathy* has also been described in cases with testicular tumors.

Metastasis is mainly reported for *Sertoli cell tumors*, with up to 15 % of neoplasms metastasizing to regional *lymph nodes*, whereas *seminomas* metastasize more rarely but often *widespread*, including the lymph nodes, lung, kidney, and *unusual sites* like the brain, eye, or skin. Sertoli cell tumors can reach considerable size, whereas interstitial tumors are mainly small and tend to be multiple. *Ectopic* or *residual testicular tissue* might also become the origin of neoplastic growth – thus, testicular tumors cannot be excluded in castrated dogs. *Sertoli cell tumors* may *invade* local *veins* and *lymphatics*, causing enlargement of the scrotal area.

Ultrasonography is recommended for all cases with suspected neoplastic growth in *cryptorchid* testes and is also useful for the exclusion of *metastases*. The presumptive diagnosis should be confirmed by fine needle aspiration and *cytology* or *histopathology*. Advanced *cytopenia* due to bone marrow suppression can lead to severe clinical symptoms, and bone marrow cytology is recommended before castration.

Gross morphology is rather distinctive in many cases of testicular tumors. *Interstitial cell tumors*

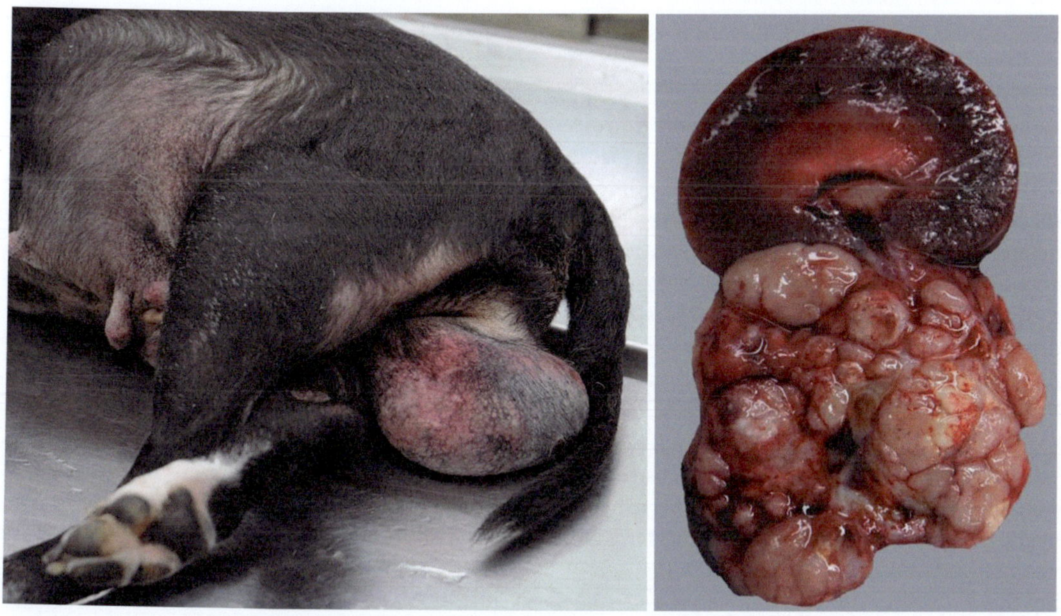

◘ **Fig. 7.2** *Left*: Sertoli cell tumor in a 14-year-old dog. Note the bilateral alopecia, hyperplasia of the mammary gland, and enlargement and hyperkeratosis of the teats, common effects caused by hormone production. *Right*: Sertoli cell tumor of a cryptorchid testis with typical fibrous appearance (With permission of (*left*) Archive of the Institute for Veterinary Pathology and (*right*) R. Klopfleisch, Freie Universität Berlin, Germany)

are often *yellow* and show multiple areas of *hemorrhage* and/or *cysts*. They often cause atrophy of the surrounding tissue. *Seminomas* tend to be *white* and *soft*, whereas *Sertoli cell tumors* are *whitish* and produce collagen, giving them a *tough desmoplastic* appearance (◘ Fig. 7.2).

▪ Cytology and Histopathology

Fine needle aspiration and cytology can confirm the presumptive diagnosis of testicular tumors, but since castration is the therapy of choice, cytology is often not necessary. There are *no* cytological or histological *markers of malignancy*. Cytological appearance is comparable to the histologic findings. Cells of *interstitial cell tumors* are round to polyhedral, with abundant, granular, or finely *vacuolated* cytoplasm which can contain yellow pigment. They may have a more mesenchymal appearance, but stroma is always scant and mitotic rate is low. A specific feature of interstitial cell tumors is the presence of *intranuclear, PAS-positive* cytoplasmic invaginations. *Seminomas* are divided into intratubular or diffuse forms and are composed of sheets of polyhedral cells with large nuclei and scant, often deeply basophilic, sometimes acidophilic cytoplasm. Special features of seminomas include accumulations of *CD8 lymphocytes* and the presence of *multinucleated* cells, and they stain positive for *vimentin* and negative for NSE. Mitoses and individual cell necrosis can be found in seminomas. *Sertoli cell tumors* can also be divided into intratubular and diffuse types, and the specific feature is a *high amount of stroma*. Neoplastic cells can resemble normal palisading Sertoli cells arranged in tubules in highly differentiated neoplasms, in which large *lipid droplets* may be present in the cytoplasm as well. Poorly differentiated Sertoli cell tumors often lose their ability to palisade and show small intracytoplasmic lipid droplets. *Sertoli cell tumors* are the only testicular neoplasms positive for *NSE*.

▪ Therapy and Prognosis

The therapy of choice is *castration*. In case of infiltrative growth, *resection of the scrotum* might be necessary. Abdominal tumors might be highly vascularized and caution is advised when removing these tumors. *The regional lymph nodes* have to be checked for metastases and need to be resected if necessary. Surgery is usually *curative*. *Chemotherapy* can be of use in metastatic tumors, although there are not many reports in veterinary medicine. The prognosis in general is good, but can be affected by *metastatic* spread or *myelosuppression*.

▪ Suggested Reading

(Banco et al. 2015; Grieco et al. 2008; Hayes et al. 1985; Hogenesch et al. 1987; Johnston et al. 1991; Liao et al. 2009; Lucas et al. 2012; Masserdotti et al. 2005; Mischke et al. 2002; Quartuccio et al. 2012; Sanpera et al. 2002; Spugnini et al. 2000; Weaver 1983; Yu et al. 2009)

7.3.1.2 Feline Testicular Tumors

Testicular tumors have only *sporadically* been described in the cat, which might be associated with the fact that most male cats are castrated at an early age. Sertoli cell tumors, seminomas, interstitial cell tumors, and mixed tumors have been diagnosed. Clinical appearance, histology, and prognosis are comparable to their canine counterparts. *Interstitial cell tumors* may be seen in young *cats*. *Castration* is usually curative.

▪ Suggested Reading

(Miller et al. 2007; Rosen and Carpenter 1993; Tucker and Smith 2008)

7.3.1.3 Equine Testicular Tumors

The most common testicular tumors of the *adult to aged* horse are *seminomas* which can become very large and metastasize widely. Notably, the most common tumors in the *young horse* are testicular *teratomas*, which rarely occur in other species. In horses, teratomas are usually *benign* and they occur in both *scrotal* and *cryptorchid* testes. They usually do not exceed 10 cm in diameter and can be composed of a *variety of tissues* including hair, adipose or sebaceous tissue, or bone. *Interstitial cell tumors* virtually occur in the *cryptorchid* testis only, and they are either well differentiated or contain spindle-shaped neoplastic cells. There are only single reports of Sertoli cell tumors in the stallion. *Hormonally induced changes* have *not* been described in stallions in detail – thus, the most prominent clinical signs are *enlargement of the testis* or symptoms ascribed to a mass effect in the abdominal cavity. *Surgery* is the therapy of choice.

▪ Suggested Reading

(Brinsko 1998; Duncan 1998; Gelberg and McEntee 1987; Govaere et al. 2010; Hunt et al. 1990; De Lange et al. 2015; Pollock et al. 2002)

7.3.1.4 Bovine Testicular Tumors

Testicular tumors are *rare* in cattle. *Interstitial cell tumors* have been reported most often, and there is a comparable higher prevalence in old *Guernseys*. Sertoli cell tumors also occur, and they can be found in young or even newborn bulls, pointing toward a role of genetic factors.

Suggested Reading

(Jensen et al. 2008; López et al. 1994)

7.3.2 Prostatic Tumors

7.3.2.1 Canine Prostatic Tumors

Box 7.11. Canine Prostatic Tumors in Four Facts

1. Rare tumors in dogs; benign prostate hyperplasia is far more common
2. More than 80 % of prostate carcinomas with metastases at the time of diagnosis, bone involvement common
3. Clinical symptoms unspecific, cytology or histopathology needed
4. Surgery often the only possible therapeutic approach but seldom curative; combination with chemotherapy is possible, but with severe side effects

Epidemiology and Pathogenesis

Tumors of the prostate do not often occur in dogs, and *benign prostatic hyperplasia* (*BPH*) is *much more common* in cases of enlarged prostate. Prostate carcinomas most often occur in *older* animals although dogs as young as 4 years can be affected. *Large breeds* tend to be overrepresented. *Adenocarcinomas* are most common, whereas transitional cell carcinomas, squamous cell carcinomas, adenomas, and mesenchymal tumors occur much less frequently. Some authors describe an increased risk for *castrated dogs*. Bouvier des Flandres dogs are significantly overrepresented in some studies. Prostatic adenocarcinomas in dogs derive from basal cells of the *ductular epithelium*. *Mixed variants* have also been reported, and as distinction is sometimes difficult, the use of the term *prostate carcinoma* is recommended. Because of the high incidence of BPH compared with rare cases of prostatic adenocarcinomas, it is questionable whether the development of a prostatic neoplasm is a multistage process. Prostatic carcinomas usually occur independently of testicular tumors.

Clinical Appearance

Although clinical signs are often those of *prostatic enlargement* which can also been seen in prostatic hyperplasia, *lameness* and *pain* in the pelvis should raise suspicion for a neoplastic disease, since *metastasis* to the *bones* (vertebra, bones of the pelvis, long bones) is common. Emaciation, hematuria, stranguria, polydipsia, and polyuria have also been described. Compared to benign prostate hyperplasia, prostatic carcinomas tend to be *more irregular in shape* and *firmer* at palpation and sometimes contain *ossifying or mineralized areas*. Firm adhesion of the prostate to the pelvis may be seen, and metastases also occur in the ribs, scapula, and digits. Cytology or histopathology is necessary to confirm the diagnosis. Since detection of neoplastic cells in the ejaculate is not evidentiary, *fine needle aspiration* under ultrasonography or *biopsies* are more useful, but care has to be taken to avoid tumor seeding. Aspiration biopsy via catheter is common and has a specificity of 98 %. *Radiography* is helpful for the detection of lung or bone metastasis. Enlargement of the *sublumbar lymph nodes* and *mineralized foci* in the prostate is nearly pathognomonic for prostatic carcinomas in *castrated* dogs, but not in uncastrated dogs. Sonography is not useful to distinguish between prostatic tumors and nonneoplastic disease but *mineralization*, *asymmetry*, and *infiltrative growth* point toward neoplasm. Prostate-specific tumor markers are not useful for tumor diagnostics in the dog.

Cytology and Histopathology

Up to 75 % of cytological diagnoses are concordant with histopathology, and in cases where cytology confirms the presence of a carcinoma, additional histopathological analysis is neither necessary nor recommended. Prostatic carcinoma cells are usually *heterogenic*, and this is the most suspicious feature, with neoplasms showing evidence of high *anisocytosis*. Inflammatory cells in cytology do not rule out neoplastic growth. Some tumor cells exhibit a *signet-ring pattern*. If they form well-differentiated acini, *mucus* can often be detected in their lumen. Up to *50* % of prostatic tumors show a *mixed morphology* with a variety of differentiation stages, including urothelial, squamoid, sarcomatoid, or glandular cells.

- **Therapy and Prognosis**

Prostatectomy is a possible therapy in prostate carcinomas but can be difficult due to *high invasiveness, metastatic spread,* and *postoperative complications* and is seldom curative. Furthermore, *incontinence* is a common sequel of prostatectomy. *Incomplete resection* of the prostate combined with *chemotherapy* prevents from incontinence in some cases, but may result in serious life-threatening side effects. *Prognosis* is thus always *guarded* or *poor*. In up to 80% of cases, *metastatic spread* is present at the time of diagnosis. Survival time without surgery or chemotherapy can be as short as 30 days after diagnosis. *Chemotherapeutic* approaches have not been regularly used, and outcome is not predictable. A combination of gemcitabine and carboplatin as well as treatment with mitoxantrone alone has been described, resulting in longer survival times. Dogs treated with piroxicam and carprofen had longer survival times than untreated dogs in one study. *NSAIDs* alone can result in significant improvement. *Radiotherapy* bears the risk of a variety of severe side effects, but in cases without side effects, survival time can be increased up to 12 months. In cases of urethral obstruction, a palliative approach is *catheterization* or *stent* implantation.

- **Suggested Reading**

(Bryan et al. 2007; Cooley and Waters 1998; Cornell et al. 2000; Dominguez et al. 2009; Freitag et al. 2007; LeRoy and Northrup 2009; Powe et al. 2004; Smith 2008; Weisse et al. 2006)

7.3.2.2 Feline Prostatic Tumors

Prostatic tumors in the cat do occur, but are *rare*. As in dogs, most tumors of the feline prostate are *malignant*, and biphasic carcinomas with more than one cell type have been reported as well. The few cases reported were *older, castrated* cats. Clinical behavior is comparable to that in the dog, with *high metastatic risk* including to the lung and abdominal organs. In contrast to prostate carcinomas in dogs, those of the cat have not been described to metastasize into bone. Clinical symptoms are comparable to those in dogs, with the exemption of bone pain, lameness, and stiff gait. *Resection* of the tumor seems to result in *longer survival time* with *fewer complications* compared to dogs, but too few cases have been described to allow for a general statement. *Chemotherapeutic* approaches with doxorubicin and cyclophosphamide have also been described in the cat, with survival times of up to 10 months.

- **Suggested Reading**

(Caney et al. 1998; Hubbard et al. 1990; LeRoy and Lech 2004; Zambelli et al. 2010)

7.3.2.3 Prostatic Tumors in Other Species

Prostatic tumors are not of relevance in other species.

7.3.3 Penile Tumors

7.3.3.1 Equine Penile Squamous Cell Carcinomas

Box 7.12. Equine Penile Squamous Cell Tumors in Four Facts

1. Most common penile or preputial tumor in the horse
2. Characteristics: cauliflower-like, ulcerated appearance, and being much larger than papillomas
3. Tend to metastasize to regional lymph nodes
4. Surgery as the therapy of choice

- **Epidemiology and Pathogenesis**

Horses affected by preputial or penile squamous cell carcinomas (SCC) are usually *older than 12 years* with a mean age of *19.5 years*, and a history of squamous papilloma at the same site is often noted; thus, this lesion might be predisposing for the development of an SCC. Most tumors arise in the glans penis, and equally to SCC in other locations, they often *ulcerate*. They can also be located at *the body of the penis* or the *inner lamina* of the *preputial fold* or at the *external fold* of the prepuce. Equine papillomavirus type 2 (EcPV2) has been identified in genital SCC as well as in normal genital mucosa, and the E6/E7 oncogenes of EcPV2 are present in the majority of neoplastic cells and in metastases.

▪ Clinical Appearance

The appearance of a penile or preputial SCC is a *large, cauliflower-like, ulcerated mass*, and they tend to be very *firm* due to an intense *desmoplastic* response. In contrast, *squamous papillomas* are usually small and exhibit a *papilliform growth* with less desmoplasia. Horses may show signs of purulent or sanguineous *discharge*. Of note, up to 25 % of penile or preputial SCC in the horse have already *metastasized* to regional *lymph nodes* at the time of diagnosis. Metastasis to the lung and liver has also been reported, but is less common.

▪ Cytology and Histopathology

Since SCC in general tend to be heavily *ulcerated* and/or *necrotic*, cytology can yield false-negative results of *suppurative* and *necrotizing inflammation* due to the high amount of *neutrophils* admixed with the tumor cells (◘ Figs. 7.3, 7.4, 7.5, and 7.6). The presence of neutrophils and the report of an ulcerative mass at the penis or prepuce of a horse should raise suspicion for SCC, and histopathology is recommended to confirm the diagnosis. The tumor is usually *heavily keratinized*, multifocally *necrotic*, and/or *mineralized*, and infiltration by neutrophils and *eosinophils* is common. SCC with *poor differentiation* tend to metastasize more often than their well-differentiated counterparts.

▪ Therapy and Prognosis

Surgery with various dimensions is the therapy of choice for penile SCC, and depending on the location and the invasiveness of the tumor, phallectomy, segmental posthectomy, phallectomy plus segmental posthectomy, or en bloc resection of the penis, prepuce, and superficial inguinal lymph nodes might be necessary. Apart from local side effects shortly after the resection, *prognosis* can be *good to fair*, but up to 19 % of horses are reported to show recurrence after resection.

▪ Suggested Reading

(Doles et al. 2001; Mair et al. 2000; van den Top et al. 2008; Vanderstraeten et al. 2011; Zhu et al. 2015)

7.3.3.2 Other Penile Tumors

Fibropapillomas in *bulls* are caused by *bovine papillomavirus-2*. They are usually multiple and can reach considerable size. They are often seen in *younger* bulls, in which they are highly cellular and contain many *mitoses*. They show benign behavior without metastasis, but large fibropapillomas can *impair retraction* of the glans, thus predisposing for infections or necrosis. Urethal obstruction and urethral disruption have been observed.

Squamous cell carcinomas (SCC) of the penis or prepuce do occur in *dogs* but are much less frequent than in horses. They are associated with *papilloma virus infection*, as are papillomas. Cases

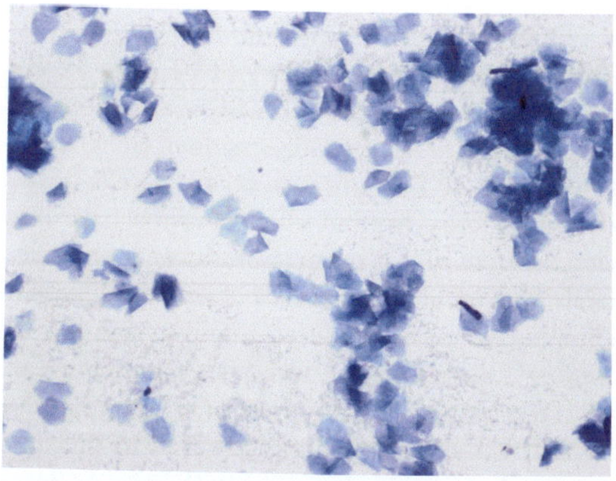

◘ **Fig. 7.3** Cytology, imprint of a normal penis, healthy horse, May-Grünwald-Giemsa, 100x. Note the numerous anucleate well-differentiated squamous epithelial cells (Photo: with permission of Dr. N. Bauer, Faculty of Veterinary Medicine, Justus-Liebig-University, Giessen, Germany)

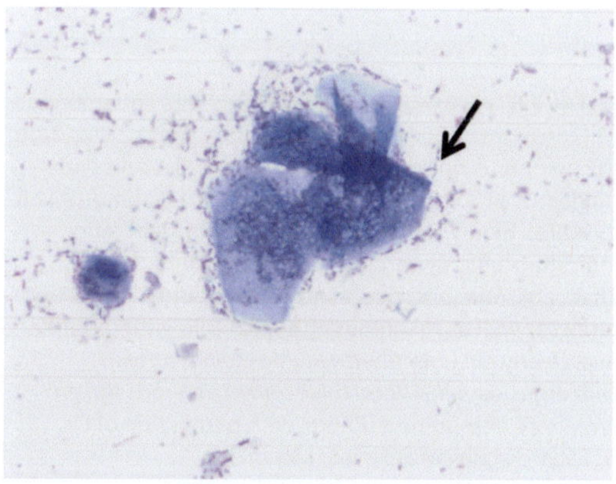

◘ **Fig. 7.4** Cytology, imprint of a normal penis, healthy horse, May-Grünwald-Giemsa, 500×. Note the anucleate well-differentiated squamous epithelial cells surrounded and covered by numerous bacterial organisms (*black arrow*) (Photo: with permission of Dr. N. Bauer, Faculty of Veterinary Medicine, Justus-Liebig-University, Giessen, Germany)

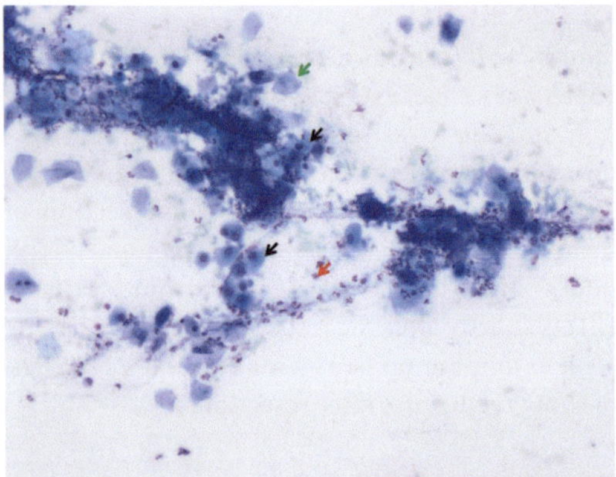

Fig. 7.5 Cytology, imprint of penis with squamous cell carcinomas, horse, May-Grünwald-Giemsa, 100×. Note the numerous nucleate squamous epithelial cells with moderate anisocytosis, anisokaryosis, and pleomorphism (*black arrow*). There are frequent, often degenerate neutrophils (*red arrow*) and few anucleate squamous epithelial cells (*green arrow*) (Photo: with permission of Dr. N. Bauer, Faculty of Veterinary Medicine, Justus-Liebig-University, Giessen, Germany)

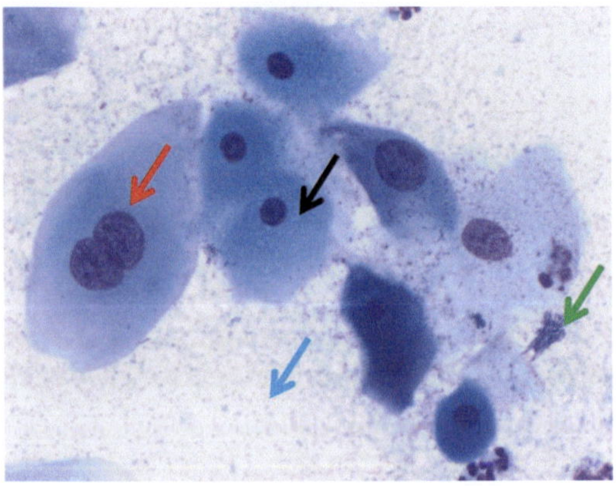

Fig. 7.6 Cytology, imprint of penis with squamous cell carcinomas, horse, May-Grünwald-Giemsa, 500×. Note the numerous nucleate squamous epithelial cells with moderate anisocytosis, anisokaryosis, and pleomorphism as well as highly variable nuclear-to-cytoplasm ratio indicating a highly variable degree of differentiation. There are some binucleate squamous epithelial cells (*red arrow*) as well as squamous epithelial cells with multiple fine, clearly circumscribed vacuoles (*black arrow*). Numerous bacterial cocci (*blue arrow*) and rods (*green arrow*) are also present (Photo: with permission of Dr. N. Bauer, Faculty of Veterinary Medicine, Justus-Liebig-University, Giessen, Germany)

of idiopathic penile squamous papillomas are described. They are usually not heavily keratinized. The mean age in dogs is *10 years. Schnauzers* are predisposed.

There are single case reports of melanomas, malignant lymphomas, mast cell tumors, plasmacytomas, hemangiosarcomas, and osteosarcomas in the canine penis. *Osteosarcomas* have a high potential for *recurrence*, and *prognosis* is usually *guarded* in these tumors. *Amputation* of the penis or the glans penis might be curative.

Suggested Reading

(Bocaneti et al. 2015; Cornegliani et al. 2007; Nasir and Campo 2008; Peppler et al. 2009; Wakui et al. 1992; Yaghoobi Yeganeh Manesh et al. 2014)

7.4 Transmissible Venereal Tumor (TVT) in Male and Female Dogs

Box 7.13 Transmissible Venereal Tumor in Five Facts

1. Tumor cells transmitted directly via coitus or sniffing
2. Arise at the outer genital of female and male dogs, but can also be located in the eye, nasal cavity, oral cavity, and skin
3. Often spontaneously regress
4. Treatment with chemotherapeutics is usually successful and results in regression
5. Surgery is not recommended

Epidemiology and Pathogenesis

Transmissible venereal tumors (TVT, syn. *Sticker sarcoma*) are transmitted directly via *cell implantation* and grow in a graft-like manner. Genetically, tumor cells of TVT are distinct from cells of the dogs they arise in, and all neoplasms have one *clonal origin*. TVT occur *worldwide* with especially high incidences in areas of *warm* and *humid* climate and are transmitted mainly via *coitus* or *sniffing*. Latency before tumor development can be 2–6 months. TVT are most often found at the *vagina* or *vestibulum* where they arise in the submucosa, but can also be found in the *oral* or *nasal cavity* and in the *skin*. In male dogs, the most common site is the *root of the penis*. *Metastasis* occurs mainly to the regional lymph nodes and is generally *rare*, but metastatic risk is *high* in *immunocompromised* individuals. Metastases to the *brain* and *eye* have been reported as well. Spontaneous *regression* accompanied by *lymphocytic* infiltration can occur and leads to lifelong *immunity*, but is not expected after 6 months of tumor growth. Tumor cells can evade the immune system by producing a tumor-associated antigen.

▪ Clinical Appearance

The most frequent clinical symptom is bloody or mucoid *discharge*. The neoplastic mass is either located at the vulva or deep in the vagina. TVT are usually focal, *multilobulated*, *glassy*, *red*, and highly *vascularized*. In male dogs, they appear as *single or multiple* nodules which are *sessile* or *pedunculated* and can reach a diameter of up to 15 cm. The surface can resemble that of a squamous cell carcinoma with cauliflower-like appearance, thus sometimes looking more malignant than they are. *Metastases* to the regional lymph nodes, eyes, central nervous system, skeletal muscle, or abdominal organs must be excluded. *Erythrocytosis* has been described as a paraneoplastic syndrome in TVT.

▪ Cytology and Histopathology

Cytology is useful for the *diagnosis* of TVT and often allows for a definitive diagnosis. The round, oval, or polygonal neoplastic cells resemble *histiocytic cells* with high amounts of bluish cytoplasm with or without vacuoles, round nuclei, and prominent nucleoli. *Variability* in cell *size* is common, and *mitotic figures* are usually *numerous*. TVT are vimentin positive and cytokeratin, CD3, CD79α, and S100 negative.

▪ Therapy and Prognosis

Chemotherapy is recommended, and good results have been obtained with vincristine alone or in combination with cyclophosphamide and methotrexate. Recurrence is very rare. Chemotherapy also leads to *remission* of *extragenital* tumors and/or metastases. Gene therapy with IL-12 or IL-2 (alone or in combination with vincristine) has been reported to be successful. In contrast, *surgery is not recommended* and usually leads to recurrence of TVT. *Prognosis* after chemotherapy is usually *good*, but is guarded in older dogs and dogs with very large tumor masses.

▪ Suggested Reading

(Amber et al. 1990; Den Otter et al. 2015; Ferreira et al. 2000; Gonzalez et al. 2000; Mozos et al. 1996; Mukaratirwa and Gruys 2003; Murchison et al. 2014; Murgia et al. 2006; Nak et al. 2005; Park et al. 2006; Strakova and Murchison 2015)

Suggested Reading

Akihara Y, Shimoyama Y, Kawasako K, Komine M, Hirayama K, Kagawa Y, Omachi T, Matsuda K, Okamoto M, Kadosawa T, Taniyama H (2007) Immunohistochemical evaluation of canine ovarian tumors. J Vet Med Sci 69(7):703–708

Amber EI, Henderson RA, Adeyanju JB, Gyang EO (1990) Single-drug chemotherapy of canine transmissible venereal tumor with cyclophosphamide, methotrexate, or vincristine. J Vet Intern Med 4(3):144–147

Ambrosio V, Borzacchiello G, Bruno F, Galati P, Roperto F (2001) Uroplakin expression in the urothelial tumors of cows. Vet Pathol 38(6):657–660

Anderson C, Pratschke K (2011) Uterine adenocarcinoma with abdominal metastases in an ovariohysterectomised cat. J Feline Med Surg 13(1):44–47

Bailey MT, Troedsson MH, Wheato JE (2002) Inhibin concentrations in mares with granulosa cell tumors. Theriogenology 57(7):1885–1895

Banco B, Antuofermo E, Borzacchiello G, Cossu-Rocca P, Grieco V (2011) Canine ovarian tumors: an immunohistochemical study with HBME-1 antibody. J Vet Diagn Invest 23(5):977–981

Banco B, Giudice C, Ghisleni G, Romussi S, Behar DK, Grieco V (2015) Immunohistochemical study of mixed germ cell sex cord stromal tumours in 13 canine testes. J Comp Pathol 152:182–187

Batchelor DJ, Bright SR, Ibarrola P, Tzannes S, Blackwood L (2006) Long-term survival after combination chemotherapy for bilateral renal malignant lymphoma in a dog. N Z Vet J 54(3):147–150

Battaglia L, Petterino C, Zappulli V, Castagnaro M (2005) Hypoglycaemia as a paraneoplastic syndrome associated with renal adenocarcinoma in a dog. Vet Res Commun 29(8):671–675

Bocaneti F, Altamura G, Corteggio A, Velescu E, Borzacchiello G (2015) Expression of bcl-2 and p53 in bovine cutaneous fibropapillomas. Infect Agent Cancer 10(1):2

Brearley MJ, Thatcher C, Cooper JE (1986) Three cases of transitional cell carcinoma in the cat and a review of the literature. Vet Rec 118(4):91–94

Brinsko SP (1998) Neoplasia of the male reproductive tract. Vet Clin North Am Equine Pract 14(3):517–533

Broome TA, Allen D, Baxter GM, Pugh DG, Mahaffey E (1992) Septic metritis secondary to torsion of a pedunculated uterine fibroleiomyoma in a filly. J Am Vet Med Assoc 200(11):1685–1688

Bryan JN, Henry CJ, Turnquist SE, Tyler JW, Liptak JM, Rizzo SA, Sfiligoi G, Steinberg SJ, Smith AN, Jackson T (2006) Primary renal neoplasia of dogs. J Vet Intern Med 20(5):1155–1160

Bryan JN, Keeler MR, Henry CJ, Bryan ME, Hahn AW, Caldwell CW (2007) A population study of neutering status as a risk factor for canine prostate cancer. Prostate 67(11):1174–1181

7

Budreckis DM, Byrne BA, Pollard RE, Rebhun RB, Rodriguez CO Jr, Skorupski KA (2015) Bacterial urinary tract infections associated with transitional cell carcinoma in dogs. J Vet Intern Med 29(3):828–833
Buijtels JJ, de Gier J, Kooistra HS, Kroeze EJ, Okkens AC (2010) Alterations of the pituitary-ovarian axis in dogs with a functional granulosa cell tumor. Theriogenology 73(1):11–19
Caney SM, Holt PE, Day MJ, Rudorf H, Gruffydd-Jones TJ (1998) Prostatic carcinoma in two cats. J Small Anim Pract 39(3):140–143
Cannon CM, Allstadt SD (2015) Lower urinary tract cancer. Vet Clin Small Anim 45:807–824
Castillo UF, Ojika M, Alonso-Amelot M, Sakagami Y (1998) Ptaquiloside Z, a new toxic unstable sesquiterpene glucoside from the neotropical bracken fern Pteridium aquilinum var. caudatum. Bioorg Med Chem 6(11):2229–2233
Cave TA, Hine R, Howie F, Thompson H, Argyle DJ (2002) Uterine carcinoma in a 10-month-old golden retriever. J Small Anim Pract 43(3):133–135
Cellio LM, Degner DA (2000) Testosterone-producing the coma in a female cat. J Am Anim Hosp Assoc 36(4):323–325
Chiang YC, Liu CH, Ho SY, Lin CT, Yeh LS (2007) Hypertrophic osteopathy associated with disseminated metastases of renal cell carcinoma in the dog: a case report. J Vet Med Sci 69(2):209–212
Choy K, Fidel J (2016) Tolerability and tumour response of a novel low-dose palliative radiation therapy protocol in dogs with transitional cell carcinoma of the bladder and urethra. Vet Radiol Ultrasound 57:341–351
Cooley DM, Waters DJ (1998) Skeletal metastasis as the initial clinical manifestation of metastatic carcinoma in 19 dogs. J Vet Intern Med 12(4):288–293
Cooper TK, Ronnett BM, Ruben DS, Zink MC (2006) Uterine myxoid leiomyosarcoma with widespread metastases in a cat. Vet Pathol 43(4):552–556
Cornegliani L, Vercelli A, Abramo F (2007) Idiopathic mucosal penile squamous papillomas in dogs. Vet Dermatol 18(6):439–443
Cornell KK, Bostwick DG, Cooley DM, Hall G, Harvey HJ, Hendrick MJ, Pauli BU, Render JA, Stoica G, Sweet DC, Waters DJ (2000) Clinical and pathologic aspects of spontaneous canine prostate carcinoma: a retrospective analysis of 76 cases. Prostate 45(2):173–183
Cota JB, Carvalho T, Pinto C, Peleteiro MC (2014) Epithelial urinary bladder tumors from cows with enzootic hematuria: structural and cell cycle-related protein expression. Vet Pathol 51(4):749–754
Crow SE, Allen DP, Murphy CJ, Culbertson R (1995) Concurrent renal adenocarcinoma and polycythemia in a dog. J Am Anim Hosp Assoc 31(1):29–33
De Lange V, Chiers K, Lefère L, Cools M, Ververs C, Govaere J (2015) Malignant seminoma in two unilaterally cryptorchid stallions. Reprod Domest Anim 50(3):510–513
Den Otter W, Hack M, Jacobs JLJ, Tan JFV, Rozendaal L, van Moorselaar RJA (2015) Effective treatment of transmissible venereal tumors in dogs with vincristine and IL2. Anticancer Res 35(2):713–717
Diez-Bru N, Garcia-Real I, Martinez EM, Rollan E, Mayenco A, Llorens P (1998) Ultrasonographic appearance of ovarian tumors in 10 dogs. Vet Radiol Ultrasound 39(3):226–233
Dobson H, Kerby MJ, Chantrey J, Smith RF (2013) Long-term outcome for two heifers with a granulosa-theca cell tumour. Vet Rec 172(22):581
Doles J, Williams JW, Yarbrough TB (2001) Penile amputation and sheath ablation in the horse. Vet Surg 30(4):327–331
Dominguez PA, Dervisis NG, Cadile CD, Sarbu L, Kitchell BE (2009) Combined gemcitabine and carboplatin therapy for carcinomas in dogs. J Vet Intern Med 23(1):130–137
Duncan RB (1998) Malignantsertoli cell tumor in a horse. Equine Vet J 30(4):355–357
Durno AS, Webb JA, Gauthier MJ, Bienzle D (2011) Polycythemia and inappropriate erythropoietin concentrations in two dogs with renal T-cell lymphoma. J Am Anim Hosp Assoc 47(2):122–128
Edmondson EF, Hess AM, Powers BE (2015) Prognostic significance of histologic features in canine renal cell carcinoma: 70 nephrectomies. Vet Pathol 52(2):260–268
El-Sheikh Ali H, Kitahara G, Nibe K, Yamaguchi R, Horii Y, Zaabel S, Osawa T (2013) Plasma anti-Müllerian hormone as a biomarker for bovine granulosa-theca cell tumors: comparison with immunoreactive inhibin and ovarian steroid concentrations. Theriogenology 80(8):940–949
Elsinghorst TA, Timmermans HJ, Hendriks HG (1984) Comparative pathology of endometrial carcinoma. Vet Q 6(4):200–208
Elzein ET, Sundberg JP, Housawi FM, Gameel AA, Ramadan RO, Hassanein MM (1991) Genital bovine papillomavirus infection in Saudi Arabia. J Vet Diagn Invest 3(1):36–38
Ferreira AJ, Jaggy A, Varejão AP, Ferreira ML, Correia JM, Mulas JM, Almeida O, Oliveira P, Prada J (2000) Brain and ocular metastases from a transmissible venereal tumour in a dog. J Small Anim Pract 41(4):165–168
Fischer AT Jr, Spier S, Carlson GP, Hackett RP (1985) Neoplasia of the equine urinary bladder as a cause of hematuria. J Am Vet Med Assoc 186(12):1294–1296
Freitag T, Jerram RM, Walker AM, Warman CG (2007) Surgical management of common canine prostatic conditions. Compend Contin Educ Vet 29(11):656–658, 660, 662–663
Fulkerson CM, Knapp DW (2015) Management of transitional cell carcinoma of the urinary bladder in dogs: a review. Vet J 205(2):217–225
Gabor LJ, Malik R, Canfield PJ (1998) Clinical and anatomical features of lymphosarcoma in 118 cats. Aust Vet J 76:725–732
Garcia Iglesias MJ, Martinez Rodriguez JM, Bravo Moral AM, EscuderoDiez A (1991) Common epithelial tumours of the ovary in cows. Res Vet Sci 50(3):358–359
Garcia-Iglesias MJ, Bravo-Moral AM, Perez-Martinez C, Ferreras-Estrada MC, Martinez-Rodriguez JM, Escudero-Diez A (1995) Incidence and pathomorphology of uterine tumours in the cow. Zentralbl Veterinarmed A 42(7):421–429
Gelberg HB, McEntee K (1985) Feline ovarian neoplasms. Vet Pathol 22(6):572–576

Gelberg HB, McEntee K (1987) Equine testicular interstitial cell tumors. Vet Pathol 24(3):231–234
Gerber K, Rees P (2009) Urinary bladder botryoid rhabdomyosarcoma with widespread metastases in an 8-month-old Labrador cross dog. J S Afr Vet Assoc 80(3):199–203
Gil da Costa RM, Santos M, Amorim I, Lopes C, Pereira PD, Faustino AM (2009) An immunohistochemical study of feline endometrial adenocarcinoma. J Comp Pathol 140(4):254–259
Glickman LT, Schofer FS, McKee LJ, Reif JS, Goldschmidt MH (1989) Epidemiologic study of insecticide exposures, obesity, and risk of bladder cancer in household dogs. J Toxicol Environ Health 28(4):407–414
Glickman LT, Raghavan M, Knapp DW, Bonney PL, Dawson MH (2004) Herbicide exposure and the risk of transitional cell carcinoma of the urinary bladder in Scottish Terriers. J Am Vet Med Assoc 224(8):1290–1297
Gonzalez CM, Griffey SM, Naydan DK, Flores E, Cepeda R, Cattaneo G, Madewell BR (2000) Canine transmissible venereal tumour: a morphological and immunohistochemical study of 11 tumours in growth phase and during regression after chemotherapy. J Comp Pathol 122(4):241–248
Govaere J, Ducatelle R, Hoogewijs M, De Schauwer C, de Kruif A (2010) Case of bilateral seminoma in a trotter stallion. Reprod Domest Anim 45(3):537–539
Govaere J, Maes S, Saey V, Blancke W, Hoogewijs M, Deschauwer C, Smits K, Roels K, Vercauteren G, de Kruif A (2011) Uterine fibrosarcoma in a Warm blood mare. Reprod Domest Anim 46(3):564–566
Grieco V, Riccardi E, Greppi GF, Teruzzi F, Iermanò V, Finazzi M (2008) Canine testicular tumours: a study on 232 dogs. J Comp Pathol 138(2–3):86–89
Hanazono K, Fukumoto S, Endo Y, Ueno H, Kadosawa T, Uchide T (2014) Ultrasonographic findings related to prognosis in canine transitional cell carcinoma. Vet Radiol Ultrasound 55(1):79–84
Haschek WM, King JM, Tennant BC (1981) Primary renal cell carcinoma in two horses. J Am Vet Med Assoc 179(10):992–994
Hayes HM Jr, Fraumeni JF Jr (1977) Epidemiological features of canine renal neoplasms. Cancer Res 37:2553–2556
Hayes HM Jr, Wilson GP, Pendergrass TW, Cox VS (1985) Canine cryptorchism and subsequent testicular neoplasia: case-control study with epidemiologic update. Teratology 32(1):51–56
Henry CJ, Turnquist SE, Smith A, Graham JC, Thamm DH, O'Brien M, Clifford CA (1999) Primary renal tumours in cats: 19 cases (1992–1998). J Feline Med Surg 1(3):165–170
HogenEsch H, Whiteley HE, Vicini DS, Helper LC (1987) Seminoma with metastases in the eyes and the brain in a dog. Vet Pathol 24(3):278–280
Hopkins NC (1986) Aetiology of enzootic haematuria. Vet Rec 118(26):715–717
Hori Y, Uechi M, Kanakubo K, Sano T, Oyamada T (2006) Canine ovarian serous papillary adenocarcinoma with neoplastic hypercalcemia. J Vet Med Sci 68(9):979–982
Hosoya K, Takagi S, Okumura M (2013) Iatrogenic tumor seeding after ureteral stenting in a dog with urothelial carcinoma. J Am Anim Hosp Assoc 49(4):262–266
Hubbard BS, Valgamott JC, Liska WD (1990) Prostatic adenocarcinoma in a cat. J Am Vet Med Assoc 197(11):1493–1494
Hunt RJ, Hay W, Collatos C, Welles E (1990) Testicular seminoma associated with torsion of the spermatic cord in two cryptorchid stallions. J Am Vet Med Assoc 197(11):1484–1486
Hurcombe SD, Slovis NM, Kohn CW, Oglesbee M (2008) Poorly differentiated leiomyosarcoma of the urogenital tract in a horse. J Am Vet Med Assoc 233(12):1908–1912
Jensen KL, Krag L, Boe-Hansen GB, Jensen HE, Lehn-Jensen H (2008) Malignant Sertoli cell tumour in a young Simmenthal bull--clinical and pathological observations. Reprod Domest Anim 43(6):760–763
Johnston GR, Feeney DA, Johnston SD, O'Brien TD (1991) Ultrasonographic features of testicular neoplasia in dogs: 16 cases (1980–1988). J Am Vet Med Assoc 198(10):1779–1784
Kelley LC, Crowell WA, Puette M, Langheinrich KA, Self AD (1996) A retrospective study of multicentric bovine renal cell tumors. Vet Pathol 33(2):133–141
Knapp DW, Ramos-Vara JA, Moore GE, Dhawan D, Bonney PL, Young KE (2014) Urinary bladder cancer in dogs, a naturally occurring model for cancer biology and drug development. ILAR J 55(1):100–118
Kobayashi M, Sakai H, Hirata A, Yonemaru K, Yanai T, Watanabe K, Yamazoe K, Kudo T, Masegi T (2004) Expression of myogenic regulating factors, Myogenin and MyoD, in two canine botryoid rhabdomyosarcomas. Vet Pathol 41(3):275–277
Krawiec DR, Heflin D (1992) Study of prostatic disease in dogs: 177 cases (1981–1986). J Am Vet Med Assoc 200(8):1119–1122
Leroy BE, Lech ME (2004) Prostatic carcinoma causing urethral obstruction and obstipation in a cat. J Feline Med Surg 6(6):397–400
Leroy BE, Northrup N (2009) Prostate cancer in dogs: comparative and clinical aspects. Vet J 180(2):149–162
Liao AT, Chu PY, Yeh LS, Lin CT, Liu CH (2009) A 12-year retrospective study of canine testicular tumors. J Vet Med Sci 71(7):919–923
Locke JE, Barber LG (2006) Comparative aspects and clinical outcomes of canine renal hemangiosarcoma. J Vet Intern Med 20(4):962–967
López A, Ikede B, Ogilvie T (1994) Unilateral interstitial (Leydig) cell tumor in a neonatal cryptorchid calf. J Vet Diagn Invest 6(1):133–135
Love NE, Walshaw R (1989) What is your diagnosis? Thick bladder wall and an irregular mixed echoic density consistent with an infiltrative bladder mass. J Am Vet Med Assoc 195(10):1409–1410
Lucas X, Rodenas C, Cuello C, Gil MA, Parrilla I, Soler M, Belda E, Agut A (2012) Unusual systemic metastases of malignant seminoma in a dog. Reprod Domest Anim 47(4):e59–e61
MacLachlan NJ (1987) Ovarian disorders in domestic animals. Environ Health Perspect 73:27–33
Mair TS, Walmsley JP, Phillips TJ (2000) Surgical treatment of 45 horses affected by squamous cell carcinoma of the penis and prepuce. Equine Vet J 32(5):406–410
Manothaiudom K, Johnston SD (1991) Clinical approach to vaginal/vestibular masses in the bitch. Vet Clin North Am Small Anim Pract 21(3):509–521

7

Masserdotti C, Bonfanti U, De Lorenzi D, Tranquillo M, Zanetti O (2005) Cytologic features of testicular tumours in dog. J Vet Med A Physiol Pathol Clin Med 52(7):339–346
McCandlish IA, Munro CD, Breeze RG, Nash AS (1979) Hormone producing ovarian tumours in the dog. Vet Rec 105(1):9–11
McCue PM (1992) Equine granulosa cell tumors. Proc Am Assoc Equine Pract 38:587–593
McCue PM, Roser JF, Munro CJ, Liu IK, Lasley BL (2006) Granulosa cell tumors of the equine ovary. Vet Clin North Am Equine Pract 22(3):799–817
McMillan SK, Boria P, Moore GE, Widmer WR, Bonney PL, Knapp DW (2011) Antitumor effects of deracoxib treatment in 26 dogs with transitional cell carcinoma of the urinary bladder. J Am Vet Med Assoc 239(8):1084–1089
Meganck V, Govaere J, Vanholder T, Vercauteren G, Chiers K, de Kruif A, Opsomer G (2011) Two atypical cases of granulosa cell tumours in Belgian Blue heifers. Reprod Domest Anim 46(4):746–749
Militerno G, Bazzo R, Bevilacqua D, Bettini G, Marcato PS (2003) Transitional cell carcinoma of the renal pelvis in two dogs. J Vet Med A Physiol Pathol Clin Med 50(9):457–459
Miller MA, Ramos-Vara JA, Dickerson MF, Johnson GC, Pace LW, Kreeger JM, Turnquist SE, Turk JR (2003) Uterine neoplasia in 13 cats. J Vet Diagn Invest 15(6):515–522
Miller MA, Hartnett SE, Ramos-Vara JA (2007) Interstitial cell tumor and Sertoli cell tumor in the testis of a cat. Vet Pathol 44(3):394–397
Mischke R, Meurer D, Hoppen HO, Ueberschär S, Hewicker-Trautwein M (2002) Blood plasma concentrations of oestradiol-17beta, testosterone and testosterone/oestradiol ratio in dogs with neoplastic and degenerative testicular diseases. Res Vet Sci 73(3):267–272
Moe L, Lium B (1997) Hereditary multifocal renal cystadenocarcinomas and nodular dermatofibrosis in 51 German shepherd dogs. J Small Anim Pract 38(11):498–505
Mooney SC, Hayes AA, Matus RE, MacEwen EG (1987) Renal lymphoma in cats. 28 cases (1977–1984). J Am Vet Med Assoc 191:1473–1477
Mozos E, Méndez A, Gómez-Villamandos JC, Martín De Las Mulas J, Pérez J (1996) Immunohistochemical characterization of canine transmissible venereal tumor. Vet Pathol 33(3):257–263
Mukaratirwa S, Gruys E (2003) Canine transmissible venereal tumour: cytogenetic origin, immunophenotype, and immunobiology. A review. Vet Q 25(3):101–111
Murchison EP, Wedge DC, Alexandrov LB, Fu B, Martincorena I, Ning Z, Tubio JMC et al (2014) Transmissible dog cancer genome reveals the origin and history of an ancient cell lineage. Science 343:437–440
Murgia C, Pritchard JK, Kim SY, Fassati A, Weiss RA (2006) Clonal origin and evolution of a transmissible cancer. Cell 126:477–487
Murphy ST, Kruger JM, Watson GL (1994) Uterine adenocarcinoma in the dog: a case report and review. J Am Anim Hosp Assoc 30(5):440–444
Mutsaers AJ, Widmer WR, Knapp DW (2003) Canine transitional cell carcinoma. J Vet Intern Med 17(2):136–144
Nak D, Nak Y, Cangul IT, Tuna B (2005) A clinico-pathological study on the effect of vincristine on transmissible venereal tumour in dogs. J Vet Med A Physiol Pathol Clin Med 52(7):366–370
Nasir L, Campo MS (2008) Bovine papillomaviruses: their role in the aetiology of cutaneous tumours of bovids and equids. Vet Dermatol 19(5):243–254
Nelissen P, White RA (2012) Subtotal vaginectomy for management of extensive vaginal disease in 11 dogs. Vet Surg 41(4):495–500
Nielsen SW, Misdorp W, McEntee K (1976a) Tumours of the ovary. Bull World Health Organ 53(2–3):203–215
Nielsen SW, Mackey LJ, Misdorp W (1976b) Tumors of the kidney. Bull World Health Organ 53(2–3):237–246
Nolan MW, Gieger TL, Vaden SL (2015) Management of transitional cell carcinoma of the urinary bladder in dogs: important challenges to consider. Vet J 205(2):126–127
Norris HJ, Taylor HB, Garner FM (1968) Equine ovarian granulosa tumours. Vet Rec 82:419–420
Osborne CA, Low DG, Perman V, Barnes DM (1968) Neoplasms of the canine and feline urinary bladder: incidence, etiologic factors, occurrence and pathologic features. Am J Vet Res 29(10):2041–2055
Park MS, Kim Y, Kang MS, Oh SY, Cho DY, Shin NS, Kim DY (2006) Disseminated transmissible venereal tumor in a dog. J Vet Diagn Invest 18(1):130–133
Pathania S, Kumar P, Devi LG, Kumar D, Dhama K, Somvanshi R (2011) Preliminary assessment of binary ethylenimine inactivated and saponized cutaneous warts (BPV-2) therapeutic vaccine for enzootic bovine haematuria in hill cows. Vaccine 29(43):7296–7302
Pathania S, Dhama K, Saikumar G, Shahi S, Somvanshi R (2012) Detection and quantification of bovine papilloma virus type 2 (BPV-2) by real-time PCR in urine and urinary bladder lesions in enzootic bovine haematuria (EBH)-affected cows. Transbound Emerg Dis 59(1):79–84
Patnaik AK, Greenlee PG (1987) Canine ovarian neoplasms: a clinicopathologic study of 71 cases, including histology of 12 granulosa cell tumors. Vet Pathol 24(6):509–514
Patnaik AK, Schwarz PD, Greene RW (2008) A histopathologic study of twenty urinary bladder neoplasms in the cat. J Small Anim Pract 27:433–445
Patrick DJ, Fitzgerald SD, Sesterhenn IA, Davis CJ, Kiupel M (2006) Classification of canine urinary bladder urothelial tumours based on the World Health Organization/International Society of Urological Pathology consensus classification. J Comp Pathol 135(4):190–199
Patterson-Kane JC, Tramontin RR, Giles RC, Harrison LR (2000) Transitional cell carcinoma of the urinary bladder in a Thoroughbred, with intra-abdominal dissemination. Vet Pathol 37:692–695
Patsikas M, Papazoglou LG, Jakovljevic S, Papaioannou NG, Papadopoulou PL, Soultani CB, Chryssogonidis IA, Kouskouras KA, Tziris NE, Charitanti AA (2014) Radiographic and ultrasonographic findings of uterine neoplasms in nine dogs. J Am Anim Hosp Assoc 50(5):330–337
Peppler C, Weissert D, Kappe E, Klump S, Kramer M, Reinacher M, Neiger R (2009) Osteosarcoma of the penile bone (os penis) in a dog. Aust Vet J 87(1):52–55
Pérez-Martínez C, Durán-Navarrete AJ, García-Fernández RA, Espinosa-Alvarez J, EscuderoDiez A, García-Iglesias

MJ (2004) Biological characterization of ovarian granulosa cell tumours of slaughtered cattle: assessment of cell proliferation and oestrogen receptors. J Comp Pathol 130(2–3):117–123

Pires I, Silva F, Queiroga FL, Rodrigues P, Henriques R, Pinto CA, Lopes C (2010) Epithelioid hemangiosarcomas of the bovine urinary bladder: a histologic, immunohistochemical, and ultrastructural examination of four tumors. J Vet Diagn Invest 22(1):116–119

Pollock PJ, Prendergast M, Callanan JJ, Skelly C (2002) Testicular teratoma in a three-day-old thoroughbred foal. Vet Rec 150(11):348–350

Powe JR, Canfield PJ, Martin PA (2004) Evaluation of the cytologic diagnosis of canine prostatic disorders. Vet Clin Pathol 33(3):150–154

Quartuccio M, Marino G, Garufi G, Cristarella S, Zanghì A (2012) Sertoli cell tumors associated with feminizing syndrome and spermatic cord torsion in two cryptorchid dogs. J Vet Sci 13(2):207–209

Ramos-Vara JA, Miller MA, Boucher M, Roudabush A, Johnson GC (2003) Immunohistochemical detection of uroplakin III, cytokeratin 7, and cytokeratin 20 in canine urothelial tumors. Vet Pathol 40(1):55–62

Reed LT, Knapp DW, Miller MA (2012) Cutaneous metastasis of transitional cell carcinoma in 12 dogs. Vet Pathol 50(4):676–681

Rhind SM, Hawe C, Dixon PM, Scudamore CL (1999) Oral metastasis of renal cell carcinoma in a horse. J Comp Pathol 120(1):97–103

Riccardi E, Grieco V, Verganti S, Finazzi M (2007) Immunohistochemical diagnosis of canine ovarian epithelial and granulosa cell tumors. J Vet Diagn Invest 19(4):431–435

Rocha TA, Mauldin GN, Patnaik AK, Bergman PJ (2000) Prognostic factors in dogs with urinary bladder carcinoma. J Vet Intern Med 14(5):486–490

Roperto S, Borzacchiello G, Brun R, Leonardi L, Maiolino P, Martano M, Paciello O, Papparella S, Restucci B, Russo V, Salvatore G, Urraro C, Roperto F (2010) A review of bovine urothelial tumours and tumour-like lesions of the urinary bladder. J Comp Pathol 142(2–3):95–108

Rosen DK, Carpenter JL (1993) Functional ectopic interstitial cell tumor in a castrated male cat. J Am Vet Med Assoc 202(11):1865–1866

Rota A, Tursi M, Zabarino S, Appino S (2013) Monophasic teratoma of the ovarian remnant in a bitch. Reprod Domest Anim 48(2):e26–e28

Sanpera N, Masot N, Janer M, Romeo C, de Pedro R (2002) Oestrogen-induced bone marrow aplasia in a dog with a Sertoli cell tumour. J Small Anim Pract 43(8):365–369

Sato T, Maeda H, Suzuki A, Shibuya H, Sakata A, Shirai W (2007) Endometrial stromal sarcoma with smooth muscle and glandular differentiation of the feline uterus. Vet Pathol 44(3):379–382

Sharma R, Bhat TK, Sharma OP (2013) The environmental and human effects of ptaquiloside-induced enzootic bovine hematuria: a tumorous disease of cattle. Rev Environ Contam Toxicol 224:53–95

Sledge DG, Patrick DJ, Fitzgerald SD, Xie Y, Kiupel M (2015) Differences in expression of uroplakin III, cytokeratin 7, and cyclooxygenase-2 in canine proliferative urothelial lesions of the urinary bladder. Vet Pathol 52(1):74–82

Smith J (2008) Canine prostatic disease: a review of anatomy, pathology, diagnosis, and treatment. Theriogenology 70(3):375–383

Spugnini EP, Bartolazzi A, Ruslander D (2000) Seminoma with cutaneous metastases in a dog. J Am Anim Hosp Assoc 36(3):253–256

Stabenfeldt GH, Hughes JP, Kennedy PC, Meagher DM, Neely DP (1979) Clinical findings, pathological changes and endocrinological secretory patterns in mares with ovarian tumours. J Reprod Fertil Suppl 27:277–285

Strakova A, Murchison EP (2015) The cancer which survived: insights from the genome of an 11000 year-old cancer. Curr Opin Genet Dev 30:49–55

Taylor AJ, Lara-Garcia A, Benigni L (2014) Ultrasonographic characteristics of canine renal lymphoma. Vet Radiol Ultrasound 55(4):441–446

Taylor SS, Goodfellow MR, Browne WJ, Walding B, Murphy S, Tzannes S, Gerou-Ferriani M, Schwartz A, Dobson JM (2009) Feline extranodal lymphoma: response to chemotherapy and survival in 110 cats. J Small Anim Pract 50:584–592

Thacher C, Bradley RL (1983) Vulvar and vaginal tumors in the dog: a retrospective study. J Am Vet Med Assoc 183(6):690–692

Tsioli VG, Gouletsou PG, Loukopoulos P, Zavlaris M, Galatos AD (2011) Uterine leiomyosarcoma and pyometra in a dog. J Small Anim Pract 52(2):121–124

Tucker AR, Smith JR (2008) Prostatic squamous metaplasia in a cat with interstitial cell neoplasia in a retained testis. Vet Pathol 45(6):905–909

Turnquist SE, Pace LW, Keegan K, Andrews-Jones L, Kreeger JM, Bailey KL, Stogsdill PL, Wilson HA (1993) Botryoid rhabdomyosarcoma of the urinary bladder in a filly. J Vet Diagn Invest 5(3):451–453

Vail DM, Moore AS, Ogilvie GK, Volk LM (1998) Feline lymphoma (145 cases): proliferation indices, cluster of differentiation, immunoreactivity, and their association with prognosis in 90 cases. J Vet Intern Med 12:349–354

Valdes-Martinez A, Cianciolo R, Mai W (2007) Association between renal hypoechoic subcapsular thickening and lymphosarcoma in cats. Vet Radiol Ultrasound 48:357–460

Valli VE, Norris A, Jacobs RM, Laing E, Withrow S, Macy D, Tomlinson J, McCaw D, Ogilvie GK, Pidgeon G et al (1995) Pathology of canine bladder and urethral cancer and correlation with tumour progression and survival. J Comp Pathol 113(2):113–130

Van den Top JG, de Heer N, Klein WR, Ensink JM (2008) Penile and preputial tumours in the horse: a retrospective study of 114 affected horses. Equine Vet J 40(6):528–532

Vanderstraeten E, Bogaert L, Bravo IG, Martens A (2011) EcPV2 DNA in equine squamous cell carcinomas and normal genital and ocular mucosa. Vet Microbiol 147(3–4):292–299

Van Mol KA, Fransen JL (1986) Renal carcinomas in a horse. Vet Rec 119(10):238–239

Vignoli M, Rossi F, Chierici C, Terragni R, DeLorenzi D, Stanga M, Olivero D (2007) Needle tract implantation

after fine needle aspiration biopsy (FNAB) of transitional cell carcinoma of the urinary bladder and adenocarcinoma of the lung. Schweiz Arch Tierheilkd 149(7):314–318
Wakui S, Furusato M, Nomura Y, Iimori M, Kano Y, Aizawa S, Ushigome S (1992) Testicular epidermoid cyst and penile squamous cell carcinoma in a dog. Vet Pathol 29(6):543–545
Walker DB, Cowell RL, Clinkenbeard KD, Turgai J (1993) Carcinoma in the urinary bladder of a cat: cytologic findings and a review of the literature. Vet Clin Pathol 22(4):103–108
Weaver AD (1983) Survey with follow-up of 67 dogs with testicular sertoli cell tumours. Vet Rec 113(5):105–107
Weisse C, Berent A, Todd K, Clifford C, Solomon J (2006) Evaluation of palliative stenting for management of malignant urethral obstructions in dogs. J Am Vet Med Assoc 229(2):226–234
Weissman A, Jiménez D, Torres B, Cornell K, Holmes SP (2013) Canine vaginal leiomyoma diagnosed by CT vaginourethrography. J Am Anim Hosp Assoc 49(6):394–397
Wilson HM, Chun R, Larson VS, Kurzman ID, Vail DM (2007) Clinical signs, treatments, and outcome in cats with transitional cell carcinoma of the urinary bladder: 20 cases (1990–2004). J Am Vet Med Assoc 231(1):101–106
Wimberly HC, Lewis RM (1979) Transitional cell carcinoma in the domestic cat. Vet Pathol 16:223–228
Wise LN, Bryan JN, Sellon DC, Hines MT, Ramsay J, Seino KK (2009) A retrospective analysis of renal carcinoma in the horse. J Vet Intern Med 23(4):913–918
Xu LR (1992) Bracken poisoning and enzootic haematuria in cattle in China. Res Vet Sci 53(1):116–121
Yaghoobi Yeganeh Manesh J, Shafiee R, Mohammad Bahrami A, Pourzaer M, Pourzaer M, Pedram B, Javanbakht J, Mokarizadeh A, Khadivar F (2014) Cyto-histopathological and outcome features of the prepuce squamous cell carcinoma of a mixed breed dog. Diagn Pathol 9:110
Yu CH, Hwang DN, Yhee JY, Kim JH, Im KS, Nho WG, Lyoo YS, Sur JH (2009) Comparative immunohistochemical characterization of canine seminomas and Sertoli cell tumors. J Vet Sci 10(1):1–7
Zambelli D, Cunto M, Raccagni R, Merlo B, Morini M, Bettini G (2010) Successful surgical treatment of a prostatic biphasic tumour (sarcomastoid carcinoma) in a cat. J Feline Med Surg 12(2):161–165
Zantingh AJ, Gaughan EM, Bain FT (2012) Case report: squamous cell carcinoma of the urinary bladder in a horse. Compend Contin Educ Vet 34(10):E1–E5
Zhu KW, Affolter VK, Gaynor AM, Dela Cruz FN Jr, Pesavento PA (2015) Equine genital squamous cell carcinoma: in situ hybridization identifies a distinct subset containing equus caballus papillomavirus 2. Vet Pathol 52(6):1067–1072
Owen L (1980) TNM classification of tumours in domestic animals, 1st edn. World Health Organization, Geneva

Hepatobiliary Tumors

Angele Breithaupt

R. Klopfleisch (ed.), *Veterinary Oncology*, DOI 10.1007/978-3-319-41124-8_8

Primary hepatic neoplasms are uncommon in most animals. A viral *etiology* has been demonstrated in woodchucks but not in cats or dogs. Trematodes, *Ancylostoma caninum* and *Trichuris vulpis,* may be involved in bile duct carcinoma development, but they are unlikely to be a major carcinogen. Toxins, including aflatoxin, induce hepatocellular carcinomas, but reports are restricted to experimental data. In contrast to humans, an association between hepatic tumors and cirrhosis or cholelithiasis is not confirmed in animals.

Nodular hyperplasia is common in older dogs and most likely does not represent a preneoplastic lesion. These nodules are found in cats and swine more rarely but not in other species and comprise nodules with regular, lobular architecture. In contrast, *regenerative hepatocellular hyperplasia* occurs in association with liver damage and thus usually with some fibrotic background.

The general macroscopic appearance is important for therapeutic approaches and prognosis and can be either *massive* (large and solitary), *nodular* (multifocal in several lobes), and *diffuse* (multifocal in all lobes or complete effacement).

Primary hepatic tumors include *hepatocellular* or *cholangiocellular* (bile duct) *adenomas* and *adenocarcinomas, mesenchymal* tumors (mostly sarcomas), and *carcinoids.*

Hepatocellular adenomas are typically massive (◘ see Fig. 8.1) but can be multiple, might reach 12 cm in diameter, and are usually not associated with clinical signs. Tumors are well demarcated and not encapsulated and are yellow to dark brown. Tumors comprise well-differentiated hepatocytes arranged in cords and trabeculae, but masses lack regular lobular architecture.

Hepatocellular adenocarcinomas appear singular, as massive, nodular, or diffuse neoplasms. Besides capsular penetration and implant metastasis, distant metastasis is rare and most likely affects hepatic lymph nodes. Not uncommonly, animals suffer from internal bleeding and less frequent from hepatic effacement or metastasis. Tumors present with less-differentiated hepatocytes, probably showing invasion into hepatic veins, vena cava, and penetration of the liver capsule, leading to implant metastasis. Consecutive capsular ruptures may lead to fatal internal bleedings. Differentiation from benign variants in cytological specimens can be difficult due to a physiological pleomorphia, but immunohistochemistry for cell proliferation markers, such as Ki67, may improve diagnostic performance.

Cholangiocellular adenomas are usually massive, pale to gray-white, well circumscribed, and more or less spherical and may be cystic, filled with watery to viscous fluid. Well-differentiated bile duct epithelium and moderate amount of fibrovascular stroma that may compress the surrounding tissue characterize this tumor type. *Cholangiocellular carcinomas* can be intrahepatic (◘ see Fig. 8.2), extrahepatic, or within the gall bladder and usually present as nodular to diffuse, pale-beige, and umbilicated mass. Metastasis to regional lymph nodes and the lung is common and implant metastasis occurs in the peritoneal cavity (◘ see Fig. 8.3). Neoplastic cells grow highly invasive in ductular, acinar, or papillary pattern, often with numerous mitosis and abundant fibrous stroma (scirrhous response).

Carcinoids are rare in cats and dogs and tend to occur at a younger age than other primary tumors.

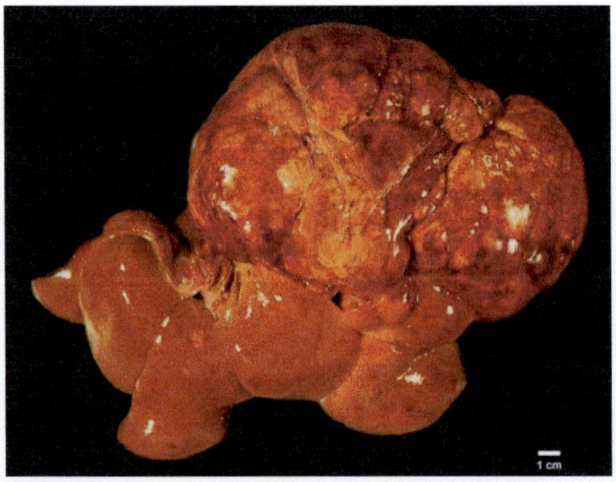

◘ **Fig. 8.1** Liver, Pekingese dog: hepatocellular adenoma, left-lateral lobe, 4 years, histopathological examination of regional lymph nodes did not show metastatic spread

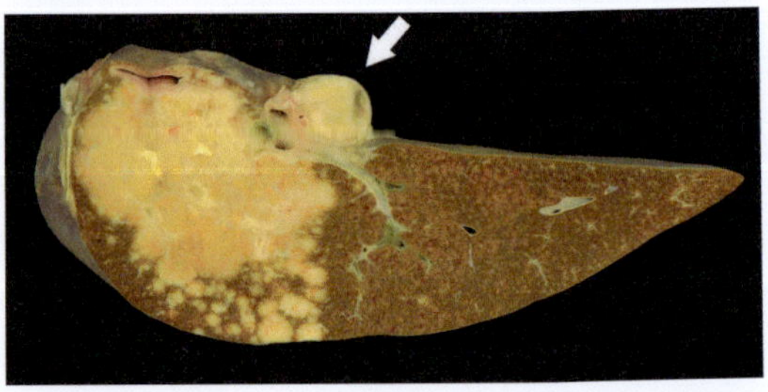

◘ **Fig. 8.2** Liver, goat: intrahepatic cholangiocellular adenocarcinoma (scirrhous), with metastasis to the hepatic lymph node (*arrow*) (Courtesy of Kristina Dietert, PhD, Freie Universität Berlin, Germany)

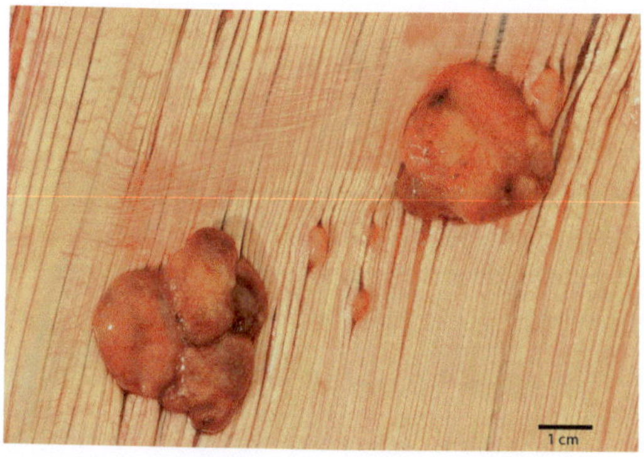

Fig. 8.3 Diaphragm, horse: multiple implant metastases of a scirrhous cholangiocellular adenocarcinoma (Courtesy of Dr. Lydia König, Freie Universität Berlin, Germany)

They arise from neuroectodermal cells and are mostly diffuse with distant metastasis to the regional lymph nodes, peritoneum, and lung. These tumors are usually not amenable to surgical resection, and the efficacy of radiotherapy and chemotherapy is not well documented, finally leading to a poor prognosis. Carcinoids are differentiated from carcinomas by the use of silver stains (reveal argyrophilic granules) or by immunohistochemistry for neurosecretory products such as serotonin.

Regarding primary hepatic *sarcomas*, hemangiosarcomas are most frequent in cats and leiomyosarcomas most common in dogs. Hemangiosarcomas are usually metastatic in dogs. In general, hepatic sarcomas behave aggressively, with metastasis to the spleen and lungs. Based on their variable origin, they may appear as ill-defined, gray-white masses (fibrosarcomas) or cavernous and blood-filled (hemangiosarcomas) masses. Particularly hemangiosarcomas may rupture and are associated with fatal internal bleeding. Hepatic sarcomas present in the typical histological pattern for either hemangiosarcomas or fibrosarcomas as in other organs and will not be discussed in detail. Prognosis is poor because metastatic disease is often present at the time of diagnosis/surgery.

Lymphomas are rarely restricted to the liver, particularly in cats, and most likely a systemic disease. Diagnosis can be challenging, particularly in diffuse infiltrating variants. For detailed information, ► see Chap. 6.

Benign tumors, including fibromas, myelolipomas, and hepatoblastomas, are very rare and will not be discussed, except for *hepatoblastomas* in horses.

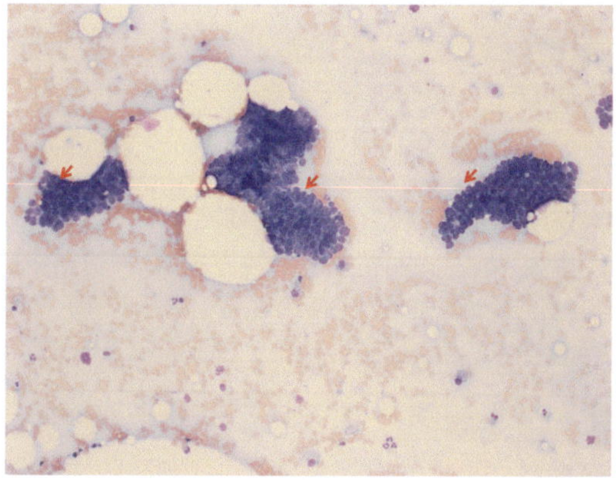

Fig. 8.4 Cytology, carcinoma, liver, dog, May-Grünwald-Giemsa 100×. The normal liver tissue is replaced by clusters of small- to medium-sized cuboidal epithelial cells with round nuclei, a high nuclear to cytoplasm ratio and fine chromatin pattern (*red arrow*). There is an acinar growth pattern. Based on the cellular morphology (relatively small cuboidal cells), a bile duct carcinoma can be suspected; however, the exact origin cannot be determined based on cytology (Photo: with permission of Dr. N. Bauer, Faculty of Veterinary Medicine, Justus-Liebig-University, Giessen, Germany)

A coagulation profile is mandatory prior to hepatic biopsy and surgery, because abnormalities of the coagulation parameters are common in liver diseases in general, particularly FXIII deficiency in cats with neoplastic disease, and hemorrhage is the most frequent complication.

For cats and dogs, a correct diagnosis can be obtained from hepatic *aspirates* but is much more reliable with *needle core biopsies*. Other authors attest that sensitivity and specificity of cytology is restricted, and histopathology of tissue samples is recommended. *Cytological diagnosis* of primary epithelial hepatic tumors is challenging: in cases of adequate samples, the identification of epithelial cells with criteria of malignancy is often possible but difficult to distinguish from metastatic epithelial disease or even from reactive hepatic or biliary cells (see Figs. 8.4 and 8.5). A differentiation between a benign mesenchymal proliferation and a malignant mesenchymal proliferation is often not possible without additional clinical data (see Fig. 8.6).

Suggested Readings

(Barr 1995; Cohen et al. 2003; Cullen and Popp 2002; Hammer and Sikkema 1995; Hayes et al. 1983; Leveille et al. 1993; Newell et al. 1998; Patnaik 1992; Patnaik et al. 1980, 1981a; Roth 2001; Stockhaus et al. 2004)

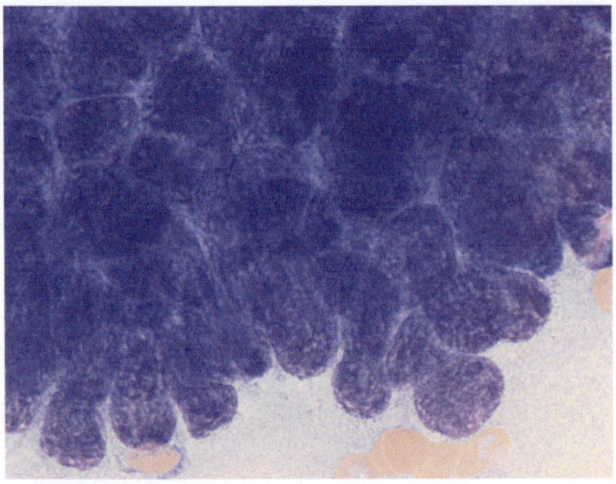

Fig. 8.5 Cytology, carcinoma, liver, dog, May-Grünwald-Giemsa 1000× (the same case as in the previous figure). There are small- to medium-sized cuboidal epithelial cells with round nuclei, a high nuclear to cytoplasm ratio and fine chromatin pattern. The cells show nuclear crowding and nuclear overlap reflecting malignancy (Photo: with permission of Dr. N. Bauer, Faculty of Veterinary Medicine, Justus-Liebig-University, Giessen, Germany)

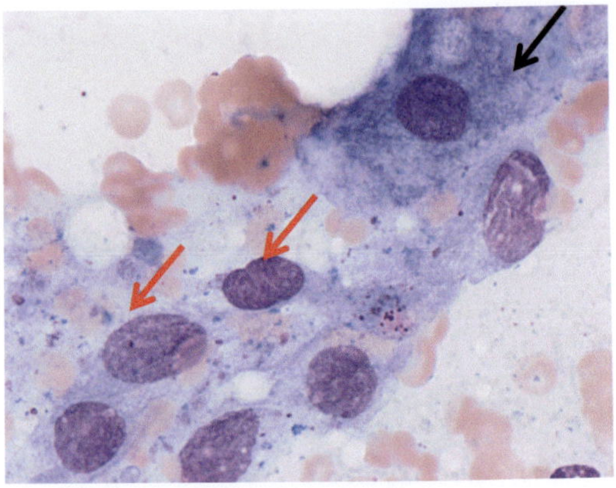

Fig. 8.6 Cytology, sarcoma, fine needle aspirate hypoechogenic liver mass of 5 × 5 × 5 mm in size, dog, May-Grünwald-Giemsa 1000×. A small cluster of moderately cohesive spindle cells with indistinct cellular borders, oval nuclei, fine chromatin, and moderate amounts of lightly basophilic cytoplasm (*red arrow*) are associated with the clusters of hepatocytes (*black arrow*). Based on cytological samples, a differentiation between a benign mesenchymal proliferation (i.e., fibrous tissue in case of liver cirrhosis) and a malignant mesenchymal proliferation (i.e., sarcoma) is generally not possible; however, in this case, the presence of a liver mass points toward a sarcoma (Photo: with permission of Dr. N. Bauer, Faculty of Veterinary Medicine, Justus-Liebig-University, Giessen, Germany)

8.1 Canine Hepatobiliary Tumors

Box 8.1. Canine Hepatobiliary Tumors in Five Facts

1. Metastatic tumors: more common than primary tumors
2. Hepatocellular tumors: common primary tumors
3. Diagnosis: sonographic examination recommended
4. Treatment of choice: surgery (lobectomy)
5. Massive hepatocellular adenocarcinomas can have a good prognosis

Epidemiology and Pathogenesis

In dogs, most tumors in the liver are secondary and metastases of tumors from non-hepatic organs or part of systemic diseases such as lymphomas, malignant histiocytosis, or mast cell tumors.

Hepatocellular carcinomas are the most common primary liver tumor in dogs. Patients average 10–11 years and there is no breed predisposition, but some authors indicate that males are overrepresented. The second most common tumors are *bile duct carcinomas*, and Labrador retrievers as well as females appear predisposed. Affected dogs average 8 years. *Bile duct adenomas* are very rare and will not be discussed in detail. *Hepatocellular adenomas* are often found incidentally and mostly do not cause clinical disease. Common metastatic tumors in dogs include lymphomas, hemangiosarcomas, and pancreas carcinomas but also mammary tumors, intestinal tumors, thyroid carcinomas, melanomas, and malignant histiocytosis, and mast cell tumors often localize in the liver.

Clinical Appearance

Hepatobiliary – primary and metastatic – tumors are associated with clinical signs in approximately 75 % of dogs, which show inappetence, weight loss, lethargy, vomiting, polydipsia–polyuria, and ascites. Ataxia and seizures may be caused by hepatic encephalopathy, paraneoplastic hypoglycemia, or central nervous system metastasis. A cranial abdominal mass is *palpable* frequently, although nodular and diffuse forms can be missed.

Morphologically, more than half of the *hepatocellular carcinomas* (*HCC*) are massive; nodular and diffuse types are less frequent. The left liver lobes are affected in more than two thirds of dogs with HCC. Metastasis to the regional lymph nodes, peritoneum, and lungs is more common in dogs with nodular and diffuse HCC.

Solid and cystic *bile duct carcinomas* have been reported, but this distinction does not influence either treatment or prognosis. Cysts may contain yellow, gelatinous material, and these tumors in general often have a high amount of fibrous tissue (scirrhous reaction). Bile duct carcinomas have an aggressive biologic behavior with common metastasis to the regional lymph nodes and lungs.

The differentiation of *hepatocellular adenomas* from *nodular hyperplasia* is difficult, even histologically. Generally, nodular hyperplasia appears multifocally with definite smaller sizes and a histologically regular lobular pattern that is characteristically lacking in adenomas.

Typically, with *laboratory tests*, several parameters might be increased including ALP (alkaline phosphatase), ALT (alanine aminotransferase), AST (aspartate aminotransferase), GGT (gamma-glutamyl transpeptidase), total bilirubin, serum bile acid, and α-fetoprotein, but they are nonspecific. Further, leukocytosis, anemia, and hypoalbuminemia are frequently present. Hypoglycemia is a paraneoplastic syndrome reported secondary to hepatic tumors.

In contrast to human cases, *α-fetoprotein* has limited value in the diagnosis and treatment monitoring of canine HCC.

Sonographic examination is recommended and can provide information about the macroscopic phenotype (massive, nodular, diffuse), the size, the location, and relationship with adjacent anatomical structures. Tumor vascularization can be determined using Doppler imaging techniques, and contrast-enhanced ultrasonography can be useful in differentiating malignant tumors from benign lesions. Limitations of sonographic diagnosis are indicated for the differentiation of nodular hyperplasia and metastatic disease and as well as visualization of infiltrating tumors, such as lymphomas.

Radiographic findings are mainly nonspecific but might be useful for evidence of lung metastasis.

▪ Cytology and Histopathology

Unspecific clinical symptoms and at least partly limited diagnostic value of imaging methods highlight the relevance of cytology and/or histopathology for diagnosis and treatment strategy. After coagulation tests *ultrasound-guided fine needle aspiration* for *cytology* or *needle core biopsy* sampling for *histopathology* is useful for diagnostic purposes. Surgical sampling of *wedge-shaped tissue* under visual control is regarded by some authors as the best diagnostic approach and enables both diagnosis and initial treatment for massive, solitary tumors in a single procedure.

▪ Therapy and Prognosis

The prognosis for dogs with liver tumors is determined by macroscopic morphology and histology: the *prognosis* is good for *massive hepatocellular* carcinoma (*HCC*) and benign tumors. Complete surgical resection is possible, and local tumor recurrence is reported in 0–13 % of dogs with massive HCC following liver lobectomy. Metastasis to other regions of the liver and lungs has been documented in 0–37 % of dogs, but most deaths are unrelated to HCC.

Prognostic factors in dogs with massive HCC include:

- Surgical treatment: the median survival time is increased four times after surgery in one study.
- Side of liver involvement: due to intraoperative death associated with right-sided tumors
- ALT and AST activity: may reflect hepatocellular injury (large tumor size or aggressiveness).
- Ratios of ALP to AST and ALT to AST

In contrast, the *prognosis* is poor for dogs with malignant tumors *other than massive HCC*. Even after lobectomy, dogs may suffer from local recurrence and metastatic disease, and other treatments are often not successful.

Liver *surgical lobectomy* is highly recommended with any hepatic tumor that has a massive morphologic appearance, and radical surgical treatments are tolerated based on the remarkable reserve capacity of this organ. *Surgical techniques* for liver lobectomy include finger fracture, mass ligation, mattress sutures, bipolar vessel sealant devices, and surgical stapling. Complications include hemorrhage, vascular compromise to adjacent liver lobes, transient hypoglycemia, and reduced hepatic function.

The role of *radiation therapy* (RT) and *chemotherapy* (CT) for HCC is neglectable. The canine liver does not tolerate high radio-therapeutic doses, and liver tumors appear to be chemoresistant, most likely due to the hepatocellular detoxification property or expression of P-glycoprotein (efflux pump associated with multidrug resistance). However, some reports (e.g., for gemcitabine) indicate encouraging results. Other treatment options include immunotherapy, hormonal therapy, and antiangiogenic agents.

▪ **Further Readings**

(Clifford et al. 2004; Cole et al. 2002; Elpiner et al. 2011; Kemp et al. 2013; Kosovsky et al. 1989; Kutara et al. 2006; Leveille et al. 1993; Nakamura et al. 2010; Patnaik et al. 1980, 1981b; Stockhaus et al. 2004; Vörös et al. 1991; Yamada et al. 1999)

8

8.2 Feline Hepatobiliary Tumors

Box 8.2. Feline Hepatobiliary Tumors in Four Facts

1. Lymphomas are the most common tumors in the liver of cats
2. Bile duct carcinomas are common non-hematopoietic hepatic tumors
3. Metastases are usually present at time of diagnosis
4. Surgery is the treatment of choice

▪ **Epidemiology and Pathogenesis**

Lymphomas are by far the most common neoplasia in the liver of cats and usually part of a multicentric disease (◘ see Fig. 8.7). Lymphomas are discussed in detail in Chap. 6.

Bile duct carcinomas are the most common non-hematopoietic hepatic tumors in cats followed by *hepatocellular carcinomas*. Benign tumors such as cystic *bile duct adenomas* or solid *hepatocellular adenomas* are also frequently described in cats. Rarely, cats present with mast cell tumors, sarcomas (most of them hemangiosarcomas), myelolipomas, and carcinoids.

▪ **Clinical Appearance**

Hepatobiliary tumors are accompanied by clinical signs in approximately 50 % of cats. Clinical signs include anorexia, depression, and weight loss, more rarely vomiting, diarrhea, polyuria and polydipsia, icterus, ascites, and abdominal pain. Paraneoplastic alopecia is recorded in a minority of cases and presents with bilateral symmetrical alopecia at the ventral thorax, abdomen, and inner thighs.

A cranial abdominal mass is *palpable* in up to three quarters of cats, but as in dogs, hepatic enlargement can be absent in nodular and diffuse forms.

Bile duct carcinomas behave aggressively, not uncommonly with implant metastasis and peritoneal carcinomatosis.

Benign tumors, such as *bile duct adenomas*, usually do not cause clinical signs until they reach critical size and compress adjacent organs.

As indicated for dogs, *radiographic* findings are mostly nonspecific – hepatomegaly with caudal displacement of the stomach – and *sonographic* examination is recommended. Again, relevant information for staging, including tumor phenotype (massive, nodular, diffuse), size, location, and association with important anatomical structures, can be specified. Also for cats, Doppler imaging techniques (for visualization of tumor vascularization) as well as contrast-enhanced sonography, for differentiating malignant tumors from benign lesions, may be used. A systematic sonography has been reported with a very high sensitivity and specificity for differentiation of benign *versus* malignant tumors and diagnosis of lymphoma in cats.

In *laboratory tests*, several parameters might be increased: the most frequent is neutrophilic leukocytosis. Some authors state ALP (alkaline phosphatase) levels are not diagnostic, and increased ALT and AST are rare in cats. Thus, reliability is questionable, possibly except for increased AST levels in visceral hemangiosarcomas. But in general, malignant tumors tend to be associated with higher liver enzyme levels compared to benign tumors. Bilirubin is elevated in some cats with hepatobiliary tumors, most markedly with bile duct carcinoma and bile duct obstructive carcinoids.

▪ **Cytology and Histopathology**

Cytology and/or histopathology is necessary for diagnosis and development of a treatment strategy. *Ultrasound-guided fine needle aspiration* for *cytology* or *needle core biopsy* sampling for *histo-*

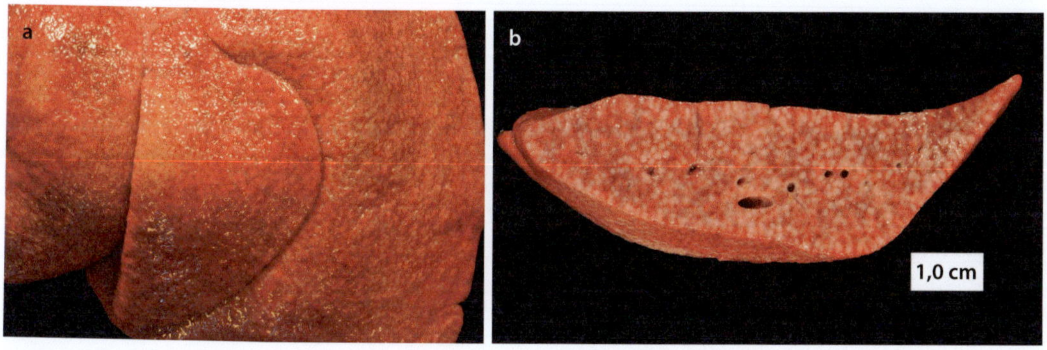

Fig. 8.7 Liver, diffuse lymphoma, cat (Courtesy of Kristina Dietert, PhD, Freie Universität Berlin, Germany)

pathology is useful for diagnostic purposes. And again, surgical sampling of *wedge-shaped tissue* under visual control is probably the best diagnostic approach and useful for initial treatment for massive, solitary tumors in a single procedure.

Fine needle aspiration (FNA) is valuable for diagnosis of most hematopoietic tumors. The differentiation of well-differentiated, low-grade lymphomas from chronic cholangiohepatitis is however challenging.

Therapy and Prognosis

The prognosis for cats is determined by macroscopic and histological findings: as in dogs, the *prognosis* is good for *massive hepatocellular carcinomas* (HCC) and *benign tumors* because complete surgical resection is usually possible.

In contrast, the *prognosis* is poor for cats with *nodular and diffuse, malignant tumors* because metastasis is more likely at time of diagnosis, and unfortunately, in the vast majority of cases in cats, tumors affect more than one liver lobe. Thus, metastases are mostly present at time of diagnosis, particularly in the lung, abdominal serosa, and liver lymph nodes.

Surgery is the treatment of choice, particularly with any massive hepatic tumor, for single bile duct adenomas or multifocal lesions confined to one or two lobes. Generally, the liver allows radical surgery due to its remarkable reserve capacity. However, one study indicated a poor outcome even for massive bile duct tumors because most patients died within 6 months due to local recurrence and metastatic disease. *Hemangiosarcomas* and *carcinoids* have a poor *prognosis* and most of the patients have to be euthanized perioperatively.

Also for cats, *surgical techniques* for liver lobectomy include finger fracture, mass ligation, mattress sutures, bipolar vessel sealant devices, and surgical stapling with the same perioperative complications (hemorrhage, vascular compromise to adjacent liver lobes, transient hypoglycemia, reduced hepatic function).

Significant data on radiation therapy and chemotherapy for cats with hepatic tumors is lacking, but some chemotherapeutics require adequate liver function and can only be used with caution such as L-asparaginase and cyclophosphamide.

Further Readings

(Balkman 2009; Cole et al. 2002; Leveille et al. 1993; Marconato et al. 2007; Newell et al. 1998; Patnaik 1992; Patnaik et al. 1975, 2005; Roth 2001; van der Luer et al. 2008)

8.3 Hepatobiliary Tumors in Horses, Ruminants, and Pigs

Box 8.3 Hepatobiliary Tumors in Horses in Two Facts

1. Hepatoblastomas are the most common hepatobiliary tumor in horses.
2. Hepatoblastomas mainly develop in young horses.

Epidemiology and Pathogenesis

Primary equine liver tumors are rare, and *hepatoblastomas* are the most common variant reported. This tumor, most likely derives from primitive hepatic precursor cells and is reported in young and adult animals (fetuses and up to 4 years of age). Metastases to distant organs have been described in some cases. Hepatoblastomas are typically single, firm, lobulated masses and may show some hemorrhages and necrosis. Histologically they can contain embryonal or fetal epithelial and mesenchymal parts and are typically *alpha-fetoprotein positive* in immunohistochemical tests.

Domestic pot-bellied pigs have an average lifespan of 20–25 years. Most tumors in pigs are therefore reported in pot-bellied pigs. One study suggests that aged pot-bellied pigs can be predisposed to hepatocellular carcinomas, with a possible male predilection. The rate of extrahepatic metastasis of hepatocellular carcinoma was over 10 %.

Reports about primary neoplasia in *ruminants* are scarce and conflicting with respect to the prevalence of hepatocellular and cholangiocellular tumors. In general, many cases are incidental findings and studies in abattoirs. Likely due to economic reasons or postmortem diagnosis, treatments generally have not been undertaken.

8

■ **Further Readings**

(Anderson and Sandison 1968; Beeler-Marfisi et al. 2010; Bettini and Marcato 1992; de Vries et al. 2013; Haddad and Habecker 2012)

Suggested Reading

Anderson LJ, Sandison AT (1968) Tumors of the liver in cattle, sheep and pigs. Cancer 21:289–301

Balkman C (2009) Hepatobiliary neoplasia in dogs and cats. Vet Clin North Am Small Anim Pract 39:617–625

Barr F (1995) Percutaneous biopsy of abdominal organs under ultrasound guidance. J Small Anim Pract 36:105–113

Beeler-Marfisi J, Arroyo L, Caswell JL, Delay J, Bienzle D (2010) Equine primary liver tumors: a case series and review of the literature. J Vet Diagn Invest 22:174–183

Bettini G, Marcato PS (1992) Primary hepatic tumours in cattle. A classification of 66 cases. J Comp Pathol 107:19–34

Clifford CA, Pretorius ES, Weisse C, Sorenmo KU, Drobatz KJ, Siegelman ES, Solomon JA (2004) Magnetic resonance imaging of focal splenic and hepatic lesions in the dog. J Vet Intern Med 18:330–338

Cohen M, Bohling MW, Wright JC, Welles EA, Spano JS (2003) Evaluation of sensitivity and specificity of cytologic examination: 269 cases (1999–2000). J Am Vet Med Assoc 222:964–967

Cole TL, Center SA, Flood SN, Rowland PH, Valentine BA, Warner KL, Erb HN (2002) Diagnostic comparison of needle and wedge biopsy specimens of the liver in dogs and cats. J Am Vet Med Assoc 220:1483–1490

Cullen JM, Popp JA (2002) Tumors in domestic animals, 4th edn. Iowa State Press, Ames

de Vries C, Vanhaesebrouck E, Govaere J, Hoogewijs M, Bosseler L, Chiers K, Ducatelle R (2013) Congenital ascites due to hepatoblastoma with extensive peritoneal implantation metastases in a premature equine fetus. J Comp Pathol 148:214–219

Elpiner AK, Brodsky EM, Hazzah TN, Post GS (2011) Single-agent gemcitabine chemotherapy in dogs with hepatocellular carcinomas. Vet Comp Oncol 9:260–268

Haddad JL, Habecker PL (2012) Hepatocellular carcinomas in Vietnamese pot-bellied pigs (Sus scrofa). J Vet Diagn Invest 24:1047–1051

Hammer AS, Sikkema DA (1995) Hepatic neoplasia in the dog and cat. Vet Clin North Am Small Anim Pract 25:419–435

Hayes HM Jr, Morin MM, Rubenstein DA (1983) Canine biliary carcinoma: epidemiological comparisons with man. J Comp Pathol 93:99–107

Kemp SD, Panciera DL, Larson MM, Saunders GK, Werre SR (2013) A comparison of hepatic sonographic features and histopathologic diagnosis in canine liver disease: 138 cases. J Vet Intern Med 27:806–813

Kosovsky JE, Manframarretta S, Matthiesen DT, Patnaik AK (1989) Results of partial-hepatectomy in 18 dogs with hepatocellular-carcinoma. J Am Anim Hosp Assoc 25:203–206

Kutara K, Asano K, Kito A, Teshima K, Kato Y, Sasaki Y, Edamura K, Shibuya H, Sato T, Hasegawa A, Tanaka S (2006) Contrast harmonic imaging of canine hepatic tumors. J Vet Med Sci 68:433–438

Leveille R, Partington BP, Biller DS, Miyabayashi T (1993) Complications after ultrasound-guided biopsy of abdominal structures in dogs and cats – 246 cases (1984–1991). J Am Vet Med Assoc 203:413–415

Marconato L, Albanese F, Viacava P, Marchetti V, Abramo F (2007) Paraneoplastic alopecia associated with hepatocellular carcinoma in a cat. Vet Dermatol 18: 267–271

Nakamura K, Takagi S, Sasaki N, Kumara WRB, Murakami M, Ohta H, Yamasaki M, Takiguchi M (2010) Contrast-enhanced ultrasonography for characterization of canine focal liver lesions. Vet Radiol Ultrasound 51:79–85

Newell SM, Selcer BA, Girard E, Roberts GD, Thompson JP, Harrison JM (1998) Correlations between ultrasonographic findings and specific hepatic diseases in cats: 72 cases (1985–1997). J Am Vet Med Assoc 213:94–98

Patnaik AK (1992) A morphologic and immunocytochemical study of hepatic neoplasms in cats. Vet Pathol 29:405–415

Patnaik AK, Hurvitz AI, Lieberman PH (1980) Canine hepatic neoplasms: a clinicopathologic study. Vet Pathol 17:553–564

Patnaik AK, Hurvitz AI, Lieberman PH, Johnson GF (1981a) Canine bile duct carcinoma. Vet Pathol 18:439–444

Patnaik AK, Lieberman PH, Erlandson RA, Antonescu C (2005) Hepatobiliary neuroendocrine carcinoma in cats: a clinicopathologic, immunohistochemical, and ultrastructural study of 17 cases. Vet Pathol 42: 331–337

Patnaik AK, Lieberman PH, Hurvitz AI, Johnson GF (1981b) Canine hepatic carcinoids. Vet Pathol 18:445–453

Patnaik AK, Liu SK, Hurvitz AI, Mcclelland AJ (1975) Nonhematopoietic neoplasms in cats. J Natl Cancer Inst 54:855–860

Roth L (2001) Comparison of liver cytology and biopsy diagnoses in dogs and cats: 56 cases. Vet Clin Pathol 30:35–38

Stockhaus C, Van den Ingh T, Rothuizen J, Teske E (2004) A multistep approach in the cytologic evaluation of liver biopsy samples of dogs with hepatic diseases. Vet Pathol 41:461–470

van der Luer R, van den Ingh T, van Hoe M (2008) Feline paraneoplastic alopecia. Tijdschr Diergeneeskd 133:182–183

Vörös K, Vrabely T, Papp L, Horvath L, Karsai F (1991) Correlation of ultrasonographic and pathomorphological findings in canine hepatic diseases. J Small Anim Pract 32:627–634

Yamada T, Fujita M, Kitao S, Ashida Y, Nishizono K, Tsuchiya R, Shida T, Kobayashi K (1999) Serum alpha-fetoprotein values in dogs with various hepatic diseases. J Vet Med Sci 61:657–659

Alimentary Tumors

Angele Breithaupt

R. Klopfleisch (ed.), *Veterinary Oncology*, DOI 10.1007/978-3-319-41124-8_9

9.1 Oropharyngeal Tumors

Oropharyngeal tumors share some similarities in terms of clinical signs, diagnostic modalities, therapy, and prognostic factors.

Typical *clinical signs* of oropharyngeal tumors are facial swellings, excessive salivation, halitosis, dysphagia, bleeding, snoring respiration, cough, anorexia, weight loss, lymphadenopathy, and changed voice. Especially tooth loss is frequently associated with neoplasia in cats and can be mistaken for a primary dental disease (see ◘ Fig. 9.1).

Diagnostic investigation includes inspection of the oral cavity and cranium to roughly estimate the tumor extension and to detect enlargement or lysis of bone, gomphiasis and tooth loss, ulceration, unilateral epiphora, sneezing and rhinorrhea, and not least mobility of the ocular bulb. Regional lymph nodes are checked for adenopathy. However, lymph node size is not an accurate predictor of metastasis. Fine-needle aspiration of the regional lymph nodes should be performed regardless of the size or degree of fixation of the lymph nodes.

Diagnostic imaging of tumors of the jaw includes computed tomography (CT) and/or magnetic resonance imaging (MRI). Radiography of the lung is useful if metastasis is suspected. Remarkably, even normal-appearing radiographs do not exclude bone invasion. Scintigraphic techniques or contrast-enhanced ultrasonography is helpful to detect the sentinel lymph nodes and guide lymph node aspirates.

Depending on the localization, sampling for *cytological or histological* investigation of the tumor should be performed on narcotized and intubated patients to prevent possible blood aspiration. Cytologic samples have a rather low sensitivity and specificity for the diagnosis of the tumors. If tumors are well demarcated and fairly resectable, intended complete resection products can be evaluated histologically and serve as basis for further specific treatment. Ideally, biopsies should extend into the bone.

Except for malignant melanomas, canine oral squamous cell carcinomas, and sarcomas, malignant oral cavity tumors rarely *metastasize*. It seems that more caudally located tumors result in a poorer prognosis compared to rostrally located tumors, possibly due to a delayed detection and/or inconvenient surgical accessibility.

Surgery and *radiotherapy* are the most common *treatments* for the local control of oral tumors. Oral tumors frequently invade underlying bone; thus, surgical resection ideally includes bone margins. Margins of at least 2 cm are recommended for all malignant cancers, partially leading to mandibulectomy, maxillectomy, and orbitectomy. *Radiotherapy* can be used with curative intent or palliatively and in combination with surgery if resection of the tumor is likely to be incomplete. Several tumors are generally radiation responsive, including melanomas and squamous cell carcinomas, whereas others are considered radiation resistant.

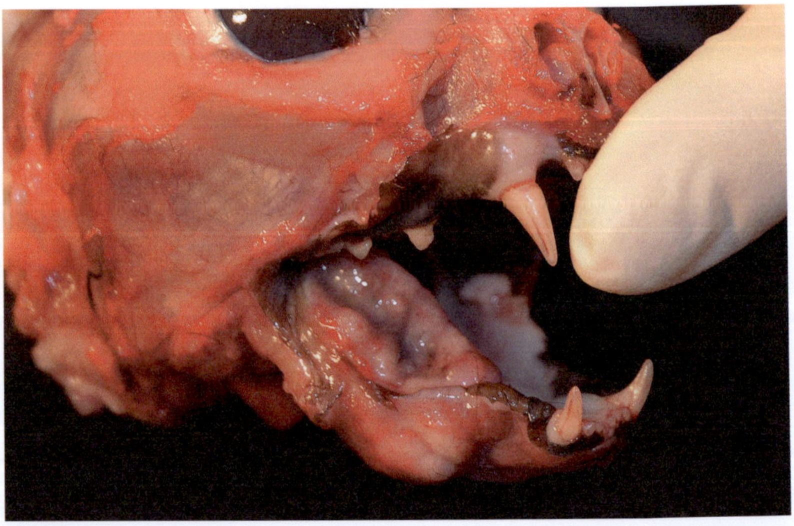

◘ **Fig. 9.1** Oral carcinoma (not further specified), cat, with tooth loss (Courtesy of Anja Meyer, PhD, Freie Universität Berlin, Germany)

The *median survival time* may be improved by combined approaches using radiotherapy, surgery, and chemotherapy, particularly for tumors suggested to be radiation resistant, including canine oral fibrosarcomas or feline oral squamous cell carcinomas. Overall, several reports indicate that histologically complete resection, smaller diameter, and a rostral location are favorable *prognostic factors* for oral tumors. Most likely, tumors with rostral location are detected earlier and with smaller size and chances are that resection is with complete surgical margins. Thus, recurrence is more likely in caudal locations and has negative effect on the survival time.

Based on these diagnostic steps, oral tumors can be clinically staged according to the WHO staging scheme (Owen 1980):

Clinical staging system for oral tumors in dogs and cats	
Primary tumor (T)	
Tis	Tumor in situ
T1	Tumor <2 cm in diameter at greatest dimension
T1a	Without evidence of bone invasion
T1b	With evidence of bone invasion
T2	Tumor 2–4 cm in diameter at greatest dimension
T2a	Without evidence of bone invasion
T2b	With evidence of bone invasion
T3	Tumor >4 cm in diameter at greatest dimension
T3a	Without evidence of bone invasion
T3b	With evidence of bone invasion
Regional lymph nodes (N)	
N0	No regional lymph node metastasis
N1	Movable ipsilateral lymph nodes
N1a	No evidence of lymph node metastasis
N1b	Evidence of lymph node metastasis
N2	Movable contralateral lymph nodes
N2a	No evidence of lymph node metastasis
N2b	Evidence of lymph node metastasis
N3	Fixed lymph nodes

Clinical staging system for oral tumors in dogs and cats			
Distant metastasis (M)			
M0	No distant metastasis		
M1	Distant metastasis [specify site(s)]		
Stage grouping	*Tumor (T)*	*Nodes (N)*	*Metastasis (M)*
I	T1	N0, N1a, N2a	M0
II	T2	N0, N1a, N2a	M0
III	T3	N0, N1a, N2a	M0
IV	Any T	N1b	M0
	Any T	N2b, N3	M0
	Any T	Any N	M1

Suggested Reading

(Herring et al. 2002; Lurie et al. 2006; Owen 1980)

9.1.1 Canine Oropharyngeal Tumors

Tumors of the oral cavity in dogs are almost evenly matched benign and malignant. Benign tumors in dogs include *epulides*, oral *papillomas*, and *plasmacytomas*. In descending order, the most common malignant canine oral tumors are malignant *melanomas*, *squamous cell carcinomas* (SCCs), and *fibrosarcomas*, although in few studies, SCCs are more common than malignant melanomas.

Other very rare tumors that will not be discussed in detail here are lingual granular cell myoblastomas, mast cell tumors, adenocarcinomas, neurofibrosarcomas, leiomyosarcomas, hemangiosarcomas and hemangiomas, rhabdomyomas and rhabdomyosarcomas, myxomas, and lipomas.

The *tonsils* are ten times more often affected in animals living in urban compared to rural areas, implying an association with environmental pollutants. Primary tumors are often SCCs (mostly unilateral) and lymphomas (often bilateral). Metastatic tumors have to be considered, particularly melanoma. In most cases, tonsillopathy is considered as systemic disease, so tonsillectomy is generally not curative but diagnostically helpful.

■ **Suggested Reading**

(Brodey 1960; Dennis et al. 2006; Todoroff and Brodey 1979)

9.1.1.1 Canine Oral Melanocytic Tumors

Box 9.1. Canine Oral Melanocytic Tumors in Six Facts

1. Oral malignant melanomas: one of the most common tumors in the oral cavity
2. Distant metastasis is common
3. Up to one third are amelanotic
4. Imunohistochemistry for detecting amelanotic melanomas: melan-A, PNL2, TRP-1, TRP-2
5. Oral melanomas have a poor prognosis
6. Prognostic factors include nuclear atypia, mitotic, and Ki67 index

9

■ **Epidemiology and Pathogenesis**

In accordance with the current World Health Organization (WHO) nomenclature, the term "melanocytoma" refers to the benign neoplasm of melanocytic origin, whereas the term "malignant melanoma (MM)" refers to the malignant variant.

Oral MM are the most common tumors of the oral cavity and predominantly occur in aged dogs (mean age 11 years). Breed predispositions are indicated for Scottish terriers, golden retrievers, poodles, and dachshunds. Melanocytomas are extremely rare in the oral cavity.

■ **Clinical Appearance**

MM appear mostly as black-brown, frequently ulcerated tumors of the gingival, labial, buccal, and palatal mucosa as well as on the tongue. One third of the tumors are amelanotic. Almost every patient develops *metastasis* in regional lymph nodes and/or the lung or less commonly in other organs including the liver, kidney, and brain. Metastasis in regional lymph nodes is not obligatorily associated with their enlargement.

For staging, there is either a four-stage scheme of the Word Heath Organization (WHO, see ◘ Table 9.1) or a more recent three-stage scheme available (see ◘ Table 9.2).

■ **Cytology and Histopathology**

Cytology and histology generally are straightforward for pigmented tumors, and even grossly nonpigmented tumors may exhibit microscopically visible melanin pigment. For malignant tumors, *cytology* in combination with immunohistochemistry, using anti-cytokeratin, anti-melan-A, and anti-vimentin antibodies, agrees very well with histopathological diagnosis. *Histopathology* is necessary to confirm malignancy. If pigment is not detectable, the diagnosis is aggravated and might merely lead to a diagnosis of (malignant) blastoma. Based on histology, recommendations for prognostication of canine melanocytic neoplasms have been worked out in detail (see below). *Immunohistochemistry* labeling with a combination of *melan-A, PNL2, TRP-1*, and *TRP-2* provides the highest sensitivity for detecting amelanotic melanomas while maintaining 100 % specificity.

◘ **Table 9.1** World Health Organization, TNM-based staging scheme for dogs with oral melanomas

T: primary tumor
T1: tumor ≤2 cm in diameter
T2: tumor 2–4 cm in diameter
T3: tumor >4 cm in diameter
N: regional lymph nodes
N0: no evidence of regional node involvement
N1: histologic/cytologic evidence of regional node involvement
N2: fixed nodes
M: distant metastasis
M0: no evidence of distant metastasis
M1: evidence of distant metastasis
Stage I = T1 N0 M0
Stage II = T2 N0 M0
Stage III = T2 N1 M0 or T3 N0 M0
Stage IV = any T, any N and M1

■ **Prognosis and Therapy**

In general, oral melanocytic neoplasms have a worse *prognosis* than cutaneous neoplasms, and distant metastasis indicates a poor prognosis. The value of staging for the prognosis of survival time and remission is debatable. In contrast, histological classification as benign or malignant is generally associated with the clinical outcome and

Table 9.2 Alternative staging system according to Hahn et al. (1994)

T	*Primary tumor*		
	T1	Tumor in situ or ≤2 cm maximum diameter (volume ≤8 cm³)	
	T2	Tumor 2–4 cm maximum diameter (volume 8–64 cm³)	
	T3	Tumor >4 cm maximum diameter (volume >64 cm³)	
	Mitotic index		
	a	≤3 per high-power field	
	b	>3 per high-power field	
	Oral cavity or oropharyngeal location		
	1	Rostral mandible/caudal maxilla	
	2	Others	
N	*Regional lymph nodes*		
	N0	No evidence of regional node involvement	
	N1	Histological evidence of regional node involvement	
	N2	Fixed nodes	
M	*Distant metastasis*		
	M0	No evidence of distant metastasis	
	M1	Distant metastasis (including distant nodes)	
Stage grouping	*T*	*N*	*M*
I	T1 a1	N0	M0
II	T1 a2, any T1 b, T2 a1	N0	M0
	Any T	N1	M0
III	Any T2 a2, any T2 b or T3	N0	M0
	Any T	N2	M0
	Any T	Any N	M1

survival. Recommended *parameters with prognostic value* include nuclear atypia, mitotic index, and Ki67 (proliferation) index. Tumor size or volume, ulceration, and lack of pigmentation are not reliably prognostic.

Due to the common invasion of oral melanomas into the periost and bone, *surgical* preservation of underlying bone by conservative excision is not recommended. To the contrary, en bloc resection is suggested. Partial mandibulectomia, maxillectomia, and also resection of the tongue are generally well tolerated in dogs.

Hypofractionized *radiotherapy* may lead to partial or complete remission, but some studies experienced a lack of positive effects of different radiotherapeutic protocols and radiosensitizing platin-based agents.

Chemotherapy is suboptimal due to an explicit low sensitivity of these tumors for chemotherapeutic drugs to date, except for rare case reports with successful treatments.

Current Research

Oral melanomas induce an immune response. This *antitumor reaction* might influence the course of disease and survival time. Immunomodulatory approaches for treatment of melanocytic tumors are under investigation.

Suggested Reading

(Blackwood and Dobson 1996; Boria et al. 2004; Burk 1996; Hahn et al. 1994; Przeździecki et al. 2015; Ramos-Vara et al. 2000; Rassnick et al. 2001; Regan et al. 2015; Smedley et al. 2011a, b; Smith et al. 2002)

9.1.1.2 Canine Oral Squamous Cell Carcinomas (SCCs)

Box 9.2. Canine Oral Squamous Cell Carcinomas in Five Facts

1. SCCs: one of the most common tumors in the oral cavity
2. Localization: gingiva, tongue, and tonsil
3. Up to one third show distant metastasis at time of diagnosis
4. Caudally located tumors have a worse prognosis
5. Radical surgery is recommended

Epidemiology and Pathogenesis

SCCs are common tumors of the oral cavity in dogs. A papillomaviral etiology has been discussed but seems unlikely. The mean age is 9 years and medium- to large-sized dogs but also West Highland white terriers may be predisposed. A breed predisposition for *tonsillar* SCC is published for German shepherds. Half of the *lingual* tumors are SCC with a potential predisposition for poodles, golden retriever, samoyeds, and female dogs with a mean age of 9.5 years.

Clinical Appearance

SCCs mostly arise in the *gingiva*, particularly rostral to premolar tooth, on the *tongue*, and *tonsils*. They appear as light-red masses, often ulcerated and bleeding, mimicking gingivitis. Invasion, osteolysis, and gomphiasis are frequent. Metastasis occurs in advanced stages, preferentially to regional (mandibular) lymph nodes. Lingual tumors occur anywhere on the tongue. Staging requires investigation of the oral cavity, pharynx, tonsils, biopsy of enlarged lymph nodes, and radiography of the lung. One third of these tumors exhibit metastasis at diagnosis.

Cytology and Histopathology

Cytology and *histology* are similar to cutaneous SCC with variably differentiated epithelial cells, keratin, keratin pearls, and frequently inflammation due to secondary infection of ulcerated tumors. Invasion of underlying bone tissue is common.

Prognosis and Therapy

SCCs occur in three distinct localizations that may correlate with prognosis: (1) gingiva including gum, labial, and buccal mucosa, (2) lingual, and (3) tonsillar. *Caudally located* gingival and lingual carcinomas are associated with a *significantly poorer prognosis* compared with more rostral tumors. Reasons may include an occult growth of the former, richer lymphatic and vascular channels of the caudal oral tissue and that rostral tumors can be resected with wider margins.

Atypical p63 labeling and *cytoplasmic E-cadherin* staining appear to be related with a higher tumor grade. Histological *grade* and *PCNA expression* may be important prognosis factors in canine SCC.

Surgery is the common approach for nontonsillar SCC. The common invasion of SCC into the periost, bone, and tongue often requires *surgical* en bloc resection or glossectomia. The recurrence rate is significantly higher after maxillectomy compared to mandibulectomy. Median *survival rates* range between few months and more than 1.5 years. Underlining the impact of histological grading, differences are most obvious regarding lingual SCCs: median survival times after surgical resection can range between 16 (grade I) and 3–4 months (grade II, III).

SCCs are sensitive for *radiotherapy*, but recurrence of tumors is nevertheless often observed. Median survival times are markedly increased if radiotherapy is combined with surgery.

Chemotherapy can be used for dogs with metastatic disease and unresectable tumors and as adjuvant treatment. The effect of chemotherapy on the metastatic rate is unknown. Few studies using piroxicam, cisplatin, or carboplatin are available. However, toxicity limits the clinical usefulness.

Current Research

Novel therapies are under investigation, including electrochemogenetherapy as well as characterization of possible papillomavirus etiologies.

Suggested Reading

(Carpenter et al. 1993; Dennis et al. 2006; Kosovsky et al. 1991; Mestrinho et al. 2014, 2015; Munday et al. 2015b, 2016; Reed et al. 2010; Wallace et al. 1992; Withrow and Holmberg 1983)

9.1.1.3 Canine Oral Sarcomas

Box 9.3. Canine Oral Sarcomas in Four Facts

1. Oral fibrosarcomas are the third most common tumor.
2. Up to one third develop distant metastasis.
3. A histologically low-grade, biologically high-grade fibrosarcoma occurs.
4. The prognosis is guarded to poor.

Epidemiology and Pathogenesis

Mesenchymal tumors comprise 12 % of all oral tumors and 20 % of all malignant tumors in the oral cavity of dogs. Fibrosarcomas are the third most common tumor in the oral cavity of dogs. Male and medium- to large-sized dogs are overrepresented. The tumors are found in dogs of all ages. Particularly, the *histologically low-grade*, *biologically high-grade fibrosarcomas* commonly occur in large breed dogs (e.g., retriever dogs) at younger ages and should not be misdiagnosed as fibromas or fibromatous epulides. Osteosarcomas and fibromas rarely occur and will not be discussed in detail.

▪ Clinical Appearance

Oral *fibrosarcomas* arise equally within the mandibula and maxilla. The gingival and palatinal mucosa are most commonly affected. Tumors have a firm consistency and are sometimes ulcerated. The tumors grow highly invasive with osteolytic activity. Up to one third of the patients develop metastases in regional lymph nodes, the lungs, and other organs, often long after assumed complete resection of the primary tumor.

Fibrosarcomas developing around the carnassial or premolar teeth and the hard palate are usually *histologically low-grade, biologically aggressive tumors.* Although well-differentiated histologically, they show a marked infiltrative growth and metastasis in the regional lymph nodes and lungs.

▪ Cytology and Histopathology

Cytology may present with less differentiated and more pleomorphic plump to spindloid cells and oval nuclei compared with well-differentiated spindle cells in fibromas. *Histology* is needed to confirm malignancy, for differentiation of other mesenchymal tumors and the evaluation of surgical margins. Fibrosarcomas may appear remarkably well-differentiated histologically, although they may behave very aggressively. Differentiation to (peripheral odontogenic) fibromas can be thus challenging even with large biopsy samples, if bone invasion and osteolytic activity are not represented in the sample.

▪ Prognosis and Therapy

The *prognosis* for dogs with oral fibrosarcomas is guarded, particularly due to a high recurrence rate and metastasis to the regional lymph nodes and to the lungs (reported in up to 27 % of patients).

Patients with *histologically low-grade, biologically high-grade fibrosarcomas* present with poorer survival rates as compared to dogs with soft tissue sarcomas of other body sites. With respect to recurrence, the *surgical* treatment should include at least 3 cm margins from the visible or palpable tumor mass, but resection of the histologically low-grade, biologically high-grade fibrosarcomas is mostly incomplete. Therefore, a combination of surgery and *radiotherapy* may improve the survival rates. Nevertheless, oral fibrosarcomas are considered radiation resistant. Data regarding systemic *chemotherapeutical* treatment of oral fibrosarcomas are sparse.

▪ Suggested Reading

(Ciekot et al. 1994; Kosovsky et al. 1991; Thrall 1981; Wallace et al. 1992)

9.1.1.4 Canine Oral Plasmacytomas

Box 9.4. Canine Oral Plasmacytomas in Four Facts

1. Oral plasmacytomas are locally invasive but rarely metastasize
2. Histological criteria of malignancy may be present – but biological behavior is generally benign
3. Prognosis is good
4. Surgery is mostly curative

Epidemiology and Pathogenesis

Oral (extramedullary) plasmacytomas account for up to 6 % of all oral neoplasia. Middle-aged dogs (7–9 years) and golden retriever dogs as well as Yorkshire terriers are overrepresented. As primary tumors, they arise from plasma cells in the soft tissue or as metastasis from primary osseous myeloma.

▪ Clinical Appearance

The tumor appears as a raised, red, lobulated mass mostly located on the gingiva or lips. They show an invasive growth pattern but rarely metastasize.

▪ Cytology and Histopathology

Cytology or histopathology is needed to differentiate the tumor from other round cell tumors and nonpigmented melanomas. *Cytologically* and *histopathologically*, this tumor is comprised of well-differentiated plasma cells. The biological behavior of these tumors is generally benign despite of their partially pleomorphic or anaplastic appearance and the presence of mitotic figures and bi- and multinucleated cells.

Prognosis and Therapy

The prognosis for oral plasmacytomas is good. *Surgical* resection is the most common therapy and may be curative. The median survival time increases significantly if the tumor is completely resected. A combination of *radiotherapy* and *chemotherapy* is recommended for unresectable tumors.

Suggested Reading

(Rakich et al. 1989; Wright et al. 2008)

9.1.1.5 Canine Oral Viral Papillomas

> **Box 9.5. Canine Oral Viral Papillomas in Three Facts**
> 1. Papilloma virus infections induce tumor development.
> 2. Tumors may interfere chewing and require resection.
> 3. Prognosis is usually excellent due to regression.

Epidemiology and Pathogenesis

Viral papillomas, induced after horizontal transmission of papillomavirus (*Papillomaviridae* family), mostly affect dogs of juvenile age. They develop on the oral mucosa and lips, among others, mostly with multiple manifestation. Canine papillomavirus type 1 (CPV1) is considered to be responsible for most oral cases; CPV13 is rarely described. Furthermore, canine papillomavirus has been proposed to be associated with oral carcinoma.

Clinical Appearance

Viral papillomatosis presents with mostly multiple, up to several cm in size, flat or pedunculated tumors with a smooth to fringy, wartlike surface. Affected dogs usually do not suffer, but tumors may interfere chewing and require resection due to recurrent bleeding.

Cytology and Histopathology

Visual examination is usually diagnostic, but a biopsy can be performed if necessary. *Cytology* is rather unspecific presenting with proliferating spindle cells. *Histologically*, a keratinizing squamous epithelium covers vascularized propria papillae. A viral etiology can be suspected due to occurrence of viral cytopathic effects including detection of "koilocytes" or basophilic intranuclear inclusion bodies.

Prognosis and Therapy

The *prognosis* is usually excellent: Papillomatosis in dogs is considered to be a self-limiting disease with *spontaneous regression* within 4–8 weeks. Regression seems to correlate with a strong antibody response. Thus, *treatment* is generally not necessary. Occasionally, papillomas persist, most likely based on immunodeficiency, and malignant progression is reported for few cases. *Resection* using cryo-, laser-, and electrosurgery is recommended in refractory cases, to prevent further transmission or if chewing is markedly interfered.

Current Research

Recent studies focus mainly on detection of new viruses and potential malignant progression as well as antitumoral immune response.

Suggested Reading

(DeBey et al. 2001; Munday et al. 2015c; Sancak et al. 2015; Watrach et al. 1970)

9.1.1.6 Canine Epulides (Fibromatous Epulides of the Periodontal Ligament)

> **Box 9.6. Canine Epulides in Four Facts**
> 1. The term "epulides" is used for fibromatous epulides of the periodontal ligament only.
> 2. Epulides have a predilection to the maxilla, rostral to the third premolar teeth.
> 3. Treatment and prognosis is similar to fibrous gingival hyperplasia.
> 4. Surgical resection is generally curative.

Epidemiology and Pathogenesis

The general term "epulis" means exophytic gingival mass but is used only for *fibromatous tumors of the periodontal ligament* (syn.:fibromatous epulis). The tumor arises from the gingival periodontal ligament. Brachycephalic breeds appear to be predisposed and tumors occur at all ages. The term peripheral odontogenic fibroma, derived from human tumor nomenclature, should be avoided. The canine tumor is comparable but not similar to the human entity. Further proliferative or hyperplastic gingival lesions occur in dogs:

- *Fibrous hyperplasia* (not longer part of fibromatous epulides): mature, low cellular, fibrous tissue, may contain epithelial nests and inflammation, and is familial in Boxer dogs
- *Pyogenic granuloma*: well-vascularized granulation tissue covered by often ulcerated gingival epithelium (pyogenic granuloma is actually a misnomer)
- *Peripheral giant cell granuloma* (not longer giant cell epulis): well-vascularized granulation tissue containing characteristic multinucleated giant cells of presumed osteoclastic origin (granuloma would therefore be a misnomer)

The fibrous hyperplasia is clinically indistinguishable from fibromatous epulis of the periodontal ligament. Treatment and prognosis are similar for both lesions, so differentiation is regarded as academic by some authors.

▪ Clinical Appearance

Epulides commonly develop at the *rostral to the third maxillary premolar teeth* and grow rather slowly, singular or multiple, and firm and rarely reach 2 cm in diameter. They are gray-pink and covered by mostly intact epithelium but may enclose or displace adjacent teeth. They are attached to the periosteum but do not invade bone.

▪ Cytology and Histopathology

Epulides are difficult to be unequivocally diagnosed *cytologically* because they can be composed of dental epithelial nests enrobed in stromal fibrous tissue that may be difficult to interpret without tissue architecture. *Histopathology* is necessary to confirm initial diagnosis and evaluation of surgical margins. The tumors comprise of regular, stellate mesenchymal cells, small fibrillary collagen fibers, and often dilated blood vessels that rarely contain red blood cells. Osteoid or bone, cementum or dentin may be present, as well as cords of odontogenic epithelium.

▪ Prognosis and Therapy

The prognosis is excellent after surgical treatment, but incomplete removal leads to recurrent growth. The risk for recurrence can be reduced by cryotherapy.

▪ Suggested Reading

(Desoutter et al. 2012; Fiani et al. 2011; Gardner 1996; Yoshida et al. 1999)

9.1.1.7 Canine Odontogenic Tumors

Box 9.7. Canine Odontogenic Tumors in Four Facts

1. Ameloblastomas mostly arise rostral, grow invasive, and do not metastasize.
2. Acanthomatous ameloblastomas are unique to the dog.
3. Odontomas mostly grow in the caudal parts and comprise of variably organized dental tissue.
4. Prognosis is favorable after complete resection.

Epidemiology and Pathogenesis

Odontogenic tumors include two categories: (1) "noninductive" types without odontogenic mesenchyma and (2) "inductive" types with the presence of odontogenic mesenchyma.

The first category comprisis *ameloblastomas* and rarely occurring amyloid-producing odontogenic tumors (APOT). For ameloblastomas, medium- to large-sized breeds are overrepresented. The mean age is 7–10 years, and these benign tumors do not metastasize.

The second category comprises *complex or compound odontomas* and the rarely occurring ameloblastic fibroma, as well as ameloblastic fibro-odontoma.

Malignant variants are extremely rare and include ameloblastic carcinomas and fibrosarcomas. All malignant tumors exhibit infiltrative growth and high mitotic activity.

▪ Clinical Appearance

Odontogenic tumors appear as slowly growing expansile or infiltrative masses that might cause dislocation of teeth, teeth loss, and bone destruction. *Ameloblastomas* typically arise in the rostral maxilla and mandibula, especially around the mandibular incisive. Tumors can be ulcerated. Despite their invasive growth, osteolysis, and teeth loss, metastasis does not occur. *Odontomas* appear mostly in the caudal parts of the mandible and maxilla.

Cytology and Histopathology

Cytology presents with clustered interdigitating neoplastic epithelial cells with some degree of anisocytosis and anisokaryosis.

Ameloblastomas appear in different histotypes, including spindle cell, basaloid, desmoplastic and keratinizing types, and most frequently *acanthomatous ameloblastoma*. This unique tumor of the dog can invade the underlying bone and is associated with cyst formation. It is composed of sheets and cords of nonkeratinizing odontogenic epithelium with prominent intercellular bridges and peripheral palisading of epithelial cells that have antibasilar nuclei.

Odontomas are benign tumors arising from the dental follicle and contain variable amounts of well-differentiated epithelial and mesenchymal dental tissues: whereas *complex odontomas* contain disorganized tissues, *compound odontomas* display completely developed teeth.

Prognosis and Therapy

A favorable prognosis after treatment is known for these benign odontogenic tumors.

Surgery is the most common therapeutic approach. Incomplete resection yields in recurrence. Especially for acanthomatous ameloblastomas, mandibulectomy or maxillectomy is required because of frequent bone invasion by this benign tumor. *Radiation* therapy is less common although ameloblastomas are highly sensitive. Many tumors however recur within the radiation field or exhibit malignant transformation. Studies on *chemotherapeutical* treatments such as intralesional bleomycin application are rather scarce.

Suggested Reading

(Fiani et al. 2011; Kelly et al. 2010; Poulet et al. 1992; Theon et al. 1997; Thrall 1984; White and Gorman 1989)

9.1.2 Feline Oropharyngeal Tumors

Oral tumors in cats are mostly malignant with *squamous cell carcinomas* (SCCs) being the most common malignancy, which will be discussed in detail. Other, more rarely occurring neoplasms include *fibrosarcomas*. *Feline inductive odontogenic tumors* are rare and affect mostly kittens as osteolytic masses of the rostral maxilla.

Reactive or hyperplastic lesions in the oral cavity of cats are *peripheral giant cell granulomas* which is the second most common oral mass after *fibromatous epulis of periodontal ligament*. Both entities appear to behave biologically similar as in dogs (see ► Sect. 9.1.1.6).

Mast cell tumors, as in dogs, should be regarded as potentially malignant with potential metastasis to regional lymph nodes.

Oral papillomas and *fibropapillomas* are very rare in cats and mostly associated with papillomavirus antigen detection. Recently, a novel papillomavirus was detected in the oral cavity of domestic cats.

Odontogenic tumors, *oral melanomas*, and *oral sarcomas* are very rare. For prognosis and possible treatment following canine tumors, see respective ► Sects. 9.1.1.1, 9.1.1.3, and 9.1.1.7).

Suggested Reading

(Dunowska et al. 2014; Gardner and Dubielzig 1995; Munday et al. 2015a; Sundberg et al. 2000)

9.1.2.1 Feline Oral Squamous Cell Carcinomas (SCCs)

Box 9.8. Feline Oral Squamous Cell Carcinomas in Four Facts

1. SCCs are the most frequent oral tumors in cats
2. Common localization: gingiva, sublingual (frenulum), and tonsil
3. Cats may develop tooth loss, exophthalmos, and lymphadenopathy
4. Oral SCCs have a poor prognosis

Epidemiology and Pathogenesis

SCC is the most frequent oral tumor in cats. One report states that the risk to develop SCC is increased with the use of flea collars and intake of canned food. The mean age is between 10 and 12 years and neither sex nor breed predispositions are proven. Recent studies do not support that papillomavirus plays a significant role in tumor development.

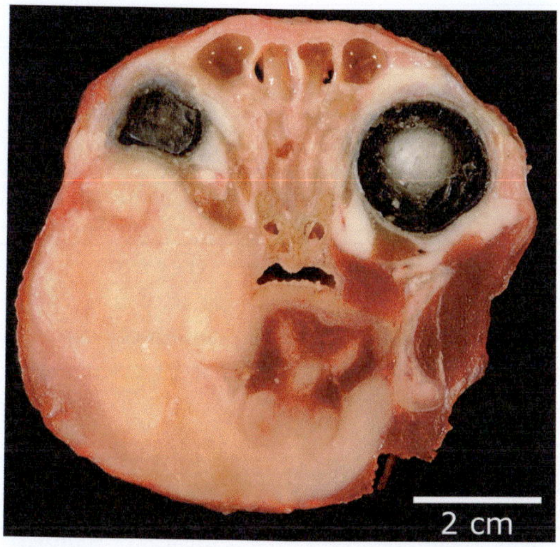

Fig. 9.2 Oral squamous cell carcinoma, cat: note marked invasive growth (Courtesy of Stefanie Binder, Freie Universität Berlin, Germany)

Clinical Appearance

SCCs occur in decreasing frequency on the (1) mandibular and maxillar *gingiva,* (2) (sub)lingual adjacent to the *lingual frenulum*, and (3) on the *tonsils*. They are mostly ulcerated and inflamed, mimicking stomatitis. An early invasion of the bone with marked osteolysis leads to loose teeth, tooth loss, and reactive bone proliferation (see Fig. 9.2). Affection of the maxilla is frequently associated with exophthalmos. Enlargement of regional lymph nodes is frequent, based mostly on associated inflammation and more rarely on metastasis. Scarce reports exist about paraneoplastic malignant hypercalcemia.

Cytology and Histopathology

Cytology typically exhibits variably differentiated epithelial cells and possibly keratin. Secondary, inflammation is frequent due to ulceration. The differentiation of SCC from epithelial hyperplasia can be difficult. *Histopathology* is necessary for final diagnosis and especially for evaluation of surgical margins.

Prognosis and Therapy

SCCs in the oral cavity have a *poor prognosis*. A multimodal treatment approach likely offers the best chance of success; however, surgery, radiation therapy, chemotherapy, and combinations of them are rarely satisfactory. *Surgical* partial mandibulectomia and maxillectomia is less well tolerated in cats than in dogs, and recurrence is common. Especially grooming might be compromised after aggressive resection and results in poor hair-coat hygiene. *Radiotherapy* does not seem to improve the survival time significantly but potentially in combination with sensitizers or with chemotherapy. Reliable data after *chemotherapeutical* treatments are scarce and mostly survival time is not essentially improved. Nonsteroidal anti-inflammatory drugs (NSAIDs) have not been described consistently effective in literature.

Current Research

There is ongoing research concerning new chemotherapeutical treatments and the role of papillomavirus in SCC.

Suggested Reading

(Bertone et al. 2003; Bilgic et al. 2015; DiBernardi et al. 2007; Hayes et al. 2007; Munday and French 2015; Northrup et al. 2006; Snyder et al. 2004; Stebbins et al. 1989)

9.1.3 Equine Oropharyngeal Tumors

Epidemiology and Pathogenesis

Tumors of the oral cavity are *uncommon* in horses and in other large animals. Fibro-osseous neoplasms including *osteomas* and *ossifying fibromas* are reported as well as *squamous cell carcinomas*. Others, such as melanomas, fibrosarcomas, and lymphomas are very rare. *Odontogenic tumors*, including ameloblastoma, ameloblastic odontoma, cementomas, and complex odontomas, are also known in horses (see Fig. 9.3).

Clinical Appearance

Oral tumors typically present with ptyalism, halitosis, quidding, tongue protrusion, nasal discharge, dysphagia, inappetence, and weight loss. Invasion of underlying bone is frequent in advanced stages.

Radiography can be used to determine tumor localization and bone lysis and endoscopy may visualize posterior masses.

Cytology and Histopathology

Depending on the tumor type, *histology* is required for definite diagnosis and evaluation of tumor margins.

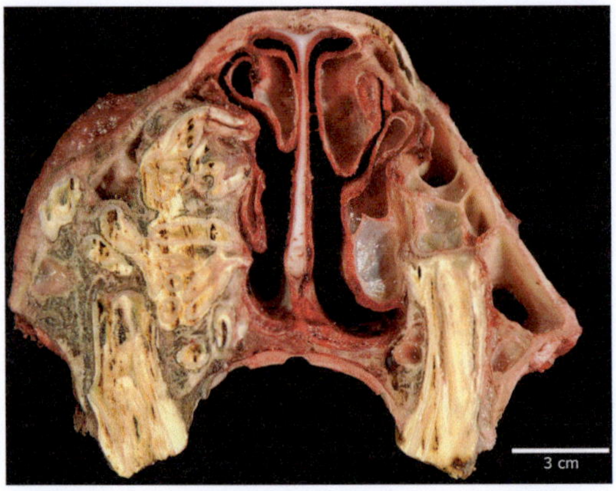

Fig. 9.3 Odontoma, zebra: note expansive growth with compression of maxillary sinuses and nasal cavity (Courtesy of Stefanie Binder, Freie Universität Berlin, Germany)

Prognosis and Therapy

The *treatment* of choice is surgical excision, probably including mandibulectomy due to recurrence after excision that is restricted to the mucosal level.

Suggested Reading

(Gardner 1994; Kreutzer et al. 2007; Morse et al. 1988)

9.1.4 Bovine Oropharyngeal Tumors

Box 9.9. Bovine Oral Tumors in Four Facts

1. Oral tumors are rare in cattle.
2. Bovine oral papillomatosis is associated with BPV-4 infection.
3. Bovine oral papillomatosis is usually self-limiting within 12 months.
4. Ameloblastomas have a favorable prognosis after resection.

Epidemiology and Pathogenesis

Large animals have a low prevalence of malignant tumors in the oral cavity. *Oral papillomatosis*, associated with *bovine papillomavirus 4* (BPV-4) infection, occurs in endemic areas such as Brazil, England, and Scotland. Squamous cell carcinomas at the same anatomical sites were also detected in some of these regions, and *bracken fern* intoxication was identified as the environmental cofactor and will not be discussed in further detail here. *Ameloblastic fibromas* are the most common odontogenic tumors of cattle. They occur at any age but may particularly arise in young cattle. Other tumors, such as oral squamous cell carcinomas, are very rare and will not be discussed in detail.

Clinical Appearance

As for all oral tumors, clinical signs include lumps, facial swellings, excessive salivation, halitosis, pain, dysphagia, bleeding, snoring respiration, cough, anorexia, weight loss, lymphadenopathy, and changed voice.

Oral papillomas are clinically and morphologically similar to the canine disease (see ► Sect. 9.1.1.5): mostly multiple, up to few centimeters in size, flat or pedunculated tumors with a smooth to fringy, wartlike surface. Lesions may extent remarkably into the esophagus and rumen.

Ameloblastic fibromas arise mostly in the vicinity of the mandibular incisors, are intraosseous, and therefore may destroy adjacent bone see (Fig. 9.4a, b).

Cytology and Histopathology

Cytology is mostly not diagnostic for papillomas. *Histopathology* is necessary for final diagnosis and evaluation of tumor margins, particularly for ameloblastic fibroma. Histopathology for papillomas is similar to lesions described in dogs (see ► Sect. 9.1.1.5).

Prognosis and Therapy

For *bovine oral papillomas*, the prognosis is usually excellent due to its *self-limiting* character. The cell-mediated immune response usually rejects the tumors within 12 months. In immunosuppressed cattle, disease may *persist* or spread remarkably.

Ameloblastic fibromas typically behave similar to ameloblastomas with a *favorable prognosis* after surgical treatment.

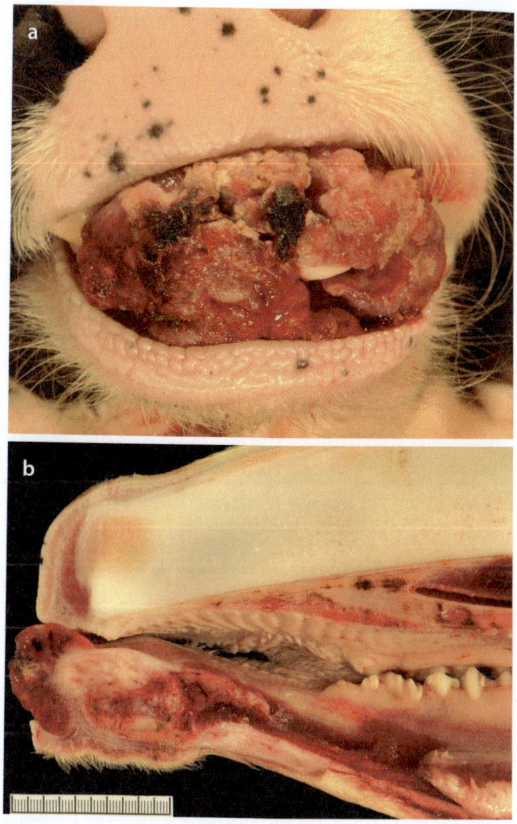

Fig. 9.4 (**a**) (frontal) and (**b**) (sagittal) Ameloblastic fibroma, mandible, calf, 3 weeks: note incorporation and dislocation of the incisor and massive granulation tissue proliferation (Courtesy of Moritz Radbruch, Freie Universität Berlin, Germany)

Suggested Reading

(Bocaneti et al. 2016; Campo et al. 1980; Masuda et al. 2011; Munday 2014; Tsirimonaki et al. 2003)

9.2 Tumors of Salivary Glands

9.2.1 Canine and Feline Salivary Gland Tumors

Salivary glands are mostly affected by sialadenitis and cysts, rarely by neoplasia. In both species, these tumors occur in aged animals (>10 years) without breed or sex predilection, and the etiology is undetermined.

Box 9.10. Canine and Feline Salivary Gland Tumors in Three Facts

1. Tumors of the salivary glands are very rare.
2. Tumors are almost always malignant.
3. Distant metastasis is frequent at time of diagnosis.

Epidemiology and Pathogenesis

Ninety-five percent of all salivary gland tumors are malignant including various *adenocarcinomas, squamous cell carcinomas, basal cell carcinomas, and anaplastic carcinomas*. Also mixed tumors of epithelial and myoepithelial origin are described. Cocker spaniel dogs and Siamese cats are potentially overrepresented. In cats, males are more frequently affected.

Clinical Appearance

Mainly, the *parotid* and *mandibular glands* are involved, inducing submandibular or periauricular unilateral lumps. Local pain, anorexia, dysphagia, bleeding, and halitosis are reported. *Metastasis* to regional lymph nodes is common, particularly in cats and distant metastasis, especially to the lung that also occur in cats and in dogs. Biopsy of enlarged lymph nodes is highly recommended. Radiography can reveal periost proliferations, osteolytic changes, calcification of the mass, and distant metastases.

Cytology and Histopathology

Cytological investigation of fine-needle aspirates can suspect salivary gland neoplasia, but *histological* confirmation is often required. It was shown that the *histological grade* was *not prognostic* for the outcome, but advanced *stage* was a negative *prognostic* factor.

Prognosis and Therapy

The *prognosis* for salivary gland cancer is unclear due to limited data. The phenotype seems not to be relevant for prognosis. Cats tend to have a more aggressive disease with more frequent metastasis to regional lymph nodes. *Surgical* therapy is aggravated due to adjacent structures that impede radical resection, but macroscopic incomplete resection yields in recurrence and a poor prognosis. Adjuvant *radiotherapy* significantly improves the survival time in dogs but not in cats.

Suggested Reading

(Brown 1989; Hammer et al. 2001; Spangler and Culbertson 1991)

9.3 Esophageal Tumors

9.3.1 Canine and Feline Esophageal Tumors

Box 9.11. Canine and Feline Esophageal Tumors in Five Facts

1. Esophageal tumors are generally rare.
2. Spirocerca lupi infection may induce mesenchymal tumors in dogs.
3. Hypertrophic osteopathy may develop in dogs.
4. Cats mostly present with SCC.
5. Tumors are often not amenable for surgical resection.

Epidemiology and Pathogenesis

Esophageal tumors are rather rare in cats and dogs. Besides primary tumors, secondary, metastatic, or invasive growth of tumors, including thymomas, chemodectomas, lymphomas, and ectopic thyroid glandular tissue, should be considered as differentials.

Primary tumors in *dogs* comprise of *squamous cell carcinomas (SCCs)* and different types of *adenocarcinomas*, *leiomyomas*, *leiomyosarcomas*, *fibrosarcomas, osteosarcomas,* and *plasmacytomas.* Affecting mostly aged dogs, there is no breed or sex predisposition. These tumors frequently grow locally invasive, and affection of the regional lymph nodes is common, either due to invasion or metastasis. *Papillomas* of the esophagus are uncommon and might be associated with oral viral papillomas (see ► Sect. 9.1.1.5). In association with nematode infections, esophageal osteosarcomas and fibrosarcomas are described. *Spirocerca lupi*-associated tumors occur in indigenous areas including Africa, Israel, and the southeastern United States. Adult nematodes are initially found within granulomas with peripheral fibroblast proliferation. Malignant progression out of these fibroblast leads to tumor development. Invasive growth and metastasis into the lung, bronchial lymph nodes, myocardium (rarely), kidneys, spleen, and adrenals is described.

Esophageal tumor in *cats* are mostly *SCC* and affect older animals.

Clinical Appearance

Animals typically show regurgitation, dysphagia, salivation, vomiting, sometimes dyspnea, and weight loss. *Palpation* of the mass can be challenging due to the common localization at the terminal esophagus and cardia.

Esophageal *SCCs* frequently arise at the level around the second rib and appear as white, nodular, and ulcerated masses. *Leiomyomas* are often found at the margin to the stomach and are mostly covered by intact, freely moveable mucosa making endoscopic biopsy unrewarding.

Hypertrophic osteopathy, spondylitis of the caudal thoracal, or more rarely lumbal vertebrae can develop as paraneoplastic syndromes associated with esophageal tumors. This reaction is most likely due to osteoproliferative growth factors secreted by esophageal tumors or their space-occupying effect.

Endoscopy is recommended and enables biopsy sampling. *Radiography* (with radiocontrast media) may be helpful to verify megaesophagus, lung metastases, and secondary aspiration pneumonia. Further, computer-assisted tomography and magnet resonance imaging can also be supportive to determine the extent of the tumor.

Cytology and Histopathology

Cytology is challenging, particularly for tumors with mesenchymal origin, and *histology* is required to confirm malignancy, particularly with *Spirocerca lupi*-associated masses. *Leiomyosarcomas* are mostly of low grade.

Prognosis and Therapy

Prognosis for malignant tumors – except for low-grade leiomyosarcoma – is very poor.

Most of the tumors are *surgically* not amenable due to their advanced stage and invasion of surrounding tissue. *Radiotherapy* is often problematic due to associated esophagitis and poor tolerance of adjacent tissue (lung, heart). *Chemotherapeutical* treatment is regarded not successful to date. *Spirocerca lupi*-associated tumors can be treated by surgery and chemotherapy (e.g., doramectin).

Suggested Reading

(Dvir et al. 2008; Farese et al. 2008; Kirberger et al. 2013; Lindsay et al. 2010; Mazaki-Tovi et al. 2002; Ranen et al. 2004; van der Merwe et al. 2008)

9.3.2 Esophageal and Forestomach Tumors in Ruminants

Esophageal and ruminal *papillomas* caused by *bovine papillomavirus-4* (BPV-4) are common in some areas, including Brazil, Bolivia, England, and Scotland. They may also affect the oral cavity. For details, see ► Sect. 9.1.4. As in the oral cavity, some cattle may develop squamous cell carcinoma associated with BPV-4 or yet undetermined cancerogens. *Fibropapillomas* are usually associated with cutaneous (fibro-) papillomas and are potentially caused by *BPV-2*, although in the alimentary tumors, BPV-2 expression could not be detected and will not be discussed in detail.

9.4 Gastrointestinal Tumors

9.4.1 Canine Gastrointestinal Tumors

▪ Epidemiology and Pathogenesis

In dogs, approximately one quarter of all gastrointestinal tumors arise within the *stomach*. The most frequent tumors are *adenocarcinomas* (see ► Sect. 9.4.1.1) and *lymphomas* (see ► Sect. 9.4.1.2), followed by *leiomyomas* and *leiomyosarcomas* (see ► Sect. 9.4.1.3). Among others, adenomas and adenomatous polyps are described and will not be discussed in detail. Dogs are typically 7–15 years of age, *adenocarcinomas* can also affect younger dogs, and *leiomyomas* often occur in very old dogs. Male dogs are overrepresented, but data are inconsistent regarding breed predisposition. The gastric mucosa of dogs is often colonized by non-*Helicobacter pylori* helicobacters (NHPH). The pathogenic significance of gastric NHPH in dogs is poorly understood and remains controversial. Most authors suggest that *Helicobacter* species are not associated with tumor development.

Small intestinal tumors occur more rarely compared to large intestinal tumors and up to 90 % are malignant *lymphomas* (see ► Sect. 9.4.1.2), which are the most common intestinal tumors in several reports, followed by *adenocarcinomas* (see ► Sect. 9.4.1.1) and *leiomyosarcomas* or *gastrointestinal stromal tumors* (see ► Sect. 9.4.1.3). Further, carcinoids and mast cell tumors are reported but will not be discussed in detail. Dogs in the middle ages are primarily affected; a predisposition for *male dogs* is inconsistently found in the literature. The relevance of chronic *lymphoplasmacytic enteritis* or inflammatory bowel disease (IBD) as a predisposing factor is under discussion.

In dogs, approximately 40 % of all intestinal tumors arise in the *large intestine*. Mean age of patients is 8.5 years. Breed predispositions are suspected for West Highland white terriers, German shepherd dog, and poodle, and male dogs are more frequently affected. The three most common tumors are benign *adenomatous polyps* (see ► Sect. 9.4.1.1), *adenocarcinomas* (mostly rectal, see ► Sect. 9.4.1.1), and *lymphomas* (see ► Sect. 9.4.1.2). Besides this, *gastrointestinal stromal tumors (GIST)*, *leiomyomas*, *leiomyosarcomas* (see ► Sect. 9.4.1.3), plasma cell tumors, carcinoids, and signet-ring cell carcinomas are reported.

▪ Clinical Appearance

Gastric tumors mostly present with blood-tinged vomiting, anorexia, and progressive weight loss, more rarely with abdominal pain. Most of the tumors arise in the distal, pylorus parts. *Ultrasound* diagnosis is recommended including imaging of lymph nodes and abdominal metastasis in combination with *endoscopy*.

For *small intestinal tumors,* patients do not show any clinical signs in 50 % of the cases, but vomiting, chronic weight loss (due to anorexia and malabsorption), abdominal pain, diarrhea, melena, and ileus are described. Abdominal *palpation* of the mass may be possible. At diagnosis, most tumors are in *advanced stages*. Metastatic spread to the mesenteric lymph nodes, omentum, spleen, liver, and lung is common.

Clinical signs of *colorectal tumors* are unspecific and match those of other large intestinal disease: tenesmus, hematochezia (bloody stool), mucous feces, diarrhea, or obstipation. In two thirds of cases, the mass can be *palpated* rectally.

Ultrasound findings typically present with bowel wall thickening and loss of normal wall layers. This method has been proven to differentiate neoplastic from nonneoplastic disease in many cases and is more sensitive than radiography for identifying a mass. It is also useful for the detection of metastasis and guidance of fine-needle aspiration/biopsy sampling.

Native *radiography* is almost always not diagnostic, but usage of contrast agent can be helpful. *Laparotomy* may be indicated in contrast to endoscopic biopsy. The macroscopic evaluation and the tissue samples obtained from laparotomy are commonly diagnostic.

Hypoproteinemia due to malabsorption is common. Dogs with non-lymphomatous neoplasia may show elevated liver enzymes, specifically alkaline phosphatase or *hypoglycemia,* particularly with smooth muscle tumors, due to insulin-like growth factor secretion.

▪ Cytology and Histopathology

Cytology and *histopathology* will be discussed for the respective tumor types (see ▶ Sects. 9.4.1.2, 9.4.1.3, 9.4.2, 9.4.2.1, 9.4.2.2, 9.4.2.3, 9.4.3, and 9.4.4).

▪ Prognosis and Therapy

For *gastric* benign tumors, complete surgery is usually curative. The *prognosis* for malignant gastric cancer is generally poor. Even after surgical resection of the tumors, most of the patients succumb within 6 months due to recurrence or metastasis. *Surgery* is the most common treatment for gastric tumors, particularly for adenomas, carcinomas, leiomyomas, and leiomyosarcomas. The procedure should include evaluation of the liver and all abdominal lymph nodes for metastasis, not least for adequate staging based on the TNM system. *Radiotherapy* with low doses may be helpful to reduce the tumor size. Generally, systemic diseases (lymphomas) require *chemotherapeutical* approaches, but dogs with gastrointestinal lymphomas generally have a worse response than do dogs with other primary locations of lymphomas. Nevertheless, resection of large-volume or ulcerative tumors may be palliative for the patient.

Generally, *intestinal* tumors have a guarded to favorable *prognosis* if resection is complete. The *prognosis* after resection of adenomas and leiomyomas is good. The survival time for sarcomas tends to be longer when compared to carcinoma. *Surgical* resection is a common treatment for intestinal tumors except for lymphomas. Resection should include tissue margins of 5 cm cranial and caudal to the tumor, which can be problematic in the proximal duodenum without resection of the bile and pancreatic duct or require anastomosis of ileum to colon. It is unclear whether *chemotherapy* is beneficial for (adjuvant) treatment of epithelial tumors; nevertheless, it is recommended after resection of solid lymphoma. *Radiotherapy* is rarely used for (adjuvant) treatment of intestinal tumors.

In the large intestine, except for lymphoma, surgical resection is generally mandatory. Depending on the localization and stage, endoscopic, laparoscopic approaches, pelvic osteotomies, or a "pull-through" technique (eversion of distal parts through the anus) can be performed. Postsurgical complications include rectal hemorrhage, wound dehiscence, tenesmus, or fecal incontinence. Non-resectable tumors can be treated by *radiotherapy*, and *chemotherapy* can improve the clinical appearance of patients.

▪ Suggested Reading

(Cohen et al. 2003; Danova et al. 2006; Eisele et al. 2010; Frank et al. 2007; Gaschen 2011; Gieger 2011; Paoloni et al. 2002; Patnaik et al. 1977, 1978, 1980; Penninck et al. 2003; Rassnick et al. 2009; Simon et al. 2005; von Babo et al. 2012; Willard 2012)

9.4.1.1 Canine Gastrointestinal Adenocarcinomas

Box 9.12. Canine Gastrointestinal Adenocarcinomas in Five Facts

1. Occur mainly in the pyloric region and great curvature of the stomach and rectum
2. Infiltrating, nonulcerating are the most common types
3. Tumor cells often induce scirrhous reaction ("leather bottle" or "linitis plastica")
4. Most tumors are metastasized at diagnosis
5. Adenomatous polyps are mostly rectal, and benign but malignant progression is possible

▪ Epidemiology and Pathogenesis

Adenocarcinomas in the gastrointestinal tract mostly affect dogs at the age of 11–12 years for gastric and 9–10 years for intestinal tumors. Male dogs may be overrepresented and German shepherds appear predisposed.

Clinical Appearance

Gastric carcinomas typically develop in the *pyloric region* and more rarely at the greater curvature. They are mostly pink to red and can be infiltrative or exophytic with or without ulceration. The *infiltrating, nonulcerating variant* is the most common type. Infiltrative variants are frequently scirrhous (with abundant fibrous tissue, "leather bottle" appearance, "linitis plastica") leading to an induration of the gastric wall. Metastasis to regional lymph nodes and more distant to the lung, liver, and spleen is commonly observed.

Intestinal adenocarcinomas grow either horizontal/cobblestone-like or circular/annular within the intestinal wall, or they vertically protrude into the lumen as pedunculated masses. The different growth patterns may relate to behavior and prognosis. They metastasize rarely but can manifest in unusual locations, including the skin or meninges. The *rectum* is the most common site and tumors are usually *palpable*; further, the colon and duodenum are common sites.

Adenomatous polyps are found in the *rectum* of dogs as solitary masses. They are usually benign and do not metastasize. Malignant progression to adenocarcinomas is possible and might be related to p53 tumor-suppressor gene mutations, but immunohistochemically detectable overexpression of p53 is not prognostic.

The most sensitive test to find rectal lesions is *digital rectal examination*. Plain *radiographs* are rarely diagnostic, but the use of contrast media may document infiltrative gastric adenocarcinomas. *Sonography* and *endoscopy* are useful for the diagnosis of gastric neoplasia. Endoscopy seems to be more accurate in identifying gastric neoplasia, particularly for lymphoma. *Percutaneous fine-needle aspiration* (FNA) of enlarged lymph nodes or thickened gastric wall is frequently diagnostic. *Endoscopy* is regarded as the most sensitive and specific way to diagnose gastric carcinomas. *Proctoscopy* (with biopsy) are recommended for more aboral lesions with rigid biopsy forceps. They enable deep-mural samples that are critical for distinguishing benign polyps from adenocarcinomas. Further aboral tumors may require ultrasonography.

Cytology and Histopathology

Cytology can be difficult to interpret. *Adenocarcinomas* are composed of variably well-differentiated neoplastic epithelial cells. Cytology however often misses the malignant cells, which are usually located deep in the intestinal wall. *Histological analysis* of *several, adequately large biopsy* samples of affected (and unaffected) regions is often necessary for final diagnosis. Histological diagnosis is aggravated by superficial samples of unaffected mucosa or due to necrosis, ulceration, and inflammation leading to false-negative biopsies.

Prognosis and Therapy

Gastrointestinal carcinomas have a poor prognosis. *Surgery* is the treatment of choice for gastric tumors. However, tumors can rarely be resected with complete margins. In addition, metastasis is often present at the time of diagnosis.

The treatment of *intestinal carcinomas* consists of surgical resection. Colon tumors are more prone to dehiscence and are often associated with fecal incontinence. If the patient does not experience complications, tumor resection may be palliative for months. *Radiation* is not commonly performed. Adjuvant *chemotherapy* can be palliative.

For adenocarcinoma, the *p53* overexpression, lower expression of *p21*, lack of *p16*, but increased *p16 index* immunoreactivity were related to histopathological characteristics of malignancy.

C2-O-sLe(x) is a suggested tumor-associated antigen that may play a role in the invasiveness and metastatic potential of certain canine gastric carcinoma types.

The expression of *gastrin* in gastric carcinomas is less common (in contrast to human tumors) and therefore not useful as prognostic marker, and the serum gastrin concentration alone is not a useful biomarker for gastric carcinomas in dogs.

Colorectal *adenocarcinomas* often express *COX-2*, suggestive for promising NSAID-based chemotherapy.

Suggested Reading

(Carrasco et al. 2011; Church et al. 1987; Hampson et al. 1990; Janke et al. 2010; Krauser 1985; Marolf et al. 2015; McEntee et al. 2002; Patnaik et al. 1977, 1980; Seim-Wikse et al. 2014; Tomlinson et al. 1982; Valerius et al. 1997; Willard 2012)

9.4.1.2 Canine Gastrointestinal Lymphomas

Box 9.13. Canine Gastrointestinal Lymphomas in Five Facts

1. Gastrointestinal lymphomas are mostly primary tumors and often T-cell derived
2. T-cell types: associated with a poor response to chemotherapy
3. T-cell types: shorter survival times and remissions
4. High-grade lymphomas are associated with higher mortality rates
5. Chemotherapy is recommended

■ Epidemiology and Pathogenesis

Lymphomas are common in the stomach and the most frequent canine intestinal tumor in most reports. It is still under debate if chronic lymphoplasmacytic gastroenteritis/inflammatory bowel disease (IBD) can progress to lymphoma.

9

■ Clinical Appearance

The majority of gastrointestinal *lymphomas* are a *primary manifestation* and not part of a multicentric tumor in dogs. The stage of the disease can be assessed by applying the clinical staging system of the WHO (World Health Organization), given in ◘ Table 6.1. For further details on different classification systems, particularly the grading system, please see ◘ Table 6.2. *Multicentric forms* present with abdominal lymphadenopathy and/or affection of the liver, spleen, and bone marrow. *Endoscopically*, lymphomas often appear in a smooth or a cobblestone pattern of a pale-white to pink mucosa, and they arise within the submucosa and the mucosa-associated lymphatic tissue (MALT). Biopsy samples from the liver spleen, and mesenteric lymph nodes should be taken to detect possible metastasis.

■ Cytology and Histopathology

Cytology can be difficult to interpret. As mentioned in other chapters, the accuracy of diagnosis for *lymphomas* is strongly correlated to the quality of the slides, i.e., the high proportion of neoplastic cells. Reactive infiltration of immune cells aggravates the diagnosis, and the differentiation of inflammation from well-differentiated small cell lymphomas is challenging. *Histopathology* may face the same problems, and several, adequately large biopsy samples should be taken.

Alimentary lymphomas in dogs are most commonly *T-cell* derived and can be classified as *small- to medium-sized* (often epitheliotropic) and *large lymphoblastic* cell types. Immunohistochemistry or special staining (e.g., CD79a as B-cell marker, CD3 as T-cell marker, Toluidine blue for detection of metachromatic granules) is recommended to distinguish tumor subtypes (B-cell origin, T-cell origin, mast cells). A grading system for lymphomas in domestic animals is given in ◘ Table 6.2. Recently, a stepwise and complex diagnostic approach using histology followed by immunophenotyping and determining the Ki67 index and finally PCR for clonality has been established to improve the accuracy of distinguishing intestinal lymphomas from IBD in dogs (see Carrasco et al. 2015).

■ Prognosis and Therapy

Gastrointestinal lymphomas are associated with a poorer prognosis compared to multicentric lymphomas. Patients with metastases commonly have a markedly shorter median survival time.

As stated in Chap. 6, in general, *high-grade lymphomas* are associated with higher mortality rates than intermediate- or low-grade lymphomas. *T-cell lymphomas*, the most common variant in dogs, are reported to have shorter survival times and remissions. Further, the T-cell phenotype of high-grade lymphoma is generally associated with a poor response to chemotherapy. Not least, the assessment of the *frequency of AgNORs* (argyrophilic nucleolar organizer regions) and the investigation of the *potential doubling time (Tpot)* can be used as predictors of outcome in dogs (see ► Chap. 6).

Chemotherapy using variations of "CHOP" combination protocols (cyclophosphamide, doxorubicin [=*h*ydroxydaunorubicin], vincristine [= Oncovin], *p*rednisone) or a modified *Madison Wisconsin protocol* is the preferred therapy (see ► Chap. 6). Dogs treated with combination chemotherapy (i.e., cyclophosphamide, doxorubicin, vincristine, L-asparaginase, prednisolone, lomustine, procarbazine, mustargen) have a more or less 50 % response rate, with a median survival time of approximately 110 days in responders. Particularly for solid forms, *surgery* may be beneficial. *Radiation* therapy may also be feasible for solitary forms or as palliative therapy.

■ Current Research

There is ongoing research focusing on new diagnostic and prognostic markers (such as antigen receptor gene rearrangements, Ki67 index) as well as chemotherapeutical protocols. Recent studies suggest that a change in the number of Foxp3-positive regulatory T cells contributes to the pathogenesis of intestinal lymphoma.

■ Suggested Reading

(Carrasco et al. 2015; Couto et al. 1989; Coyle and Steinberg 2004; Frank et al. 2007; Gieger 2011; Maeda et al. 2016; Ohmura et al. 2015; Rassnick et al. 2009; Simon et al. 2006, 2008)

9.4.1.3 Canine Gastrointestinal Spindle Cells Tumors (Leiomyomas, Myosarcomas, and Gastrointestinal Stromal Tumors (GIST))

Box 9.14. Canine Gastrointestinal Leiomyomas, Myosarcomas and GIST in Three Facts

1. The clinical relevance of differentiating GISTs from leiomyosarcomas is unclear.
2. GIST arise predominantly in the stomach and large intestine.
3. GIST are positive for CD117 (c-Kit) and CD34 and negative for SMA and desmin.

Epidemiology and Pathogenesis

Leiomyomas and *leiomyosarcomas* are primarily tumors in aged dogs (>10 years). These tumors grow slowly and metastasize late if at all. *Gastrointestinal stromal tumors (GIST)* arise from the cells of Cajal, the so-called intestinal pace makers, and can be differentiated from other mesenchymal tumors, particularly leiomyosarcomas. The clinical importance of this differentiation is uncertain at this time.

■ Clinical Appearance

Leiomyomas are more common in the stomach, arise extraluminal, often solitary within the muscular wall and may project into the lumen. They are covered by intact mucosa and can reach large size until the dog shows clinical disease (see ◘ Fig. 9.5).

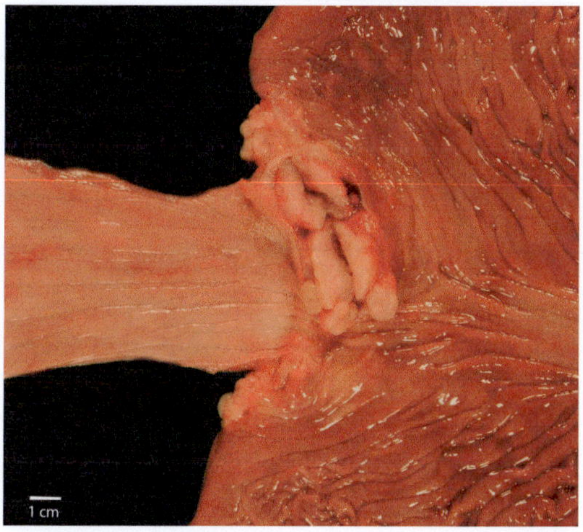

◘ **Fig. 9.5** Gastric leiomyoma in the cardiac region, dog, adult (Courtesy of Dr. Marie von Deetzen, Freie Universität Berlin, Germany)

Leiomyosarcomas arise typically in the intestine and grow slowly and infiltrative. Dogs often present with anorexia, lethargy, vomiting, weight loss, abdominal distention, and diarrhea. Perforation of the intestinal wall may be present. Paraneoplastic hypoglycemia is frequently reported with both leiomyomas and myosarcomas. *GIST* are found in the stomach and intestine with some preference to the large bowel. They grow slowly and only late stages exhibit metastasis to mesenteric lymph nodes, seldomly to the liver and spleen.

Plain *abdominal* radiographs may indicate an abdominal mass, but *ultrasonography* is more reliable. *Endoscopically*, these tumors mostly appear as hard masses covered with normal mucosa.

■ Cytology and Histopathology

Cytology of fine-needle aspirates is generally not helpful for tumor diagnosis. *Histology* is necessary for final diagnosis and examination of tumor margins. *Immunohistochemistry* is necessary to differentiate GIST, leiomyomas, or sarcomas. *GIST* are positive for *c-Kit* (CD117) and *CD34*, while leiomyomas and *leiomyosarcomas* are negative for these antigens but positive for *smooth muscle actin* and/or *desmin*.

■ Prognosis and Therapy

Leiomyomas have a good prognosis and surgery is usually curative.

Surgical excision is the common treatment for intestinal *leiomyosarcoma*. The *prognosis* is relatively good. The median survival time varies greatly between 1 and 2 years. Even with detectable metastasis at the time of surgery, long mean survival times are documented. Anyhow, metastatic rates are low to moderate. Long-term survival is reported possibly with early, complete surgical excision.

GIST appear to have longer median survival times compared to leiomyosarcomas, but data are inconsistent. *GIST* can have a mutation in the c-KIT oncogene. Inhibitors of tyrosine kinase show promising effects, but until now, reliable data are missing. *Proliferation markers* (Ki67, AgNor) seem to have prognostic relevance for GIST.

Suggested Reading

(Cohen et al. 2003; Frost et al. 2003; Gillespie et al. 2011; Gregory-Bryson et al. 2010; Hayes et al. 2013; LaRock and Ginn 1997; Maas et al. 2007; Russell et al. 2007; Willard 2012)

9.4.2 Feline Gastrointestinal Tumors

Epidemiology and Pathogenesis

Gastric tumors are rare in cats. The most common tumors are *lymphomas* (see ► Sect. 9.4.2.1), followed by *adenocarcinomas* (see ► Sect. 9.4.2.2) and leiomyomas; the latter will not be discussed in detail.

The role of *Helicobacter* sp. in the development of gastric tumors is still under discussion.

Small intestinal tumors in cats include in decreasing order of frequency *lymphomas*, *adenocarcinomas*, and *mast cell tumors (MCTs)*. Mean ages of cats range between 10 and 12 years, but (most likely FeLV positive) patients can be younger. A gender predisposition is discordantly reported. Siamese cats are overrepresented for intestinal adenocarcinomas and lymphomas. There is no association between retroviral infection and nonlymphomatous intestinal neoplasia in cats. Other neoplasias are rare and will not be discussed in detail.

In cats, 10–15 % of all gastrointestinal tumors arise in the *large intestine*. Mean age of these cats is 12.5 years; no sex and breed predispositions are proven so far. The most frequent types are *adenocarcinomas*, *lymphomas*, and *MCTs*. Colorectal lymphomas are usually not associated with FeLV, but some cats have been positive for FIV.

Clinical Appearance

Cats with *gastric tumors* most commonly present with vomiting, hematemesis, anorexia, and less frequently weight loss. A gastric mass is difficult to *palpate*, but *endoscopy*, *ultrasonography*, and *radiography* may help to visualize a distinct mass or thickened gastric wall with loss of physiologic layering.

For *intestinal tumors*, weight loss due to anorexia and/or malabsorption and vomiting are reported. For detailed diagnostic approaches, see in the following chapters on specific tumors.

Cytology and Histopathology

Cytology and *histopathology* will be discussed for specific tumor types in the following chapters.

Suggested Reading

(Bridgeford et al. 2008; Canejo-Teixeira et al. 2014; Gabor et al. 1998; Patnaik et al. 1976; Rissetto et al. 2011; Slawienski et al. 1997)

9.4.2.1 Feline Gastrointestinal Lymphomas

Box 9.15. Feline Gastrointestinal Lymphomas in Five Facts

1. Most frequent intestinal tumors
2. Cats <4 years usually have FeLV-associated lymphomas, which are rare
3. Cats >8 years usually have non-FeLV-associated lymphomas, which are more common
4. Well-differentiated/low-grade/lymphocytic types have a better prognosis
5. Poorly differentiated/high-grade/lymphoblastic types have poorer progression

Epidemiology and Pathogenesis

For detailed information about feline lymphomas in general and particularly the association with feline leukemia virus (FeLV) and feline immunodeficiency virus (FIV), see also Chap. 6. Lymphomas in cats are associated with a bimodal age distribution. The first peak, at <4 years of age, is mostly FeLV associated and less common. The second peak, at >8 years of age, is usually not FeLV associated and more common. Siamese cats and males have been associated with a higher risk to develop lymphomas.

Gastric lymphomas area relatively uncommon manifestation with a predominance of large B-cell lymphoblastic lymphomas.

Lymphomas are the *most frequent intestinal tumors* in cats with an increasing incidence, and most of them are FeLV- and FIV-negative. The differentiation from chronic inflammatory bowel disease can be challenging. Some authors suggest that inflammatory bowel disease is a prelymphoma entity.

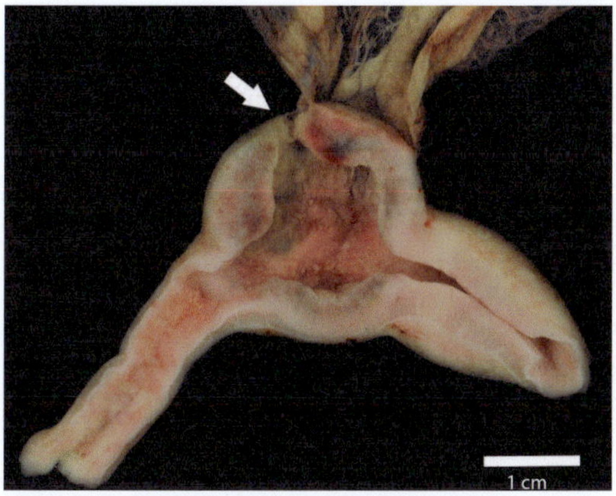

Fig. 9.7 Alimentary lymphoma, cat: note the ulceration (*arrow*) (Courtesy of Anja Ostrowski, PhD, Freie Universität Berlin, Germany)

Clinical Appearance

In general, *solid forms* are differentiated from *diffuse forms* with mural infiltrations. Solid tumors may lead to obstruction and are often ulcerated (see Figs. 9.6 and 9.7). With systemic affection, enlarged abdominal lymph nodes, liver, spleen, and kidneys are found.

Vomiting is a common clinical sign of *gastric lymphomas*. The tumors can present as either a diffuse infiltration or a discrete, solid mass; the latter is more common. *Palpation* of gastric masses is challenging, but a mass or thickened gastric wall might be visible with *ultrasonography*

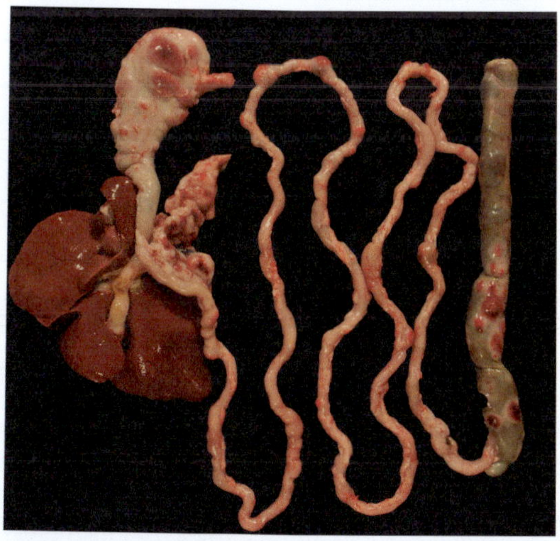

Fig. 9.6 Alimentary lymphoma, cat: manifestation in the stomach and intestine (Courtesy of Kristina Dietert, PhD, Freie Universität Berlin, Germany)

or *radiography*, particularly using contrast media. *Endoscopy* is a useful technique to visualize the tumor and enable sampling.

Intestinal lymphomas cause weight loss, sometimes associated with diarrhea and vomiting. Large intestinal involvement causes more frequently diarrhea and can also cause weight loss. *Ultrasound* is suitable for imaging and guidance of fine-needle aspiration. Tumors characteristically present with intestinal wall thickening and loss of normal wall layers. *Endoscopic* evaluation of tumors is restricted to duodenal masses. Plain abdominal *radiographs* may reveal an abdominal mass, but the use of contrast media may be more useful. Thoracic radiographs complete evaluation of the patient for metastatic disease.

The progression of disease depends on the type of lymphoma with *well-differentiated, lymphocytic forms* progressing slower (months) than *poorly differentiated, lymphoblastic forms* (days or weeks). Two different *staging systems* are commonly used and given in Chap. 6, including the WHO staging of lymphomas in domestic animals (Owen 1980, see Table 6.1) and the system for staging of feline lymphomas established by Mooney and Hayes (1986, see Table 6.3).

Cytology and Histopathology

Cytology and histology of feline lymphomas are given in detail in Chap. 6 including figures (cytology) and apply also for lymphomas in the stomach and the lower gastrointestinal tract.

In general, *cytology* is likely diagnostic with samples from the actual tumor with adequate numbers of neoplastic cells and less reliable with samples of the tumor boarder or necrotic tumor parts with low numbers of neoplastic cells, abundant reactive lymphocytic background, and if neoplastic cells are well-differentiated (see Fig. 9.8)

Histopathology is also restricted by these factors, but the evaluation and effacement of the tissue architecture can be helpful. Due to the fact that well-differentiated neoplastic lymphocytes can mimic nonneoplastic lymphocytes, and less differentiated neoplastic lymphocytes resemble lymphoblasts, the interpretation of the growth pattern is important. In challenging cases, it is highly recommended to include *immunohistochemistry* for CD3/CD79a (T-cell/B-cell marker) and the *assessment of clonality* (reactive, polyclonal lymphocytes vs. neoplastic, monoclonal lymphocytes) to support the diagnosis. *Three histological grades* are recognized: low-, intermediate-, and high-grade lymphomas. Recent reports have shown a predominance of high-grade lymphomas arising in the *stomach.*

B- and T-cell tumors are almost equally frequent. Recent investigations indicate a predominance of *mucosal T-cell lymphoma* types in the intestinal tract in general, particularly in the *jejunum* and a B-cell-type predominance in the stomach. The authors suggested that cases of T-cell lymphoma can be misinterpreted as inflammatory bowel disease. Finally, a diagnostic algorithm to differentiate lymphomas from inflammation in feline small intestinal biopsy samples has been established (see Kiupel et al. 2011).

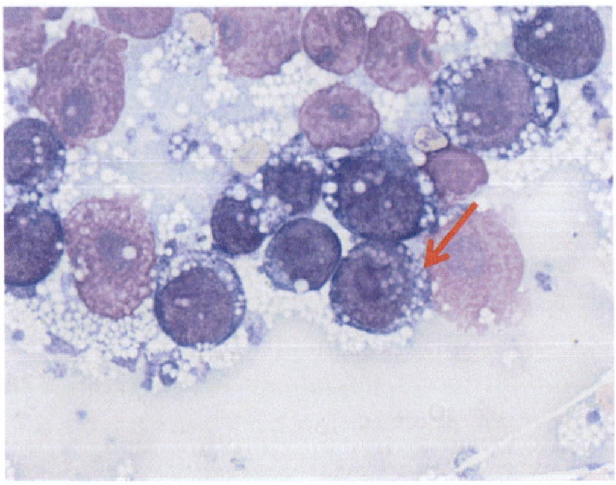

Fig. 9.8 Cytology, high-grade B-cell lymphoma (Burkitt-like lymphoma), intestinal wall, cat, May-Grünwald-Giemsa 1000×. There are numerous, medium-sized to large lymphatic blasts with round eccentrically located nucleus, fine chromatin pattern, mainly indistinct nucleoli and moderate amounts of a basophilic cytoplasm containing many small vacuoles (*red arrow*) (Photo: with permission of Dr. N. Bauer, Faculty of Veterinary Medicine, Justus-Liebig-University, Giessen, Germany)

Prognosis and Therapy

Detailed information on prognosis specific for *gastric lymphomas* is not available, but reports indicate that gastric lymphomas can experience survival times comparable to other types of feline lymphomas with chemotherapy.

Median survival times for *gastrointestinal lymphomas* vary from 2 to 24 months; a specific location has not been shown to be prognostic, and the most consistent prognostic factor appears to be the response to treatment. Further, *low-grade lymphomas* seem to have a better prognosis (median survival of, e.g., 17 months) than *high-grade lymphomas* (2.7 months). Other prognostic factors, such as substage, immunophenotype, and pretreatment with steroids, inconsistently predict the outcome. A prognostic value of the *immunophenotyping* (i.e., B- or T-cell lymphomas) could not be confirmed in general. Recent studies on gastrointestinal lymphomas however suggest that *low-grade T-cell lymphomas* (small cell type) are associated with prolonged survival (median 18.9 months); cats with *transmural T-cell lymphomas* (particularly large granular lymphocyte type) had a much shorter median survival time (1.5 months). Further, the presence of secondary leukemia may have an adverse effect on prognosis.

Feline lymphomas are mostly a systemic disease, requiring *chemotherapy.* So again, modifications of the CHOP protocol (cyclophosphamide, doxorubicin [=*h*ydroxydaunorubicin], vincristine [=Oncovin], prednisone) are useful, except for the therapy of well-differentiated types. Based on the occurrence of solitary form, particularly in the stomach (and lower intestinal tract), *radiation therapy* can be useful.

Whereas *well-differentiated/lymphocytic/small cell lymphomas* may show a high responsiveness and remission rate with prednisone and chlorambucil treatment and a median survival times of nearly 2 years, *poorly differentiated/lymphoblastic lymphomas* appear less responsive with lower remission rate and median survival times of less than 3 months. Adjuvant *surgery* seems not to improve survival compared to chemotherapy alone.

▪ Current Trends in Research

Hematopoietic tumors represent the bulk of neoplastic diseases in cats; thus, ongoing research focuses on the improvement of therapy and diagnosis as well as factors and markers that might be prognostic.

▪ Suggested Reading

(Grover 2005; Gustafson et al. 2014; Kiupel et al. 2011; Lingard et al. 2009; Moore et al. 2012; Patterson-Kane et al. 2004; Pohlman et al. 2009; Rissetto et al. 2011; Roccabianca et al. 2006; Willard 2012)

9.4.2.2 Feline Gastrointestinal Adenocarcinomas

Box 9.16. Feline Gastrointestinal Adenocarcinomas in Three Facts

1. Mostly arise in the small intestine.
2. Distant metastasis is usually present at diagnosis.
3. Typical "bottle neck" appearance due to circular stricture.

Epidemiology and Pathogenesis

Adenocarcinomas primarily affect older cats, of which 50 % are older than 11 years. There is no gender predisposition, but Siamese cats are overrepresented. In decreasing order of occurrence, adenocarcinomas arise in the *jejunum*, *ileum*, *ileocecal region*, and *duodenum*. At diagnosis, metastasis is present in mesenteric lymph nodes, peritoneum (carcinomatosis), liver, and lung in most patients.

▪ Clinical Appearance

Cats with intestinal carcinomas may present with anorexia, vomiting, obstruction, diarrhea, weight loss, bleeding, and/or intussusception. In approximately 50 % of cases, cats have a *palpable* mass in the abdomen that is also visible on *radiographics*. Mostly, usage of contrast agent visualizes a partial or complete obstruction. Typically, the tumor leads to a circular stricture with an orally located dilation, called "bottle neck appearance" see (◘ Fig. 9.9).

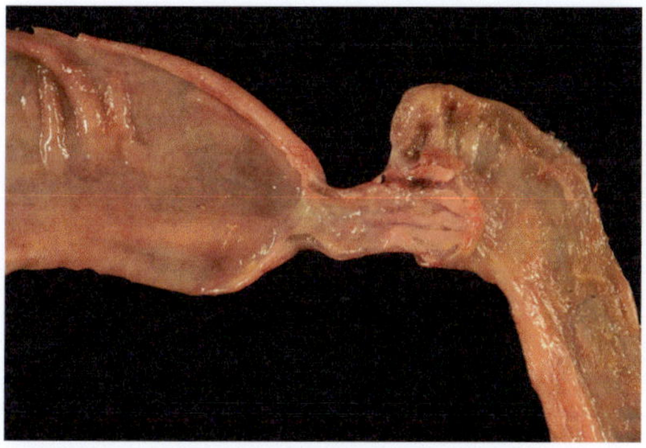

◘ **Fig. 9.9** Intestinal adenocarcinoma, cat: note the typical "bottle neck appearance" (Courtesy of Dr. Stefanie Eggert, Freie Universität Berlin, Germany)

▪ Cytology and Histopathology

As mentioned for canine adenocarcinomas, *cytology* can be difficult to interpret. *Adenocarcinomas* usually have the general characteristics of neoplastic epithelial cells, but cytological samples often do not include tumor cells because of their deep location.

For *histopathology*, several adequately large biopsy samples should be taken. Histological diagnosis is aggravated due to the often unaffected mucosa in only superficial samples or due to necrosis, ulceration, and inflammation leading to false-negative biopsies. Samples of mesenteric or ileocecal lymph nodes are recommended for detection of metastasis.

Several *histologic* subtypes of *adenocarcinomas* are described including solid (low grade), papillary, or tubular and finally mucinous. Fibrous, cartilaginous, or osseous metaplasia is frequent. Histology is needed for final diagnosis on evaluation of surgical margins.

▪ Prognosis and Therapy

The prognosis of gastric adenocarcinomas is unclear due to the small number of reported cases but most likely is guarded to poor. Prognosis for adenocarcinomas might depend on the location or the histological phenotype. Median survival times vary (weeks to years) depending on the progress of the disease.

Surgery is the common treatment and in many cases possible with complete surgical margins.

For adenocarcinomas, solid masses should be treated surgically with at least 5 cm of unaffected margins.

To date adjuvant *chemotherapy* is not proven to be beneficial. Long-term survival is rare but possible as long as metastasis is not evident.

Suggested Reading

(Birchard et al. 1986; Cribb 1988; Kosovsky et al. 1988; Patnaik et al. 1976; Willard 2012)

9.4.2.3 Feline Gastrointestinal Mast Cell Tumors (MCTs)

Box 9.17. Feline Gastrointestinal Mast Cell Tumors in Four Facts

1. MCTs have to be differentiated from feline gastrointestinal eosinophilic sclerosing fibroplasia.
2. MCT should be considered malignant since metastasis is common at time of diagnosis.
3. Prognosis is poor.
4. Surgery is the treatment of choice.

9

Epidemiology and Pathogenesis

Intestinal *MCTs* are the third most common tumors in the intestinal tract of cats and preferentially affect aged animals. Tumors have to be differentiated from *feline gastrointestinal eosinophilic sclerosing fibroplasia.* The latter is an ulcerated, intramural mass occurring usually in the stomach (pyloric region) or ileocecal junction and may also affect adjacent lymph nodes.

Clinical Appearance

Cats with intestinal MCT present with intermittent vomiting, diarrhea, weight loss, anorexia, and depression. The most common *location* for MCT is the small bowel. Usually there are no eosinophilia or circulating mast cells present in the blood. *Metastasis* to the lymph nodes, liver, or spleen is common at time of diagnosis. Diagnostic *ultrasound* typically depicts a noncircumferential eccentric wall thickening or very asymmetric, circumferential, eccentric wall thickening, often with loss of physiological wall layering (see Fig. 9.10).

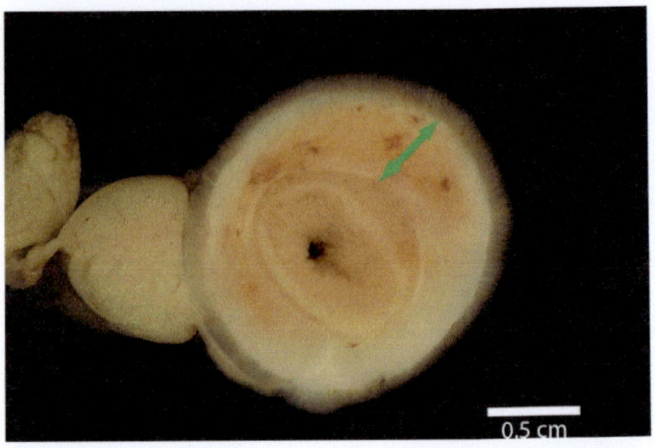

Fig. 9.10 Intestinal mast cell tumor, cat: note diffuse infiltration (*arrow*) of the intestinal wall (Courtesy of Dr. Marie von Deetzen, Freie Universität Berlin, Germany)

Cytology and Histopathology

Cytology may not be diagnostic, and *histology* of biopsy sample is the most effective diagnostic approach. Mucosal ulceration is rare in feline primary intestinal mast cell tumors. Neoplastic cells are usually less well differentiated than the cutaneous counterpart and may require special staining (even metachromatic staining is often difficult to identify) or immunohistochemistry. Sheets of round cells often infiltrate the muscularis and propria with associated fibrosis. Eosinophilic infiltrates are uncommon.

Prognosis and Therapy

In general, these tumors should be considered *malignant.* Survival time is <4 months. *Metastasis* is common at time of diagnosis. *Surgery* is the treatment of choice for MCT. The overall postsurgical prognosis is however poor. Medical management with histamine block (H_1 and H_2 blockers) should be considered. To date, receptor tyrosine kinase inhibitors have not been tested in large prospective trials.

Suggested Reading

(Bortnowski and Rosenthal 1992; Craig et al. 2009; Henry and Herrera 2013; Laurenson et al. 2011; Linton et al. 2015; Sato and Solano 2004)

9.4.3 Equine Gastrointestinal Tumors

Box 9.18. Equine Gastrointestinal Tumors in Four Facts

1. Squamous cell carcinoma (SCC) is the most common gastric tumor.
2. SCCs arise usually in the nonglandular part of the stomach.
3. SCCs usually have a marked stromal component (scirrhous growth).
4. Most common intestinal tumors are lymphomas of the small intestine.

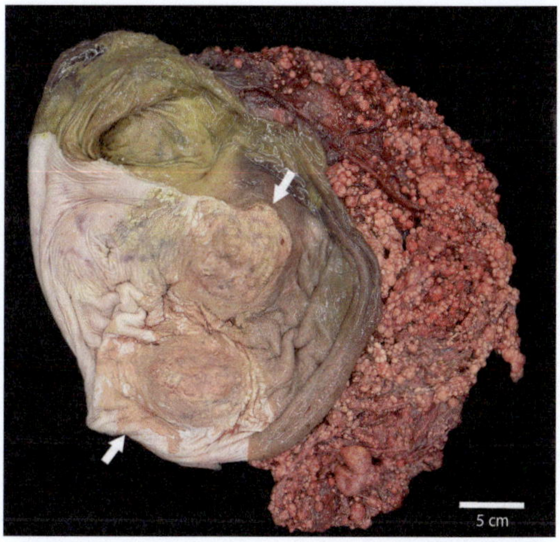

Fig. 9.11 Gastric squamous cell carcinoma, horse: note the large primary tumor (between *arrows*) and numerous serosal metastatic tumors with scirrhous reaction (Courtesy of Philipp Olias, PhD, Freie Universität Berlin, Germany)

▪ Epidemiology and Pathogenesis

The most common *gastric tumors* are *squamous cell carcinomas (SCCs)*. Adenocarcinomas, leiomyosarcomas, gastrointestinal stromal tumors, papillomas, and benign polyps are rarely reported and will not be discussed in detail. *SCCs* are frequently located in the nonglandular mucosa. A breed or sex predilection has not been identified. Adult to aged horses are most commonly affected, and the mean age ranges between 7 and 18 years.

The alimentary form of *lymphomas* is the most common equine *intestinal neoplasm*. Typically, affected horses are 8 years and older. Other possible but rare equine intestinal neoplasms are adenocarcinomas, leiomyomas, leiomyosarcomas, myxosarcomas, ganglioneuromas, nerve sheath tumors, and carcinoids and will not be discussed in detail.

▪ Clinical Appearance

For *gastric SCC*, acute onset of disease or several years of mild signs are reported, mostly nonspecific, and include inappetence, weight loss, abdominal pain, hypoalbuminemia/hyperglobulinemia, and anemia due to internal bleeding. The peritoneal fluid can be analyzed and is often abnormal but unspecifically resemble non-septic exudates. Rectal palpation may reveal abdominal masses. *Endoscopy* and transabdominal *ultrasound* examination can be very helpful for visualization and determination of the tumor size, but normal findings do not rule out gastric neoplasia. Tumors are often in an advanced stage at the time of diagnosis. The tumors are usually well-demarcated cauliflower-like and can be very large. The muscular wall is often thickened, with a firm (scirrhous) texture. The *scirrhous reaction* may extent on the gastric serosa (see ◘ Fig. 9.11). Hematogenous metastasis to the liver and more rarely the lung, kidney, and other organs is rarely observed. The primary tumor can be ulcerated and may extend into the esophagus, leading to obstruction.

The most common location for *gastrointestinal lymphomas* is the small intestine. *Ultrasound* can be a sensitive diagnostic tool. Annular small intestinal thickening seems to be characteristic for lymphomas. Mesenteric lymphadenopathy is frequent. *Rectal biopsy* may be a sensitive and specific indicator of infiltrative disease in advanced clinical cases, but results in some studies indicate poor sensitivity. Furthermore, *exploratory abdominal surgery* may be valuable for establishing a definitive diagnosis and may enable therapeutic excision if a localized lesion can be identified. *Metastasis* is commonly observed at the time of diagnosis.

Cytology and Histopathology

For *SCC*, neoplastic cells are often found in the peritoneal fluid and enable minimal invasive evaluation. *Cytologically*, the neoplasms are typical squamous cell carcinomas with variably differentiated epithelial cells and keratin. *Histologically*, SCCs show invasion of the gastric wall and grow in cords or nests of cells, often with marked desmoplasia (scirrhous) and prominent intercellular bridges. Immunohistochemistry for cytokeratin may be useful for poorly differentiated cells.

As mentioned for *lymphomas* in general, it is a diagnostic challenge to differentiate lymphomas from inflammatory bowel disease and may require immunohistochemistry (CD79a, CD3) for B-cell and T-cell identification.

Prognosis and Therapy

Treatment is aggravated in horses because of the poor accessibility and the usually advanced stage of disease. The *survival time* after diagnosis of gastric neoplasia in horses is usually short. *Radiation therapy* and *chemotherapy* can be of benefit, such as piroxicam and COX inhibitors for *SCC*. However, the prognosis for long-term survival in horses with intestinal neoplasia is grave.

Suggested Reading

(Olsen 1992; Recknagel et al. 2012; Reef et al. 1984; Taylor et al. 2009; Vandenhoven and Franken 1983)

9.4.4 Bovine Abomasal and Intestinal Tumors

Box 9.19. Bovine Abomasal and Intestinal Tumors in Five Facts

1. Lymphoma is the most common abomasal tumor.
2. BLV can cause abomasal B-cell lymphomas in adult cattle.
3. Prognosis is poor; treatment is not economically beneficial.
4. Prevention of infection and elimination of infected cattle is the main prevention strategy.

Epidemiology and Pathogenesis

Neoplasia of the *abomasum* is generally rare in cattle. The most common tumors in the abomasum are *lymphomas*. Rarely carcinomas, sarcomas and adenomas occur but will not be discussed in detail. Lymphomas may also affect the intestine, but this is very rare. *Bovine leukemia virus* (BLV) causes B-cell lymphomas (*enzootic bovine leukosis*) particularly in adult cattle (>2 years of age). This virus is transmitted horizontally by bloodsuckling arthropods and by lymphocyte contaminated needles. Approximately *98 % of serologically BLV-positive cattle do not develop tumors.*

Intestinal neoplasias include polyps and adenocarcinomas that may be associated with *papillomavirus* infection or intoxication with *bracken fern* and will not be discussed in detail.

Clinical Appearance

Cattle may present with anorexia, weight loss, decreased milk production, and rarely fever. The most sensitive *antemortem diagnostic tests* include examinations of peripheral lymph node wedge biopsies and percutaneous aspirate or biopsy of a mass. The positive *predictive value of BLV serology is very low*. Further, transabdominal ultrasonography may reveal abnormal thickening and loss of the typical layered appearance. Ulceration of the mucosa can lead to hemorrhage, melena, and anemia; occasionally abomasal reflux and hypochloremic alkalosis can be found.

Besides the *abomasum*, typical manifestations of BLV-associated tumors include lymph nodes (e.g., retrobulbar, pharyngeal), the heart, the uterus, the epidural space, and the liver and spleen. *The sporadic, non-BLV associated variant* may affect the lymph nodes, the thymus, or the skin.

Cytology and Histopathology

As stated above *cytological* and *histological* examinations of peripheral lymph node *wedge biopsies*, and *percutaneous aspirate or biopsy* of a mass are the *most sensitive antemortem tests*. Cytologic examination of *fine-needle aspirates* (FNA) appear less sensitive but highly specific, and due to the fact that FNA is quick, uncomplicated, and relatively cheap to perform, this test might also be useful. As mentioned in other chapters, the accuracy of diagnosis is strongly associated with the quality of the slides (high proportion of neoplastic cells from the actual tumor mass). Aspiration of reactive infiltration of immune cells at the tumor borders aggravate the diagnosis. The differentiation of inflammation from well-differentiated small cell lymphomas is challenging.

Prognosis and Therapy

Abomasal lymphomas have a relatively poor prognosis. Treatment of *enzootic bovine leukosis* is not economically sustainable except for animals with high genetic value. Therefore, the strategy is to identify and eliminate BLV-infected cattle to *prevent transmission*, i.e., by the single-use needles and syringes or reduction of insect contact. An efficient vaccine is not available.

Current Research

New, effective vaccines, as well as competitive infection with deletant viruses are evaluated.

Suggested Reading

(Bertone 1990; Buczinski et al. 2011; Burton et al. 2010; Gutierrez et al. 2014; Rodriguez et al. 2011)

Suggested Reading

Bertone AL (1990) Neoplasms of the bovine gastrointestinal-tract. Vet Clin North Am Food Anim Pract 6:515–524

Bertone ER, Snyder LA, Moore AS (2003) Environmental and lifestyle risk factors for oral squamous cell carcinoma in domestic cats. J Vet Intern Med 17:557–562

Bilgic O, Duda L, Sanchez MD, Lewis JR (2015) Feline oral squamous cell carcinoma: clinical manifestations and literature review. J Vet Dent 32:30–40

Birchard SJ, Couto CG, Johnson S (1986) Nonlymphoid intestinal neoplasia in 32 dogs and 14 cats. J Am Anim Hosp Assoc 22:533–537

Blackwood L, Dobson JM (1996) Radiotherapy of oral malignant melanomas in dogs. J Am Vet Med Assoc 209:98–102

Bocaneti F, Altamura G, Corteggio A, Velescu E, Roperto F, Borzacchiello G (2016) Bovine papillomavirus: new insights into an old disease. Transbound Emerg Dis 63:14–23

Boria PA, Murry DJ, Bennett PF, Glickman NW, Snyder PW, Merkel BL, Schlittler DL, Mutsaers AJ, Thomas RM, Knapp DW (2004) Evaluation of cisplatin combined with piroxicam for the treatment of oral malignant melanoma and oral squamous cell carcinoma in dogs. J Am Vet Med Assoc 224:388–394

Bortnowski HB, Rosenthal RC (1992) Gastrointestinal mast-cell tumors and eosinophilia in 2 cats. J Am Anim Hosp Assoc 28:271–275

Bridgeford EC, Marini RP, Feng Y, Parry NMA, Rickman B, Fox JG (2008) Gastric Helicobacter species as a cause of feline gastric lymphoma: a viable hypothesis. Vet Immunol Immunopathol 123:106–113

Brodey RS (1960) A clinical and pathologic study of 130 neoplasms of the mouth and pharynx in the dog. Am J Vet Res 21:787–812

Brown NO (1989) Salivary gland diseases. Diagnosis, treatment, and associated problems. Probl Vet Med 1:281–294

Buczinski S, Belanger AM, Francoz D (2011) Ultrasonographic appearance of lymphomatous infiltration of the abomasum in cows with lymphoma. J Am Vet Med Assoc 238:1044–1047

Burk RL (1996) Radiation therapy in the treatment of oral neoplasia. Vet Clin North Am Small Anim Pract 26:155–163

Burton AJ, Nydam DV, Long ED, Divers TJ (2010) Signalment and clinical complaints initiating hospital admission, methods of diagnosis, and pathological findings associated with bovine lymphosarcoma (112 cases). J Vet Intern Med 24:960–964

Campo MS, Moar MH, Jarrett WFH, Laird HM (1980) A new papillomavirus associated with alimentary cancer in cattle. Nature 286:180–182

Canejo-Teixeira R, Oliveira M, Pissarra H, Niza MMRE, Vilela CL (2014) A mixed population of Helicobacter pylori, Helicobacter bizzozeronii and "Helicobacter heilmannii" in the gastric mucosa of a domestic cat. Ir Vet J 67(1):25

Carpenter LG, Withrow SJ, Powers BE, Ogilvie GK, Schwarz PD, Straw RC, Larue SM, Berg J (1993) Squamous-cell carcinoma of the tongue in 10 dogs. J Am Anim Hosp Assoc 29:17–24

Carrasco V, Canfran S, Rodriguez-Franco F, Benito A, Sainz A, Rodriguez-Bertos A (2011) Canine gastric carcinoma: immunohistochemical expression of cell cycle proteins (p53, p21, and p16) and heat shock proteins (Hsp27 and Hsp70). Vet Pathol 48:322–329

Carrasco V, Rodriguez-Bertos A, Rodriguez-Franco F, Wise AG, Maes R, Mullaney T, Kiupel M (2015) Distinguishing intestinal lymphoma from inflammatory bowel disease in canine duodenal endoscopic biopsy samples. Vet Pathol 52:668–675

Church EM, Mehlhaff CJ, Patnaik AK (1987) Colorectal adenocarcinoma in dogs: 78 cases (1973–1984). J Am Vet Med Assoc 191:727–730

Ciekot PA, Powers BE, Withrow SJ, Straw RC, Ogilvie GK, LaRue SM (1994) Histologically low-grade, yet biologically high-grade, fibrosarcomas of the mandible and maxilla in dogs: 25 cases (1982–1991). J Am Vet Med Assoc 204:610–615

Cohen M, Post GS, Wright JC (2003) Gastrointestinal leiomyosarcoma in 14 dogs. J Vet Intern Med 17:107–110

Couto CG, Rutgers HC, Sherding RG, Rojko J (1989) Gastrointestinal lymphoma in 20 dogs – a retrospective study. J Vet Intern Med 3:73–78

Coyle KA, Steinberg H (2004) Characterization of lymphocytes in canine gastrointestinal lymphoma. Vet Pathol 41:141–146

Craig LE, Hardam EE, Hertzke DM, Flatland B, Rohrbach BW, Moore RR (2009) Feline gastrointestinal eosinophilic sclerosing fibroplasia. Vet Pathol 46:63–70

Cribb AE (1988) Feline gastrointestinal adenocarcinoma: a review and retrospective study. Can Vet J 29:709–712

Danova NA, Robles-Emanuelli JC, Bjorling DE (2006) Surgical excision of primary canine rectal tumors by an anal approach in twenty-three dogs. Vet Surg 35:337–340

DeBey BM, Bagladi-Swanson M, Kapil S, Oehme FW (2001) Digital papillomatosis in a confined Beagle. J Vet Diagn Invest 13:346–348

Dennis MM, Ehrhart N, Duncan CG, Barnes AB, Ehrhart EJ (2006) Frequency of and risk factors associated with lingual lesions in dogs: 1,196 cases (1995–2004). J Am Vet Med Assoc 228:1533–1537

Desoutter AV, Goldschmidt MH, Sanchez MD (2012) Clinical and histologic features of 26 canine peripheral giant cell granulomas (formerly giant cell epulis). Vet Pathol 49:1018–1023

DiBernardi L, Dore M, Davis JA, Owens JG, Mohammed SI, Guptill CF, Knapp DW (2007) Study of feline oral squamous cell carcinoma: potential target for cyclooxygenase inhibitor treatment. Prostaglandins Leukot Essent Fatty Acids 76:245–250

Dunowska M, Munday JS, Laurie RE, Hills SFK (2014) Genomic characterisation of Felis catus papillomavirus 4, a novel papillomavirus detected in the oral cavity of a domestic cat. Virus Genes 48:111–119

Dvir E, Kirberger RM, Mukorera V, van der Merwe LL, Clift SJ (2008) Clinical differentiation between dogs with benign and malignant spirocercosis. Vet Parasitol 155:80–88

Eisele J, McClaran JK, Runge JJ, Holt DE, Culp WT, Liu S, Long F, Bergman PJ (2010) Evaluation of risk factors for morbidity and mortality after pylorectomy and gastroduodenostomy in dogs. Vet Surg 39:261–267

Farese JP, Bacon NJ, Ehrhart NP, Bush J, Ehrhart EJ, Withrow SJ (2008) Oesophageal leiomyosarcoma in dogs: surgical management and clinical outcome of four cases. Vet Comp Oncol 6:31–38

Fiani N, Verstraete FJM, Kass PH, Cox DP (2011) Clinicopathologic characterization of odontogenic tumors and focal fibrous hyperplasia in dogs: 152 cases (1995–2005). J Am Vet Med Assoc 238:495–500

Frank JD, Reimer SB, Kass PH, Kiupel M (2007) Clinical outcomes of 30 cases (1997–2004) of canine gastrointestinal lymphoma. J Am Anim Hosp Assoc 43:313–321

Frost D, Lasota J, Miettinen M (2003) Gastrointestinal stromal tumors and leiomyomas in the dog: a histopathologic, immunohistochemical, and molecular genetic study of 50 cases. Vet Pathol 40:42–54

Gabor LJ, Malik R, Canfield PJ (1998) Clinical and anatomical features of lymphosarcoma in 118 cats. Aust Vet J 76:725–732

Gardner DG (1994) Ameloblastomas in the horse – a critical-review and report of an additional example. J Oral Pathol Med 23:41–44

Gardner DG (1996) Epulides in the dog: a review. J Oral Pathol Med 25:32–37

Gardner DG, Dubielzig RR (1995) Feline inductive odontogenic-tumor (inductive fibroameloblastoma) – a tumor unique to cats. J Oral Pathol Med 24:185–190

Gaschen L (2011) Ultrasonography of small intestinal inflammatory and neoplastic diseases in dogs and cats. Vet Clin North Am Small Anim Pract 41:329–344

Gieger T (2011) Alimentary lymphoma in cats and dogs. Vet Clin North Am Small Anim Pract 41:419–432

Gillespie V, Baer K, Farrelly J, Craft D, Luong R (2011) Canine gastrointestinal stromal tumors: immunohistochemical expression of CD34 and examination of prognostic indicators including proliferation markers Ki67 and AgNOR. Vet Pathol 48:283–291

Gregory-Bryson E, Bartlett E, Kiupel M, Hayes S, Yuzbasiyan-Gurkan V (2010) Canine and human gastrointestinal stromal tumors display similar mutations in c-KIT exon 11. BMC Cancer 10:559

Grover S (2005) Gastrointestinal lymphoma in cats. Comp Cont Educ Pract Vet 27:741–751

Gustafson TL, Villamil A, Taylor BE, Flory A (2014) A retrospective study of feline gastric lymphoma in 16 chemotherapy-treated cats. J Am Anim Hosp Assoc 50:46–52

Gutierrez G, Rodriguez SM, de Brogniez A, Gillet N, Golime R, Burny A, Jaworski JP, Alvarez I, Vagnoni L, Trono K, Willems L (2014) Vaccination against delta-retroviruses: the bovine leukemia virus paradigm. Viruses 6:2416–2427

Hahn KA, Denicola DB, Richardson RC, Hahn EA (1994) Canine oral malignant-melanoma – prognostic utility of an alternative staging system. J Small Anim Pract 35:251–256

Hammer A, Getzy D, Ogilvie G, Upton M, Klausner J, Kisseberth WC (2001) Salivary gland neoplasia in the dog and cat: survival times and prognostic factors. J Am Anim Hosp Assoc 37:478–482

Hampson ECGM, Wilkinson GT, Sutton RH, Turner SA (1990) Cutaneous metastasis of a colonic-carcinoma in a dog. J Small Anim Pract 31:155–158

Hayes AM, Adams VJ, Scasey TJ, Murphy S (2007) Survival of 54 cats with oral squamous cell carcinoma in United Kingdom general practice. J Small Anim Pract 48:394–399

Hayes S, Yuzbasiyan-Gurkan V, Gregory-Bryson E, Kiupel M (2013) Classification of canine nonangiogenic, nonlymphogenic, gastrointestinal sarcomas based on microscopic, immunohistochemical, and molecular characteristics. Vet Pathol 50:779–788

Henry C, Herrera C (2013) Mast cell tumors in cats: clinical update and possible new treatment avenues. J Feline Med Surg 15:41–47

Herring ES, Smith MM, Robertson JL (2002) Lymph node staging of oral and maxillofacial neoplasms in 31 dogs and cats. J Vet Dent 19:122–126

Janke L, Carlson CS, St Hill CA (2010) The novel carbohydrate tumor antigen C2-O-sLe x is upregulated in canine gastric carcinomas. Vet Pathol 47:455–461

Kelly JM, Belding BA, Schaefer AK (2010) Acanthomatous ameloblastoma in dogs treated with intralesional bleomycin. Vet Comp Oncol 8:81–86

Kirberger RM, Clift SJ, van Wilpe E, Dvir E (2013) Spirocerca lupi-associated vertebral changes: a radiologic-pathologic study. Vet Parasitol 195:87–94

Kiupel M, Smedley RC, Pfent C, Xie Y, Xue Y, Wise AG, DeVaul JM, Maes RK (2011) Diagnostic algorithm to differentiate lymphoma from inflammation in feline small intestinal biopsy samples. Vet Pathol 48:212–222

Kosovsky JF, Matthiesen DT, Patnaik AK (1988) Small intestinal adenocarcinoma in cats – 32 cases (1978–1985). J Am Vet Med Assoc 192:233–235

Kosovsky JK, Matthiesen DT, Marretta SM, Patnaik AK (1991) Results of partial mandibulectomy for the treatment of oral tumors in 142 dogs. Vet Surg 20:397–401

Krauser K (1985) Neoplasien des Magens beim Hund. Berl Münch Tierärztl Wschr 98:48–53

Kreutzer R, Wohlsein P, Staszyk C, Nowak M, Sill V, Baumgartner W (2007) Dental benign cementomas in three horses. Vet Pathol 44:533–536

LaRock RG, Ginn PE (1997) Immunohistochemical staining characteristics of canine gastrointestinal stromal tumors. Vet Pathol 34:303–311

Laurenson MP, Skorupski KA, Moore PF, Zwingenberger AL (2011) Ultrasonography of intestinal mast cell tumors in the cat. Vet Radiol Ultrasound 52:330–334

Lindsay N, Kirberger R, Williams M (2010) Imaging diagnosis-spinal cord chondrosarcoma associated with spirocercosis in a dog. Vet Radiol Ultrasound 51:614–616

Lingard AE, Briscoe K, Beatty JA, Moore AS, Crowley AM, Krockenberger M, Churcher RK, Canfield PJ, Barrs VR (2009) Low-grade alimentary lymphoma: clinicopathological findings and response to treatment in 17 cases. J Feline Med Surg 11:692–700

Linton M, Nimmo JS, Norris JM, Churcher R, Haynes S, Zoltowska A, Hughes S, Lessels NS, Wright M, Malik R (2015) Feline gastrointestinal eosinophilic sclerosing fibroplasia: 13 cases and review of an emerging clinical entity. J Feline Med Surg 17:392–404

Lurie DM, Seguin BD, Schneider PD, Verstraete FJ, Wisner ER (2006) Contrast-assisted ultrasound for sentinel lymph node detection in spontaneously arising canine head and neck tumors. Invest Radiol 41:415–421

Maas CP, ter Haar G, van der Gaag I, Kirpensteijn J (2007) Reclassification of small intestinal and cecal smooth muscle tumors in 72 dogs: clinical, histologic, and immunohistochemical evaluation. Vet Surg 36: 302–313

Maeda S, Ohno K, Fujiwara-Igarashi A, Uchida K, Tsujimoto H (2016) Changes in Foxp3-positive regulatory T cell number in the intestine of dogs with idiopathic inflammatory bowel disease and intestinal lymphoma. Vet Pathol 53:102–112

Marolf AJ, Bachand AM, Sharber J, Twedt DC (2015) Comparison of endoscopy and sonography findings in dogs and cats with histologically confirmed gastric neoplasia. J Small Anim Pract 56:339–344

Masuda EK, Kommers GD, Martins TB, Barros CSL, Piazer JVM (2011) Morphological factors as indicators of malignancy of squamous cell carcinomas in cattle exposed naturally to bracken fern (Pteridium aquilinum). J Comp Pathol 144:48–54

Mazaki-Tovi M, Baneth G, Aroch I, Harrus S, Kass PH, Ben-Ari T, Zur G, Aizenberg I, Bark H, Lavy E (2002) Canine spirocercosis: clinical, diagnostic, pathologic, and epidemiologic characteristics. Vet Parasitol 107:235–250

McEntee MF, Cates JM, Neilsen N (2002) Cyclooxygenase-2 expression in spontaneous intestinal neoplasia of domestic dogs. Vet Pathol 39:428–436

Mestrinho LA, Faísca P, Peleteiro MC, Niza MM (2014) PCNA and grade in 13 canine oral squamous cell carcinomas: association with prognosis. Vet Comp Oncol. doi: 10.1111/vco.12134. [Epub ahead of print]

Mestrinho LA, Pissarra H, Faisca PB, Braganca M, Peleteiro MC, Niza MM (2015) p63 and E-cadherin expression in canine oral squamous cell carcinoma. Vet Pathol 52:614–620

Moore PF, Rodriguez-Bertos A, Kass PH (2012) Feline gastrointestinal lymphoma: mucosal architecture, immunophenotype, and molecular clonality. Vet Pathol 49:658–668

Mooney SC, Hayes AA (1986) Lymphomas in the cat: an approach to diagnosis and management. Semin Vet Med Surg (Small Anim) 1 (1):51–57

Morse CC, Saik JE, Richardson DW, Fetter AW (1988) Equine juvenile mandibular ossifying fibroma. Vet Pathol 25:415–421

Munday JS (2014) Bovine and human papillomaviruses: a comparative review. Vet Pathol 51:1063–1075

Munday JS, French AF (2015) Felis catus papillomavirus types 1 and 4 are rarely present in neoplastic and inflammatory oral lesions of cats. Res Vet Sci 100:220–222

Munday JS, Fairley RA, Mills H, Kiupel M, Vaatstra BL (2015a) Oral papillomas associated with felis catus papillomavirus type 1 in 2 domestic cats. Vet Pathol 52: 1187–1190

Munday JS, French A, Harvey CJ (2015b) Molecular and immunohistochemical studies do not support a role for papillomaviruses in canine oral squamous cell carcinoma development. Vet J 204:223–225

Munday JS, Tucker RS, Kiupel M, Harvey CJ (2015c) Multiple oral carcinomas associated with a novel papillomavirus in a dog. J Vet Diagn Invest 27:221–225

Munday JS, Dunowska M, Laurie RE, Hills S (2016) Genomic characterisation of canine papillomavirus type 17, a possible rare cause of canine oral squamous cell carcinoma. Vet Microbiol 182:135–140

Northrup NC, Selting KA, Rassnick KM, Kristal O, O'Brien MG, Dank G, Dhaliwal RS, Jagannatha S, Cornell KK, Gieger TL (2006) Outcomes of cats with oral tumors treated with mandibulectomy: 42 cases. J Am Anim Hosp Assoc 42:350–360

Ohmura S, Leipig M, Schopper I, Hergt F, Weber K, Rutgen BC, Tsujimoto H, Hermanns W, Hirschberger J (2015) Detection of monoclonality in intestinal lymphoma with polymerase chain reaction for antigen receptor gene rearrangement analysis to differentiate from enteritis in dogs. Vet Comp Oncol. doi: 10.1111/vco.12151. [Epub ahead of print]

Olsen SN (1992) Squamous-cell carcinoma of the equine stomach – a report of 5 cases. Vet Rec 131:170–173

Owen LN (1980) World Health Organisation TNM Classification of tumors in domestic animals. Geneva

Paoloni MC, Penninck DG, Moore AS (2002) Ultrasonographic and clinicopathologic findings in 21 dogs with intestinal adenocarcinoma. Vet Radiol Ultrasound 43:562–567

Patnaik AK, Liu SK, Johnson GF (1976) Feline intestinal adenocarcinoma. A clinicopathologic study of 22 cases. Vet Pathol 13:1–10

Patnaik AK, Hurvitz AI, Johnson GF (1977) Canine gastrointestinal neoplasms. Vet Pathol 14:547–555

Patnaik AK, Hurvitz AI, Johnson GF (1978) Canine gastric adenocarcinoma. Vet Pathol 15:600–607

Patnaik AK, Hurvitz AI, Johnson GF (1980) Canine intestinal adenocarcinoma and carcinoid. Vet Pathol 17:149–163

Patterson-Kane JC, Kugler BP, Francis K (2004) The possible prognostic significance of immunophenotype in feline alimentary lymphoma: a pilot study. J Comp Pathol 130:220–222

Penninck D, Smyers B, Webster CR, Rand W, Moore AS (2003) Diagnostic value of ultrasonography in differentiating enteritis from intestinal neoplasia in dogs. Vet Radiol Ultrasound 44:570–575

Pohlman LM, Higginbotham ML, Welles EG, Johnson CM (2009) Immunophenotypic and histologic classification of 50 cases of feline gastrointestinal lymphoma. Vet Pathol 46:259–268

Poulet FM, Valentine BA, Summers BA (1992) A survey of epithelial odontogenic-tumors and cysts in dogs and cats. Vet Pathol 29:369–380

Przeździecki R, Czopowicz M, Sapierzyński R (2015) Accuracy of routine cytology and immunocytochemistry in preoperative diagnosis of oral amelanotic melanomas in dogs. Vet Clin Pathol 44:597–604

Rakich PM, Latimer KS, Weiss R, Steffens WL (1989) Mucocutaneous plasmacytomas in dogs: 75 cases (1980–1987). J Am Vet Med Assoc 194:803–810

Ramos-Vara JA, Beissenherz ME, Miller MA, Johnson GC, Pace LW, Fard A, Kottler SJ (2000) Retrospective study of 338 canine oral melanomas with clinical, histologic, and immunohistochemical review of 129 cases. Vet Pathol 37:597–608

Ranen E, Lavy E, Aizenberg Z, Perl S, Harrus S (2004) Spirocercosis-associated esophageal sarcomas in dogs – a retrospective study of 17 cases (1997–2003). Vet Parasitol 119:209–221

Rassnick KM, Ruslander DM, Cotter SM, Al-Sarraf R, Bruyette DS, Gamblin RM, Meleo KA, Moore AS (2001) Use of carboplatin for treatment of dogs with malignant melanoma: 27 cases (1989–2000). J Am Vet Med Assoc 218:1444–1448

Rassnick KM, Moore AS, Collister KE, Northrup NC, Kristal O, Chretin JD, Bailey DB (2009) Efficacy of combination chemotherapy for treatment of gastrointestinal lymphoma in dogs. J Vet Intern Med 23:317–322

Recknagel S, Nicke M, Schusser GF (2012) Diagnostic assessment of peritoneal fluid cytology in horses with abdominal neoplasia. Tierarztl Prax Ausg G Grosstiere Nutztiere 40:85–93

Reed SD, Fulmer A, Buckholz J, Zhang B, Cutrera J, Shiomitsu K, Li S (2010) Bleomycin/interleukin-12 electrochemogenetherapy for treating naturally occurring spontaneous neoplasms in dogs. Cancer Gene Ther 17:571–578

Reef VB, Dyson SS, Beech J (1984) Lymphosarcoma and associated immune-mediated hemolytic-anemia and thrombocytopenia in horses. J Am Vet Med Assoc 184:313–317

Regan D, Guth A, Coy J, Dow S (2015) Cancer immunotherapy in veterinary medicine: current options and new developments. Vet J 207:20–28

Rissetto K, Villamil JA, Selting KA, Tyler J, Henry CJ (2011) Recent trends in feline intestinal neoplasia: an epidemiologic study of 1,129 cases in the veterinary medical database from 1964 to 2004. J Am Anim Hosp Assoc 47:28–36

Roccabianca P, Vernau W, Caniatti M, Moore PF (2006) Feline large granular lymphocyte (LGL) lymphoma with secondary leukemia: primary intestinal origin with predominance of a CD3/CD8 alpha alpha phenotype. Vet Pathol 43:15–28

Rodriguez SM, Florins A, Gillet N, de Brogniez A, Sanchez-Alcaraz MT, Boxus M, Boulanger F, Gutierrez G, Trono K, Alvarez I, Vagnoni L, Willems L (2011) Preventive and therapeutic strategies for bovine leukemia virus: lessons for HTLV. Viruses 3:1210–1248

Russell KN, Mehler SJ, Skorupski KA, Baez JL, Shofer FS, Goldschmidt MH (2007) Clinical and immunohistochemical differentiation of gastrointestinal stromal tumors from leiomyosarcomas in dogs: 42 cases (1990–2003). J Am Vet Med Assoc 230:1329–1333

Sancak A, Favrot C, Geisseler MD, Muller M, Lange CE (2015) Antibody titres against canine papillomavirus 1 peak around clinical regression in naturally occurring oral papillomatosis. Vet Dermatol 26:57–59

Sato AF, Solano M (2004) Ultrasonographic findings in abdominal mast cell disease: a retrospective study of 19 patients. Vet Radiol Ultrasound 45:51–57

Seim-Wikse T, Kolbjornsen O, Jorundsson E, Benestad SL, Bjornvad CR, Grotmol T, Kristensen AT, Skancke E (2014) Tumour gastrin expression and serum gastrin concentrations in dogs with gastric carcinoma are poor diagnostic indicators. J Comp Pathol 151:207–211

Simon D, Meneses F, Nolte I (2005) Möglichkeiten der Diagnostik von Tumorerkrankungen am Magen-Darm-Trakt. Tierärztl Prax K 33:401–406

Simon D, Nolte I, Eberle N, Abbrederis N, Killich M, Hirschberger J (2006) Treatment of dogs with lymphoma using a 12-week, maintenance-free combination chemotherapy protocol. J Vet Intern Med 20:948–954

Simon D, Moreno SN, Hirschberger J, Moritz A, Kohn B, Neumann S, Jurina K, Scharvogel S, Schwedes C, Reinacher M, Beyerbach M, Nolte I (2008) Efficacy of a continuous, multiagent chemotherapeutic protocol versus a short-term single-agent protocol in dogs with lymphoma. J Am Vet Med Assoc 232:879–885

Slawienski MJ, Mauldin GE, Mauldin GN, Patnaik AK (1997) Malignant colonic neoplasia in cats: 46 cases (1990–1996). J Am Vet Med Assoc 211:878–881

Smedley RC, Lamoureux J, Sledge DG, Kiupel M (2011a) Immunohistochemical diagnosis of canine oral amelanotic melanocytic neoplasms. Vet Pathol 48:32–40

Smedley RC, Spangler WL, Esplin DG, Kitchell BE, Bergman PJ, Ho HY, Bergin IL, Kiupel M (2011b) Prognostic markers for canine melanocytic neoplasms: a comparative review of the literature and goals for future investigation. Vet Pathol 48:54–72

Smith SH, Goldschmidt MH, McManus PM (2002) A comparative review of melanocytic neoplasms. Vet Pathol 39:651–678

9

Snyder LA, Bertone ER, Jakowski RM, Dooner MS, Jennings-Ritchie J, Moore AS (2004) p53 expression and environmental tobacco smoke exposure in feline oral squamous cell carcinoma. Vet Pathol 41:209–214

Spangler WL, Culbertson MR (1991) Salivary gland disease in dogs and cats: 245 cases (1985–1988). J Am Vet Med Assoc 198:465–469

Stebbins KE, Morse CC, Goldschmidt MH (1989) Feline oral neoplasia: a ten-year survey. Vet Pathol 26:121–128

Sundberg JP, Van Ranst M, Montali R, Homer BL, Miller WH, Rowland PH, Scott DW, England JJ, Dunstan RW, Mikaelian I, Jenson AB (2000) Feline papillomas and papillomaviruses. Vet Pathol 37:1–10

Taylor SD, Haldorson GJ, Vaughan B, Pusterla N (2009) Gastric neoplasia in horses. J Vet Intern Med 23: 1097–1102

Teske E, van Heerde P, Rutteman GR, Kurzman ID, Moore PF, MacEwen EG (1994) Prognostic factors for treatment of malignant lymphoma in dogs. J Am Vet Med Assoc 205:1722–1728

Theon AP, Rodriguez C, Griffey S, Madewell BR (1997) Analysis of prognostic factors and patterns of failure in dogs with periodontal tumors treated with megavoltage irradiation. J Am Vet Med Assoc 210:785–788

Thrall DE (1981) Orthovoltage radiotherapy of oral fibrosarcomas in dogs. J Am Vet Med Assoc 179:159–162

Thrall DE (1984) Orthovoltage radiotherapy of acanthomatous epulides in 39 dogs. J Am Vet Med Assoc 184: 826–829

Todoroff RJ, Brodey RS (1979) Oral and pharyngeal neoplasia in the dog – retrospective survey of 361 cases. J Am Vet Med Assoc 175:567–571

Tomlinson MJ, Mckeever PJ, Nordine RA (1982) Colonic adenocarcinoma with cutaneous metastasis in a dog. J Am Vet Med Assoc 180:1344–1345

Tsirimonaki E, O'Neil BW, Williams R, Campo MS (2003) Extensive papillomatosis of the bovine upper gastrointestinal tract. J Comp Pathol 129:93–99

Vail DM, Kisseberth WC, Obradovich JE, Moore FM, London CA, MacEwen EG, Ritter MA (1996) Assessment of potential doubling time (Tpot), argyrophilic nucleolar organizer regions (AgNOR), and proliferating cell nuclear antigen (PCNA) as predictors of therapy response in canine non-Hodgkin's lymphoma. Exp Hematol 24:807–815

Valerius KD, Powers BE, McPherron MA, Hutchison JM, Mann FA, Withrow SJ (1997) Adenomatous polyps and carcinoma in situ of the canine colon and rectum: 34 cases (1982–1994). J Am Anim Hosp Assoc 33:156–160

Valli VE, Kass PH, San Myint M, Scott F (2013) Canine lymphomas: association of classification type, disease stage, tumor subtype, mitotic rate, and treatment with survival. Vet Pathol 50:738–748

van der Merwe LL, Kirberger RM, Clift S, Williams M, Keller N, Naidoo V (2008) Spirocerca lupi infection in the dog: a review. Vet J 176:294–309

Vandenhoven R, Franken P (1983) Clinical aspects of lymphosarcoma in the horse – a clinical report of 16 cases. Equine Vet J 15:49–53

von Babo V, Eberle N, Mischke R, Meyer-Lindenberg A, Hewicker-Trautwein M, Nolte I, Betz D (2012) Canine non-hematopoietic gastric neoplasia. Epidemiologic and diagnostic characteristics in 38 dogs with post-surgical outcome of five cases. Tierarztl Prax Ausg K Kleintiere Heimtiere 40:243–249

Wallace J, Matthiesen DT, Patnaik AK (1992) Hemimaxillectomy for the treatment of oral tumors in 69 dogs. Vet Surg 21:337–341

Watrach AM, Small E, Case MT (1970) Canine papilloma – progression of oral papilloma to carcinoma. J Natl Cancer Inst 45:915–920

White RA, Gorman NT (1989) Wide local excision of acanthomatous epulides in the dog. Vet Surg 18:12–14

Willard MD (2012) Alimentary neoplasia in geriatric dogs and cats. Vet Clin North Am Small Anim Pract 42: 693–706

Withrow SJ, Holmberg DL (1983) Mandibulectomy in the treatment of oral-cancer. J Am Anim Hosp Assoc 19:273–286

Wright ZM, Rogers KS, Mansell J (2008) Survival data for canine oral extramedullary plasmacytomas: a retrospective analysis (1996–2006). J Am Anim Hosp Assoc 44:75–81

Yoshida K, Yanai T, Iwasaki T, Sakai H, Ohta J, Kati S, Minami T, Lackner AA, Masegi T (1999) Clinicopathological study of canine oral epulides. J Vet Med Sci 61:897–902

Tumors of the Exocrine Pancreas

Stephanie Plog

R. Klopfleisch (ed.), *Veterinary Oncology*, DOI 10.1007/978-3-319-41124-8_10

10.1 Canine Exocrine Pancreas Tumors

Box 10.1. Canine Exocrine Pancreatic Neoplasms in Five Facts

1. Nonneoplastic benign nodular hyperplasia much more common than true neoplasms
2. Neoplasms mainly highly malignant adenocarcinomas
3. Widespread metastases at the time of diagnosis
4. Partial pancreatectomy possibly, chemotherapy not useful
5. Prognosis poor

▪ Epidemiology and Pathogenesis

Tumors of the exocrine pancreas are very *rare* in dogs. The vast majority of tumors are of *epithelial* origin, originating from ductal or acinar cells. Females seem to be overrepresented, but information about breed dispositions and possible etiologic components are contradictory. The mean *age* is 10 years, but cases in younger dogs have been described as well. Pancreatic *adenocarcinomas* are very *aggressive*, and *metastases* to the lymph nodes, liver, and peritoneum or distant metastases are present at the time of diagnosis in most of the cases.

Pancreatic *adenomas* are extremely rare and present as solitary, noninvasive nodules. In contrast, nodular *hyperplasia* of the pancreas is very common and is a frequent incidental finding, especially in older dogs. Adenomas and nodular hyperplasias are usually smaller than adenocarcinomas.

▪ Clinical Appearance

Clinical signs are *unspecific* and include signs of pancreatic *insufficiency* like vomitus, anorexia, and lethargy. The tumor is usually not palpable, but abdominal distension is seen in some cases with plant metastases and ascites. There may be signs of *diabetes mellitus* or *jaundice* due to destruction of the endocrine pancreas or obstruction of the bile duct, respectively. In a few cases, steatitis, panniculitis, and epidermal necrosis have been described. *Bloodwork* might reveal enhanced lipase and amylase values, but a normal range does not exclude a neoplasm. *Ultrasonography* is useful for identifying the pancreatic mass, which is often located centrally or in the *duodenal part* of the pancreas and may also detect local and distant metastases. Computer tomography (CT) is another useful diagnostic approach in localizing the tumor, and contrast-enhanced ultrasonography was shown to be of use for differentiation between endocrine and exocrine pancreatic tumors. Diagnostic (and palliative, if applicable) *laparotomy* is recommended when other diagnostic methods are not specific enough. Pancreatic *carcinomas* appear as *solitary*, often *invasive* single nodules or invade the organ more diffusely. They show prominent fibrous tissue, and hemorrhage, necrosis, and mineralization are common. Many *small nodules* in the pancreas as detected by ultrasonography or laparotomy may point more toward a benign *hyperplasia* than toward a malignant process.

▪ Cytology and Histopathology

Ultrasound-guided *fine needle aspiration* of the pancreatic tumor or, less often, tumor cells in the abdominal fluid can be helpful for the diagnosis. *Poorly differentiated epithelial cells*, occasionally forming acini, but often poorly cohesive, with often numerous and atypical mitoses, can be identified in the cytological smear. There is a high correlation of cytological and histopathological results. However, histopathology is needed for the assessment of invasion and margins. The most common histopathological form is the small tubular type of pancreatic adenocarcinomas. Even well-differentiated tumors can metastasize widely, and *prognosis* is *not dependent* on any histological *subclassification*.

▪ Therapy and Prognosis

Partial *pancreatectomy* is the method of choice in dogs with non overt metastatic spread, but there is a high complication rate, and partial *duodenectomy* might be necessary in addition. *Chemotherapeutic* approaches with *cisplatin* have been described but are usually only effective for amelioration of clinical signs caused by metastases. The prognosis is *poor* due to the *high metastatic rate* and the side effects caused by pancreatic destruction, and survival time is often only in some days.

▪ Suggested Reading

(Allen et al. 1989; Bennett et al. 2001; Cave et al. 2007; Chang et al. 2007; Cobb and Merrell 1984; Cordner et al 2015; Dennis et al. 2008; Kircher and Nielsen 1976; Newman et al. 2005; Priester 1974; Quigley et al. 2001; Vanderperren et al. 2014)

10.2 Feline Exocrine Pancreas Tumors

Box 10.2. Feline Exocrine Pancreatic Neoplasms in Five Facts

1. Nonneoplastic benign nodular hyperplasia far more common than true neoplasms
2. True neoplasms mainly highly malignant adenocarcinomas
3. Often widespread metastases at the time of diagnosis
4. Partial pancreatectomy possibly, chemotherapy might be beneficial
5. Prognosis poor

▪ Epidemiology and Pathogenesis

Pancreatic tumors are *rare* in cats, and nodular *hyperplasias* are more common. Most are of epithelial origin and malignant, similar to the dog. The mean *age* is 12 years, but cases in younger cats are described as well. Pancreatic adenocarcinomas are extremely *aggressive*, and metastases to the lymph nodes, liver, and peritoneum or distant metastases are present at the time of diagnosis in most cases. Pancreatic adenomas are rare.

▪ Clinical Appearance

The clinical signs of an exocrine pancreatic neoplasm are similar to that in dogs (▶ see Sect. 10.1), which means they are often *unspecific*. A clinical sign particularly seen in cats is *paraneoplastic alopecia* at the ventrum, head, and limbs with characteristic *glistening appearance* of the skin. However, this is not considered a specific sign for pancreatic neoplasms since it can also occur with other tumors. Metabolic *epidermal necrosis* has also been described. In some cases abdominal masses are *palpable* in cats with pancreatic tumors. Ultrasonographically, a single *pancreatic nodule* with a *diameter >2 cm* is suspicious for a malignant tumor. Diabetes mellitus is not uncommon in cats with pancreatic neoplasia but is an unspecific sign.

▪ Cytology and Histopathology

Cytological and histopathological appearance of feline pancreatic adenocarcinomas is similar to that in the dog (▶ see Sect. 10.1).

▪ Therapy and Prognosis

Partial *pancreatectomy* is the method of choice in cats with non-overt metastatic spread, but there is a high complication rate, and partial *duodenectomy* might be necessary in addition. *Chemotherapeutic* approaches with *gemcitabine* and *carboplatin* seem to yield better results in cats than in dogs, with *survival times* up to 165 days and complete remission in a minority of cats. The prognosis is nevertheless *poor* due to the high metastatic rate and the side effects caused by pancreatic destruction. Abdominal effusion at time of diagnosis seems to worsen the prognosis, and prednisone therapy alone is not beneficial.

▪ Suggested Reading

(Banner et al. 1979; Bennett et al. 2001; Fabbrini et al. 2005; Hecht et al. 2007; Kircher and Nielsen 1976; Knell and Venzin 2012; Linderman et al. 2013; Lobetti 2015; Marconato et al. 2007; Martinez-Ruzafa et al. 2009; Priester 1974; Seaman 2004; Tasker et al. 1999; Turek 2003; Yoshimura et al. 2013)

10.3 Exocrine Pancreas Tumors in Horses and Cattle

Exocrine pancreas tumors are *very rare* in horses and cattle, but if *adenocarcinomas* occur, they also metastasize widely, comparable to those in dogs and cats. Nodular *hyperplasia* is far more common than true pancreatic neoplasms. Endocrine tumors of the pancreas seem to outnumber exocrine tumors at least in cattle (▶ see Chap. 12 for endocrine pancreatic tumors).

▪ Suggested Reading

(de Brot et al. 2014; Kelley et al. 1996; Lucena et al. 2011; Rendle et al. 2006)

Suggested Reading

Allen SW, Cornelius LM, Mahaffey EA (1989) A comparison of two methods of partial pancreatectomy in the dog. Vet Surg 18(4):274–278

Banner BF, Alroy J, Kipnis RM (1979) Acinar cell carcinoma of the pancreas in a cat. Vet Pathol 16(5):543–547

Bennett PF, Hahn KA, Toal RL, Legendre AM (2001) Ultrasonographic and cytopathological diagnosis of exocrine pancreatic carcinoma in the dog and cat. J Am Anim Hosp Assoc 37(5):466–473

Cave TA, Evans H, Hargreaves J, Blunden AS (2007) Metabolic epidermal necrosis in a dog associated with pancreatic adenocarcinoma, hyperglucagonemia, hyperinsulinemia and hypoaminoacidemia. J Small Anim Pract 48(9):522–526

Chang SC, Liao JW, Lin YC, Liu CI, Wong ML (2007) Pancreatic acinar cell carcinoma with intracranial metastasis in a dog. J Vet Med Sci 69(1):91–93

Cobb LF, Merrell RC (1984) Total pancreatectomy in dogs. J Surg Res 37(3):235–240

Cordner AP, Sharkey LC, Armstrong PJ, McAteer KD (2015) Cytologic findings and diagnostic yield in 92 dogs undergoing fine-needle aspiration of the pancreas. J Vet Diagn Invest 27(2):236–240

de Brot S, Junge H, Hilbe M (2014) Acinar cell carcinoma of exocrine pancreas in two horses. J Comp Pathol 150(4):388–392

Dennis MM, O'Brien TD, Wayne T, Kiupel M, Williams M, Powers BE (2008) Hyalinizing pancreatic adenocarcinoma in six dogs. Vet Pathol 45(4):475–483

Fabbrini F, Anfray P, Viacava P, Gregori M, Abramo F (2005) Feline cutaneous and visceral necrotizing panniculitis and steatitis associated with a pancreatic tumour. Vet Dermatol 16(6):413–419

Hecht S, Penninck DG, Keating JH (2007) Imaging findings in pancreatic neoplasia and nodular hyperplasia in 19 cats. Vet Radiol Ultrasound 48(1):45–50

Kelley LC, Harmon BG, McCaskey PC (1996) A retrospective study of pancreatic tumors in slaughter cattle. Vet Pathol 33(4):398–406

Kircher CH, Nielsen SW (1976) Tumours of the pancreas. Bull World Health Organ 53(2–3):195–202

Knell S, Venzin C (2012) Partial pancreatectomy and splenectomy using a bipolar vessel sealing device in a cat with an anaplastic pancreatic carcinoma. Schweiz Arch Tierheilkd 154(7):298–301

Linderman MJ, Brodsky EM, de Lorimier LP, Clifford CA, Post GS (2013) Feline exocrine pancreatic carcinoma: a retrospective study of 34 cases. Vet Comp Oncol 11(3):208–218

Lobetti R (2015) Lymphocytic mural folliculitis and pancreatic carcinoma in a cat. J Feline Med Surg 17(6):548–550

Lucena RB, Rissi DR, Kommers GD, Pierezan F, Oliveira-Filho JC, Macêdo JT, Flores MM, Barros CS (2011) A retrospective study of 586 tumours in Brazilian cattle. J Comp Pathol 145(1):20–24

Marconato L, Albanese F, Viacava P, Marchetti V, Abramo F (2007) Paraneoplastic alopecia associated with hepatocellular carcinoma in a cat. Vet Dermatol 18(4):267–271

Martinez-Ruzafa I, Dominguez PA, Dervisis NG, Sarbu L, Newman RG, Cadile CD, Kitchell BE (2009) Tolerability of gemcitabine and carboplatin doublet therapy in cats with carcinomas. J Vet Intern Med 23(3):570–577

Newman SJ, Steiner JM, Woosley K, Barton L, Williams DA (2005) Correlation of age and incidence of pancreatic exocrine nodular hyperplasia in the dog. Vet Pathol 42(4):510–513

Priester WA (1974) Data from eleven United States and Canadian colleges of veterinary medicine on pancreatic carcinoma in domestic animals. Cancer Res 34(6):1372–1375

Quigley KA, Jackson ML, Haines DM (2001) Hyperlipasemia in 6 dogs with pancreatic or hepatic neoplasia: evidence for tumor lipase production. Vet Clin Pathol 30(3):114–120

Rendle DI, Hewetson M, Barron R, Baily JE (2006) Tachypnoea and pleural effusion in a mare with metastatic pancreatic adenocarcinoma. Vet Rec 159(11):356–359

Seaman RL (2004) Exocrine pancreatic neoplasia in the cat: a case series. J Am Anim Hosp Assoc 40(3):238–245

Tasker S, Griffon DJ, Nuttall TJ, Hill PB (1999) Resolution of paraneoplastic alopecia following surgical removal of a pancreatic carcinoma in a cat. J Small Anim Pract 40(1):16–19

Turek MM (2003) Cutaneous paraneoplastic syndromes in dogs and cats: a review of the literature. Vet Dermatol 14(6):279–296

Vanderperren K, Haers H, Van der Vekens E, Stock E, Paepe D, Daminet S, Saunders JH (2014) Description of the use of contrast-enhanced ultrasonography in four dogs with pancreatic tumours. J Small Anim Pract 55(3):164–169

Yoshimura H, Matsuda Y, Kawamoto Y, Michishita M, Ohkusu-Tsukada K, Takahashi K, Naito Z, Ishiwata T (2013) Acinar cell cystadenoma of the pancreas in a cat. J Comp Pathol 149(2–3):225–228

10

Skeletal Tumors

Robert Klopfleisch

R. Klopfleisch (ed.), *Veterinary Oncology*, DOI 10.1007/978-3-319-41124-8_11

11.1 Canine Bone and Joint Tumors

Osteosarcomas are the most important bone tumors of the dog. They make up almost 90 % of all bone tumors. *Chondrosarcomas* are the second most common tumors representing 5 % of bone tumors. Fibrosarcomas, hemangiosarcomas, and osteochondromas are rare and mostly represent the remaining tumors. *Synovial cell sarcomas* are the most important joint-associated tumor in dogs.

11.1.1 Canine Osteosarcomas

Box 11.1. Canine Osteosarcomas in Ten Facts

1. Appendicular osteosarcomas of the limbs most common
2. Axial osteosarcomas of calvarium, ribs, spine, and pelvis with a higher incidence in small dogs
3. All osteosarcomas of highly invasive local growth
4. 90 % of appendicular osteosarcomas with distant metastases
5. Axial osteosarcomas with less frequent (30–50 %) distant metastases
6. Direct hematogenous spread, lymph node metastases not commonly present
7. Surgery (amputation/limb sparing) treatment modality of choice
8. Adjuvant chemotherapy necessary to decelerate growth of metastases
9. Radiotherapy mainly used for pain palliation
10. Plethora of prognostic factors

Epidemiology and Pathogenesis

Osteosarcomas are the most frequent bone tumor of dogs. They constitute up to *90 % of all bone tumors* and 5 % of all malignant tumors in dogs. They occur mostly in middle aged to old dogs with a median *age* of 7 years. They are however also occasionally found in young dogs around the age of 2 years. Osteosarcomas are tumors of larger

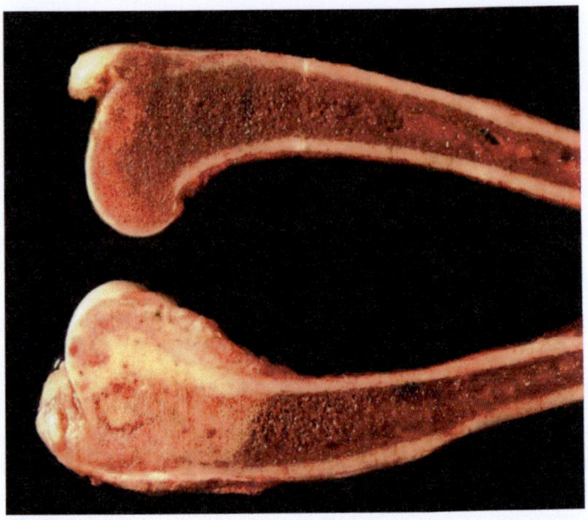

Fig. 11.1 Osteosarcoma of the humerus of a dog (lower humerus, upper contralateral humerus not affected)

dogs with that only 5 % of all canine osteosarcomas present in dogs with a *body weight* <15 kg. German shepherds, Great Danes, Rottweiler, Doberman, greyhounds, and golden retriever are repeatedly reported to be *breeds* with an increased risk to develop osteosarcomas. *Larger size* and *higher weight* are nevertheless reported to be a stronger predisposing factor than breed. Deeper analysis of the genetic basis of inheritance of osteosarcoma predisposition identified a *polygenic spectrum of germline risk factors* pointing to specific pathways of bone differentiation and growth. There is no confirmed *gender* predisposition.

Osteosarcomas are coarsely separated by their anatomical location into *appendicular osteosarcomas* of the limbs (Fig. 11.1) and *axial osteosarcomas* of the spine and flat bones of the skull and pelvis. Approximately 75 % of canine osteosarcomas develop in the *appendicular skeleton*, i.e., the limbs, which constitute 95 % of osteosarcomas in large breeds. Appendicular tumors usually develop in the *metaphyseal bone*, and *front limbs* are more often affected by osteosarcomas than diaphyseal bone and hind limbs. Osteosarcomas in the front limbs are usually developing in the proximal humerus and the distal radius but rarely adjacent to the elbow joint. Appendicular osteosarcomas are locally aggressive with invasion of surrounding bony and soft tissue structures. In addition, *metastasis is observed in 90 % of dogs* with appendicular osteosarcomas. In contrast, *axial osteosarcomas* of the head, spine, ribs, and pelvis represent 60 % of osteosarcomas in smaller breeds. They are also locally aggressive with invasion of surrounding structures and have a *metastatic rate of 30 %*.

There is ongoing research on the *etiology* of osteosarcomas in the dog. The predisposition of large and heavyweight dogs has led to the hypothesis that *repeated microfractures* and tissue damage may induce appendicular osteosarcomas. This hypothesis has not been confirmed by comparing CT scans, which found no significant differences in the presence of microfractures in the nonneoplastic bones of large and small dogs. Sequence and expression level analysis of several genes has been conducted to identify the molecular mechanisms of osteosarcoma carcinogenesis. *Defects in p53 function and p53 overexpression* and thus deficient DNA repair and apoptosis induction have been identified as a potential cause for canine osteosarcomas. Loss of the phosphatase and tensin homolog (*PTEN*), a tumor suppressor gene, has been identified in up to 50 % of osteosarcoma samples in diverse studies. Overexpression or excessive signaling of the proto-oncogene tyrosine kinase receptor *MET*, the insulin-like growth factor 1 (*IGF1*) and its receptor (*IGF1R*), the transforming growth factor beta 1 (*TGFb1*), and the membrane-cytoskeleton linker *ezrin* have also been identified as a potential cause of canine osteosarcoma development and metastasis.

Clinical Appearance

Dogs with *appendicular osteosarcomas* are mostly first presented due to severe *lameness* and *pain* in the affected bone. The pain is caused by microfractures, pathologic fractures of the cortical bone, or periosteal irritation. Swelling is usually seen only at late stages of tumor development. Dogs with tumors in the axial skeleton present with clinical signs, which obviously depend on the affected bone. Osteosarcomas are aggressive tumors with *invasion and lysis of the preexisting bony structures*. Although they often develop in the metaphyseal bone and thus close to joints, they usually never cross joints to invade the neighboring bone. Approximately *90 % of osteosarcomas metastasize early and hematogenously*. At primary presentation less than 10 % of dogs with osteosarcomas have detectable metastases in the lung (Fig. 11.2) or other distant organs. However, 90 % of the dogs will have metastatic disease 1 year after immediate amputation without adjuvant therapy. Lymphogenic spread with detection of swelling and *metastases to the regional lymph node is rare* and present in less than 10 % of dogs with osteosarcoma.

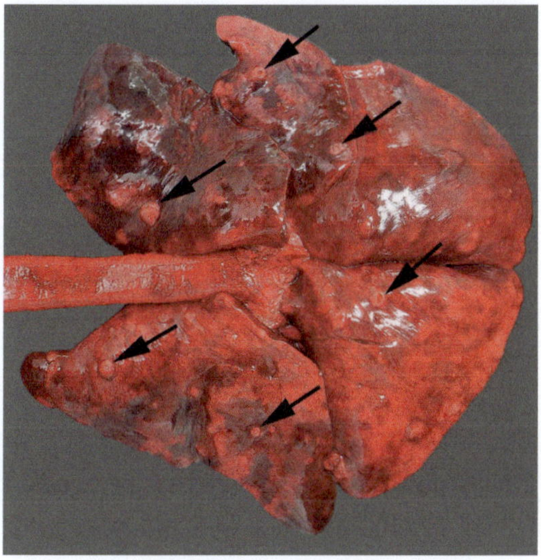

Fig. 11.2 Lung metastases (*arrows*) of an appendicular osteosarcoma of a dog (Photo with permission of S. Plog, PhD, IDEXX, Wetherby, UK and the Archive of the Institute of Veterinary Pathology, Freie Universität Berlin, Germany)

Non-appendicular, axial osteosarcomas are of similar *local aggressive* behavior and also frequently *metastasize. Osteosarcomas of the skull* are locally aggressive but have a *lower metastatic rate* of approximately 33 %.

Radiographs of the affected bones are of particular relevance for the diagnosis of osteosarcomas (Fig. 11.3). Osteosarcomas are variable in their radiographic appearance and present either as predominantly lytic tumors with loss of bone structure or as proliferative tumors with detection of a neoplastic mass. However, *cortical lysis* is usually present, leading to discontinuity and pathologic fracture of the cortical bone. Palisading, perpendicular radiating new bone formation from the cortical bone into the surrounding soft tissue, also called *sunburst phenomenon,* is often seen. The new bone formation may also lead to triangular elevation of the periost with decreasing height toward the periphery of the tumor, which is called

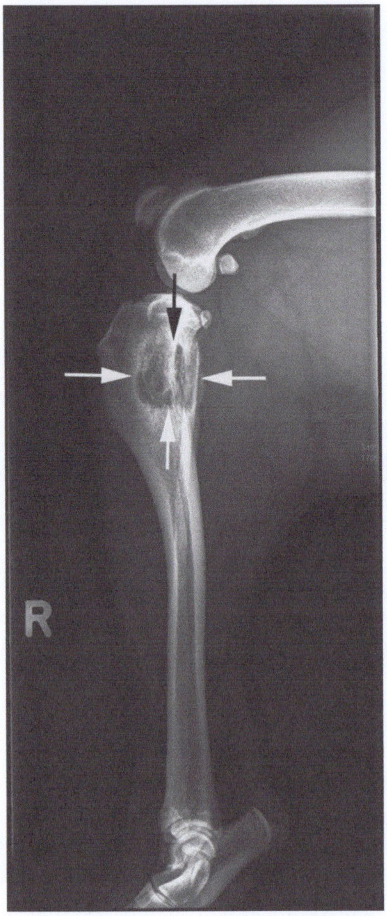

Fig. 11.3 Radiograph of an osteosarcoma (*arrows*) in the proximal tibia of a dog (Photo with permission of Dr. Lottermoser, Small Animal Clinic Sörensen, Berlin, Germany)

Codman's triangle. Codman's triangles are however also seen in nonneoplastic diseases with focal new bone formation. Magnetic resonance imaging (*MRI*) and computed tomography (*CT*) are increasingly used to obtain more detailed information on the extent of tumor invasion and boarders. Both are also more sensitive in the detection of lung metastases. Clinical examination, radiographs, CT, and MRI are usually sufficiently specific to lead to a tentative diagnosis of osteosarcoma. However, a final diagnosis which excludes other causes of bone lysis and new bone formation like osteomyelitis requires a biopsy.

The *Enneking staging system* (Enneking et al. 1980) is commonly used for canine osteosarcomas. It is a *5-tier system* based on the surgical grade, the surgical site (invasiveness) of the primary tumors, and the presence of metastases (Table 11.1). In this system *tumor grade* defines the biologic aggressiveness of the tumor. Low-grade tumors are histologically well-differentiated tumors with a low risk of metastasis (<25 %), while high-grade lesions have a significantly higher incidence of metastases, are histologically poorly differentiated, and show a high mitotic rate, necrosis, and microvascular invasion. *Tumor site* defines what kind of surgical margin is appropriate for the tumor. The prime factor is therefore if the tumor is within a well-delineated anatomic compartment or if it is diffusely infiltrating adjacent compartments which are adventitial planes and spaces like cortical bone, articular cartilage, or periosteal soft tissue. Two stages are subdivided: intracompartmental or extracompartmental tumors. Finally, the presence of local or distant metastases is embraced in the staging system.

Bone alkaline phosphatase (bALP) is often increased in the serum of dogs with osteosarcomas, and increased serum levels are associated with shorter median survival times (5.5 versus 12.5 months) and a worse prognosis than in dogs with normal levels.

Cytology and Histopathology

Cytology of osteosarcomas requires aspiration of cells *from the middle and lytic areas* of the tumor since tissue samples from the periphery of the tumor usually contain nonspecific and nonneoplastic reactive bone proliferation. A *bone marrow biopsy needle* may be used for a better penetration of the cortical bone and to allow for larger tissue samples than with standard aspiration needles. Ultrasound guidance is recommended to increase the accuracy of the diagnosis. A correct cytologic diagnosis of an osteosarcoma however requires an experienced and well-trained cytologist to avoid false-negative diagnoses. Osteosarcoma samples contain single or clustered round, plump, or fusiform mesenchymal cells. Individual neoplastic cells may display anisocytosis, anisokaryosis, and karyomegaly. Osteoclast-type cells are larger, multinucleate cells. Osteoid islands may be observed in some of the tumor cell clusters and is very helpful in the diagnosis of osteosarcomas. Osteoid is

Table 11.1 Enneking staging for malignant musculoskeletal tumors (Enneking et al. 1980)

Stage	Tumor grade	Tumor site	Metastasis
IA	Low (G1)	Intracompartmental (T1)	No metastasis (M0)
IB	Low (G1)	Extracompartmental (T2)	No metastasis (M0)
IIA	High (G2)	Intracompartmental (T1)	No metastasis (M0)
IIB	High (G2)	Extracompartmental (T2)	No metastasis (M0)
III (MST 3–76 days)	Any (G)	Any (T)	Regional/distant metastasis (M1)

MST median survival time

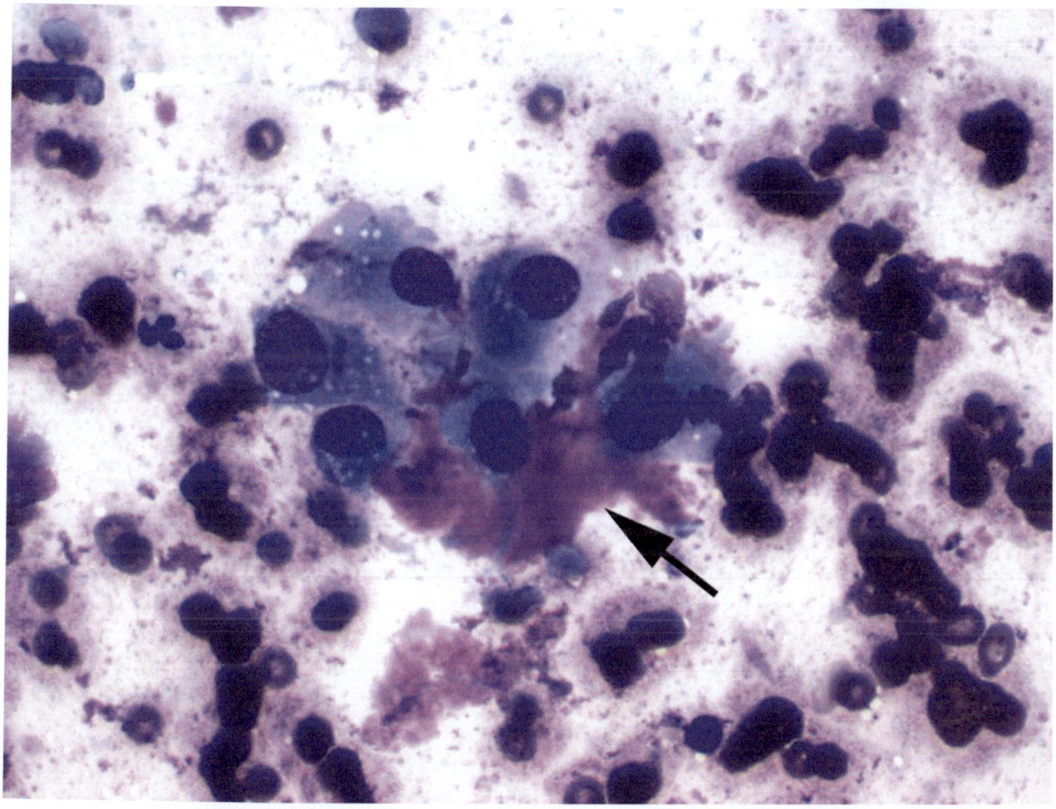

Fig. 11.4 Fine needle aspiration from an appendicular osteosarcoma of a dog (*arrow*: Osteoid island)

amorphous to fibrillar and bright pink in Wright's-stained cytology specimens (Fig. 11.4).

Alkaline phosphatase staining of the aspirated cells may increase the specificity and sensitivity of diagnosis.

Histopathology of osteosarcomas requires a more invasive biopsy taking. The skin incision for biopsy taking should be placed so that it can be excised with the rest of the tumor later on, since there is suspicion that biopsy taking may displace tumor cells into the biopsy canal. *Open incisional biopsies* with surgical incision of the skin and periosteal soft tissue allow for a targeted extraction of tumor tissue but

Table 11.2 Grading system for canine osteosarcoma (Kirpensteijn et al. 2002)

Tumor grade	Metastases/ vessel invasion	Pleomorphism	Mitoses[a]	Tumor matrix	Tumor cells	Necrosis
I	None	1 (25 %)	1 (<10)	1 (50 %)	1 (25 %)	0–1 (25 %)
II	None	2 (25–50 %)	2 (10–20)	2 (25–50 %)	2 (25–50 %)	2 (25–50 %)
III	None	3 (50 %)	3 (>20)	3 (25 %)	3 (50 %)	3 (50 %)
III	Present	Irrelevant				

[a]Per three 400× microscopic fields

are associated with an increased risk of local infection, hematoma formation, and pathologic fracture. *Closed needle biopsies* using a bone marrow biopsy needle or *trephine biopsies* using a Michele trephine have the advantage of smaller wounds with a decreased risk of infection. Both trephine and needle biopsies have a diagnostic accuracy of over 90 %, which is less than for incisional biopsies. A grading system has been developed by Kirpensteijn et al. 2002 (Table 11.2).

▪ Therapy

The therapy of osteosarcomas is primarily focusing on local tumor control but always has to include adjuvant treatment of already present metastases or prevention of most probably developing metastases. *Surgery with adjuvant chemotherapy is the main treatment option for osteosarcomas.* The efficacy of radiotherapy is still in debate but seems to be helpful in some aspects, for instance, for pain palliation or in a curative approach using stereotactic and extracorporeal radiation therapy.

Amputation of the affected limb including scapula or – for proximal femoral tumors – part of the pelvis is the gold standard for appendicular osteosarcomas due to their aggressive local behavior. Even large and heavyweight dogs usually compensate the loss of a limb well, although osteoarthritis may progress more rapidly in the joints of the remaining limbs.

Limb-sparing surgery is an alternative if the owner declines amputation or if the dog is affected by other orthopedic or neurological disorders, which preclude three-leg locomotion. Limb sparing is however only an option if complete excision of the tumor with *potentially tumor-free margins* is possible. Due to the common metaphyseal location of appendicular osteosarcomas, free tumor margins usually require an arthrodesis which restricts limb-sparing surgery to few mainly distal tumors of the ulna and radius. Partial resection of weight-bearing bones requires replacement with allograft, metal endoprosthesis, circular external fixators, or free or roll-in bone autografts. Another possible but rarely used method is *extracorporeal tumor sterilization* of the affected bone fragment. These approaches remove the bone segment with the tumor and pasteurize it at 65 °C for 40 min or irradiate it outside of the body (extracorporeal radiation) and reimplant it. All of these approaches preserve limb function in 80 % of the cases. However, *complications* like infections (up to 50 %), implant rejection (up to 40 %), and tumor recurrence (up to 25 %) are common. Independent from the type of surgery, survival times of dogs treated with surgery alone are <6 months on average. The most common cause of *death or euthanasia* is the development of metastases.

Adjuvant chemotherapy is therefore commonly used to prevent or slow down the development of metastases. Although chemotherapy has some proven efficacy, the prognosis for dogs with osteosarcomas is still poor even with adjuvant chemotherapy. Cisplatin, carboplatin, and doxorubicin alone or in combination with each other are the most commonly applied anticancer drugs for canine osteosarcomas. *Single-agent cisplatin* adjuvant treatment increases median survival times to 11 months (compared to 4 months without treatment). It however seems to slow down but not to prevent metastasis since most of the dogs with these therapy protocols die due to metastases although at a later time point. *Single-agent carboplatin* for adjuvant treatment also increases median survival times to 10 months but usually does not prevent metastasis development. *Single-agent doxorubicin* has similar efficacy to prolong median survival times to up to 12 months (4 months without treatment). *Combination therapy* of carboplatin and doxorubicin may have the same effect on survival, prolonged survival, or decreased survival times when compared to monotherapy depending on the study. Diverse attempts to improve chemotherapy protocols by addition of bisphosphonate-containing pamidronate, gemcitabine, suramin, and other substances did not significantly improve survival times. Dogs treated with *local application of a biodegradable cisplatin polymer* into the lesion after limb-sparing surgery has a proven efficacy and bisects the likelihood for local recurrence of the tumors.

Radiation therapy is currently mainly applied as a palliative treatment for canine osteosarcomas since it alleviates pain and mildly increases survival times from 2 to 4 months after diagnosis. Palliative radiotherapy of the primary tumors is usually *combined with systemic chemotherapy* to slow down the growth of micrometastases and increases the survival times to up to 6 months. *Stereotactic radiosurgery* using linear accelerators has been used in few dogs to locally treat canine osteosarcomas in a limb-sparing approach. It involves precise delivery of a single large dose of radiation to the designated *non-resected tumor* in situ. Results suggest that stereotactic radiosurgery may provide long-term local tumor control when combined with chemotherapy for *small tumors in early developmental stages* without extensive bone lysis.

▪ Prognostic Factors and Markers

Numerous positive and negative prognostic factors for dogs with osteosarcomas have been published, and most important factors are summarized in ◘ Table 11.3.

11.1.2 Canine Chondrosarcomas

Box 11.2. Canine Chondrosarcomas in Five Facts

1. Nasal cavity as the most common site but every bony structure may be affected.
2. Locally aggressive but growth much slower than for osteosarcomas.
3. Metastases in ~33 % of all cases but very rare for nasal chondrosarcomas.
4. Surgery often results in long-term tumor control.
5. Metastases may develop years after resection of the primary tumor.

▪ Epidemiology and Pathogenesis

Chondrosarcomas are low malignant tumors developing from chondrocytes or their precursors. With a share of *5 % of all canine bone tumors*, they are the second most common bone tumor after osteosarcomas. The etiology and causes of canine chondrosarcomas are unknown. Mean *age* of dogs with first diagnosis is 9 years, but they may develop at any age. The nasal cavity is the most frequently observed *anatomic location*, but chondrosarcomas of the rib (◘ Fig. 11.5), the limbs, the pelvis, and the skull are also frequently described. Large but not giant *breeds* are predisposed with a particular predilection of boxer, golden retriever, and German shepherds. Boxers

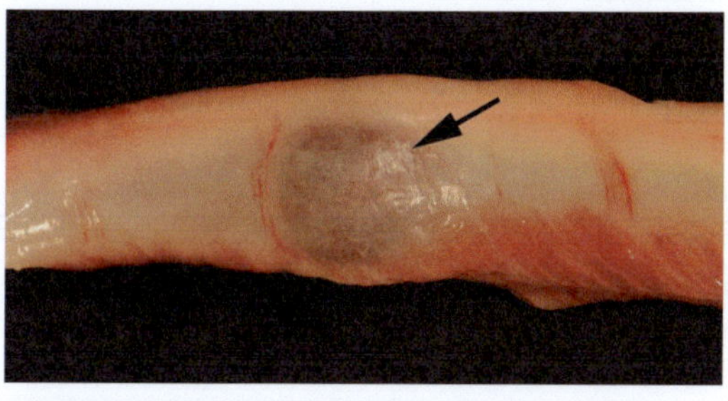

◘ **Fig. 11.5** Chondroma (*arrow*) of the rib in a dog (Photo with permission of A. Ostrowski, PhD and the Archive of the Institute for Veterinary Pathology, Freie Universität Berlin)

Table 11.3 Prognostic factors for canine osteosarcomas

Factor	Details	Influenced clinical features (control group)
Increased ALP serum levels	Meta-analysis of several studies	156 d shorter survival times
Location at the proximal humerus	Meta-analysis of several studies	132 d shorter survival times
Location proximal from the tarsal/carpal joint	OSA	Worse prognosis
Mandibular OSA	Mandibular OSA	Better prognosis than all other OSA
Tumor grade[a]	OSA	Grade III with poor prognosis
Tumor grade[a]	Mandibular OSA	MST grade I: 648 Grade III: 306
Tumor grade[a]	Appendicular OSA treated with carboplatin	MST grade I: 162 days Grade II: 298 days Grade III: 162 days
Wound infection	Appendicular OSA after limb-sparing surgery	MST ~550 days (~400 days)
Tumor-free margins	Surgery and diverse adjuvant treatments of OSA of the maxilla, mandible, and calvarium	Hazard ratios for PFI 40 %/OST 50 % (100 % with tumor in margins)
Teleangiectic histologic type	Ulnar osteosarcomas	Osteosarcoma seven times more likely to be cause of death
Lymph node metastasis	Appendicular OSA	MST 59 days (MST 318 days)
Ezrin expression	OSA	DFI 188 d (DFI 116 d)
Low survivin expression	OSA	DFI 5 months (DFI 10 months)
Strong Cox2 expression	OSA	MST 35 months (MST 12 months without Cox2 expression)

[a]Tumor grading by Kirpensteijn et al. (2002)
ALP alkaline phosphatase, *d* days, *DFI* disease-free survival, *MST* median survival, *OSA* appendicular osteosarcoma, *OST* overall survival time, *PFI* progression-free interval

are predisposed to develop chondrosarcomas of the ribs and the pelvis.

Clinical Appearance

In comparison with osteosarcomas, chondrosarcomas have a *less aggressive biologic behavior*. First *clinical signs* usually develop slowly over weeks to months. The dominant clinical signs obviously depend on the location of the tumor and may consist of nasal discharge due to sinonasal chondrosarcomas but *usually are firm swellings*, which grow rather slowly. The *metastatic rate is <33 %* of all cases and therefore significantly lower than for osteosarcomas, and nasal chondrosarcomas metastasize even less often. A characteristic feature of chondrosarcomas is the *late development of metastases*. They are usually clinically relevant not before months to years after resection of the primary tumor.

Radiographically, chondrosarcomas present with a mix of osteolysis of cortical bone and detectable tumor mass formation, similar to osteosarcomas.

Cytology and Histopathology

Cytologically, chondrosarcomas are characterized by amorphous chondroid material containing clusters of chondroblasts with round hyperchromatic nuclei and scanty cytoplasm, pleomorphic mesenchymal cells with round nuclei and vacuolated cytoplasm, and groups of immature cartilaginous cells with single or double nuclei and fibrillar or filmy cytoplasm. *Histologically*, chondrosarcomas are characterized by dedifferentiated, moderately pleomorphic chondrocytes and synthesis of typical cartilaginous matrix. The differentiation of tumor cells can however vary within and between tumors. A *tumor grading system* has been proposed by Farese et al. (2009) and seems to be of prognostic relevance at least for appendicular chondrosarcomas of the limb after amputation (Table 11.4). Unfortunately, not all histologic features included in the scoring system are sufficiently specified in the original publication. Furthermore, other studies postulated that in chondrosarcomas *tumor location is more relevant than tumor grading*, and chondrosarcomas of the limb have the best prognosis.

Therapy

Surgery is the treatment of choice for chondrosarcomas at any anatomic location and often

Table 11.4 Grading system for canine appendicular chondrosarcomas (Evans et al. 1977; Rozemann et al. 2006; Farese et al. 2009)

Histologic criteria	Points	Features
A. Matrix production	1	Chondroid to myxoid
	2	More myxoid
	3	No matrix
B. Architecture	1	Not specified
	2	Not specified
	3	Not specified
C. Degree of pleomorphism	1	Few larger, pleomorphic nuclei
	2	Increased number of pleomorphic nuclei
	3	Larger nuclei with higher pleomorphism
D. Cellularity	1	Few cells located in lacuna
	2	Increased cellularity toward the periphery
	3	Spindle-shaped cells in highly cellular areas
E. Necrosis	1	Not specified
	2	Not specified
	3	Not specified
F. Mitosis	1	0 mitoses/10 HPF
	2	<2 mitoses/10 HPF
	3	>2 mitoses/10 HPF
Total score (sum A–E and F)	<6 and mitosis = 1	*Grade 1* (survival after amputation: 6 years)
Total score (sum A–E and F)	7–10 and mitosis = 1–2	*Grade 2* (survival after amputation: 2.7 years)
Total score (sum A–E or F)	11–16 or mitosis = 3	*Grade 2* (survival after amputation: 0.9 years)

HPF high power field, size not specified

results in long-term tumor control. Median survival times of up to several years even without any adjuvant chemotherapy or radiotherapy have been reported but seem to depend on the anatomic location. Complete surgical removal of *nasal cavity chondrosarcomas* is usually not possible. Survival times with surgery alone vary between 5 months and <2 years and may be increased by the application of adjuvant radiation therapy to >2 years. *En bloc* resection of *chondrosarcomas of the ribs* without any adjuvant therapy is associated with reported survival times of 5 years or more. Most of the animals however died or were euthanized due to tumor recurrence or metastasis, which developed years after resection of the primary tumor. Similarly, resection of *chondrosarcomas of the pelvis* by hemipelvectomy is associated with survival times between 5 months and 8 years, and the reason for euthanasia is usually development of late distant metastases.

Adjuvant chemotherapy protocols for chondrosarcomas are unknown, and their necessity is questionable due to the long survival times with surgery only.

Adjuvant radiation therapy has been used for cases of incompletely resected nasal chondrosarcomas.

11.1.3 Canine Synovial Cell Sarcomas

Epidemiology and Pathogenesis

Synovial cell sarcomas are the most common joint tumors in the dog. They are derived from synovioblastic mesenchymal cells in the soft tissue surrounding the joints. They are therefore usually integrated into the large group of soft tissue sarcomas. Synovial cell sarcomas *have to be differentiated from CD18-positive periarticular histiocytic sarcomas*, which are occasionally considered as a synovial cell sarcoma subtype. They are however localized histiocytic tumors. There is a *breed* predilection for synovial cell sarcomas for large breeds and a *gender* predisposition for males. The median *age* of dogs at first diagnosis is 8 years (range 1–14 years). The stifle joint is the most commonly affected *anatomic location* followed by the ankle and the elbow joint. There are no known molecular mechanisms of synovial cell sarcoma carcinogenesis.

Box 11.3. Canine Synovial Cell Sarcomas in Five Facts

1. Malignant tumors derived from periarticular stromal cells
2. Are usually separated from periarticular histiocytic sarcomas of histiocytic origin
3. Approximately 50 % of tumors with distant metastasis
4. Amputation of the limb as proximal as possible as treatment of choice
5. Effect of adjuvant therapy not systematically tested

Clinical Appearance

Primary clinical signs of dogs with synovial cell sarcomas are *lameness* and *swelling* of the joint. The tumors usually *grow invasively* and *slowly* over weeks to months along preexisting fascia and ligaments. They may destroy the subchondral bone of all participating joints. *Radiographically*, synovial cell sarcomas are radiolucent soft tissue tumors, which may be associated with varying degrees of osteolysis. *Metastasis* is detected in up to 30 % of dogs at primary tumor diagnosis. Final stages of the disease are associated with metastasis to the regional lymph node or lung in up to 50 % of dogs. Dogs with metastatic disease have a *median survival times* of <6 months compared to >3 years of dogs without metastasis. A staging system has been developed for canine synovial cell sarcomas by Vail et al. 1994 (■ Table 11.5).

Cytology and Histopathology

Aspirations from synovial cell sarcomas are usually highly cellular. In biphasic tumors they contain cuboidal to pleomorphic epithelial cells and fibroblast-like spindle cells with ovoid nuclei and finely granular cytoplasm. They are commonly aggregated in small clusters with ragged edges. Monophasic synovial cell sarcomas contain only spindles cells and are thus

Table 11.5 Staging system for canine synovial cell sarcomas (Vail et al. 1994)

Primary tumor	T1	Well defined, no invasion of surrounding tissues
	T2	Invasion of soft tissues
	T3	Invasion of joints and bones
Regional lymph node metastasis	N0	No metastases
	N1	Metastases
Distant metastasis	M0	No metastases
	M1	Metastases
		MDFI/MST (months)
Stage 1	T3, N0, M0	>48/n.d.
Stage 2	>T3, N0, M0	3/3

MDFI median disease-free interval, *MST* median survival time, *n.d.* not described

difficult to be differentiated from (other) soft tissue sarcomas.

Histologically, the tumors may be composed of a single population of spindloid cells (monophasic tumors) or a mixed population of spindloid and epithelioid cells (biphasic). Monophasic tumors are difficult to be differentiated from fibrosarcomas. The presence of epithelioid cells has been associated with a better prognosis compared to monophasic tumors. Epithelioid components are however extremely rare in canine synovial cell sarcomas in contrast to their human counterpart. A grading system has been proposed by Vail et al. (1994) and is occasionally used for prognostic evaluation. Grade III synovial cell sarcomas are associated with survival times of 7 months, while grade I or II synovial cell sarcomas have median survival times of 4 and 3 years, respectively.

▪ Therapy

Amputation of the limb as proximal as possible is the treatment of choice for synovial cell sarcomas. It is associated with median survival times of 1–3 years after amputation. *Limb-sparing surgery* is usually not performed due to the common affection of bony structures and soft tissue components of all bones participating in the joint. Marginal, limb-sparing tumor resection is associated with survival times of approximately 1.5 years compared to approximately 2.5 years with limb amputation.

Adjuvant chemotherapy using vincristine, doxorubicin, and cyclophosphamide in different combinations and *adjuvant radiotherapy* may increase survival times although clinical studies confirming these effects are lacking.

▪ Prognostic Factors and Molecular Markers

Negative prognostic factors for survival are the presence of metastasis, invasion of bony structures, >30 % of areas with necrosis, and monophasic tumors. *Immunohistochemistry for CD18* can be used to identify histiocytic sarcoma.

▪ Suggested Reading

(Hodge et al. 2011; Morello et al. 2003; Ryseff and Bohn 2012; Szewczyk et al. 2015; Venzin et al. 2012)

11.2 Feline Bone and Joint Tumors

Primary bone tumors are rare in cats. Most of them are however malignant and 80 % of them are *osteosarcomas*. Chondrosarcomas, fibrosarcomas, and hemangiosarcomas represent the rest of bone tumors but can be considered as very rare. Synovial cell sarcomas are also very rare in cats.

11.2.1 Feline Osteosarcomas

Box 11.4. Feline Osteosarcomas in Five Facts

1. Less common than in dogs
2. Axial and appendicular osteosarcomas with similar frequency
3. Locally aggressive tumors with a metastatic rate of <10 %
4. Resection as treatment option of choice
5. Adjuvant radiation therapy most probably of positive effect for survival

Epidemiology and Pathogenesis

Osteosarcomas are rare malignant tumors, which are derived from mesenchymal cells of the bone. They are less common than canine osteosarcomas but constitute 80 % of malignant bone tumors. They may occur at any age but are most commonly seen at an *age* of 9–10 years. A *breed* predisposition is suspected for Siamese cats. Osteosarcomas in the cat are almost evenly distributed in the skeletal system. *Appendicular osteosarcomas* of the limbs are only minimally more frequent than *axial osteosarcomas* of the flat bones of the skull, the ribs, the pelvis, and the scapula. Approximately *two thirds* of the axial osteosarcomas *develop in cranial and the mandibular bones*. There is a fraction of osteosarcomas, which develop in areas with known fracture and osteosynthesis years ago.

Clinical Appearance

Cats with osteosarcomas usually present with progressive lameness, local swelling, deformity, and pathologic fractures. Osteosarcomas of the head are usually diagnosed due to dental problems or ulcerative lesions in the oral cavity. *Radiographically*, feline appendicular osteosarcomas usually present with strong osteolysis and only few areas of proliferation. The *sunburst phenomenon*, which is characterized by perpendicular radiating new bone formation from the cortical bone, and the *Codman's triangle*, a subperiosteal new bone formation with triangular shape, are less commonly seen than in the dog. *Axial osteosarcomas* more often represent as proliferative than osteolytic lesions. Feline osteosarcomas are first and foremost locally aggressive and invasive tumors. With a metastatic rate of <10 %, metastasis is far less common than in the dog.

Cytology and Histopathology

Cytology, see chapter on canine osteosarcomas.

Histologically, several histological subtypes have been described for feline osteosarcomas, but a correlation with survival and biologic behavior is lacking. In contrast, the *grading system* for dogs by Kirpensteijn and colleagues (2002) has been adapted to feline osteosarcomas (Dimopoulou et al. 2008. Higher histologic grade is described to be associated with a 48 % increase in hazard for shorter disease-free survival of cats with osteosarcomas.

Therapy

Tumor resection with wide tumor margins is the treatment of choice for feline osteosarcomas at any anatomic location. Due to the low metastatic rate, complete surgical excision with tumor-free margins is one of the most important prognostic factors for survival time, disease, and recurrence-free survival. *Amputation* of the limbs with *appendicular osteosarcomas* can be associated with long survival times of up to 4 years without adjuvant therapy. In contrast, *axial osteosarcomas* are associated with survival times of <6 months most probably due to incomplete resection in these more difficult locations.

Adjuvant and *stereotactic radiotherapy* may be of benefit for incompletely resectable or resected axial osteosarcoma, but there is a lack of systematic evaluation of therapy protocols.

Adjuvant chemotherapy is usually of no additional effect on survival in cats due to the low metastatic rate.

Suggested Reading

(Bitetto et al. 1987; Bray et al. 2014; Dimopoulou et al. 2008; Hahn and McEntee 1997; Heldmann et al. 2000; Helm and Morris 2012; Liu et al. 1974; McEntee 1997; Okada et al. 2009; Quigley and Leedale 1983; Sonnenschein et al. 2012)

Suggested Reading

Alexander K, Joly H, Blond L, D'Anjou MA, Nadeau ME, Olive J, Beauchamp G (2012) A comparison of computed tomography, computed radiography, and film-screen radiography for the detection of canine pulmonary nodules. Vet Radiol Ultrasound 53:258–265

Amsellem PM, Selmic LE, Wypij JM, Bacon NJ, Culp WT, Ehrhart NP, Powers BE, Stryhn H, Farese JP (2014) Appendicular osteosarcoma in small-breed dogs: 51 cases (1986–2011). J Am Vet Med Assoc 245: 203–210

Armbrust LJ, Biller DS, Bamford A, Chun R, Garrett LD, Sanderson MW (2012) Comparison of three-view thoracic radiography and computed tomography for detection of pulmonary nodules in dogs with neoplasia. J Am Vet Med Assoc 240:1088–1094

Ballegeer EA, Adams WM, Dubielzig RR, Paoloni MC, Klauer JM, Keuler NS (2010) Computed tomography characteristics of canine tracheobronchial lymph node metastasis. Vet Radiol Ultrasound 51:397–403

Barrett LE, Pollard RE, Zwingenberger A, Zierenberg-Ripoll A, Skorupski KA (2014) Radiographic characterization of primary lung tumors in 74 dogs. Vet Radiol Ultrasound 55:480–487

Bettini G, Marconato L, Morini M, Ferrari F (2009) Thyroid transcription factor-1 immunohistochemistry: diagnostic

tool and malignancy marker in canine malignant lung tumours. Vet Comp Oncol 7:28–37
Bitetto WV, Patnaik AK, Schrader SC, Mooney SC (1987) Osteosarcoma in cats: 22 cases (1974–1984). J Am Vet Med Assoc 190:91–93
Bongiovanni L, Mazzocchetti F, Malatesta D, Romanucci M, Ciccarelli A, Buracco P, De Maria R, Palmieri C, Martano M, Morello E, Maniscalco L, Della Salda L (2012) Immunohistochemical investigation of cell cycle and apoptosis regulators (survivin, beta-catenin, p53, caspase 3) in canine appendicular osteosarcoma. BMC Vet Res 8:78
Bray JP, Worley DR, Henderson RA, Boston SE, Mathews KG, Romanelli G, Bacon NJ, Liptak JM, Scase TJ (2014) Hemipelvectomy: outcome in 84 dogs and 16 cats. A veterinary society of surgical oncology retrospective study. Vet Surg 43:27–37
Brodey RS, Misdorp W, Riser WH, van der Heul RO (1974) Canine skeletal chondrosarcoma: a clinicopathologic study of 35 cases. J Am Vet Med Assoc 165:68–78
Culp WT, Olea-Popelka F, Sefton J, Aldridge CF, Withrow SJ, Lafferty MH, Rebhun RB, Kent MS, Ehrhart N (2014) Evaluation of outcome and prognostic factors for dogs living greater than one year after diagnosis of osteosarcoma: 90 cases (1997–2008). J Am Vet Med Assoc 245: 1141–1146
D'Costa S, Yoon BI, Kim DY, Motsinger-Reif AA, Williams M, Kim Y (2012) Morphologic and molecular analysis of 39 spontaneous feline pulmonary carcinomas. Vet Pathol 49:971–978
Dimopoulou M, Kirpensteijn J, Moens H, Kik M (2008) Histologic prognosticators in feline osteosarcoma: a comparison with phenotypically similar canine osteosarcoma. Vet Surg 37:466–471
Eberle N, Fork M, von Babo V, Nolte I, Simon D (2011) Comparison of examination of thoracic radiographs and thoracic computed tomography in dogs with appendicular osteosarcoma. Vet Comp Oncol 9:131–140
Enneking WF, Spanier SS, Goodman MA (1980) A system for the surgical staging of musculoskeletal sarcoma. Clin Orthop Relat Res 153:106–120
Evans HL, Ayala AG, Romsdahl MM (1977) Prognostic factors in chondrosarcoma of bone: a clinicopathologic analysis with emphasis on histologic grading. Cancer 40(2): 818–831.
Farese JP, Kirpensteijn J, Kik M, Bacon NJ, Waltman SS, Seguin B, Kent M, Liptak J, Straw R, Chang MN, Jiang Y, Withrow SJ (2009) Biologic behavior and clinical outcome of 25 dogs with canine appendicular chondrosarcoma treated by amputation: a Veterinary Society of Surgical Oncology retrospective study. Vet Surg 38:914–919
Goldfinch N, Argyle DJ (2012) Feline lung-digit syndrome: unusual metastatic patterns of primary lung tumours in cats. J Feline Med Surg 14:202–208
Gottfried SD, Popovitch CA, Goldschmidt MH, Schelling C (2000) Metastatic digital carcinoma in the cat: a retrospective study of 36 cats (1992–1998). J Am Anim Hosp Assoc 36:501–509
Hahn KA, McEntee MF (1997) Primary lung tumors in cats: 86 cases (1979–1994). J Am Vet Med Assoc 211:1257–1260
Hahn KA, McEntee MF (1998) Prognosis factors for survival in cats after removal of a primary lung tumor: 21 cases (1979–1994). Vet Surg 27:307–311
Hahn KA, McGavin MD, Adams WH (1997) Bilateral renal metastases of nasal chondrosarcoma in a dog. Vet Pathol 34:352–355
Heldmann E, Anderson MA, Wagner-Mann C (2000) Feline osteosarcoma: 145 cases (1990–1995). J Am Anim Hosp Assoc 36:518–521
Helm J, Morris J (2012) Musculoskeletal neoplasia: an important differential for lumps or lameness in the cat. J Feline Med Surg 14:43–54
Hodge SC, Degner D, Walshaw R, Teunissen B (2011) Vascularized ulnar bone grafts for limb-sparing surgery for the treatment of distal radial osteosarcoma. J Am Anim Hosp Assoc 47:98–111
Karlsson EK, Sigurdsson S, Ivansson E, Thomas R, Elvers I, Wright J, Howald C, Tonomura N, Perloski M, Swofford R, Biagi T, Fryc S, Anderson N, Courtay-Cahen C, Youell L, Ricketts SL, Mandlebaum S, Rivera P, von Euler H, Kisseberth WC, London CA, Lander ES, Couto G, Comstock K, Starkey MP, Modiano JF, Breen M, Lindblad-Toh K (2013) Genome-wide analyses implicate 33 loci in heritable dog osteosarcoma, including regulatory variants near CDKN2A/B. Genome Biol 14:R132
Kim J, Kwon SY, Cena R, Park S, Oh J, Oui H, Cho KO, Min JJ, Choi J (2014) CT and PET-CT of a dog with multiple pulmonary adenocarcinoma. J Vet Med Sci 76:615–620
Kirpensteijn J, Kik M, Rutteman GR, Teske E (2002) Prognostic significance of a new histologic grading system for canine osteosarcoma. Vet Pathol 39(2):240–246.
Kujawa A, Olias P, Bottcher A, Klopfleisch R (2014) Thyroid transcription factor-1 is a specific marker of benign but not malignant feline lung tumours. J Comp Pathol 151:19–24
Lee JH, Lee JH, Yoon HY, Kim NH, Sur JH, Jeong SW (2012) Hypertrophic osteopathy associated with pulmonary adenosquamous carcinoma in a dog. J Vet Med Sci 74:667–672
Liu SK, Dorfman HD, Patnaik AK (1974) Primary and secondary bone tumours in the cat. J Small Anim Pract 15: 141–156
MacEwen EG, Pastor J, Kutzke J, Tsan R, Kurzman ID, Thamm DH, Wilson M, Radinsky R (2004) IGF-1 receptor contributes to the malignant phenotype in human and canine osteosarcoma. J Cell Biochem 92:77–91
Maniscalco L, Iussich S, Morello E, Martano M, Gattino F, Miretti S, Biolatti B, Accornero P, Martignani E, Sanchez-Cespedes R, Buracco P, De Maria R (2014) Increased expression of insulin-like growth factor-1 receptor is correlated with worse survival in canine appendicular osteosarcoma. Vet J 205(2):272–280
Maritato KC, Schertel ER, Kennedy SC, Dudley R, Lamm C, Barnhart M, Kass P (2014) Outcome and prognostic indicators in 20 cats with surgically treated primary lung tumors. J Feline Med Surg 16:979–984
Mayhew PD, Hunt GB, Steffey MA, Culp WT, Mayhew KN, Fuller M, Johnson LR, Pascoe PJ (2013) Evaluation of short-term outcome after lung lobectomy for resection of primary lung tumors via video-assisted thoracoscopic surgery or open thoracotomy in medium- to large-breed dogs. J Am Vet Med Assoc 243:681–688
McCleese JK, Bear MD, Kulp SK, Mazcko C, Khanna C, London CA (2013) Met interacts with EGFR and Ron in canine osteosarcoma. Vet Comp Oncol 11:124–139

McEntee MC (1997) Radiation therapy in the management of bone tumors. Vet Clin North Am Small Anim Pract 27:131–138

McNiel EA, Ogilvie GK, Powers BE, Hutchison JM, Salman MD, Withrow SJ (1997) Evaluation of prognostic factors for dogs with primary lung tumors: 67 cases (1985–1992). J Am Vet Med Assoc 211:1422–1427

Morello E, Vasconi E, Martano M, Peirone B, Buracco P (2003) Pasteurized tumoral autograft and adjuvant chemotherapy for the treatment of canine distal radial osteosarcoma: 13 cases. Vet Surg 32:539–544

Neihaus SA, Locke JE, Barger AM, Borst LB, Goring RL (2011) A novel method of core aspirate cytology compared to fine-needle aspiration for diagnosing canine osteosarcoma. J Am Anim Hosp Assoc 47:317–323

Okada M, Kitagawa M, Nagasawa A, Itou T, Kanayama K, Sakai T (2009) Magnetic resonance imaging and computed tomography findings of vertebral osteosarcoma in a cat. J Vet Med Sci 71:513–517

Polton GA, Brearley MJ, Powell SM, Burton CA (2008) Impact of primary tumour stage on survival in dogs with solitary lung tumours. J Small Anim Pract 49:66–71

Popovitch CA, Weinstein MJ, Goldschmidt MH (1994) Chondrosarcoma: a retrospective study of 97 dogs (1987–1990). J Am Anim Hosp Assoc 30:81–85

Portela RF, Fadl-Alla BA, Pondenis HC, Byrum ML, Garrett LD, Wycislo KL, Borst LB, Fan TM (2014) Pro-tumorigenic effects of transforming growth factor beta 1 in canine osteosarcoma. J Vet Intern Med 28:894–904

Quigley PJ, Leedale AH (1983) Tumors involving bone in the domestic cat: a review of fifty-eight cases. Vet Pathol 20:670–686

Rozeman LB, Cleton-Jansen AM, Hogendoorn PC (2006) Pathology of primary malignant bone and cartilage tumours. Int Orthop 30(6):437–444

Ryseff JK, Bohn AA (2012) Detection of alkaline phosphatase in canine cells previously stained with Wright-Giemsa and its utility in differentiating osteosarcoma from other mesenchymal tumors. Vet Clin Pathol 41:391–395

Sabattini S, Mancini FR, Marconato L, Bacci B, Rossi F, Vignoli M, Bettini G (2014) EGFR overexpression in canine primary lung cancer: pathogenetic implications and impact on survival. Vet Comp Oncol 12:237–248

Schmidt AF, Nielen M, Klungel OH, Hoes AW, de Boer A, Groenwold RH, Kirpensteijn J, Investigators VSSO (2013) Prognostic factors of early metastasis and mortality in dogs with appendicular osteosarcoma after receiving surgery: an individual patient data meta-analysis. Prev Vet Med 112:414–422

Sonnenschein B, Dickomeit MJ, Bali MS (2012) Late-onset fracture-associated osteosarcoma in a cat. Vet Comp Orthop Traumatol 25:418–420

Sylvestre AM, Cockshutt JR (1992) A case series of 25 dogs with chondrosarcoma. Vet Comp Ortho Traumatol 1:17–21

Szewczyk M, Lechowski R, Zabielska K (2015) What do we know about canine osteosarcoma treatment? Review. Vet Res Commun 39:61–67

Theon AP, Madewell BR, Harb MF, Dungworth DL (1993) Megavoltage irradiation of neoplasms of the nasal and paranasal cavities in 77 dogs. J Am Vet Med Assoc 202:1469–1475

Vail DM, Powers BE, Getzy DM, Morrison WB, McEntee MC, O'Keefe DA, Norris AM, Withrow SJ (1994) Evaluation of prognostic factors for dogs with synovial sarcoma: 36 cases (1986-1991). J Am Vet Med Assoc 205(9):1300–1307

Venzin C, Grundmann S, Montavon P (2012) Endoprosthesis (EN) in frontlimb-sparing surgery for distal radial tumours in the dog: preliminary results. Schweiz Arch Tierheilkd 154:337–343

Wood EF, O'Brien RT, Young KM (1998) Ultrasound-guided fine-needle aspiration of focal parenchymal lesions of the lung in dogs and cats. J Vet Intern Med 12:338–342

Endocrine Tumors

Robert Klopfleisch

R. Klopfleisch (ed.), *Veterinary Oncology*, DOI 10.1007/978-3-319-41124-8_12

12.1 Tumors of the Pituitary Gland

The pituitary gland is composed of three lobes: anterior, intermediate, and posterior. The *anterior pituitary lobe* is most often affected by endocrine tumors which may secrete or hamper the secretion of hormones physiologically secreted by the endocrine cells of this lobe: growth hormone (GH), thyroid-stimulating hormone (TSH), adrenocorticotropic hormone (ACTH), prolactin (PRL), luteinizing hormone (LH), and many more. The *intermediate pituitary lobe* secretes melanocyte-stimulating hormone (MSH), and the *posterior pituitary lobe* secretes but does not synthesize antidiuretic hormone (ADH). Both maybe affected secondarily by compression by anterior lobe tumors but are usually not affected by primary tumors.

Tumors of the anterior pituitary lobe are coarsely divided into corticotroph and somatotroph tumors depending on the cell of origin and the hormone secreted by the tumor cells. *Corticotroph tumors* are derived from pituitary corticotroph cells and mainly *secrete ACTH* and thus influence the metabolism of the cortical cells of the adrenal gland. *Somatotroph tumors* are derived from pituitary somatotropic cells and *secrete GH*, which indirectly influences diverse tissues including the muscle, bone, liver, and kidney.

12

12.1.1 Canine Pituitary Corticotroph Tumors

Box 12.1. Canine Pituitary Tumors in Seven Facts

1. Usually slowly and expansively growing nonmetastatic tumors
2. Clinical signs mostly based on hypercortisolism due to ACTH hypersecretion by tumor cells
3. Neurological signs rare and not present until advanced stages of tumor growth
4. Screening tests for hypercortisolism: ACTH stimulation, LDDST, and cortisol/creatinine ratio
5. Differentiation tests: endogenous ACTH measurement, HDDST
6. Medical treatment with trilostane and mitotane treatment of choice
7. Transsphenoidal hypophysectomy and radiotherapy also described

Epidemiology and Pathogenesis

Adrenocorticotropic hormone (ACTH)-secreting pituitary tumors (PT) are tumors of dogs >9 years of *age* (Fig. 12.1). There is a *breed* predisposition for dachshunds, poodle, and terriers and a *gender* predisposition for females, which are slightly overrepresented with approximately 60 % of cases. The molecular basis and causes for PT development in the dog is unknown.

ACTH-secreting PT are the *cause of 85 % of cases of hypercortisolism* (syn. hyperadrenocorticism, Cushing's syndrome) in the dog. The continuously and excessively secreted ACTH induces bilateral hyperplasia of the adrenal gland cortex and excess secretion of cortisol (hypercortisolemia). The consequences of hypercortisolism are also the most important clinical signs in dogs with ACTH-secreting PT, while neurologic signs due to invasive or expansive tumor growth are rare. Approximately *60 % of PT are noninvasive expansively growing tumors*, 30 % are locally invasive adenomas, while *only 6 % of the tumors are adenocarcinomas with metastasis.*

Clinical Appearance

Clinical signs associated with PT in dogs are in almost all cases caused by ACTH-stimulated

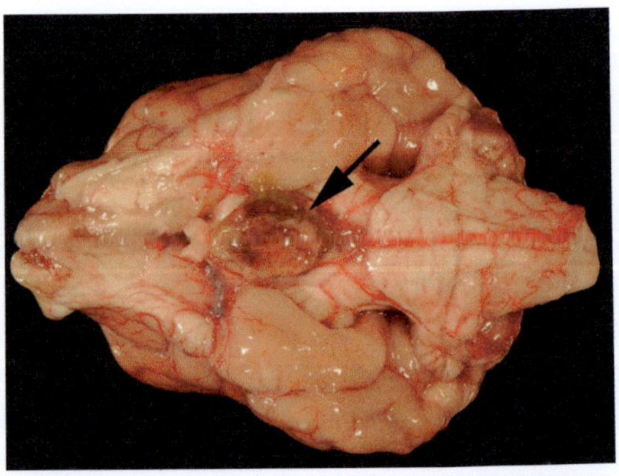

Fig. 12.1 Pituitary corticotroph adenoma (*arrow*) of a dog (Photo with permission of K. Dietert, PhD and the Archive of the Institute of Veterinary Pathology, Freie Universität Berlin, Germany)

hypercortisolism. Clinical neurologic signs due to the space-occupying growth of the tumor are rare and usually present only in advanced stages of the disease. Typical *clinical signs of hypercortisolism* are *polyuria/polydipsia*, *abdominal enlargement*, *muscle weakness*, *alopecia* (▫ Fig. 12.2), *calcinosis cutis* (▫ Fig. 12.3), *dermal thinning*, decreased immune status with common urinary tract infections, and poor wound healing, all of which are the result of the metabolic effects of increased levels of circulating glucocorticoids. Diabetes mellitus due to insulin resistance may develop in <10 % of dogs with PT, which is in contrast to >80 % of cats with ACTH-secreting PT. *Neurologic signs* commonly develop when tumors reach a size of >1 cm. The clinical signs described above should lead to the tentative diagnosis of PT-associated hypercortisolism in dogs not receiving exogenous glucocorticoids. Further laboratory and imaging is however necessary to confirm the diagnosis.

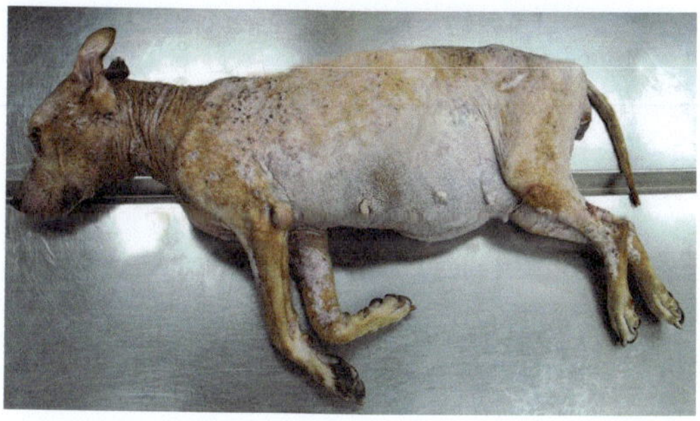

▫ **Fig. 12.2** Alopecia and cutaneous calcification in a dog with pituitary corticotroph adenoma (Photo with permission of K. Dietert, PhD and the Archive of the Institute of Veterinary Pathology, Freie Universität Berlin, Germany)

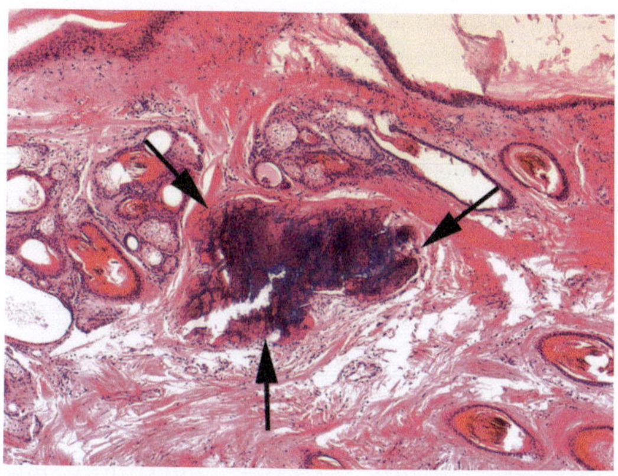

▫ **Fig. 12.3** Subcutaneous mineralization in a dog with pituitary corticotroph adenoma

Standard blood tests of dogs with hypercortisolism are characterized by neutrophilia, monocytosis, lymphopenia, eosinopenia, hypercho lesterolemia, and increased alkaline phosphatase (ALP) levels.

Three main *screening tests* are commonly used to verify the diagnosis of hypercortisolism. They have a moderate specificity and sensitivity to differentiate PT-associated from adrenal gland tumor-associated hypercortisolism. *The ACTH stimulation test* assesses the reaction of the adrenal glands to ACTH. After injection of ACTH, the *blood levels of cortisol at least triple* within 60–90 min in dogs with hypercortisolism. The *low-dose dexamethasone suppression test (LDDST)* is assessing the reactivity of the adrenal glands to exogenous low doses of dexamethasone. In healthy dogs this leads to suppression of endogenous cortisol levels *<10 ng/ml after 8 h*. In addition, a delayed decrease by less than 50 % of the basal concentration of endogenous blood glucocorticoids after 4 h is occasionally considered indicative for an adrenal gland tumor-dependent hypercortisolism. The *urine cortisol/creatinine ratio* is a highly sensitive but moderately specific test for hypercortisolism. A *ratio of >16* is indicative for hypercortisolism. However, other diseases and stress may also lead to increased ratios.

In the case of positive test results in any of the screening tests, *differentiation tests* are used to differentiate adrenal gland tumor – from PT-dependent hypercortisolism. The *high-dose dexamethasone suppression test (HDDST)* assesses the responsiveness of the adrenal glands to injections of high doses of dexamethasone. In dogs with PT-dependent hypercortisolism, this should lead to a reaction of the nonneoplastic adrenal gland with decreased levels of endogenous glucocorticoids <1.5 µg/dl after 8 h while a lack of a drop in glucocorticoid secretion is seen in dogs with hormonally active, neoplastic adrenal glands. The measurement of *endogenous ACTH* is the *definitive method to discriminate adrenal gland – from PT-dependent hypercortisolism*. It is increased in dogs with pituitary but not in dogs with adrenal hypercortisolism.

Computed tomography (CT) and *magnetic resonance imaging (MRI)* are helpful in the diagnosis and differentiation of adrenal gland tumor-dependent and PT-dependent hypercortisolism. They are however not routinely used in the diagnosis of pituitary-dependent hypercortisolism, most probably due to their high cost and the restricted access to surgical or radiotherapy treatment options. In addition, almost 50 % of all PT are too small to be identified radiologically even with CT and MRI.

Cytology and Histopathology

Cytologic preparations of pituitary tumors are usually not available due to restricted access to the cranial cavity. *Histologic analysis* is restricted to postmortem diagnostics.

Therapy

The treatment of PT in the dog is usually based on medical treatment modalities although studies on the efficacy of surgery and radiotherapy are also available.

Medical therapy is based on two drugs, mitotane and trilostane. *Trilostane* competitively inhibits 3β-hydroxysteroid dehydrogenase, which is essential for cortisol synthesis. It has to be given for the rest of the dog's life and its effect has to be tested by ACTH stimulation tests continuously but at prolonged intervals. *Mitotane* (Lysodren) is a cytotoxic, adrenocorticolytic agent, which destroys the zona fasciculata and reticularis of the adrenal gland. Two approaches are described: nonselective complete and selective incomplete adrenocorticolysis. *Selective adrenocorticolysis* intends to destroy a part of the adrenal cortex but leaves a functional residual tissue to maintain a basal secretion of glucocorticoids. *Nonselective, complete adrenocorticolysis* completely destroys all of the adrenal cortex, which leaves the dog dependent on glucocorticoid and mineralocorticoid supplementation for the rest of his life. There is no significant difference in *survival times* of dogs treated with trilostane (MST 662 days, range 8–1971 days) or mitotane (MST 708 days, range 33–1399 days).

Surgery for hypophysectomy is the treatment of choice for human patients with PT but only available in very few veterinary medical centers worldwide and thus is a very uncommon treatment modality. *Transsphenoidal hypophysectomy* is associated with an overall success rate of 65 % and 4-year survival rates of approximately 70 %.

Radiation therapy is a promising therapy option for PT inducing with neurologic tumors. The success rate negatively correlates with tumor size. Early detection and treatment of small PT is therefore necessary for optimal treatment outcome. However, *excessive ACTH secretion is unlikely to be cured* with radiotherapy alone, and adjuvant medical therapy is necessary to control clinical disease. Two studies found that irradiation increases mean survival time up to 4 years compared to 1.5 years in nonirradiated dogs.

12.1.2 Feline Pituitary Corticotroph Tumors

Box 12.2. Feline Pituitary Corticotroph Tumors in Eight Facts

1. Rare tumors in cats
2. Associated with typical signs of Cushing's syndrome
3. Approx. 80 % of cases also with diabetes mellitus
4. Neurological signs not until advanced stages of tumor growth
5. Screening tests for hypercortisolism: ACTH stimulation, LDDST, and cortisol/creatinine ratio
6. Differentiation tests: endogenous ACTH measurement, HDDST
7. Bilateral adrenalectomy as common treatment modality
8. First promising studies on efficacy of medical treatment with trilostane and mitotane
9. Hypophysectomy and radiotherapy also described

Epidemiology and Pathogenesis

Feline pituitary corticotroph tumors (PT) are rare tumors in cats as is pituitary-dependent hypercortisolism in general (Fig. 12.4). However, if present, hypercortisolism is based on hypersecretion by PT in 85 %, while only 15 % are caused by adrenal gland tumors. Cats developing PT-dependent hypercortisolism are usually around the *age* of 10 years but can be older or younger. There is no *breed* or *gender* predisposition. Feline PT are usually adenomas, and carcinomas are very rarely reported. PT in cats are usually *corticotroph*, but there is also a significant fraction of *somatotroph feline PT with growth hormone (GH) secretion* and *associated signs of acromegaly*. Additionally, several case reports describe multi-hormonal somato- and corticotroph feline PT with a wide variety of associated metabolic changes in affected cats.

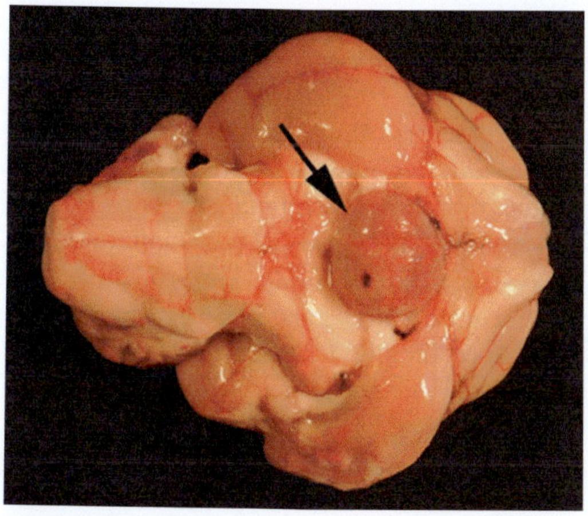

■ Fig. 12.4 Pituitary corticotroph adenoma in a cat (Photo with permission of A. Meyer, PhD, IDEXX Ludwigshafen and the Archive of the Institute of Veterinary Pathology, Freie Universität Berlin, Germany)

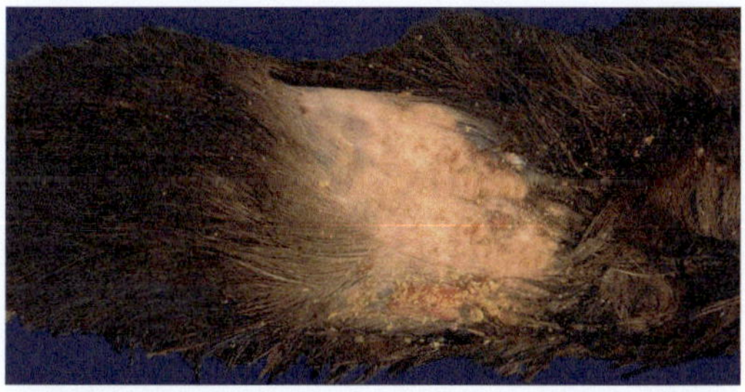

■ Fig. 12.5 Alopecia and scaling in a cat with pituitary corticotroph adenoma in a cat (Photo with permission of the Archive of the Institute of Veterinary Pathology, Freie Universität Berlin, Germany)

■ Clinical Appearance

Clinical signs of cats with PT-dependent hypercortisolism include the *typical signs of Cushing's syndrome*: polyuria/polydipsia, potbellied appearance, muscle atrophy, alopecia/unkempt hair coat, and fragile skin (■ Fig. 12.5). Approximately 80 % of cats with hypercortisolism develop an *insulin-resistant diabetes mellitus* compared to only 10 % of dogs with hypercortisolism. Severe *systemic hypertension* has been reported to be associated with PT-dependent hypercortisolism in few cats. *Neurological signs* due to expansive or invasive tumor growth are in cats.

The clinical signs described above should lead to the tentative diagnosis of PT-associated hypercortisolism in cats not receiving exogenous glucocorticoids. Further laboratory and imaging is however necessary to confirm the diagnosis.

Laboratory testing of cats with PT-dependent hypercortisolism often reveals *hyperglycemia and glucosuria* due to diabetes mellitus but only occasionally hypercholesterolemia, increased alanine aminotransferase (ALT), and alkaline phosphatase (ALP) levels.

Three main screening tests are commonly used to verify the diagnosis of hypercortisolism. They have a moderate specificity and sensitivity to differentiate PT-associated from adrenal gland tumor-associated hypercortisolism. *The ACTH stimulation test* is of moderate specificity and sensitivity to diagnose feline hypercortisolism. It assesses the reaction of the adrenal glands to exogenous adrenocorticotropic hormone (ACTH). After injection of ACTH, the *blood levels of cortisol significantly increase* within 30–60 min above the basal values in cats with hypercortisolism. The *low-dose dexamethasone suppression test (LDDST)* is of higher specificity and sensitivity and assesses the reactivity of the adrenal glands toward exogenous low doses of dexamethasone. Cats with hypercortisolism show a decreased suppression of cortisol after 8 h. The *urine cortisol/creatinine ratio* is a highly sensitive but moderately specific test for hypercortisolism. A *ratio of >30* is indicative for hypercortisolism. However, other diseases and stress may also lead to increased ratios.

In the case of positive test results in any of the screening test, *differentiation tests* are used to differentiate adrenal – from pituitary-dependent hypercortisolism. The *high-dose dexamethasone suppression test (HDDST)* assesses the responsiveness of the adrenal gland to injections of high doses of dexamethasone. In cats with pituitary-dependent hypercortisolism, this may lead to a reaction of the nonneoplastic adrenal gland with decreased levels of endogenous glucocorticoids after 8 h while a lack of drop in glucocorticoid secretion is seen in cats with hormonally active, neoplastic adrenal glands. The measurement of *endogenous ACTH* is the *definitive laboratory method to discriminate adrenal from pituitary* hypercortisolism. These are increased in feline with pituitary but not in cats with adrenal hypercortisolism.

Imaging with *computed tomography (CT)* and *magnetic resonance imaging (MRI)* are helpful in the diagnosis and differentiation of adrenal-dependent and pituitary-dependent hypercortisolism. They are however not routinely used in the diagnosis of pituitary-dependent hypercortisolism, most probably due to their high cost and the restricted access to surgical or radiotherapy treatment options. In addition, approximately 50 % of PT in cats are histologically perceivable only but not detectable by CT or MRI.

▪ Cytology and Histopathology

Cytologic biopsies of pituitary tumors are usually not available due to the restricted access to the cranial cavity. *Histologic analysis* is restricted to postmortem diagnosis.

▪ Therapy

There are only few reports on *medical treatment* of PT-dependent hypercortisolism in cats. The efficacy of *mitotane*, a cytotoxic, adrenocorticolytic agent, which destroys the zona fasciculata and reticularis of the adrenal gland, was evaluated with contradictory results on its efficacy for the treatment of feline hypercortisolism. Recent studies and case reports indicate that *trilostane* therapy, which competitively inhibits 3β-hydroxysteroid dehydrogenase and therefore cortisol synthesis, may ameliorate clinical signs in cats with hypercortisolism.

Surgical bilateral adrenalectomy with consecutive glucocorticoid and mineralocorticoid replacement therapy has been described as the method of choice for cats with hypercortisolism. *Transsphenoidal hypophysectomy* has also been described in few studies as effective for the treatment of feline hypercortisolism.

12.1.3 Feline Pituitary Somatotroph Tumors (Feline Acromegaly)

Box 12.3. Feline Pituitary Somatotroph Tumors in Six Facts

1. Rare tumor type
2. Clinical symptoms dominated by the secretion of growth hormone
3. Clinical symptoms include abnormal growth of limbs, mandibles, and organomegaly
4. Most cats also develop insulin-resistant diabetes mellitus
5. Somatostatin analogues and radiotherapy as treatment of choice
6. Transsphenoidal surgery only available in few veterinary medical centers

▪ Epidemiology and Pathogenesis

Feline pituitary somatotroph tumors (PT) are rare tumors in cats. In contrast to the corticotroph tumors described above, they are secreting excessive *growth hormone (GH, syn. somatotropin)* instead of adrenocorticotroph hormone (ACTH). The effects of excessive GH secretion are mediated by induction of insulin-like growth factor 1 (IGF-1) synthesis. GH and IGF-1 together stimulate the proliferation and division of chondroblasts and osteoblasts and thus *bone growth* mainly in the limbs and the cranium. In addition, all cats with PT-dependent GH secretion develop *diabetes mellitus* due to peripheral insulin resistance, which is based on a post-insulin receptor signaling block in target cells. Although these tumors and the associated acromegaly is considered to be rare, recent studies suggest that a significant proportion of up to 33 % of cases of feline diabetes mellitus may be associated with undetected somatotroph PT. Cats developing GH-secreting PT are on average *10 years old*. There is a *gender* predisposition for males but no *breed* predisposition has been described. Feline somatotroph PT are *usually adenomas*, and carcinomas are very rarely reported. There is discussion whether some of GH-secreting pituitary lesions are rather hyperplasia but not adenomas. Additionally, several case reports describe multihormonal, mixed somato-, and corticotroph feline PT with a wide variety of associated metabolic changes in affected cats.

▪ Clinical Appearance

Cats with somatotroph PT are usually initially presented due to *clinical signs of diabetes mellitus* including polydipsia/polyuria. In contrast to diabetes mellitus of other causes, acromegaly-associated diabetes mellitus is often characterized by *weight gain*. *Signs of acromegaly* include broadening of the face, protrusion of the mandible, increased interdental spaces, enlarged feet, and a general coarse physique, which are developing slowly and may be overseen by the owner. Organomegaly of the kidney, liver, and heart is also present in most cats, occasionally with systolic cardiac murmur and cardiac failure.

Laboratory tests of cats with somatotroph tumors are dominated by *blood values typical for diabetes mellitus* including hyperglycemia, glucosuria, and increased fructosamine and liver enzyme levels. Measurement of blood levels of

GH and IGF-1 have been described for final confirmation of acromegaly. *Serum GH* measurement is nevertheless of reduced specificity and sensitivity since PT GH secretion is intermittent and the peptide has a short half-life. *Serum IGF-1* measurement is moderately specific and more sensitive for the detection of somatotroph PT since its levels are stable for 24 h after induction by GH. A very recent study indicated that *serum ghrelin*, a growth hormone secretagogue, is decreased in cats with acromegaly and its increase may be a marker of treatment effect. Neurological signs are rarely reported for cats with somatotroph PT maybe due to their slow growth rate.

Imaging with *computed tomography (CT)* and *magnetic resonance imaging (MRI)* may directly identify somatotroph PT as masses in the pituitary. However, a proportion of the tumors seem to be too small to be recognized even with these high-resolution imaging technologies.

■ Cytology and Histopathology

Cytologic biopsies of pituitary tumors are usually not available due to the restricted access to the cranial cavity. *Histologic analysis* is restricted to confirmation of the diagnosis postmortem.

■ Therapy

Reports on treatment of somatotroph PT are rare due to the small number of cases. *Medical treatment* of the diabetic signs by *insulin therapy* is the only treatment available and affordable for most owners. Due to the fluctuation in insulin resistance in cats with somatotroph PT, glucose levels should be carefully monitored and insulin doses adapted correspondingly to avoid hypoglycemia. The application of *somatostatin analogues*, which bind to the somatostatin receptor and suppresses release of GH, has been tested in cats with acromegaly. One of these, octreotide, has been shown to be effective to suppress GH release at least in some cats.

Transsphenoidal surgery to remove the PT is the treatment of choice in humans but requires specialized surgeons, which are available in only few veterinary medical centers worldwide.

Radiation therapy of feline somatotroph PT is momentarily considered the treatment of choice. Several studies report on the efficacy of radiation therapy for feline PT but usually lack information on long-term follow-up of these cats.

Treatment-independent *survival time* of cats with PT-associated acromegaly is 1.5–3 years. The most common *cause of death* in these animals is renal failure.

12.1.4 Equine Pituitary Corticotroph Tumors

Box 12.4. Equine Pituitary Corticotroph Tumors in Seven Facts

1. Clinical disease named "pituitary pars intermedia dysfunction" (PPID)
2. Caused by ACTH-secreting pituitary adenomas or hyperplasia due to neurodegenerative loss of hypothalamic dopaminergic pituitary inhibition
3. Pathognomonic clinical signs of hirsutism and hyperhidrosis
4. Most animals with insulin resistance and laminitis
5. Dopamine D2 receptor agonist pergolide as treatment of choice

■ Epidemiology and Pathogenesis

There is a profound basis of knowledge on the pathogenesis of pituitary hyperplasia and tumors (PT) in horses with *pituitary pars intermedia dysfunction* (*PPID*, syn. equine Cushing's disease). *Age* is the most important risk factor for development of PPID, which is a disease of horse older than 15 years, but younger animals may also be affected occasionally. Studies indicate that up to 30 % of aged horses may have at least mild forms of the disease. Pony *breeds* and Morgans seem to be more often affected.

PPID is associated with changes of the pars intermedia of the pituitary gland. This is in contrast to canine Cushing's disease, which is caused by tumors of the pars distalis. In healthy horses, almost all *ACTH* is synthesized by the pars distalis, while the pars intermedia is not significantly contributing to serum ACTH levels. With increasing age, there is however a slow progressive loss of hypothalamic control of cells, melanotrope cells, in the pars distalis due to oxidative stress-induced *neurodegeneration of dopamine-secreting cells* in the hypothalamus. Subsequently, there is a *hyperplasia or benign neoplastic proliferation (adenomas)* of the pars intermedia and an excessive secretion of hormones including adrenocorticotropic hormone (ACTH), endorphins, and melanocortins. The adenomas may also compress the hypothalamus and the optic chiasm in the affected horse.

▪ Clinical Appearance

There are several typical clinical signs associated with PPID. *Hirsutism* is a pathognomonic clinical sign of PPID in horses. It is characterized by an excessive hair growth and abnormal retention of the winter hair coat in summer, which leads to abnormally long and occasionally curly hair. The pathogenesis of hirsutism is supposed to be based on the increased serum levels of melanocortin, which is physiologically involved in the development of winter hair coat. *Hyperhidrosis*, excessive sweating, is also a typical finding for many but not all horses with PPID. The mechanism behind this clinical sign is also unknown. *Skeletal muscle atrophy* (sarcopenia), *polyuria/polydipsia*, *insulin resistance*, and *laminitis* are other prominent features of many but not all horses with PPID but may also be seen with other endocrinopathies like the equine metabolic syndrome. *Abnormal distribution of fat deposits* above the eyes in the supraorbital fossa, along the crest of the neck, over the tail head, and in the mammary region is also observed in some horses with PPID. Horses with PPID may also become lethargic due to their abnormal metabolism, and the horses may also develop neurological signs of ataxia, blindness, and seizures most probably due to the expansive growth of the tumors.

The most common findings in general *laboratory tests of horses with PPID are hyperglycemia due to insulin resistance* and less often increased hepatic enzyme activities due to steroid-induced hepatopathies.

Common *specific diagnostic tests for PPID* include dexamethasone suppression test, endogenous plasma α-melanocyte-stimulating hormone (α-MSH) concentrations, and thyroid-releasing hormone (TRH) stimulation tests. None of these tests is specific due to seasonal variation in hormone secretion, overlaps with other diseases, and the slow progressive nature of the disease with inconsistent correlation of hormonal serum levels with clinical signs of PPID.

Dexamethasone suppression test (DST) has been considered the most sensitive and specific test for PPID. Application of dexamethasone suppresses ACTH and consecutively cortisol secretion in the pars distalis of the pituitary due to negative feedback mechanism by cortisol receptors. ACTH secretion by melanotrope cells of the pars intermedia is not controlled by a negative feedback mechanism, and horses with PPID do not have decreased cortisol levels 24 h after dexamethasone injection. Sensitivity of DST is high in animals with overt clinical signs.

Increased *endogenous plasma α-MSH concentration* has been shown to be correlated with PPID. The α-MSH concentration is however also fluctuating seasonally with higher concentrations in autumn. In addition, *measurement of endogenous ACTH* has been proposed as a potential approach to diagnose PPID, but its level seems to be influenced by many factors including stress and exercise.

The *TRH stimulation test*, which is based on the observation that administration of TRH increases cortisol levels in horses with PPID, not in healthy horses, by up to 50 %, has been proposed to be sensitive and convenient. However, false-positive results have been revealed in every third healthy horse.

Contrast-enhanced magnetic resonance imaging (MRI) has the capability to image the equine pituitary gland in resolutions high enough to visualize details of the changes in the pars intermedia. Due to its high costs and the lack of availability, MRI is however rarely used for the diagnosis of PPID.

▪ Cytology and Histopathology

Cytologic biopsies of pituitary tumors are usually not available due to the restricted access to the cranial cavity. *Histologic analysis* is restricted to confirmation of the diagnosis postmortem.

▪ Therapy

Several *medical therapy modalities* have been reported, including cyproheptadine (serotonin antagonist), bromocriptine (dopaminergic agonist), trilostane (3β-hydroxysteroid dehydrogenase inhibitor), and pergolide (dopaminergic agonist). *Pergolide, a dopamine D2 receptor agonist*, is the treatment of choice for horse with PPID. It acts by replacing the lost dopaminergic inhibitory signals and thus suppresses ACTH secretion by the hyperplastic or neoplastic pars intermedia of the pituitary gland. Amelioration of clinical signs may take however months after first administration of pergolide. Administered has to be maintained lifelong but may allow animals an acceptable quality of life for years.

Survival times of animals with PPID independent from therapy protocol was 4.5 years for 50 % of horses with the majority of owners satisfied with quality of life of their animals.

12.2 Adrenal Gland Tumors

Adrenal gland tumors (AGT) are commonly seen only in cats, dogs, and cattle and are a frequent disease in ferrets. AGT in the horse and other animals are very rare. AGT are coarsely separated into adrenocortical and adrenomedullary tumors, both of which may be endocrinological functional or nonfunctional. Adrenocortical tumors may secrete excessive cortisol or less often androstenedione, progesterone, 17-hydroxyprogesterone, testosterone, and estradiol, while adrenomedullary tumors (pheochromocytomas) usually secrete excessive amounts of catecholamines. Pheochromocytomas are of any relevance only in dogs and very rare in other animals.

12.2.1 Canine Adrenocortical Tumors

Box 12.5. Canine Adrenocortical Tumors in Six Facts

1. Cause of 15 % of cases of hypercortisolism
2. Excessively secret cortisol, approx. 20 % invade vena cava and metastasize
3. Clinical signs include alopecia, polyuria/polydipsia, pendulous abdomen, and muscle atrophy
4. Important hormonal tests are LDDST, cortisol/creatinine ratio, and endogenous ACTH
5. Adrenalectomy as treatment of choice, high intraoperative complication rate
6. Trilostane and mitotane as efficient medical therapies

Epidemiology and Pathogenesis

Primary adrenal gland tumors (AGT) are rather rare tumors in the dog with a prevalence <5 % (Fig. 12.6). Of these, *adrenocortical tumors* (ACT) of the adrenal cortex are more common than tumors of the medulla, and secondary tumors are almost as common in the canine adrenal gland as are primary tumors. The *incidence of adrenocortical adenomas and carcinomas* is reported to be either similar or four times higher than for adenomas. Approximately 20 % of tumors show invasion of vessels, and approx. 50 % of carcinomas metastasize to the liver, lung, and other distant organs (Fig. 12.7). ACT are seen in dogs at an average *age* of 11 years. There is a slight *gender* predisposition for males and a *breed* predisposition for large breeds including German shepherds, poodles, Labrador retrievers, and terriers.

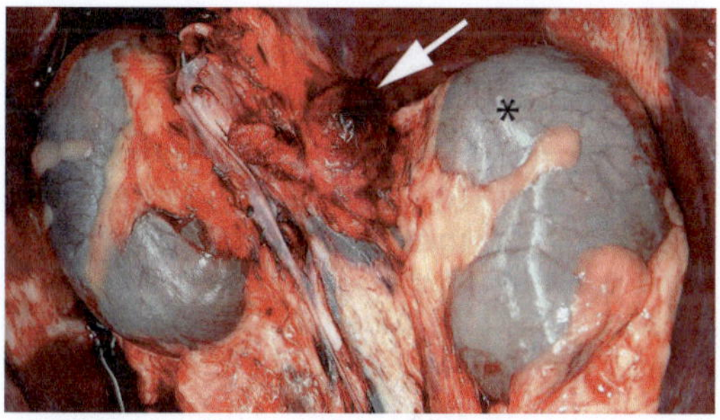

Fig. 12.6 Adrenocortical tumor (*arrow*) in a dog (Photo with permission of Dr. P. Schlieben, PhD, LUA Frankfurt/Oder, Germany and the Archive of the Freie Universität Berlin, Germany). * Kidney

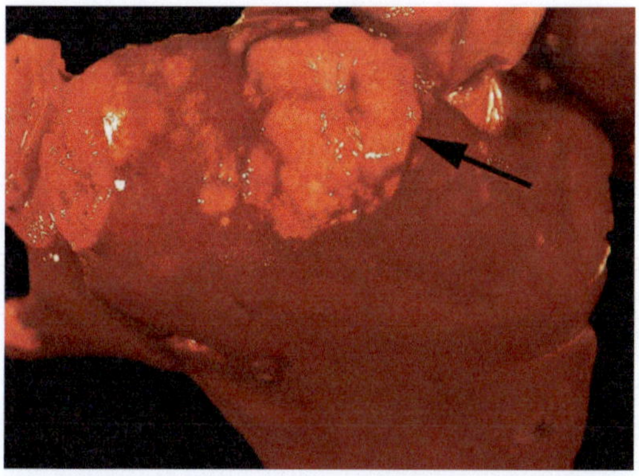

Fig. 12.7 Liver metastases (*arrow*) of an adrenocortical carcinoma in a dog (Photo with permission of Dr. P. Schlieben, PhD, LUA Frankfurt/Oder, Germany and the Archive of the Freie Universität Berlin, Germany)

ACT may be *endocrinologically functional* or nonfunctional, but data on the prevalence of either form are not available although it seems that nonfunctional tumors are rare. Endocrinologic functional, excessively *cortisol-secreting ACT* are the cause for <15 % of hypercortisolism (*Cushing's syndrome*) in dogs, while >80 % of cases of hypercortisolism are caused by pituitary gland tumors (▶ see Sect. 12.1.1). The molecular pathogenesis of ACT in the dog is unknown.

▪ Clinical Appearance

Clinical signs, imaging, and hormonal testing are central in the ultimate diagnosis of ACT. All of them are however not fully specific and sensitive. The complete picture of clinical signs, imaging results, and hormonal testing have thus to be considered for diagnosis.

Clinical signs of ACT are the *classical signs of hypercortisolism* with polyuria/polydipsia, polyphagia, pendulous abdomen, muscle weakness, lethargy, and bilaterally symmetric alopecia. *Laboratory tests* usually show neutrophilia, lymphopenia, monocytosis, and eosinopenia. In addition, increased serum alkaline phosphatase activity, elevated cortisol serum levels, decreased urine specific gravity, hyperglycemia, lipemia, and increased serum cholesterol is observed. Clinical signs are usually milder in ACT-associated than in pituitary tumor-dependent hypercortisolism.

Specific screening tests for the diagnosis of adrenocortical hypercortisolism include the measurement of serum cortisol, *low-dose dexamethasone suppression test* (LDDST), the *cortisol/creatinine ratio*, and measurement of *endogenous ACTH* (▶ see Sect. 12.1.1 for detailed description). Low endogenous ACTH levels are a valuable sign, which indicates ACT – rather than pituitary tumor-dependent hypercortisolism.

Ultrasonography is often used for evaluation of shape and size of adrenal glands in animals with suspected hypercortisolism. Mineralization has been identified as a moderately specific feature of ACT but is not specific for either adenomas or carcinomas. Identification of vascular invasion or metastasis is the only reliable clinical finding for the confirmation of malignancy.

Computed tomography (CT) and enhanced CT have been described to provide an accurate impression of size and invasive character of ACT. There are only few reports on the value of magnetic resonance imaging (*MRI*) for the diagnosis of ACT.

▪ Cytology and Histopathology

The presence of an ACT can be determined by *cytology* in most cases. Cytology is however not routinely recommended because of the high risk of complications including massive hemorrhage and the difficulty to reliably differentiate between benign and malignant tumors. *At necropsy* or after adrenalectomy, adrenocortical *adenomas* are macroscopically usually <2 cm in diameter, well-circumscribed, solitary yellow nodules which expand the cortex and compress adjacent normal cortex and medulla. *Adenocarcinomas* are usually >2 cm large, yellow to red friable masses with areas of necrosis, often poorly circumscribed, and invading surrounding tissues and vessels. They metastasize primarily to the liver, lung, kidney, and mesenteric lymph nodes. *Histologically, adenomas* contain polygonal cells with cytoplasmic vacuolation, fibrin thrombi, and hematopoiesis. *Adenocarcinomas* are characterized by capsular invasion, peripheral fibrosis, trabecular growth pattern, hemorrhage, necrosis, cellular pleomorphism, and a high mitotic rate. Carcinomas also show a higher Ki-67 rate than adenomas. In animals with endocrinologically functional ACT, the *contralateral adrenal gland* is atrophic and lacks cortical parenchyma.

▪ Therapy

Adrenalectomy is the treatment of choice for canine ACT. Advanced surgical skills are required for tumors with invasion of the phrenicoabdominal vein. Due to the atrophy of the contralateral adrenal, animals often require cortisol substitution for several weeks postoperatively. There is a high postoperative complication and mortality rate of 20 % due to hemorrhage, pancreatitis, and thromboembolism. Patients surviving the first weeks after surgery have a median survival time between 1 and 2 years. *Laparoscopic adrenalectomy* has recently been introduced and may be associated with less postoperative complications.

Medical therapy using *trilostane*, which competitively inhibits 3β-hydroxysteroid dehydrogenase that is essential for cortisol synthesis, is an alternative for animals for which surgery is not possible. It however requires lifelong administration. *Mitotane* (Lysodren) is another drug for the treatment of hypercortisolism. It is cytotoxic and adrenocorticolytic and destroys the zona fasciculata and reticularis of the adrenal gland. Complete destruction of the adrenal cortex may induce complete tumor remission but requires lifelong cortisol and mineralocorticoid substitution. One study reported median *survival times* of approx. 1 year and 3 months with after trilostane or mitotane treatment, respectively. Another recent study found a similar survival time of approx. 16 months of dogs treated with either drug.

Prognostic Factors and Markers

Most important *negative prognostic factors* for canine ACT are histologic signs of malignancy, vascular invasion, and metastases. Lethargy, thrombocytopenia, hypokalemia, and increased AST have been identified as negative preoperative prognostic factors. Another report found invasion of the caudal vena cava to be associated with a higher postoperative mortality rate.

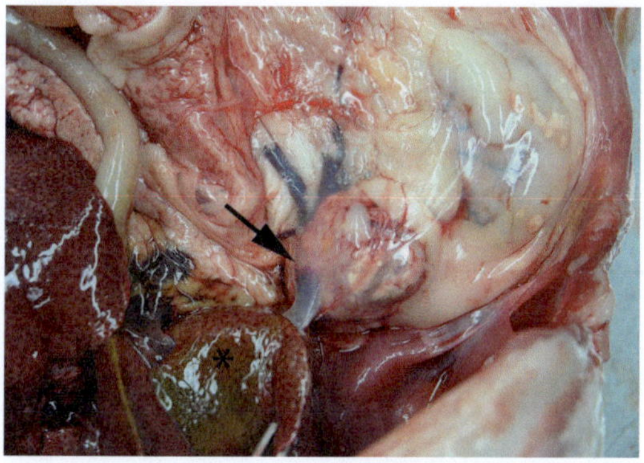

Fig. 12.8 Metastatic adrenocortical tumor with invasion of the vena cava (*arrow*) in a cat (Photo with permission of S. Plog, PHD, IDEXX Wetherby, UK and the Archive of the Freie Universität Berlin, Germany)

12.2.2 Feline Adrenocortical Tumors

Box 12.6. Feline Adrenocortical Tumors in Seven Facts

1. Rare tumors in cat
2. Cause for 15 % hypercortisolism cases (alopecia, polyuria/polydipsia, pendulous abdomen)
3. More often cause of Conn's syndrome (hyperaldosteronism, hypertension, hypokalemia)
4. LDDST, cortisol/creatinine ratio, and endogenous ACTH as hormonal tests for hypercortisolism
5. Plasma aldosterone/renin ratio is the laboratory test for hyperaldosteronismus
6. Adrenalectomy is the treatment of choice but with high intraoperative complication rate
7. Trilostane and mitotane are efficient medical therapies

Epidemiology and Pathogenesis

Primary adrenal gland tumors (AGT) are rare tumors in cats with a prevalence <1 % of feline tumors. Adrenocortical tumors (ACT) are more common than tumors of the medulla. Adrenocortical adenomas and carcinomas seem to have the same incidence but conclusive epidemiological data are lacking due to the rarity of the tumors. ACT are usually diagnosed in cats at an average *age* of 12 years. There is no known *breed* or *gender* predisposition. The pathogenesis of ACT in the cat is unknown. ACT may be endocrinologically functional or nonfunctional, but data on the prevalence of either forms are not available. AGT may invade the vena cava and metastasize to distant organs (Fig. 12.8).

Primary hyperaldosteronism (syn. Conn's syndrome) is the most frequently described clinical syndrome associated with feline ACT. *Conn's syndrome* is characterized by excessive autonomous secretion of mainly aldosterone but also other mineralocorticoids by ACT or nodular hyperplasia. Increased aldosterone levels lead to increased water and sodium retention and increased potassium excretion, which together lead to systemic *arterial hypertension* and/or *hypokalemia* and chronic renal failure. The median age of cats with hyperaldosteronism is 13 years (range 5–20 years). No breed or sex predisposition has been documented.

Hypercortisolism is less common in cats than in dogs, but the distribution between the pituitary tumor-dependent form (approx. 85 %) and the ACT-dependent form (15 %) is almost similar.

■ Clinical Appearance

Clinical signs, imaging, and hormonal testing are central in the ultimate diagnosis of ACT. All of them are however not fully specific and sensitive. The complete picture of clinical signs, imaging results, and hormonal testing have thus to be considered for diagnosis.

Clinical signs of cats with ACT-associated *primary hyperaldosteronism* are based on the excessive secretion of mineralocorticoids like aldosterone and thus hypokalemia and/or systemic arterial hypertension. Most affected cats also show muscular weakness and/or ocular signs of arterial hypertension. The *plasma aldosterone/renin ratio* is currently considered as the best screening test for feline primary hyperaldosteronism. However, imaging is required to differentiate between adrenocortical neoplasia and bilateral hyperplasia.

Clinical signs of cats with ACT-associated *hypercortisolism* are classical signs of Cushing's syndrome with polyuria/polydipsia, polyphagia, pendulous abdomen, muscle weakness, lethargy, and bilateral symmetric alopecia. *Laboratory tests* usually show neutrophilia, lymphopenia, monocytosis, and eosinopenia. In addition, increased serum alkaline phosphatase (ALP) activity, elevated cortisol serum levels, decreased urine specific gravity, hyperglycemia, lipemia, and increased serum cholesterol are observed. Clinical signs are usually milder in ACT-associated than pituitary-dependent hypercortisolism.

Specific screening tests for the diagnosis of ACT hypercortisolism include the measurement of serum cortisol, *low-dose dexamethasone suppression test* (LDDST), the *urine cortisol/creatinine ratio, ACTH stimulation test*, and measurement of *endogenous ACTH* (▶ see Sect. 12.1.1 for detailed description). Low endogenous ACTH level is a sensitive sign which indicates ACT – rather than pituitary-dependent hypercortisolism.

Ultrasonography is often used for evaluation of shape and size of adrenal glands in animals with suspected hypercortisolism. Bilateral enlargement is indicative for pituitary tumor-dependent hypercortisolism, while tumors are usually unilateral masses. Ultrasonography is also helpful in the identification of invasion of the causal vena cava and thus identification of malignancy. An ultimate differentiation of adrenocortical from adrenomedullary and adenomas from carcinomas is however not possible.

There are few reports on the value and results of *computed tomography* (CT) or *magnetic resonance imaging* (MRI) for the diagnosis of feline ACT. However, it can be assumed that feline ACT may appear similar to canine ACT (▶ see Sect. 12.2.1).

■ Cytology and Histopathology

The presence and origin of an AGT can be determined by *cytology* in most cases. Cytology is however not reliable in distinguishing benign from malignant neoplasia. Cytology of the well-vascularized tumors is also not routinely recommended because of the high risk of complications including massive hemorrhage. There is a lack of literature on histologic features of malignancy of ACT in cats; it can however be assumed that histologic features may be *similar to canine ACT* (▶ see Sect. 12.2.1).

■ Therapy

There is only limited literature on treatment of feline ACT. *Adrenalectomy* is the current treatment of choice for ACT in cats. The *postoperative complication rate* and mortality in cats after adrenalectomy is controversially discussed. Some studies report good outcomes with survival times of approx. 3 years, while others postulate high postoperative complication rates of 40 % with hemorrhage and sepsis being the most common cause of death. Unilateral adrenalectomy is associated with higher survival rates than bilateral. However, cats with immediate survival of surgery have a generally good long-term prognosis with survival for up to 5 years.

Medical treatment of hyperaldosteronism is advised in cases where tumors are non-resectable or comorbidities and distant metastases hamper adrenalectomy. The *mineralocorticoid receptor blocker spironolactone* is most often used in cats but is most often not able to lead to a complete remission of clinical signs.

Both trilostane and mitotane have been used for *medical treatment of adrenal hypercortisolism* in cats. *Trilostane* is well tolerated in cats and ameliorates clinical signs including diabetes mellitus. Median survival times were reported to be approx. 2 years (range 80–1278 days).

12.2.3 Adrenocortical Tumors in the Ferret (Adrenocortical Disease, ACD)

Box 12.7. Adrenocortical Tumors in Ferrets in Six Facts

1. Adrenocortical disease characterized by hypersecretion of sex steroids
2. Adrenal proliferation most probably induced by increased pituitary secretion of FSH and LH
3. Neutering and prolonged photoperiods of major impact for development
4. Hair loss, vulvar swelling, stranguria, and palpable adrenal glands are common clinical signs
5. Adrenalectomy is the treatment of choice with fair prognosis after perioperative survival
6. GnRH agonists, melatonin, and GnRH-vaccines are potential medical therapies

▪ Epidemiology and Pathogenesis

Adrenocortical disease (ACD), i.e., *hyperadrenocorticism*, is one of the most important diseases in ferrets with a prevalence of the disease of up to 70 % of pet ferrets. ACD in ferrets is caused by adrenocortical adenomas (~10 %), hyperplasia (~45 %), or adenocarcinomas (~45 %), all of which may *release excess sex steroids* (estradiol-17b, androstenedione, dehydroepiandrosterone, 17-hydroxyprogesterone, and progesterone) *but not cortisol*. The left adrenal gland may be more often affected. There is a slight *gender* predisposition for females, and the median *age* of first clinical signs is 4 years (range 8 months – 9 years). *Metastasis* of adenocarcinomas is rare and usually found at late stages of the disease.

The exact *etiology* of ACD in ferrets is unknown. There seems to be a *genetic basis* since the disease is more prevalent in the more inbred ferrets in the United States than the more outbred ferrets in Europe. For instance, abnormally increased expression of the *tumor suppressor gene* GATA-4 has been identified in adrenocortical tumors but not in adrenal hyperplasia.

The most important hypotheses on the development of ACD in ferrets, however, focus on non-genetic, *environmental causes* of disease. *Sterilization* in general and particularly early sterilization of ferrets at an age of 4–6 weeks is thought to majorly contribute to disease development. It is thought that the hypothalamus of neutered ferrets continue to secrete gonadotropin-releasing hormone (GnRH), which stimulates pituitary secretion of luteinizing hormone (LH) and follicle-stimulating hormone (FSH). Both hormones stimulate proliferation and secretion of sex hormones (estradiol) by the adrenal cortex. Adrenal secretion does however not induce a negative feedback in the hypothalamus, which continuously releases GnRH and thus stimulates adrenocortical proliferation. *Unphysiologically long photoperiods* of >8 h of indoor pet ferrets are believed to contribute to development of ACD. Ferrets are highly sensitive to photoperiod length, and the light cycles seem to strongly stimulate GnRH and LH production.

▪ Clinical Appearance

Clinical signs of ACD in ferrets are centered on the excess sex steroid secretion by the adrenal tumor but less often by its space-occupying growth or metastasis. Progressive and symmetric *alopecia* is present in >90 % of affected ferrets. *Vulvar swelling* (70 %) in spayed females, increased *aggression* or sexual behavior in spayed females and neutered males, *stranguria* in males secondary to urethral obstruction from prostate hyperplasia, *palpable adrenal glands*, and *anemia* are other common clinical signs.

Clinical diagnosis of ACD is supported by *hormone measurement*. Affected animals have increased serum levels of estradiol, androstenedione, and 17-hydroxyprogesterone. Plasma cortisol concentrations are usually not increased in ferrets with ACD.

Abdominal ultrasound is also highly sensitive to identify adrenal masses. These are often cystic or mineralized and may compress or invade the vena cava. *Radiographs* are usually not sensitive enough to identify smaller masses.

▪ Cytology and Histopathology

Grossly, affected glands may be cystic, discolored, enlarged, or irregular. Additionally, atrophy of the contralateral gland may occur. *Cytology* of the primary adrenal mass is usually not performed in ferrets. However, cornification of preputial epithelial cells from preputial lavage was correlated with an increase in serum 17-hydroxyprogesterone concentration as well as clinical signs of adrenocortical disease in castrated male ferrets. *Histopathology* is necessary for the ultimate differentiation of hyperplasia, adenomas, or carcinomas. The presence of necrosis, cellular atypia, and a high mitotic rate are proposed markers of malignancy for adrenal tumors in the ferret.

Therapy

Adrenalectomy of the diseased adrenal gland is considered the treatment of choice for animals suitable for surgery and associated with a *good prognosis*. The survival time after surgery was influenced by the success of complete resection but not by the histologic features of the tumor and the adrenal gland affected (right, left, or bilateral). Other authors however state that complete bilateral adrenalectomy is not recommended because it may lead to hypoadrenocorticism. In addition, surgical resection is associated with the typical high surgical risks of adrenalectomy like hemorrhage particularly in old and debilitated ferrets.

Several effective *medical therapies* for hyperadrenocorticism have been introduced in the recent years. They ameliorate the clinical signs of hyperadrenocorticism but do not resolve the underlying cause of disease, the adrenocortical neoplasms.

Prolonged administration of high levels of *gonadotropin-releasing hormone (GnRH) agonists* leuprolide and deslorelin is able to downregulate the release of follicle-stimulating hormone (FSH) and luteinizing hormone (LH) by the pituitary gland, which in turn decreases secretion of sex steroids by the adrenal gland.

The exact function of *melatonin* and the mechanism by which melatonin affects LH and FSH secretion is unknown. The administration of melatonin has however been described to have suppressive effects on sex steroid release, which may lead to an amelioration of clinical signs in ferrets with ACD at least for few months. It is speculated that the exogenous melatonin administration may substitute for decreased endogenous melatonin due to prolonged photoperiods.

In an experimental approach, the efficacy of an *anti-GnRH vaccine* for the prevention and treatment of ACD in ferrets has been tested. It is assumed that the production of antibodies against GnRH is suppressing the production and release of LH. Vaccination indeed ameliorated ACD symptoms. In addition, vaccination also significantly reduced the incidence of ACD when animals were vaccinated at an age <3 years.

12.2.4 Canine Adrenomedullary Tumors (Pheochromocytomas)

Box 12.8. Canine Pheochromocytomas in Five Facts

1. Mostly malignant tumors of the chromaffin cells of the adrenal medulla
2. Often incidental necropsy findings
3. May be clinical relevant due to invasive/expansive growth or catecholamine release
4. Adrenalectomy is the treatment of choice but associated with high complication rate
5. Preoperative α-adrenergic antagonist necessary to reduce risk of intraoperative complications

Epidemiology and Pathogenesis

Pheochromocytomas (PCT) are tumors of the chromaffin cells of the adrenal medulla, but chromaffin cells are present and may give rise to PCT in many other body locations. Endocrinologically functional PCT are rare in dogs but may secrete *epinephrine* and/or *norepinephrine* intermittently. The median *age* of dogs with first diagnosis of this tumor is 11 years. There is no *breed* or *gender* predisposition.

PCT are uncommon tumors of dogs *and very rare in cats*. They are slowly growing tumors but nevertheless generally considered as malignant tumors due to the detection of peritumoral *vessel invasion* in >80 % of cases and the detection of *metastasis* to the regional lymph nodes, liver, lung, spleen, and kidney in 40 % of cases.

Clinical Appearance

PCT are *often incidental findings at necropsy* without prior clinical signs. If clinical signs are present, they may be either caused by expansive or invasive growth of the tumors or less often by their secretion of epinephrine or norepinephrine.

Clinical signs due to space-occupying tumor masses or local vascular invasion can be vomiting, abdominal pain and abdominal distension, and hemoperitoneum due to tumor rupture. Invasion and thrombosis of the vena cava or extramural compression may also occlude venous return from the posterior extremities and cause edema.

Clinical signs due to catecholamine release are rare in dogs and are usually intermittent. Clinical signs may be present several times a day or only from time to time and diagnosis may therefore be challenging for the clinician. Most common clinical signs include episodic weakness and collapse, anxiety, tachycardia, cardiac arrhythmias, hypertension, hyperthermia, and sweating.

Abdominal ultrasonography is usually very helpful in the identification of the up to 10 cm in diameter large PCT and the evaluation of vascular invasion and metastatic disease. Ultrasonography is however not able to ultimately differentiate PCT from adrenocortical and secondary tumors.

Magnetic resonance imaging (MRI) and *computed tomography* (CT) are more sensitive than ultrasonography for the diagnosis of even small adrenal masses and potential metastases but are also not able to discriminate the different types of adrenal tumors.

Standard laboratory tests are usually unremarkable in dogs with PCT. The few available studies on specific *biochemical tests* for dogs with PCT indicate that an increased *urinary metanephrine/creatinine ratio* is a specific and sensitive marker of PCT. The influence on stress and the intermittent secretion of catecholamine has however not finally been analyzed.

▪ Cytology and Histopathology

The presence of an adrenal tumor can be determined by *cytology* in most cases. Cytology is however not routinely recommended because of the high risk of complications and the difficulty to reliably differentiate between benign and malignant tumors. Reliable *histopathologic markers of malignancy* are vascular invasion and local and distant metastasis while tumor cell shape is not significantly different in benign and malignant PCT. *Immunohistochemically*, PCT are positive for chromogranin A, synaptophysin, N-CAM (CD56), and protein gene product 9.5 (PGP 9.5). *Grossly*, pheochromocytomas are usually unilateral or bilateral, dark reddish-brown, up to 10 cm large, soft, well-demarcated nodules, central in the adrenal gland. Areas of necrosis and hemorrhage are common.

▪ Therapy

Adrenalectomy is the treatment of choice for canine PCT. Preoperative administration of the *α-adrenergic antagonist phenoxybenzamine* for up to 3 weeks drastically reduces intraoperative complication rate caused by massive catecholamine release, like hyper-/hypotension or cardiac arrhythmias from 48 to 13 %.

▪ Prognostic Factors and Markers

The general prognosis for dogs with PCT is fair. The most important prognostic factor is *perioperative survival.* Of the 70–80 % of animals surviving the immediate postoperative phase, most animals survive for up to 1–3 years. Other prognostic factors are tumor size >5 cm, vessel invasion, and presence of metastases.

12.3 Thyroid Gland Tumors

12.3.1 Canine Thyroid Gland Tumors

Box 12.9. Canine Thyroid Gland Tumors in Six Facts

1. Rare tumors in dogs
2. 90 % are invasive, malignant carcinomas
3. >50 % with metastasis into the lung and other organs
4. 60 % euthyroid, 30 %hypothyroid, and 10 % hyperthyroid dogs with thyroid gland tumors
5. Thyroidectomy for moveable and irradiation or radioactive iodide for fixed tumors as treatment of choice
6. Treatment associated with survival times of 1–3 years depending on tumor stage

▪ Epidemiology and Pathogenesis

Thyroid gland tumors are rare tumors in dogs (< 4 % of all tumors). *Up to 90 % of clinically apparent tumors are carcinomas,* while adenomas are more common incidental findings at necropsy. Thyroid tumors are tumors of dogs with a median *age* of 10 years. There is a *breed* predilection for golden retrievers, beagles, boxers, and Siberian huskies. There is no *gender* predisposition and no predisposition of either left or right thyroid gland. More than 50 % of tumors involve both glands. *Metastasis* is common at initial diagnosis and the great majority of carcinomas, particularly large and bilateral tumors and mostly present in the lungs. Only approx. 20 % are endocrinologically functional and induce hyperthyroidism. The etiology and carcinogenesis of canine thyroid tumors are almost completely unknown. *Iodine deficiency, nuclear radiation*, and an upregulation of the *PI3K/Akt pathway* have been identified as potential carcinogenic factors.

▪ Clinical Appearance

Most dogs are presented clinically because of the consequences of the *space-occupying growth of the tumor* (◘ Fig. 12.9). These dogs usually have a *palpable ventral cervical mass*, which in some cases is associated with coughing, dyspnea, dysphagia, dysphonia, laryngeal paralysis, and Horner's syndrome. Acute severe hemorrhage can occur due to rupture of the well-vascularized tumors or invasion of the cervical vasculature. *Metastasis* is present in approx. 50 % of dogs at the time of first diagnosis and correlated with tumor volume. A volume >20 cm^3 is associated with a metastatic rate of 75 % or higher. Tumors often show direct hematogenous spread to the lungs and less often lymphogenic spread to enlarged cervical lymph nodes.

The majority of canine *thyroid tumors are nonfunctional*. Approx. 60 % of patients are euthyroid, 30 % are hypothyroid due to destruction of normal thyroid parenchyma, and 10 % are hyperthyroid. Clinical signs of *hyper- and hypothyroidism* are therefore uncommon but, if present, very helpful in the diagnosis of canine thyroid tumors. Typical *signs of hypothyroidism* are hair thinning/alopecia, excess shedding or scaling, weight gain, reduced activity, skin infections, and subcutaneous accumulation of mucopolysaccharides (myxedema). Many hyperthyroid dogs are asymptomatic, but typical *signs of hyperthyroidism* are weight loss, polyuria/polydipsia, polyphagia, hyperthermia, aggressiveness, tachycardia, panting, and restlessness.

Three-view thoracic *radiographs*, cervical *ultrasonography, magnetic resonance imaging (MRI)*, and *computed tomography (CT)* are used to confirm the presence and evaluate the invasiveness of the thyroid tumor. One study found com-

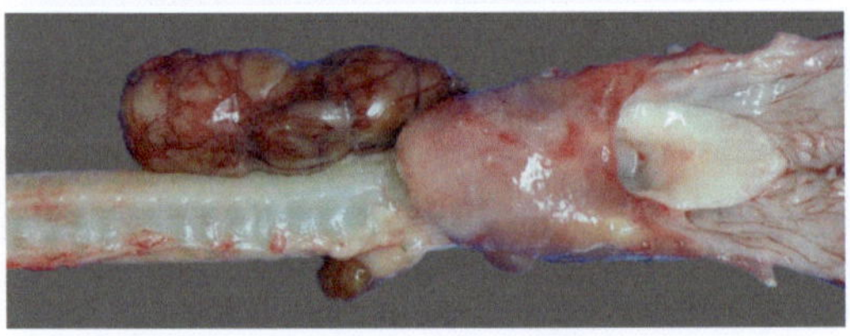

◘ **Fig. 12.9** Thyroid gland adenoma in a dog (Photo with permission of the Archive of the Institute of Veterinary Pathology, Freie Universität Berlin, Germany)

◘ **Table 12.1** WHO staging for canine thyroid tumors (Owen et al. 1980)

Category/ stage	Description
Tumor (T)	
T0	No tumor
T1a/T1b	Tumor <2 cm, T1a tumor not fixed, T1b tumor fixed
T2a/T2b	Tumor 2–5 cm, T2a tumor not fixed, T2b tumor fixed
T3a/T3b	Tumor >5 cm, T3a tumor not fixed, T3b tumor fixed
Lymph node (N)	
N0	No lymph node metastasis
N1a/N1b	Ipsilateral lymph node involved, N1a not fixed, N1b fixed
N2a/N2b	Bilateral lymph nodes involved, N2a not fixed, N2b fixed
Distant metastasis (M)	
M0	No metastasis
M1	Metastasis
Stage	
I	T1 with N0, M0
II	T0 or T1 with N1 T2 with N0 or N1a
III	T3 with M0 T0–T2 with N1b orN2b
IV	Each T/N with M1

puted tomography had the highest specificity (100 %) and MRI to have the highest sensitivity (93 %) in diagnosing thyroid carcinoma, while ultrasound was considerably less useful. MRI detected tumor invasion most sensitively, while palpation was not an accurate predictor of local invasion. *Scintigraphy* using 99mTc-pertechnetate is performed in a few medical centers to identify local residual disease after surgery or metastatic disease.

The commonly used WHO staging of canine thyroid tumors (Owen et al. 1980) is based on clinical signs, cytology/histopathology results, and clinical imaging including scintigraphy (◘ Table 12.1).

Cytology and Histopathology

Accuracy of *cytology* in dogs with thyroid masses is reported to be problematic. Cytology is often able to confirm the thyroid origin of the tumors but definitive identification of malignancy is difficult (◘ Fig. 12.10). Incisional biopsies and examination of the tumor edges may improve accuracy. However, malignant thyroid tumors are usually highly vascularized, and hemodilution is a common problem for cytologic diagnosis and a significant risk in core needle biopsy procedures.

Histopathologically, adenomas are expansively growing and encapsulated with well-differentiated tumors cells. Carcinomas have an increased cellularity, cellular pleomorphism, and invasion of the fibrous capsule and surrounding vessels. Solid, non-follicular growth, vessel invasion, and a high cellular pleomorphism have been associated with a worse prognosis. The thyroid origin of highly dedifferentiated tumors and their metastases can be confirmed using immunohistochemistry for thyroglobulin and TTF-1 (thyroid transcription factor).

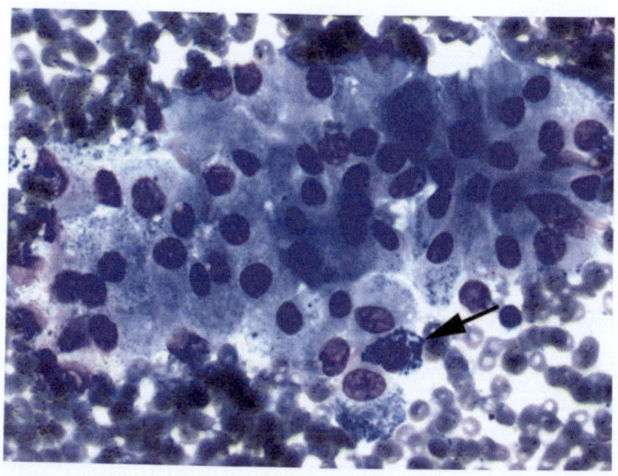

◘ **Fig. 12.10** Cytology of a thyroid gland adenoma in a dog

Therapy

The choice of the appropriate therapy modality is primarily influenced by the movability and invasive character of the tumor as identified by palpation and clinical imaging.

Surgery is the treatment of choice for *freely movable tumors* without extensive invasion of surrounding structures (approx. 50 % of all tumors). Severe hemorrhage is a common *intraoperative risk* during excision of the well-vascularized thyroid tumors. In addition, bilateral thyroidectomy may lead to hypocalcemia due to hypoparathyroidism. Hypothyroidism is another common *postoperative risk*. Median survival of dogs after excision of freely movable tumors is approx. 3 years.

Thyroidectomy is *not recommended for fixed tumors*. Therapeutic management is based on *radiation therapy* to reduce tumor size to a level acceptable for surgery in these animals. Radiation therapy is associated with progression-free survival rates of approx. 70 % after 3 years. Radiation therapy has also been successfully used for palliation of metastatic disease with survival times of up to 6 months.

Radioactive ^{131}I has been used for thyroid ablation in dogs with unresectable thyroid tumors. The radioactive iodine is preferably accumulating in hyper- and neoplastic thyroid cells and kills these cells usually after one administration and after few days. Nonneoplastic, usually atrophic thyroid cells are mostly spared by the effect and may be reactivated and establish a normal hormonal hemostasis. Survival times of up to 3 years have been reported for stage II and III tumors and 1 year for metastatic stage IV tumors. Severe myelosuppression was observed as a major side effect of ^{131}I in some dogs.

Chemotherapy is recommended for stage III and IV tumors due to their high risk for distant metastases. The few studies available indicate that doxorubicin or cisplatin induce a partial response in approx. 50 % of animals. Other studies however found no effect of adjuvant chemotherapy on survival.

12.3.2 Feline Thyroid Gland Tumors

Box 12.10. Feline Thyroid Gland Tumors in Five Facts

1. Most common endocrine tumor in the cat
2. Most tumors are benign hyperplasias or adenomas
3. Only 3 % carcinomas with a metastatic rate of 70 %
4. Most tumors are functional and majority of affected cats have hyperthyroidism
5. Radioactive ^{131}I therapy and thyroidectomy as therapy of choice

▪ Epidemiology and Pathogenesis

Hyperthyroidism with elevated serum concentrations of thyroxine (T4) and triiodothyronine (T3) is the *most common endocrine disorder in cats*. It is caused by primary thyroid proliferation of which multinodular *adenomatous hyperplasia* and less often *single adenomas* make up the vast majority. It is assumed but not finally proven that adenomas may develop directly from hyperplastic follicular cells. *Carcinomas* make up only <3 % of all cases but have a metastatic rate of up to 70 %. Thyroid tumors in the cat are *almost always endocrinologically functional*, in contrast to dogs, which have more often carcinomas but mostly nonfunctional tumors. Thyroid tumors are a disease of older cats with a median *age* of 13 years at first presentation. There is no *breed* or *gender* predisposition.

Several dietary, environmental, and inflammatory *risk factors* are suspected to be involved in the etiology of feline thyroid hyperplasia and neoplasia, but final proof for their relevance is lacking. Mutations in the thyroid-stimulating hormone (TSH) receptor, a G-protein inhibitory protein of the TSH-receptor-signaling pathway, have been identified, but their relevance is not proven.

▪ Clinical Appearance

Most feline thyroid tumors are benign but functional, and clinical signs are thus caused most often by the hormonal imbalance and only rarely by the space-occupying mass or metastasis.

The most common *clinical signs due to tumor-associated hyperthyroidism* are weight loss, polyphagia, polydipsia, polyuria, vomiting, diarrhea, presence of a palpable thyroid nodule, cardiac left ventricular hypertrophy, tachycardia, gallop rhythm, and poor hair coat.

Standard laboratory tests in cats with hyperthyroidism may show lympho- and eosinopenia, azotemia, and hypokalemia. Definitive diagnosis of hyperthyroidism is confirmed by *hormonal tests*. Increased *serum total T4 level* is present in 90 % of cats, while T3 levels are less often increased. Cats with suspected hyperthyroidism but normal total T4 level should be measured again after some days. *Free T4* and *TSH measurement* may be helpful in the diagnosis of occult hyperthyroidism in cats with normal T4 levels.

Ultrasonography and *computed tomography* (CT) are used for the identification of the tumor mass. Adenomas are usually well circumscribed and occasionally cystic structures, while carcinomas are poorly circumscribed and of highly variable texture.

Tc-pertechnetate scintigraphy is used when ultrasonography and CT fail to detect a suspected functional tumor. Scintigraphy is able to detect rare ectopic thoracic thyroid tumors or metastases.

Palpable ventral cervical masses are associated with *mass effects* like coughing, dyspnea, dysphagia, dysphonia, or laryngeal paralysis. Horner's syndrome is only seen in cats with invasive carcinomas and thus rare.

▪ Cytology and Histopathology

There is a lack of reports on the sensitivity and specificity of *cytology* for the diagnosis of feline thyroid tumors. *Histolopathologically*, adenomatous hyperplasia is of variable appearance with either small regular to large irregular follicles with papillary projections into the lumen. They are however not encapsulated and do not compress the adjacent thyroid tissue. *Adenomas* are classified as follicular, papillary, or cystic. *Carcinomas* are mostly solid accumulations of pleomorphic cells with invasion of the surrounding tissues.

▪ Therapy

There are three main therapy modalities for feline thyroid tumors: radioactive ^{131}I therapy, thyreostatic drugs, and thyroidectomy.

If available, *radioactive* ^{131}*I therapy* is considered the therapy of choice for feline hyperthyroidism. The radioactive iodine is preferably accumulating in hyperplastic and neoplastic thyroid cells and kills these cells usually after one administration and after a few days. Nonneoplastic usually atrophic thyroid cells are mostly spared by the effect and may be reactivated and establish a normal hormonal hemostasis. Median survival time of ^{131}I-treated cats may be up to 4 years and relapse rates are <5 %.

Medical therapy using thiamiden, which inhibits thyroid hormone synthesis, is used for preoperative amelioration of clinical signs. It reduces serum T4 concentrations in the long term. It does however not reduce tumor size and usually not able to treat carcinoma-associated hyperthyroidism.

Thyroidectomy is another effective treatment of feline thyroid tumors and hyperthyroidism. Careful analysis of the size of the tumor by ultrasonography, CT, and scintigraphy is necessary for complete removal of the tumor. *Cardiac arrhythmias* are a common intraoperative complication during thyroidectomy and may require administration of β-adrenergic blockers. Amelioration of clinical signs of hyperthyroidism may however take several weeks after thyroidectomy. Removal of parathyroid glands may lead to hypoparathyroidism and hypocalcemia.

12.4 Parathyroid Gland Tumors

Parathyroid tumors are uncommon tumors of older dogs and very rare tumors in old cats. They develop from parathyroid chief cells and may secrete excess parathyroid hormone (PTH), thus leading primary hyperparathyroidism and to hypercalcemia.

12.4.1 Canine Parathyroid Gland Tumors

Box 12.11. Canine Parathyroid Gland Tumors in Five Facts

1. Mostly adenomas, carcinomas very rare
2. Almost always functional with increased parathormone secretion and hypercalcemia
3. Usually identified due to clinical signs while tumors too small to be palpated
4. Parathyroidectomy as treatment of choice
5. Generally very good prognosis for survival

Epidemiology and Pathogenesis

Canine parathyroid tumors are usually single, well-circumscribed benign *adenomas* of the parathyroid chief cells. Malignant *carcinomas* are very rare and may metastasize to the regional lymph nodes or the lung. The median *age* at primary diagnosis is 11 years, and there is a *breed* predisposition for keeshond dogs and German shepherds but no *gender* predisposition.

Almost all canine parathyroid tumors derived from the chief cells are *functional tumors*, which excessively *secrete parathyroid hormone (PTH)* and thus lead to clinically apparent *hypercalcemia due to primary hyperparathyroidism*. PTH leads to increased serum calcium concentrations due to osteolysis by indirect (/osteoblast-mediated) activation of osteoclasts, which may lead to fibrous osteodystrophy, increased resorption of calcium (Ca) in the distal renal tubuli, and increased intestinal Ca uptake by increased levels of activated vitamin D.

Clinical Appearance

The most important *clinical signs* of parathyroid tumors are evoked by the *hyperparathyroidism* and *rarely by mass effects*. They consist of hypercalcemia, polyuria/polydipsia, weakness, decreased appetite, weight loss, and neuromuscular signs like trembling, cardiac arrhythmia, or smooth muscle paralysis. In addition, increased serum Ca concentrations often lead to urolithiasis and lower urinary tract infections. However, hypercalcemia due to hyperparathyroidism is often an incidental finding during routine health check. The tumors are usually too small to be palpable. Hypercalcemia is verified by the presence of *increased serum ionized calcium* and *normal to low serum phosphate* concentrations and *increased serum PTH levels*.

Ultrasonography is helpful for presurgical identification and localization of parathyroid tumors larger than 3 mm.

■ **Cytology and Histopathology**

Parathyroid tumors are often difficult to be unequivocally identified by fine needle aspiration. However, if successfully targeted, *cytology* of *adenomas* is characterized by oval, uniform nuclei in a light eosinophilic cytoplasm. *Carcinoma* cells may be more pleomorphic but are often cytologically similar. *Histopathologically, adenomas* are usually well-circumscribed accumulations of closely packed chief cells with lightly eosinophilic cytoplasm, a thin fibrous capsule, and mild compression of adjacent tissues. *Carcinomas* are usually unencapsulated with more pleomorphic cells and invasion of adjacent tissues and vessels.

■ **Therapy**

Parathyroidectomy is the treatment of choice for canine parathyroid tumors. Alternatively, percutaneous *ultrasound-guided ethanol or heat ablation* is also described in dogs. However, the success rates are highest and the complication rate was lowest for parathyroidectomy while ablation performs nevertheless well. Approximately 10% of patients have tumors in more than one gland and up to three of the four parathyroid glands can be removed without the *complication of hypoparathyroidism*. Hyperparathyroidism is nevertheless associated with atrophy of the nonneoplastic parathyroid glands, which may lead to *temporary postsurgical hypocalcemia* even if only one parathyroid gland is resected. Serum ionized calcium levels have thus to be monitored postsurgically for at least 1 week.

■ **Prognostic Factors and Markers**

The long-term *prognosis* after surgery or ablation *is very good* even for nonmetastatic carcinomas. The recurrence rate is <10% in treated dogs.

12.5 Insulinomas (Beta Cell Tumors)

Insulinomas are the most common tumor of ferrets with an incidence of up to 25% in older ferrets. In contrast, insulinomas are uncommon tumors of dogs and only rarely diagnosed in cats (◘ Fig. 12.11). Tumors of the other pancreatic island cells like glucagonomas and gastrinomas are rare in animals.

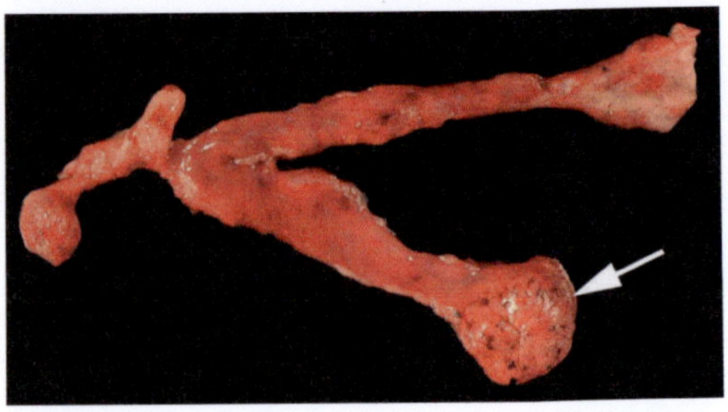

◘ **Fig. 12.11** Insulinoma in the pancreas (*arrow*) of a cat (Photo with permission of A. Schmidt, PhD, IDEXX Ludwigshafen, Germany and the Archive of the Institute of Veterinary Pathology, Freie Universität Berlin, Germany)

12.5.1 Canine Insulinomas

Box 12.12. Canine Insulinomas in Six Facts

1. Rare tumors in dogs
2. Mostly functional with excessive insulin secretion
3. Approx. 50% of tumors with metastasis to the liver and lung
4. Intermittent neurological signs of hypoglycemia are the typical clinical sign
5. Tumors often too small for clinical imaging
6. Surgery as treatment of choice with survival times of few months to 2 years depending on clinical stage

■ **Epidemiology and Pathogenesis**

Canine insulinomas are rare tumors of the pancreatic beta cells. There is a *breed* predilection for medium to large dogs and particularly for retrievers, German shepherds, Irish setters, and boxers. The median *age* at first presentation is 9 years (range 3–15 years). There is no *gender* predilection. Most of the insulinomas are functional with *excess secretion of insulin* and associated hypoglycemia. There is controversy about the morphologic classification of benign and malignant insulinomas. However, approx. 50% of canine insulinomas have developed *metastasis* to the regional lymph nodes and the liver but only rarely to the lungs at the time of diagnosis. The *molecular pathogenesis* for the development of canine insulinomas is largely unknown, but somatostatin receptor, growth hormone, and insulin-like growth factor expression have been discussed as potential factors in their development.

Clinical Appearance

The *diagnostic hallmark* of dogs with insulinomas is a normal to elevated blood insulin concentration in the presence of low blood glucose levels. The *clinical signs* are therefore mostly the results of *hypoglycemia in the nervous system*, including muscle tremor, weakness, ataxia, collapse, disorientation, behavioral changes, and seizures. Clinical signs are often of short duration (seconds to minutes) and intermittent or episodic.

The diagnosis of an insulinoma is confirmed by *blood tests* for detection of normal or *elevated serum insulin concentration (hyperinsulinism) during hypoglycemia* (blood glucose <3 mmol/l). *Low fructosamine* concentration can be used as an indicator of chronic hypoglycemia.

Ultrasonography is often used for imaging of insulinomas for confirmation of the diagnosis and preparation of surgery. However, it has a sensitivity of only approx. 50 % since most insulinomas are too small to be depicted and false-negative results are common. *Computed tomography (CT)* is of higher sensitivity (70 %) to detect canine insulinomas. *Radiographs* are usually unremarkable.

A *staging system* of the World Health Organization (WHO, Owen et al. 1980) is currently used for canine pancreatic tumors (Table 12.2).

Cytology and Histopathology

In *ultrasound-guided fine needle aspirate cytology*, benign insulinomas are characterized by well-differentiated, non-pleomorphic tumors cells in typical neuroendocrine clusters with indistinct cytoplasmic borders, numerous vacuoles, and mildly anisokaryotic nuclei with one nucleolus. Carcinomas may contain more pleomorphic cells but definitive identification of malignancy is usually not possible by cytology. A recent study also confirmed the good diagnostic yield and low rate of clinical complications of pancreatic fine needle aspirations in dogs, which had a high correlation with consecutive histology results.

Table 12.2 WHO staging for canine pancreatic tumors (Owen et al. 1980)

Category/stage	Description
Tumor (T)	
T1	Tumor present
Lymph node (N)	
N0	No lymph node metastasis
N1a/N1b	Regional lymph node involved
N2a/N2b	Distant lymph node involved
Distant metastasis (M)	
M0	No metastasis
M1	Distant metastasis
Stage	
I	T1, N0, M0
II	T1, N1, M0
III	T1, N1, M1 or T1, N0, M1

Histopathologically, adenomas are characterized by well-differentiated round to polygonal cells with distinct cell borders and pale eosinophilic finely granular cytoplasm. The cells are arranged in typical endocrine nests and packets. Carcinomas are usually larger than adenomas, invade the fibrous capsule, and contain densely packed, more pleomorphic cells. Hemorrhage and necrosis may be present.

Therapy

Surgical tumor excision is the treatment of choice for canine insulinomas, together with acute treatment of hypoglycemia by intravenous dextrose administration. Approximately 50 % of canine insulinomas have metastasized at the time of diagnosis. This *high risk of metastatic* disease should be actively communicated to the dog owners. Suspected metastases in the regional lymph node or liver should be resected. The most common postoperative complications are pancreatitis and persistent hypoglycemia. The *median survival times* following surgery vary between several months and up to 2 years in various studies. The prognosis also depends on the clinical stage of the disease. Half of the dogs with stage I tumors are free of hypoglycemia 14 months after surgery, while only <20 % of dogs in stages II and III are euglycemic at this time. In addition, stage III tumors are associated with a significantly shorter survival time with approx. 50 % fatalities due to metastasis after 6 months.

Medical therapy of the neoplastic disease is occasionally used in dogs. *Streptozotocin*, a drug specifically cytotoxic for pancreatic beta cells, has been used in dogs. Adverse effects like high nephrotoxicity and moderate efficacy are however hampering its clinical use. Furthermore, *octreotide*, a somatostatin analogue, may suppress insulin synthesis in dogs with insulinomas.

▪ Prognostic Factors and Markers

On univariate analysis, the presence of nuclear atypia is significantly predictive only for disease-free interval (DFIs) of canine insulinomas, while tumor size, TNM stage, necrosis, and Ki67 index are significant for prognosis of both DFI and survival time. On multivariate analysis, tumor size and Ki67 index are predictive for survival time and tumor size is predictive for DFI.

12.5.2 Insulinomas in the Ferret

Box 12.13. Insulinomas in Ferrets in Seven Facts

1. Most common tumor in the ferret
2. Mostly biologically benign but almost always excessively secreting insulin
3. Intermittent neurological signs of hypoglycemia
4. Low blood glucose levels with concurrent high insulin levels diagnostic
5. Most tumors too small to be identified by clinical imaging
6. Surgical excision as treatment of choice
7. Dietary changes and diazoxide as palliative treatment

▪ Epidemiology and Pathogenesis

Insulinomas are the *most frequent tumor in ferrets* with an incidence of 25 % of all tumors. The *black-footed ferret is an exception* and is only rarely affected by the tumor. Insulinomas in the ferret are *usually functional* and thus excessively secrete insulin and induce hypoglycemia-associated clinical signs. The tumors are tumors of the middle-aged to old ferret with a median age of 4 years but may develop very early in life. Insulinomas in the ferret are *more often benign* in terms of general biologic behavior than malignant. They may grow modestly invasive but only *rarely metastasize* to the regional lymph nodes, liver, and spleen, which is in contrast to the often metastatic canine insulinomas. There is no gender predisposition.

▪ Clinical Appearance

Clinical signs are dominated by *hypoglycemia* and only rarely by mass effects of the tumor. They include lethargy, dullness, stargazing, muscle weakness, and ataxia. Seizures are less common than in dogs. The tumors seem to *secrete insulin intermittently*, which is also reflected in the episodic character of the clinical signs. The clinical signs however disappear after intravenous administration of glucose, which is not seen with other neurological diseases.

Laboratory tests of ferrets with insulinomas show a *fasting blood glucose concentration <70 mg/dL. Increased serum insulin concentrations* (>35 mU/ml) with concurrent hypoglycemia strongly support the diagnosis of an insulinoma. Measurement of serum insulin concentration in the ferret is however validated in only few laboratories.

Ultrasonography may be helpful in the diagnosis of insulinomas. However, most insulinomas are small with few millimeters in diameter, and ultrasonography has thus only a moderate sensitivity with many false-negative results.

▪ Cytology and Histopathology

There is no available literature on the *cytology* of insulinomas in the ferret but due to the high overlap in histopathology, their cytologic appearance should be similar to that in dogs. *Histopathologically*, insulinomas may be hyperplasia or adenomas or carcinomas. They are usually arranged in the typical neuroendocrine nests and consist of polyhedral cells in a fine fibrovascular stroma. Infiltrative or unencapsulated carcinomas are rather rare. Immunohistochemical detection of insulin and chromogranin A maybe helpful in the diagnosis of the rare anaplastic tumors.

Therapy

Surgical excision is considered the treatment of choice for insulinomas in ferrets. Survival times are longer than with medical therapy. However, clinical signs often recur and many animals remain hypoglycemic after assumed complete removal of the tumor.

Diet modification and *medical therapy* have been reported to be *effective for palliative therapy. Glucocorticoids* are able to increase hepatic gluconeogenesis and increase peripheral insulin resistance. *Diazoxide* directly inhibits pancreatic insulin secretion by influencing the beta cell calcium hemostasis and increasing hepatic gluconeogenesis.

Dietary modification should aim at avoidance of rapid increase of blood glucose which induces even higher insulin levels in hypoglycemic ferrets with insulinomas. *High-protein but low-carb diet* is recommended.

Suggested Reading

Abraham LA, Helmond SE, Mitten RW, Charles JA, Holloway SA (2002) Treatment of an acromegalic cat with the dopamine agonist L-deprenyl. Aust Vet J 80:479–483

Anderson CR, Birchard SJ, Powers BE, Belandria GA, Kuntz CA, Withrow SJ (2001) Surgical treatment of adrenocortical tumors: 21 cases (1990-1996). J Am Anim Hosp Assoc 37:93–97

Antinoff N, Hahn K (2004) Ferret oncology: diseases, diagnostics, and therapeutics. Vet Clin North Am Exot Anim Pract 7(579–625):vi

Arenas C, Melian C, Perez-Alenza MD (2014) Long-term survival of dogs with adrenal-dependent hyperadrenocorticism: a comparison between mitotane and twice daily trilostane treatment. J Vet Intern Med/Am Coll Vet Inter Med 28:473–480

Arenas C, Perez-Alenza D, Melian C (2013) Clinical features, outcome and prognostic factors in dogs diagnosed with non-cortisol-secreting adrenal tumours without adrenalectomy: 20 cases (1994-2009). Vet Rec 173:501

Aronsohn MG, Schunk KL, Carpenter JL, King NW (1984) Clinical and pathologic features of thymoma in 15 dogs. J Am Vet Med Assoc 184:1355–1362

Ash RA, Harvey AM, Tasker S (2005) Primary hyperaldosteronism in the cat: a series of 13 cases. J Feline Med Surg 7:173–182

Atwater SW, Powers BE, Park RD, Straw RC, Ogilvie GK, Withrow SJ (1994) Thymoma in dogs: 23 cases (1980-1991). J Am Vet Med Assoc 205:1007–1013

Barber LG (2007) Thyroid tumors in dogs and cats. Vet Clin North Am Small Anim Pract 37(755–773):vii

Barber PJ (2004) Disorders of the parathyroid glands. J Feline Med Surg 6:259–269

Barrera JS, Bernard F, Ehrhart EJ, Withrow SJ, Monnet E (2013) Evaluation of risk factors for outcome associated with adrenal gland tumors with or without invasion of the caudal vena cava and treated via adrenalectomy in dogs: 86 cases (1993-2009). J Am Vet Med Assoc 242:1715–1721

Beech J, Boston RC, McFarlane D, Lindborg S (2009) Evaluation of plasma ACTH, alpha-melanocyte-stimulating hormone, and insulin concentrations during various photoperiods in clinically normal horses and ponies and those with pituitary pars intermedia dysfunction. J Am Vet Med Assoc 235:715–722

Benchekroun G, de Fornel-Thibaud P, Rodriguez Pineiro MI, Rault D, Besso J, Cohen A, Hernandez J, Stambouli F, Gomes E, Garnier F, Begon D, Maurey-Guenec C, Rosenberg D (2010) Ultrasonography criteria for differentiating ACTH dependency from ACTH independency in 47 dogs with hyperadrenocorticism and equivocal adrenal asymmetry. J Vet Intern Med/Am Coll Vet Intern Med 24:1077–1085

Bennett KR, Gaunt MC, Parker DL (2015) Constant rate infusion of glucagon as an emergency treatment for hypoglycemia in a domestic ferret (Mustela putorius furo). J Am Vet Med Assoc 246:451–454

Berg RIM, Nelson RW, Feldman EC, Kass PH, Pollard R, Refsal KR (2007) Serum insulin-like growth factor-I concentration in cats with diabetes mellitus and acromegaly. J Vet Intern Med 21:892–898

Bertazzolo W, Didier M, Gelain ME, Rossi S, Crippa L, Avallone G, Roccabianca P, Bonfanti U, Giori L, Fracassi F (2014) Accuracy of cytology in distinguishing adrenocortical tumors from pheochromocytoma in companion animals. Vet Clin Pathol/Am Soc Vet Clin Pathol 43:453–459

Boag AK, Neiger R, Church DB (2004) Trilostane treatment of bilateral adrenal enlargement and excessive sex steroid hormone production in a cat. J Small Anim Pract 45:263–266

Bonczynski J (2007) Primary hyperparathyroidism in dogs and cats. Clin Tech Small Anim Pract 22:70–74

Brearley MJ, Polton GA, Littler RM, Niessen SJM (2006) Coarse fractionated radiation therapy for pituitary tumours in cats: a retrospective study of 12 cases. Vet Comp Oncol 4:209–217

Buishand FO, Kik M, Kirpensteijn J (2010) Evaluation of clinico-pathological criteria and the Ki67 index as prognostic indicators in canine insulinoma. Vet J 185:62–67

Buishand FO, van Erp MG, Groenveld HA, Mol JA, Kik M, Robben JH, Kooistra HS, Kirpensteijn J (2012) Expression of insulin-like growth factor-1 by canine insulinomas and their metastases. Vet J 191:334–340

Buishand FO, Visser J, Kik M, Grone A, Keesler RI, Briaire-de Bruijn IH, Kirpensteijn J (2014) Evaluation of prognostic indicators using validated canine insulinoma tissue microarrays. Vet J 201:57–63

Caplan ER, Peterson ME, Mullen HS, Quesenberry KE, Rosenthal KL, Hoefer HL, Moroff SD (1996) Diagnosis and treatment of insulin-secreting pancreatic islet cell tumors in ferrets: 57 cases (1986-1994). J Am Vet Med Assoc 209:1741–1745

Cavalcanti JV, Moura MP, Monteiro FO (2014) Thymoma associated with exfoliative dermatitis in a cat. J Feline Med Surg 16:1020–1023
Caywood DD, Klausner JS, O'Leary TP (1988) Pancreatic insulin-secreting neoplasms: clinical, diagnostic, and prognostic features in 73 dogs. J Am Anim Hosp Assoc 24:577–584
Chen S (2008) Pancreatic endocrinopathies in ferrets. Vet Clin North Am Exot Anim Pract 11(107–123):vii
Chen S (2010) Advanced diagnostic approaches and current medical management of insulinomas and adrenocortical disease in ferrets (Mustela putorius furo). Vet Clin North Am Exot Anim Pract 13:439–452
Combes A, Pey P, Paepe D, Rosenberg D, Daminet S, Putcuyps I, Bedu AS, Duchateau L, de Fornel-Thibaud P, Benchekroun G, Saunders JH (2013) Ultrasonographic appearance of adrenal glands in healthy and sick cats. J Feline Med Surg 15:445–457
Cordner AP, Sharkey LC, Armstrong PJ, McAteer KD (2015) Cytologic findings and diagnostic yield in 92 dogs undergoing fine-needle aspiration of the pancreas. J Vet Diagn Invest Off Publ Am Assoc Vet Lab Diagn Inc 27:236–240
Daminet S, Kooistra HS, Fracassi F, Graham PA, Hibbert A, Lloret A, Mooney CT, Neiger R, Rosenberg D, Syme HM, Villard I, Williams G (2014) Best practice for the pharmacological management of hyperthyroid cats with antithyroid drugs. J Small Anim Pract 55:4–13
Daniel G, Mahony OM, Markovich JE, Appleman E, Monaghan KN, Lawrence YA, Fiocchi EH, Weaver K, Johnston A, Barton B (2015) Clinical findings, diagnostics and outcome in 33 cats with adrenal neoplasia (2002-2013). J Feline Med Surg 18(2):77–84
Daniel GB, Neelis DA (2014) Thyroid scintigraphy in veterinary medicine. Semin Nucl Med 44:24–34
Davis MK, Schochet RA, Wrigley R (2012) Ultrasonographic identification of vascular invasion by adrenal tumors in dogs. Vet Radiol Ultrasound Off J Am Coll Vet Radiol Int Vet Radiol Assoc 53:442–445
de Brito Galvao JF, Chew DJ (2011) Metabolic complications of endocrine surgery in companion animals. The Veterinary clinics of North America. Small Animal Pract 41:847–868, v
Diez de Castro E, Lopez I, Cortes B, Pineda C, Garfia B, Aguilera-Tejero E (2014) Influence of feeding status, time of the day, and season on baseline adrenocorticotropic hormone and the response to thyrotropin releasing hormone-stimulation test in healthy horses. Domest Anim Endocrinol 48:77–83
Dirtu AC, Niessen SJM, Jorens PG, Covaci A (2013) Organohalogenated contaminants in domestic cats' plasma in relation to spontaneous acromegaly and type 2 diabetes mellitus: a clue for endocrine disruption in humans? Environ Int 57–58:60–67
Djajadiningrat-Laanen S, Galac S, Kooistra H (2011) Primary hyperaldosteronism: expanding the diagnostic net. J Feline Med Surg 13:641–650
Edinboro CH, Scott-Moncrieff JC, Glickman LT (2010) Feline hyperthyroidism: potential relationship with iodine supplement requirements of commercial cat foods. J Feline Med Surg 12:672–679
Ehrhart N, Withrow SJ, Ehrhart EJ, Wimsatt JH (1996) Pancreatic beta cell tumor in ferrets: 20 cases (1986-1994). J Am Vet Med Assoc 209:1737–1740
Elliott DA, Feldman EC, Koblik PD, Samii VF, Nelson RW (2000) Prevalence of pituitary tumors among diabetic cats with insulin resistance. J Am Vet Med Assoc 216:1765–1768
Feldman EC, Hoar B, Pollard R, Nelson RW (2005) Pretreatment clinical and laboratory findings in dogs with primary hyperparathyroidism: 210 cases (1987-2004). J Am Vet Med Assoc 227:756–761
Feldman EC, Nelson RW, Feldman MS, Farver TB (1992) Comparison of mitotane treatment for adrenal tumor versus pituitary-dependent hyperadrenocorticism in dogs. J Am Vet Med Assoc 200:1642–1647
Feldman EC, Wisner ER, Nelson RW, Feldman MS, Kennedy PC (1997) Comparison of results of hormonal analysis of samples obtained from selected venous sites versus cervical ultrasonography for localizing parathyroid masses in dogs. J Am Vet Med Assoc 211:54–56
Fineman LS, Hamilton TA, de Gortari A, Bonney P (1998) Cisplatin chemotherapy for treatment of thyroid carcinoma in dogs: 13 cases. J Am Anim Hosp Assoc 34:109–112
Fischetti AJ, Gisselman K, Peterson ME (2012) Ct and Mri evaluation of skull bones and soft tissues in six cats with presumed acromegaly versus 12 unaffected cats. Vet Radiol Ultrasound 53:535–539
Friedrich-Rust M, Glasemann T, Polta A, Eichler K, Holzer K, Kriener S, Herrmann E, Nierhoff J, Bon D, Bechstein WO, Vogl T, Zeuzem S, Bojunga J (2011) Differentiation between benign and malignant adrenal mass using contrast-enhanced ultrasound. Ultraschall in der Medizin 32:460–471
Fukazawa K, Kayanuma H, Kanai E, Sakata M, Shida T, Suganuma T (2009) Insulinoma with basal ganglion involvement detected by magnetic resonance imaging in a dog. J Vet Med Sci/Jap Soc Vet Sci 71:689–692
Gilson SD, Withrow SJ, Wheeler SL, Twedt DC (1994) Pheochromocytoma in 50 dogs. J Vet Int Med/Am Coll Vet Int Med 8:228–232
Goldstein LJ, Galski H, Fojo A, Willingham M, Lai SL, Gazdar A, Pirker R, Green A, Crist W, Brodeur GM et al (1989) Expression of a multidrug resistance gene in human cancers. J Natl Cancer Inst 81:116–124
Gostelow R, Bridger N, Syme HM (2013) Plasma-free metanephrine and free normetanephrine measurement for the diagnosis of pheochromocytoma in dogs. J Vet Int Med/Am Coll Vet Int Med 27:83–90
Goutal CM, Brugmann BL, Ryan KA (2012) Insulinoma in dogs: a review. J Am Anim Hosp Assoc 48:151–163
Greco DS (2012) Feline acromegaly. Top Companion Anim M 27:31–35
Gregori T, Mantis P, Benigni L, Priestnall SL, Lamb CR (2015) Comparison of computed tomographic and pathologic findings in 17 dogs with primary adrenal neoplasia. Vet Radiol Ultrasound Off J Am Coll Vet Radiol Int Vet Radiol Assoc 56:153–159
Ham K, Greenfield CL, Barger A, Schaeffer D, Ehrhart EJ, Pinkerton M, Valli VE (2009) Validation of a rapid parathyroid hormone assay and intraoperative measurement of parathyroid hormone in dogs with benign naturally occurring primary hyperparathyroidism. Vet Surg 38:122–132
Helm JR, McLauchlan G, Boden LA, Frowde PE, Collings AJ, Tebb AJ, Elwood CM, Herrtage ME, Parkin TD, Ramsey IK

(2011) A comparison of factors that influence survival in dogs with adrenal-dependent hyperadrenocorticism treated with mitotane or trilostane. J Vet Intern Med/Am Coll Vet Int Med 25:251–260

Herrera MA, Mehl ML, Kass PH, Pascoe PJ, Feldman EC, Nelson RW (2008) Predictive factors and the effect of phenoxybenzamine on outcome in dogs undergoing adrenalectomy for pheochromocytoma. J Vet Intern Med/Am Coll Vet Int Med 22:1333–1339

Hibbert A, Gruffydd-Jones T, Barrett EL, Day MJ, Harvey AM (2009) Feline thyroid carcinoma: diagnosis and response to high-dose radioactive iodine treatment. J Feline Med Surg 11:116–124

Higgs P, Hibbert A (2012) Managing hyperthyroidism in cats. Vet Rec 171:225–226

Hunt GB, Churcher RK, Church DB, Mahoney P (1997) Excision of a locally invasive thymoma causing cranial vena cava syndrome in a dog. J Am Vet Med Assoc 210:1628–1630

Hurty CA, Flatland B (2005) Feline acromegaly: a review of the syndrome. J Am Anim Hosp Assoc 41:292–297

Iseri T, Yamada K, Chijiwa K, Nishimura R, Matsunaga S, Fujiwara R, Sasaki N (2007) Dynamic computed tomography of the pancreas in normal dogs and in a dog with pancreatic insulinoma. Vet Radiol Ultrasound Off J Am Coll Vet Radiol Int Vet Radiol Assoc 48:328–331

Javadi S, Slingerland LI, van de Beek MG, Boer P, Boer WH, Mol JA, Rijnberk A, Kooistra HS (2004) Plasma renin activity and plasma concentrations of aldosterone, cortisol, adrenocorticotropic hormone, and alpha-melanocyte-stimulating hormone in healthy cats. J Vet Intern Med/Am Coll Vet Int Med 18:625–631

Jensen KB, Forcada Y, Church DB, Niessen SJM (2015) Evaluation and diagnostic potential of serum ghrelin in feline hypersomatotropism and diabetes mellitus. J Vet Intern Med 29:14–20

Kaser-Hotz B, Rohrer CR, Stankeova S, Wergin M, Fidel J, Reusch C (2002) Radiotherapy of pituitary tumours in five cats. J Small Anim Pract 43:303–307

Kent MS, Bommarito D, Feldman E, Theon AP (2007) Survival, neurologic response, and prognostic factors in dogs with pituitary masses treated with radiation therapy and untreated dogs. J Vet Intern Med/Am Coll Vet Int Med 21:1027–1033

Kooistra HS (2014) Feline hyperthyroidism: a common disorder with unknown pathogenesis. Vet Rec 175:456–457

Kyles AE, Feldman EC, De Cock HE, Kass PH, Mathews KG, Hardie EM, Nelson RW, Ilkiw JE, Gregory CR (2003) Surgical management of adrenal gland tumors with and without associated tumor thrombi in dogs: 40 cases (1994-2001). J Am Vet Med Assoc 223:654–662

Labelle P, Kyles AE, Farver TB, De Cock HE (2004) Indicators of malignancy of canine adrenocortical tumors: histopathology and proliferation index. Vet Pathol 41:490–497

Lamb CR, Ciasca TC, Mantis P, Forcada Y, Potter M, Church DB, Niessen SJ (2014) Computed tomographic signs of acromegaly in 68 diabetic cats with hypersomatotropism. J Feline Med Surg 16:99–108

Lamb CR, Simpson KW, Boswood A, Matthewman LA (1995) Ultrasonography of pancreatic neoplasia in the dog: a retrospective review of 16 cases. Vet Rec 137:65–68

Lang JM, Schertel E, Kennedy S, Wilson D, Barnhart M, Danielson B (2011) Elective and emergency surgical management of adrenal gland tumors: 60 cases (1999-2006). J Am Anim Hosp Assoc 47:428–435

Larson RN, Schmiedt CW, Wang A, Lawrence J, Howerth EW, Holmes SP, Grey SW (2013) Adrenal gland function in a dog following unilateral complete adrenalectomy and contralateral partial adrenalectomy. J Am Vet Med Assoc 242:1398–1404

Lautenschlaeger IE, Hartmann A, Sicken J, Mohrs S, Scholz VB, Neiger R, Kramer M (2013) Comparison between computed tomography and (99m)TC- pertechnetate scintigraphy characteristics of the thyroid gland in cats with hyperthyroidism. Vet Radiol Ultrasound Off J Am Coll Vet Radiol Int Vet Radiol Assoc 54:666–673

Li X, Fox JG, Padrid PA (1998) Neoplastic diseases in ferrets: 574 cases (1968-1997). J Am Vet Med Assoc 212:1402–1406

Liles SR, Linder KE, Cain B, Pease AP (2010) Ultrasonography of histologically normal parathyroid glands and thyroid lobules in normocalcemic dogs. Vet Radiol Ultrasound Off J Am Coll Vet Radiol Int Vet Radiol Assoc 51:447–452

Littler RM, Polton GA, Brearley MJ (2006) Resolution of diabetes mellitus but not acromegaly in a cat with a pituitary macroadenoma treated with hypofractionated radiation. J Small Anim Pract 47:392–395

Llabres-Diaz FJ, Dennis R (2003) Magnetic resonance imaging of the presumed normal canine adrenal glands. Vet Radiol Ultrasound Off J Am Coll Vet Radiol Int Vet Radiol Assoc 44:5–19

Lo AJ, Holt DE, Brown DC, Schlicksup MD, Orsher RJ, Agnello KA (2014) Treatment of aldosterone-secreting adrenocortical tumors in cats by unilateral adrenalectomy: 10 cases (2002-2012). J Vet Int Med/Am Coll Vet Int Med 28:137–143

Long CD, Goldstein RE, Hornof WJ, Feldman EC, Nyland TG (1999) Percutaneous ultrasound-guided chemical parathyroid ablation for treatment of primary hyperparathyroidism in dogs. J Am Vet Med Assoc 215:217–221

Madarame H, Kayanuma H, Shida T, Tsuchiya R (2009) Retrospective study of canine insulinomas: eight cases (2005-2008). J Vet Med Sci/Jap Soc Vet Sci 71:905–911

Maggio F, DeFrancesco TC, Atkins CE, Pizzirani S, Gilger BC, Davidson MG (2000) Ocular lesions associated with systemic hypertension in cats: 69 cases (1985-1998). J Am Vet Med Assoc 217:695–702

Massari F, Nicoli S, Romanelli G, Buracco P, Zini E (2011) Adrenalectomy in dogs with adrenal gland tumors: 52 cases (2002-2008). J Am Vet Med Assoc 239:216–221

Mastro LM, Adams AA, Urschel KL (2015) Pituitary pars intermedia dysfunction does not necessarily impair insulin sensitivity in old horses. Domest Anim Endocrinol 50:14–25

Mayer MN, Treuil PL (2007) Radiation therapy for pituitary tumors in the dog and cat. Can Vet J La revue veterinaire canadienne 48:316–318

Mc Gowan TW, Pinchbeck GP, Mc Gowan CM (2013) Evaluation of basal plasma alpha-melanocyte-stimulating hormone and adrenocorticotrophic hormone concentrations for the diagnosis of pituitary pars intermedia dysfunction from a population of aged horses. Equine Vet J 45:66–73

McFarlane D (2011) Equine pituitary pars intermedia dysfunction. Vet Clin North Am Equine Pract 27:93–113
McGowan TW, Pinchbeck GP, McGowan CM (2013) Prevalence, risk factors and clinical signs predictive for equine pituitary pars intermedia dysfunction in aged horses. Equine Vet J 45:74–79
Meij BP, Auriemma E, Grinwis G, Buijtels JJCWM, Kooistra HS (2010) Successful treatment of acromegaly in a diabetic cat with transsphenoidal hypophysectomy. J Feline Med Surg 12:406–410
Meleo KA (1997) The role of radiotherapy in the treatment of lymphoma and thymoma. Vet Clin North Am Small Anim Pract 27:115–129
Milovancev M, Schmiedt CW (2013) Preoperative factors associated with postoperative hypocalcemia in dogs with primary hyperparathyroidism that underwent parathyroidectomy: 62 cases (2004-2009). J Am Vet Med Assoc 242:507–515
Moore AS, Nelson RW, Henry CJ, Rassnick KM, Kristal O, Ogilvie GK, Kintzer P (2002) Streptozocin for treatment of pancreatic islet cell tumors in dogs: 17 cases (1989-1999). J Am Vet Med Assoc 221:811–818
Moore LE, Biller DS, Smith TA (2000) Use of abdominal ultrasonography in the diagnosis of primary hyperaldosteronism in a cat. J Am Vet Med Assoc 217(213–215):197
Moore SA, O'Brien DP (2008) Canine pituitary macrotumors. Compendium 30:33–40; quiz 41
Morrison SA, Randolph J, Lothrop CD (1989) Hypersomatotropism and insulin-resistant diabetes-mellitus in a Cat. J Am Vet Med Assoc 194:91–94
Myers NC 3rd, Bruyette DS (1994) Feline adrenocortical diseases: part I--hyperadrenocorticism. Semin Vet Med Surg 9:137–143
Naan EC, Kirpensteijn J, Dupre GP, Galac S, Radlinsky MG (2013) Innovative approach to laparoscopic adrenalectomy for treatment of unilateral adrenal gland tumors in dogs. Vet Surg 42:710–715
Nakamura K, Lim SY, Ochiai K, Yamasaki M, Ohta H, Morishita K, Takagi S, Takiguchi M (2015) Contrast-enhanced ultrasonographic findings in three dogs with pancreatic insulinoma. Vet Radiol Ultrasound Off J Am Coll Vet Radiol Int Vet Radiol Assoc 56:55–62
Neiger R, Witt AL, Noble A, German AJ (2004) Trilostane therapy for treatment of pituitary-dependent hyperadrenocorticism in 5 cats. J Vet Int Med/Am Coll Vet Int Med 18:160–164
Nichols R (1997) Complications and concurrent disease associated with canine hyperadrenocorticism. Vet Clin North Am Small Anim Pract 27:309–320
Niessen S (2010) Feline acromegaly: an essential differential diagnosis for the difficult diabetic. J Feline Med Surg 12:15–23
Niessen SJ, Khalid M, Petrie G, Church DB (2007a) Validation and application of a radioimmunoassay for ovine growth hormone in the diagnosis of acromegaly in cats. Vet Rec 160:902–907
Niessen SJ, Petrie G, Gaudiano F, Khalid M, Smyth JB, Mahoney P, Church DB (2007b) Feline acromegaly: an underdiagnosed endocrinopathy? J Vet Int Med/Am Coll Vet Int Med 21:899–905
Niessen SJM, Church DB, Forcada Y (2013) Hypersomatotropism, acromegaly, and hyperadrenocorticism and feline diabetes mellitus. Vet Clin N Am-Small 43:319–350
Norman EJ, Mooney CT (2000) Diagnosis and management of diabetes mellitus in five cats with somatotrophic abnormalities. J Feline Med Surg 2:183–190
Northrup NC, Rassnick KM, Gieger TL, Kosarek CE, McFadden CW, Rosenberg MP (2013) Prospective evaluation of biweekly streptozotocin in 19 dogs with insulinoma. J Vet Int Med/Am Coll Vet Int Med 27:483–490
Owen LN (1980) Skeletal tumors. In: TNM classification of tumours in domestic, 1st edn. World Health Organization, Geneva, pp 66–67
Pack L, Roberts RE, Dawson SD, Dookwah HD (2001) Definitive radiation therapy for infiltrative thyroid carcinoma in dogs. Vet Radiol Ultrasound 42:471–474
Peterson M (2012) Hyperthyroidism in cats: what's causing this epidemic of thyroid disease and can we prevent it? J Feline Med Surg 14:804–818
Peterson ME (2007) Acromegaly in cats: are we only diagnosing the tip of the iceberg? J Vet Int Med/Am Coll Vet Int Med 21:889–891
Peterson ME (2013a) Feline focus: diagnostic testing for feline thyroid disease: hyperthyroidism. Compendium 35, E3
Peterson ME (2013b) More than just T(4): diagnostic testing for hyperthyroidism in cats. J Feline Med Surg 15:765–777
Peterson ME, Broome MR (2015) Thyroid scintigraphy findings in 2096 cats with hyperthyroidism. Vet Radiol Ultrasound Off J Am Coll Vet Radiol Int Vet Radiol Assoc 56:84–95
Peterson ME, Taylor RS, Greco DS, Nelson RW, Randolph JF, Foodman MS, Moroff SD, Morrison SA, Lothrop CD (1990) Acromegaly in 14 cats. J Vet Intern Med 4:192–201
Peterson ME, Ward CR (2007) Etiopathologic findings of hyperthyroidism in cats. The Veterinary clinics of North America. Small Anim Pract 37:633–645, v
Pey P, Rossi F, Vignoli M, Duchateau L, Marescaux L, Saunders JH (2014) Use of contrast-enhanced ultrasonography to characterize adrenal gland tumors in dogs. Am J Vet Res 75:886–892
Phair KA, Carpenter JW, Schermerhorn T, Ganta CK, DeBey BM (2011) Diabetic ketoacidosis with concurrent pancreatitis, pancreatic beta islet cell tumor, and adrenal disease in an obese ferret (Mustela putorius furo). J Am Assoc Lab Anim Sci JAALAS 50:531–535
Pollard RE, Bohannon LK, Feldman EC (2015) Prevalence of incidental thyroid nodules in ultrasound studies of dogs with hypercalcemia (2008-2013). Vet Radiol Ultrasound Off J Am Coll Vet Radiol Int Vet Radiol Assoc 56:63–67
Pollard RE, Long CD, Nelson RW, Hornof WJ, Feldman EC (2001) Percutaneous ultrasonographically guided radiofrequency heat ablation for treatment of primary hyperparathyroidism in dogs. J Am Vet Med Assoc 218:1106–1110
Pollard RE, Reilly CM, Uerling MR, Wood FD, Feldman EC (2010) Cross-sectional imaging characteristics of pituitary adenomas, invasive adenomas and adenocarcinomas in dogs: 33 cases (1988-2006). J Vet Int Med/Am Coll Vet Int Med 24:160–165

Polton GA, White RN, Brearley MJ, Eastwood JM (2007) Improved survival in a retrospective cohort of 28 dogs with insulinoma. J Small Anim Pract 48:151–156
Popovitch CA, Weinstein MJ, Goldschmidt MH (1994) Chondrosarcoma: a retrospective study of 97 dogs (1987–1990). J Am Anim Hosp Assoc 30:81–85
Posch B, Dobson J, Herrtage M (2011) Magnetic resonance imaging findings in 15 acromegalic cats. Vet Radiol Ultrasound 52:422–427
Radlinsky MG (2007) Thyroid surgery in dogs and cats. Vet Clin N Am-Small 37:789–798
Rasmussen SH, Andersen HH, Kjelgaard-Hansen M (2014) Combined assessment of serum free and total T4 in a general clinical setting seemingly has limited potential in improving diagnostic accuracy of thyroid dysfunction in dogs and cats. Vet Clin Pathol/Am Soc Vet Clin Pathol 43:1–3
Rasor L, Pollard R, Feldman EC (2007) Retrospective evaluation of three treatment methods for primary hyperparathyroidism in dogs. J Am Anim Hosp Assoc 43:70–77
Robben JH, Pollak YW, Kirpensteijn J, Boroffka SA, van den Ingh TS, Teske E, Voorhout G (2005) Comparison of ultrasonography, computed tomography, and single-photon emission computed tomography for the detection and localization of canine insulinoma. J Vet Int Med/Am Coll Vet Int Med 19:15–22
Robben JH, van den Brom WE, Mol JA, van Haeften TW, Rijnberk A (2006) Effect of octreotide on plasma concentrations of glucose, insulin, glucagon, growth hormone, and cortisol in healthy dogs and dogs with insulinoma. Res Vet Sci 80:25–32
Rosenstein DS (2000) Diagnostic imaging in canine pheochromocytoma. Vet Radiol Ultrasound Off J Am Coll Vet Radiol Int Vet Radiol Assoc 41:499–506
Salesov E, Boretti FS, Sieber-Ruckstuhl NS, Rentsch KM, Riond B, Hofmann-Lehmann R, Kircher PR, Grouzmann E, Reusch CE (2015) Urinary and plasma catecholamines and metanephrines in dogs with pheochromocytoma, hypercortisolism, nonadrenal disease and in healthy dogs. J Vet Int Med/Am Coll Vet Int Med 29:597–602
Sangster JK, Panciera DL, Abbott JA (2013) Cardiovascular effects of thyroid disease. Compendium 35, E5
Scavelli TD, Peterson ME, Matthiesen DT (1986) Results of surgical treatment for hyperadrenocorticism caused by adrenocortical neoplasia in the dog: 25 cases (1980-1984). J Am Vet Med Assoc 189:1360–1364
Schaefer C, Goldstein RE (2009) Canine primary hyperparathyroidism. Compendium 31:382–389; quiz 390
Schulman RL (2010) Feline primary hyperaldosteronism. Vet Clin North Am Small Anim Pract 40:353–359
Schultz RM, Wisner ER, Johnson EG, MacLeod JS (2009) Contrast-enhanced computed tomography as a preoperative indicator of vascular invasion from adrenal masses in dogs. Vet Radiol Ultrasound Off J Am Coll Vet Radiol Int Vet Radiol Assoc 50:625–629
Schwartz P, Kovak JR, Koprowski A, Ludwig LL, Monette S, Bergman PJ (2008) Evaluation of prognostic factors in the surgical treatment of adrenal gland tumors in dogs: 41 cases (1999-2005). J Am Vet Med Assoc 232:77–84
Schwedes CS (1997) Mitotane (o, p'-DDD) treatment in a cat with hyperadrenocorticism. J Small Anim Pract 38:520–524
Scott-Moncrieff JC (2012) Thyroid disorders in the geriatric veterinary patient. Vet Clin North Am Small Anim Pract 42(707–725):vi–vii
Sellon RK, Fidel J, Houston R, Gavin PR (2009) Linear-accelerator-based modified radiosurgical treatment of pituitary tumors in cats: 11 cases (1997-2008). J Vet Intern Med 23:1038–1044
Shiel RE, Mooney CT (2007) Testing for hyperthyroidism in cats. Vet Clin North Am Small Anim Pract 37(671–691):vi
Shilo Y, Pypendop BH, Barter LS, Epstein SE (2011) Thymoma removal in a cat with acquired myasthenia gravis: a case report and literature review of anesthetic techniques. Vet Anaesth Analg 38:603–613
Singh A, Boston SE, Poma R (2010) Thymoma-associated exfoliative dermatitis with post-thymectomy myasthenia gravis in a cat. Can Vet J La revue veterinaire canadienne 51:757–760
Skelly BJ, Franklin RJ (2007) Mutations in genes causing human familial isolated hyperparathyroidism do not account for hyperparathyroidism in Keeshond dogs. Vet J 174:652–654
Slingerland LI, Voorhout G, Rijnberk A, Kooistra HS (2008) Growth hormone excess and the effect of octreotide in cats with diabetes mellitus. Domest Anim Endocrinol 35:352–361
Spadavecchia C, Jaggy A (2008) Thymectomy in a cat with myasthenia gravis: a case report focusing on perianaesthetic management. Schweiz Arch Tierheilkd 150:515–518
Syme HM, Fletcher MG, Bailey SR, Elliott J (2007) Measurement of aldosterone in feline, canine and human urine. J Small Anim Pract 48:202–208
Taeymans O, Dennis R, Saunders JH (2008) Magnetic resonance imaging of the normal canine thyroid gland. Vet Radiol Ultrasound 49:238–242
Tobin RL, Nelson RW, Lucroy MD, Wooldridge JD, Feldman EC (1999) Outcome of surgical versus medical treatment of dogs with beta cell neoplasia: 39 cases (1990-1997). J Am Vet Med Assoc 215:226–230
Trepanier LA (2006) Medical management of hyperthyroidism. Clin Tech Small Anim Pract 21:22–28
Trepanier LA (2007) Pharmacologic management of feline hyperthyroidism. Vet Clin North Am Small Anim Pract 37(775–788):vii
Trifonidou MA, Kirpensteijn J, Robben JH (1998) A retrospective evaluation of 51 dogs with insulinoma. Vet Q 20(Suppl 1):S114–S115
Turrel JM, McEntee MC, Burke BP, Page RL (2006) Sodium iodide I 131 treatment of dogs with nonresectable thyroid tumors: 39 cases (1990-2003). Javma-J Am Vet Med A 229:542–548
van Sluijs FJ, Sjollema BE, Voorhout G, van den Ingh TS, Rijnberk A (1995) Results of adrenalectomy in 36 dogs with hyperadrenocorticism caused by adreno-cortical tumour. Vet Q 17:113–116
Vanderperren K, Haers H, Van der Vekens E, Stock E, Paepe D, Daminet S, Saunders JH (2014) Description of the use of contrast-enhanced ultrasonography in four dogs with pancreatic tumours. J Small Anim Pract 55:164–169

Volckaert V, Vandermeulen E, Dobbeleir A, Duchateau L, Saunders JH, Peremans K (2015) Effect of thyroid volume on radioiodine therapy outcome in hyperthyroid cats. J Feline Med Surg 18(2):144–149

Voorhout G, Stolp R, Rijnberk A, van Waes PF (1990) Assessment of survey radiography and comparison with x-ray computed tomography for detection of hyperfunctioning adrenocortical tumors in dogs. J Am Vet Med Assoc 196:1799–1803

Wagner RA, Piche CA, Jochle W, Oliver JW (2005) Clinical and endocrine responses to treatment with deslorelin acetate implants in ferrets with adrenocortical disease. Am J Vet Res 66:910–914

Weiss CA, Scott MV (1997) Clinical aspects and surgical treatment of hyperadrenocorticism in the domestic ferret: 94 cases (1994-1996). J Am Anim Hosp Assoc 33:487–493

Weiss CA, Williams BH, Scott MV (1998) Insulinoma in the ferret: clinical findings and treatment comparison of 66 cases. J Am Anim Hosp Assoc 34:471–475

Nervous System Tumors

Robert Klopfleisch

R. Klopfleisch (ed.), *Veterinary Oncology*, DOI 10.1007/978-3-319-41124-8_13

Nervous system tumors are of relevance in dogs and cats. These tumors are only rarely reported and, if present, not treated in other animals. A specific feature of all central nervous (CNS) tumors is that the common *criteria used for differentiation of benign and malignant tumors* do not implicitly apply. Every CNS tumor has to be considered malignant, independent from its invasiveness and metastatic character. Even slowly and noninvasively growing tumors may increase intracranial pressure or lead to compression of highly relevant brain areas and thus to neurological signs and death. Clinical symptoms are usually not specific for a certain tumor type and very much depend on the location of the tumor. Seizures and changes in consciousness and behavior are most commonly observed. *Metastasis* to organs outside the brain is very rare for all CNS tumors. Secondary tumors, i.e., metastases to the brain, occur occasionally. The most common second CNS tumors are hemangiosarcomas; mammary, pulmonary, and prostatic carcinomas; malignant melanomas; and lymphomas.

Meningioma and gliomas (i.e., astrocytomas and oligodendrogliomas) are the most common tumors of the CNS in most species and will be discussed in detail in this chapter. There are however several other tumor types, which are rather rare in veterinary oncology and therefore not discussed in this chapter. These include:

13

- *Choroid plexus papillomas and carcinomas*, which originate from cells of the choroid plexus. They compress the adjacent neuropil and are often associated with hydrocephalus due to excessive liquor production and obstipation of the draining channels. Intracranial metastasis into other ventricular structures can be observed, but metastasis to extracranial organs is uncommon.
- *Ependymomas*, which originate from the ependymal cells lining the ventricular system of the brain. Similar to choroid plexus tumors, they may lead to hydrocephalus due to liquor drainage block.
- *Primitive neuroectodermal tumors* are rare tumors of young animals. They are usually invasive and fast-growing neoplasias.

13.1 Canine Nervous System Tumors

A wide variety of nervous system tumors has been described in dogs. Of these, glioma of astrocytic or oligodendrocytic origin, meningiomas, and peripheral nerve sheath tumors are diagnosed with a higher frequency.

13.1.1 Canine Gliomas

Box 13.1. Canine Gliomas in Five Facts

1. Are separated into astrocytomas (glioblastomas) and oligodendrogliomas
2. Similar incidence to meningiomas
3. Mostly aged and brachycephalic dogs, i.e., boxers
4. Gliomas are associated with a poor prognosis (untreated <1 month median survival time)
5. Combination of surgery and postsurgical radiotherapy may lead to increased survival

Epidemiology and Pathology

Gliomas are common brain tumors in dogs. They are differentiated into astrocytomas and oligodendrogliomas. Both tumor types are mostly observed in dogs at the *age* of 7–10. There is a *breed* predisposition for large and brachycephalic breeds, i.e., boxers. *Astrocytomas* derive from astrocytes and are graded based on their histologic appearance into *well differentiated* (low grade), *anaplastic* (medium grade) and *glioblastomas* (high grade) (◘ Fig. 13.1). Astrocytomas grow invasively, metastasize within the CNS but do not metastasize to organs outside the CNS. Mutations in the p53, retinoblastoma, and p16 genes have been reported in astrocytomas. *Oligodendrogliomas* are derived from oligodendrocytic cells. They are commonly observed in the frontal and pyriform lobes, thalamus, and the white matter of cerebrum but may also occur in the spinal cord (◘ Fig. 13.2). The etiology and pathogenesis of these tumors is unclear.

Clinical Appearance

Clinical signs associated with canine gliomas depend on tumor location within the brain. Independent from the location, most dogs have a history of seizures and slow progressive behavioral changes. All aged dogs with these symptoms are therefore potentially affected by a CNS tumor.

Magnetic resonance imaging (MRI) is the diagnostic modality of choice for CNS tumors. It

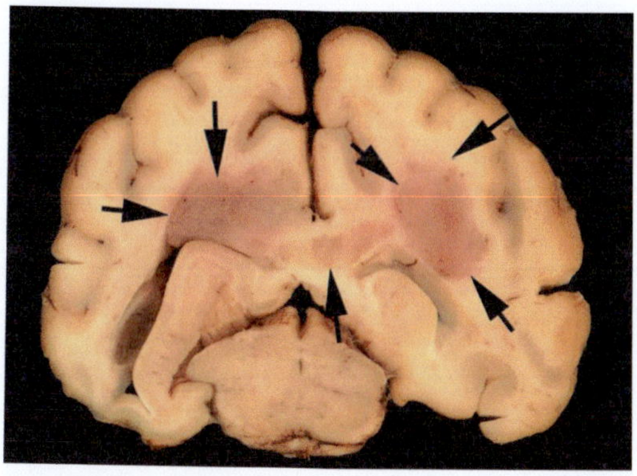

Fig. 13.1 Middle grade astrocytoma in a dog (*arrows*). Astrocytomas are usually poorly defined and *white to pink*. High-grade glioblastoma are often characterized by necrosis and hemorrhage

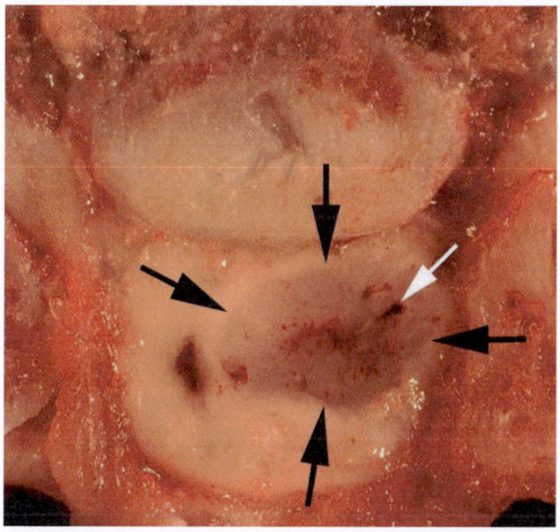

Fig. 13.2 Oligodendroglioma in the spinal cord of a dog (*black arrows*). At necropsy oligodendrogliomas are usually well demarcated and gelatinous tumors compressing the surrounding neuropil. Intra-tumoral hemorrhage is also a common finding (*white arrow*)

allows evaluating the location and extent of the tumor. Contrast agents can be used and accumulate within or around the tumor and increase the sensitivity of tumor detection. However, the unequivocal differentiation of glioma from non-neoplastic disease is not possible due to overlapping features. Combination of the imaging data with clinical signs and epidemiology however gives a good hint on the nature of the lesion.

Cerebrospinal fluid analysis, *standard blood tests*, and thoracic radiographs are not diagnostic for CNS tumors but helpful to exclude concurrent diseases.

Cytology and Histopathology

Intravitam *biopsy taking* of suspected intracranial tumors is uncommon because of the associated high surgical efforts and the high morbidity and mortality of these attempts. *Histologic analysis* is therefore mostly restricted to postmortem diagnosis. However, a recent study showed that *frame-based stereotactic brain biopsies* (*FBSB*), which uses MRI and CT images to establish stereotactic planes to allow for biopsy taking without intraoperative image guidance, are safe and provide neuropathological diagnoses.

Therapy

A recent meta-analysis identified radiotherapy and surgery to have a beneficial effect. Interestingly, there is little difference between the outcome after radiotherapy and surgery alone.

Radiotherapy is the treatment of choice for canine brain tumors. Fractionated radiation therapy protocols can be associated with survival times of up to 10 months, while dogs without treatment have survival times of less than a month. *Stereotactic radiosurgery (SRS)* is a new treatment option for CNS tumors. It includes the delivery of a single high dose of ionizing radiation to a defined anatomic target. Administration of the high dose of radiation is ablating the tumor similar to a surgical resection. The linear accelerators used in this approach are therefore often named radio knives.

Surgical excision of gliomas or parts of them requires advanced surgical skills. Complete or partial resection depends on the location of the tumor. The invasive character and the difficulties to unequivocally define the tumor margins hamper complete resection in almost all cases. However, partial resection may have a short-term palliative effect by decreasing intracranial pressure. Combination of surgery with postsurgical radiotherapy may increase the survival time, but larger clinical studies on this question are currently not available.

The knowledge on the effects of *chemotherapeutic agents* is restricted to few case reports. Lomustine, carmustine, and hydroxyurea may have a palliative and life-prolonging effect.

Prognosis

The prognosis for canine gliomas is poor. Untreated dogs die or are euthanized within less than a month after diagnosis. Surgery and radiotherapy may prolong post-diagnosis survival times up to several months but require specialized clinical skills and are associated with a high mortality rate.

13.1.2 Canine Meningiomas

Box 13.2. Canine Meningioma in Five Facts

1. Are tumor of aged, dolichocephalic dogs.
2. Growth mostly expansive but occasionally infiltrative.
3. Fast-growing meningiomas and meningiomas growing around cranial/spinal nerve roots can cause clinical signs.
4. Surgery is often successful for meningiomas of the forebrain.
5. Additional or exclusive radiotherapy is recommended for invasive meningiomas and meningiomas on the cerebellum, brain stem, or distal brain surfaces.

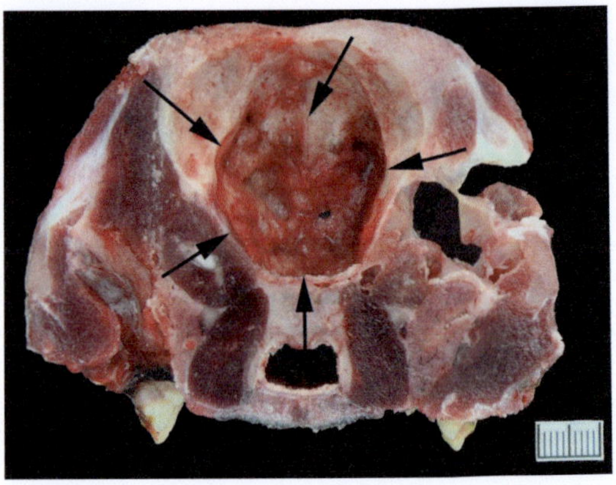

Fig. 13.3 Infiltrative meningioma in the frontal/rostral region of the calvarium of a dog

Epidemiology and Pathology

Meningiomas are as common as gliomas in dogs. They are derived from cap cells covering the arachnoid granulations of the dura mater and common tumors in dogs older than *8 years*. Dolichocephalic *breeds* and golden retriever have a breed predisposition. There is no sex predisposition. Meningiomas are often slow growing, discrete, expansile neoplasms developing of the calvarium and here mostly of the olfactory/frontal region (Fig. 13.3). Canine meningiomas may be quite invasive associated with clinical signs. Metastases are very rare.

Clinical Appearance

Clinical signs associated with meningiomas are usually slowly progressing due to the low growth rate of most meningiomas. Altered consciousness, seizures, vestibular dysfunction, and cranial nerve deficits are the most common clinical signs associated with canine meningiomas. Some meningiomas are incidental findings at necropsy.

Magnetic resonance imaging (MRI) is the diagnostic modality of choice for intracranial tumors. It allows evaluating the location and extent of the tumor. Contrast agents can be used and accumulate within or around the tumor and increase the sensitivity of tumor detection. However, the unequivocal differentiation of the diverse CNS tumor types from each other and from nonneoplastic disease is not always possible due to overlapping features. Typical MRI feature of meningiomas is displacement instead of invasion of adjacent superficial brain structures, occasionally cystic spaces or mineralization and the "dural tail," which describes a taillike extension from the main meningioma mass along the neuropil surface.

Cerebrospinal fluid analysis, standard blood tests and thoracic radiographs are not diagnostic for meningiomas but helpful to exclude concurrent diseases.

Cytology and Histopathology

Intravitam *biopsy taking* of suspected brain tumors is uncommon because of the associated high surgical efforts and the high mortality associated with these attempts. *Histologic analysis* is therefore restricted to postmortem diagnostics but allows for a final diagnosis. However, a recent study showed that *frame-based stereotactic brain biopsies* (*FBSB*), which uses MRI and CT images to establish stereotactic planes to allow for biopsy taking without intraoperative image guidance, are safe and provide neuropathological diagnoses. Several histologic subtypes are described, but their clinical relevance is unclear. There are attempts to include a histologic grading into the histopathologic diagnosis of canine meningiomas, which is however of minor clinical relevance yet.

Therapy

Surgical excision is the method of choice for meningiomas located on the cerebral cortical surface. Survival times of 7 months and more have been reported. Canine meningiomas however tend to be more infiltratively growing than feline meningiomas. Some authors therefore recommend surgery only in combination with postsurgical radiotherapy.

Radiotherapy is the treatment of choice for canine meningiomas not located on the cerebral cortical surface. Fractionated radiation therapy protocols can be associated with survival times of few months to several years. In contrast, dogs without treatment have survival times of less than a month. Combination of surgery with postsurgical radiotherapy may increase the survival time up to 2–7 years.

The knowledge on the effects of *chemotherapeutic agents* is restricted to few case reports. Treatment with hydroxyurea and glucocorticoids only is associated with survival times of up to 6 months.

▪ Prognosis

The prognosis for canine meningiomas is better than for glioma tumors but still poor if clinical signs are present. As mentioned above, treatment may prolong survival times. In addition, cranial location on the forebrain is associated with survival times of 7 years, while caudal or distal meningiomas are associated with survival times of less than 2 years. The impact of general histologic subtyping for prognosis is not fully confirmed. However, signs of malignancy and infiltrative growth are associated with significantly shorter survival times.

13.1.3 Canine Peripheral Nerve Sheath Tumors (PNST)

Box 13.3. Canine Peripheral Nerve Sheath Tumors (PNST) in Six Facts

1. Are differentiated into peripheral nervous system and subcutaneous PNST.
2. Can occur at any spinal or cranial nerve and their peripheral ramifications.
3. Associated with hypoesthesia, lameness, and paralysis.
4. Surgery is the treatment of choice.
5. Full resection is difficult to achieve due to their infiltrative growth.
6. Prognosis is guarded to poor.

▪ Epidemiology and Pathology

There is still some controversy on the definition of *peripheral nerve sheath tumors (PNST)*. The narrowest definition only includes tumors unequivocally arising from *Schwann cells* or their precursors around the cranial and spinal nerves and often the brachial plexus. There is however a discussion on whether or not some or most of the canine subcutaneous *soft tissue sarcomas (STS)* are actually also PNST, although their "nerve of origin" is usually unknown. In this chapter, we discuss only PNST in the narrow, i.e., tumors arising around spinal and cranial nerves and the brachial plexus. The reader is referred to Chap. 4 on subcutaneous STS for more information on subcutaneous PNST.

PNST occur in middle-aged to old dogs without a specific breed predisposition. Occasionally, PNST are subclassified into schwannoma, neurofibroma, and neurofibrosarcoma. This separation is however clinically irrelevant. PNST cells are characterized by a typical ultrastructure and expression genes like nerve growth factor receptor (NGFR), S100, PGP9.5, GLI1, and CLEC3B.

▪ Clinical Appearance

Clinical signs associated with PNST depend on tumor location but often include hypoesthesia, paresis, and paralysis. Brachial plexus tumors of decent size may be palpable. Magnetic resonance imaging is the imaging modality of choice for the detection of PNST. Smaller tumors may not be apparent as a mass but associated with mild disturbance of the physiologic arrangement of the surrounding nerves and other tissues.

▪ Cytology and Histopathology

Cytologic preparations of PNST are characterized by loosely cohesive clusters and fascicular arrangement of spindle cells with rounded ends, a mild nuclear pleomorphic and a fibrillary background. *Histologically*, PNST are well circumscribed and contain spindle to ovoid cells with small amounts of eosinophilic cytoplasm. There are more tightly packed cells in the so-called Antoni A patterns and parallel rows of palisading nuclei (Verocay-like bodies). Whorling of the neoplastic spindle cells often whorl (fingerprint pattern) around capillaries and/or collagen, and myxoid areas are common.

▪ Therapy

Surgical excision is the treatment of choice for canine PNST. This may include limb amputation for brachial plexus PNST and laminectomy for spinal nerve PNST. Resection is mostly not complete due to infiltrative character of PNST. *Postoperative radiotherapy* may therefore be helpful to ablate remaining tumor cells. Comprehensive clinical studies on this topic are however lacking.

▪ Prognosis

PNST of the spinal and cranial nerves and the brachial plexus have a *guarded to poor prognosis* due to their infiltrative characters. In contrast, subcutaneous PNST have a much better prognosis because they are more often completely resectable.

13.2 Feline Nervous System Tumors

Nervous system tumors *are rare in cats* with the exception of meningiomas of older cats. Gliomas, ependymomas, and intracranial lymphomas are occasionally reported. Peripheral nerve sheath tumors (PNST) are exceptional cases.

13.2.1 Feline Gliomas

Box 13.4. Feline Gliomas in Three Facts

1. Are rare (<10 % of intracranial tumors).
2. Clinical signs depend on location, but altered consciousness and seizures are most common.
3. Few case report on successful treatment with surgery or radiotherapy.

▪ Epidemiology and Pathology

Gliomas are rare brain tumors in cats, representing less than 10 % of all brain tumors (85 % meningiomas). They are separated into astrocytomas and oligodendrogliomas. *Astrocytomas* are derived from astrocytes and graded based on their histologic appearance as *well differentiated* (low grade), *anaplastic* (medium grade), and *glioblastoma* (high grade). Astrocytomas grow invasively, metastasize within the CNS, but do not metastasize to organs outside the CNS. *Oligodendrogliomas* are derived from oligodendrocytic cells. The etiology and pathogenesis of gliomas in the cat are unclear.

There are only few case reports on feline gliomas. These are mostly reports of tumors in cats older than 10 years of *age*, and the reported *tumor locations* are mostly in the forebrain.

▪ Clinical Appearance

Clinical signs associated with gliomas in cats depend on the location of the tumor within the brain. However, most cats have altered consciousness, such as depression; stupor, or coma; circling; seizures; ataxia; and behavioral changes.

Magnetic resonance imaging (MRI) is the diagnostic modality of choice for brain tumors. It allows to evaluate the location and extent of the tumor. Contrast agents can be used and accumulate within or around the tumor and increase the sensitivity of tumor detection. However, the unequivocal differentiation of glioma from nonneoplastic disease is not possible due to overlapping features. Combination of the tumor location with clinical signs however gives a good hint on the nature of the lesion.

Cerebrospinal fluid analysis, standard blood tests, and thoracic radiographs are not diagnostic for brain tumors but helpful to exclude concurrent diseases.

▪ Cytology and Histopathology

Intravitam *biopsy taking* of suspected brain tumors is uncommon because of the associated high surgical efforts and the high morbidity and mortality of these attempts. *Histologic analysis* is therefore mostly restricted to postmortem diagnosis. However, a recent study (in dogs) showed that *frame-based stereotactic brain biopsies (FBSB)*, which uses MRI and CT images to establish stereotactic planes to allow for exact biopsy taking without intraoperative image guidance, are safe and provide neuropathological diagnoses.

▪ Therapy

A recent meta-analysis identified *radiotherapy* and *surgery* to have a beneficial effect for canine tumors. Similar data are lacking for the cat.

There are single case reports on the effect of surgery, radiotherapy, and even chemotherapy. The number of reported cases is nevertheless too little to give an educated recommendation on therapy. Most authors however expect at least similar responses of feline gliomas compared to canine glioma.

Prognosis

The prognosis for untreated feline gliomas is poor with survival times of few weeks. Two case reports however show a remission for a 4 years' period after surgery or radiotherapy in two cats with gliomas.

13.2.2 Feline Meningiomas

Box 13.5. Feline Meningiomas in Four Facts

1. A common tumor of older cats
2. Often incidental necropsy findings but may induce altered consciousness, seizures, and behavioral changes
3. Surgical excision treatment of choice with acceptable success rate
4. Little to no information on radiotherapy/chemotherapy success available

Epidemiology and Pathology

Meningiomas are the *most common feline nervous system tumor* (85 % of all intracranial tumors). Approximately 20 % of the cats with meningioma have multiple meningiomas. Meningiomas are derived from cap cells covering the arachnoid granulations of the dura mater and occur mostly in cats older than *9 years*. There is a mild sex predisposition for male cats. Feline meningiomas are mostly slow growing, discrete, expansile nonmetastatic neoplasms developing on the surface of the cerebrum. Feline meningiomas are often an incidental finding during necropsy of older cats without any history of neuronal signs (Fig. 13.4).

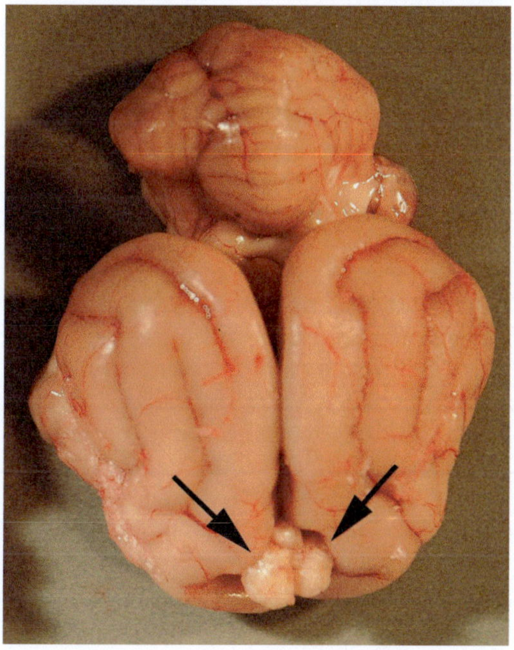

Fig. 13.4 Meningioma in a cat. The tumor was an incidental finding in an older cat without any neurologic disturbances

Clinical Appearance

Clinical signs associated with meningiomas are usually slowly progressing due to the low growth rate of most meningiomas. Altered consciousness, seizures, behavioral changes, and occasionally cranial nerve deficits are the most commonly observed clinical signs.

Magnetic resonance imaging (MRI) is the diagnostic modality of choice for intracranial tumors. It allows to evaluate the location and extent of the tumor. Contrast agents can be used and accumulate within or around the tumor and increase the sensitivity of tumor detection. However, the unequivocal differentiation of the diverse CNS tumor types from each other and from nonneoplastic disease is not always possible due to overlapping features. Typical MRI feature of meningiomas is displacement instead of invasion of adjacent, superficial brain structures, occasionally cystic spaces, or mineralization and the "dural tail," which describes a taillike extension from the main meningioma mass along the neuropil surface.

Cerebrospinal fluid analysis, standard blood tests, and thoracic radiographs are not diagnostic for meningiomas but helpful to exclude concurrent diseases.

Cytology and Histopathology

Intravitam *biopsy taking* of suspected brain tumors is uncommon because of the associated high surgical efforts and the high morbidity and mortality of these attempts. *Histologic analysis* is therefore restricted to postmortem diagnostics but allows for a final diagnosis. However, a recent study (in dogs) showed that *frame-based stereotactic brain biopsies* (*FBSB*), which uses MRI and CT images to establish stereotactic planes to allow for biopsy taking without intraoperative image guidance, are safe and provide neuropathological diagnoses. Feline meningiomas are much less diverse in their histologic appearance and are mostly composed of *long spindle to epitheloid cells* arranged in long fascicles or whorls.

- **Therapy**

Surgical excision is the method of choice for feline meningiomas because tumors in this species are mostly well circumscribed. It is associated with median survival times of more than 2 years. A postsurgical recurrence has been reported for 20 % of cases.

There is no educated information on the relevance of *radiotherapy* or chemotherapy on the outcome of feline meningiomas.

- **Prognosis**

The prognosis for feline meningiomas is guarded. Due to their slow growth and well-defined tumor boarders, feline meningiomas may stay clinically inapparent or have an 80 % chance of complete resection.

Suggested Reading

Adamo PF, Forrest L, Dubielzig RR (2004) Canine and feline meningiomas: diagnosis, treatment and prognosis. Compend Contin Educ Pract Vet 27:951–966

Axlund TW, McGlasson ML, Smith AN (2002) Surgery alone or in combination with radiation therapy for treatment of intracranial meningiomas in dogs: 31 cases (1989-2002). J Am Vet Med Assoc 221:1597–1600

Bagley RS, Gavin PR (1998) Seizures as a complication of brain tumors in dogs. Clin Tech Small Anim Pract 13:179–184

Bagley RS, Gavin PR, Moore MP, Silver GM, Harrington ML, Connors RL (1999) Clinical signs associated with brain tumors in dogs: 97 cases (1992-1997). J Am Vet Med Assoc 215:818–819

Bentley RT (2015) Magnetic resonance imaging diagnosis of brain tumors in dogs. Vet J 205:204–216

Bentley RT, Ober CP, Anderson KL, Feeney DA, Naughton JF, Ohlfest JR, O'Sullivan MG, Miller MA, Constable PD, Pluhar GE (2013) Canine intracranial gliomas: relationship between magnetic resonance imaging criteria and tumor type and grade. Vet J 198:463–471

Brearley MJ, Jeffery ND, Phillips SM, Dennis R (1999) Hypofractionated radiation therapy of brain masses in dogs: a retrospective analysis of survival of 83 cases (1991-1996). J Vet Intern Med 13:408–412

Dennis MM, McSporran KD, Bacon NJ, Schulman FY, Foster RA, Powers BE (2011) Prognostic factors for cutaneous and subcutaneous soft tissue sarcomas in dogs. Vet Pathol 48:73–84

Ettinger SN (2003) Principles of treatment for soft-tissue sarcomas in the dog. Clin Tech Small Anim Pract 18:118–122

Forterre F, Jaggy A, Rohrbach H, Dickomeit M, Konar M (2009) Modified temporal approach for a rostrotemporal basal meningioma in a cat. J Feline Med Surg 11:510–513

Graham JP, Newell SM, Voges AK, Roberts GD, Harrison JM (1998) The dural tail sign in the diagnosis of meningiomas. Vet Radiol Ultrasound 39:297–302

Gupta K, Dey P, Vashisht R (2004) Fine-needle aspiration cytology of malignant peripheral nerve sheath tumors. Diagn Cytopathol 31:1–4

Hu H, Barker A, Harcourt-Brown T, Jeffery N (2015) Systematic review of brain tumor treatment in dogs. J Vet Intern Med 29:1456–1463

Ijiri A, Yoshiki K, Tsuboi S, Shimazaki H, Akiyoshi H, Nakade T (2014) Surgical resection of twenty-three cases of brain meningioma. J Vet Med Sci 76:331–338

Klopfleisch R, Meyer A, Lenze D, Hummel M, Gruber AD (2013) Canine cutaneous peripheral nerve sheath tumours versus fibrosarcomas can be differentiated by neuroectodermal marker genes in their transcriptome. J Comp Pathol 148:197–205

Klopp LS, Rao S (2009) Endoscopic-assisted intracranial tumor removal in dogs and cats: long-term outcome of 39 cases. J Vet Intern Med 23:108–115

Kraft S, Ehrhart EJ, Gall D, Klopp L, Gavin P, Tucker R, Bagley R, Kippenes H, DeHaan C, Pedroia V, Partington B, Olby N (2007) Magnetic resonance imaging characteristics of peripheral nerve sheath tumors of the canine brachial plexus in 18 dogs. Vet Radiol Ultrasound 48:1–7

Lipsitz D, Higgins RJ, Kortz GD, Dickinson PJ, Bollen AW, Naydan DK, LeCouteur RA (2003) Glioblastoma multiforme: clinical findings, magnetic resonance imaging, and pathology in five dogs. Vet Pathol 40:659–669

Lu D, Pocknell A, Lamb CR, Targett MP (2003) Concurrent benign and malignant multiple meningiomas in a cat: clinical, MRI and pathological findings. Vet Rec 152:780–782

MacLeod AG, Dickinson PJ, LeCouteur RA, Higgins RJ, Pollard RE (2009) Quantitative assessment of blood volume and permeability in cerebral mass lesions using dynamic contrast-enhanced computed tomography in the dog. Acad Radiol 16:1187–1195

Mariani CL, Schubert TA, House RA, Wong MA, Hopkins AL, Barnes Heller HL, Milner RJ, Lester NV, Lurie DM, Rajon DA, Friedman WA, Bova FJ (2015) Frameless stereotactic radiosurgery for the treatment of primary intracranial tumours in dogs. Vet Comp Oncol 13:409–423

Meyer A, Klopfleisch R (2014) Multiple polymerase chain reaction markers for the differentiation of canine cutaneous peripheral nerve sheath tumours versus canine fibrosarcomas. J Comp Pathol 150:198–203

Motta L, Mandara MT, Skerritt GC (2012) Canine and feline intracranial meningiomas: an updated review. Vet J 192:153–165

Nafe LA (1979) Meningiomas in cats: a retrospective clinical study of 36 cases. J Am Vet Med Assoc 174:1224–1227

Oliveira M, De La Fuente C, Pumarola M, Anor S (2014) Imaging diagnosis: cranial cervical intraspinal schwannoma in a dog. Vet Radiol Ultrasound 55:300–304

Pang DS, Allaire J, Rondenay Y, Kaartinen J, Cuvelliez SG, Troncy E (2009) The use of lingual venous blood to determine the acid-base and blood-gas status of dogs under anesthesia. Vet Anaesth Analg 36:124–132

Platt SR, Alleman AR, Lanz OI, Chrisman CL (2002) Comparison of fine-needle aspiration and surgical-tissue biopsy in the diagnosis of canine brain tumors. Vet Surg 31:65–69

Polizopoulou ZS, Koutinas AF, Souftas VD, Kaldrymidou E, Kazakos G, Papadopoulos G (2004) Diagnostic correlation of CT-MRI and histopathology in 10 dogs with brain neoplasms. J Vet Med A 51:226–231

Rodenas S, Pumarola M, Gaitero L, Zamora A, Anor S (2011) Magnetic resonance imaging findings in 40 dogs with histologically confirmed intracranial tumours. Vet J 187:85–91

Rose S, Long C, Knipe M, Hornof B (2005) Ultrasonographic evaluation of brachial plexus tumors in five dogs. Vet Radiol Ultrasound 46:514–517

Rossmeisl JH (2014) New treatment modalities for brain tumors in dogs and cats. Vet Clin North Am Small Anim Pract 44:1013–1038

Rossmeisl JH Jr, Jones JC, Zimmerman KL, Robertson JL (2013) Survival time following hospital discharge in dogs with palliatively treated primary brain tumors. J Am Vet Med Assoc 242:193–198

Rossmeisl JH, Andriani RT, Cecere TE, Lahmers K, LeRoith T, Zimmerman KL, Gibo D, Debinski W (2015) Frame-based stereotactic biopsy of canine brain masses: technique and clinical results in 26 cases. Front Vet Sci 2:20

Shihab N, Summers BA, Benigni L, McEvoy AW, Volk HA (2013) Imaging diagnosis-malignant peripheral nerve sheath tumor presenting as an intra-axial brain mass in a young dog. Vet Radiol Ultrasound 54:278–282

Snyder JM, Shofer FS, Van Winkle TJ, Massicotte C (2006) Canine intracranial primary neoplasia: 173 cases (1986-2003). J Vet Intern Med 20:669–675

Song RB, Vite CH, Bradley CW, Cross JR (2013) Postmortem evaluation of 435 cases of intracranial neoplasia in dogs and relationship of neoplasm with breed, age, and body weight. J Vet Intern Med 27:1143–1152

Stoica G, Kim HT, Hall DG, Coates JR (2004) Morphology, immunohistochemistry, and genetic alterations in dog astrocytomas. Vet Pathol 41:10–19

Sturges BK, Dickinson PJ, Bollen AW, Koblik PD, Kass PH, Kortz GD, Vernau KM, Knipe MF, Lecouteur RA, Higgins RJ (2008) Magnetic resonance imaging and histological classification of intracranial meningiomas in 112 dogs. J Vet Intern Med 22:586–595

Suzuki S, Uchida K, Nakayama H (2014) The effects of tumor location on diagnostic criteria for canine malignant peripheral nerve sheath tumors (MPNST) and the markers for distinction between canine MPNST and canine perivascular wall tumors. Vet Pathol 51:722–736

Tamura S, Tamura Y, Ohoka A, Hasegawa T, Uchida K (2007) A canine case of skull base meningioma treated with hydroxyurea. J Vet Med Sci 69:1313–1315

Tamura M, Hasegawa D, Uchida K, Kuwabara T, Mizoguchi S, Ochi N, Fujita M (2013a) Feline anaplastic oligodendroglioma: long-term remission through radiation therapy and chemotherapy. J Feline Med Surg 15:1137–1140

Tamura S, Hori Y, Tamura Y, Uchida K (2013b) Long-term follow-up of surgical treatment of spinal anaplastic astrocytoma in a cat. J Feline Med Surg 15:921–926

Tomek A, Cizinauskas S, Doherr M, Gandini G, Jaggy A (2006) Intracranial neoplasia in 61 cats: localisation, tumour types and seizure patterns. J Feline Med Surg 8:243–253

Troxel MT, Vite CH, Van Winkle TJ, Newton AL, Tiches D, Dayrell-Hart B, Kapatkin AS, Shofer FS, Steinberg SA (2003) Feline intracranial neoplasia: retrospective review of 160 cases (1985-2001). J Vet Intern Med 17:850–859

Troxel MT, Vite CH, Massicotte C, McLear RC, Van Winkle TJ, Glass EN, Tiches D, Dayrell-Hart B (2004) Magnetic resonance imaging features of feline intracranial neoplasia: retrospective analysis of 46 cats. J Vet Intern Med Am Coll Vet Intern Med 18:176–189

Wisner ER, Dickinson PJ, Higgins RJ (2011) Magnetic resonance imaging features of canine intracranial neoplasia. Vet Radiol Ultrasound 52:S52–S61

York D, Higgins RJ, LeCouteur RA, Wolfe AN, Grahn R, Olby N, Campbell M, Dickinson PJ (2012) TP53 mutations in canine brain tumors. Vet Pathol 49:796–801

Young BD, Levine JM, Porter BF, Chen-Allen AV, Rossmeisl JH, Platt SR, Kent M, Fosgate GT, Schatzberg SJ (2011) Magnetic resonance imaging features of intracranial astrocytomas and oligodendrogliomas in dogs. Vet Radiol Ultrasound 52:132–141

Respiratory System Tumors

Robert Klopfleisch

R. Klopfleisch (ed.), *Veterinary Oncology*, DOI 10.1007/978-3-319-41124-8_14

14.1 Nasal Cavity Tumors

Tumors of the nasal cavity or nasal sinus usually have a varied cellular origin. Despite this difference in histopathology, they often have similar clinical presentations and are therefore treated with identical therapeutic protocols, regardless of cell type. Histologically, the tumor types found in the nasal and sinus cavities include: adenocarcinomas and anaplastic carcinomas derived from the nasal mucosa, squamous cell carcinoma derived from nasal squamous epithelium, and sarcomas (fibrosarcomas, chondrosarcoma, osteosarcoma). Due to their different histologic origins, they are associated with slightly different prognoses. Epithelial tumors have a median survival time of 9–13 months, while fibrosarcomas are associated with a survival of up to 24 months. Lymphoma is the most common tumor of the nasal cavity in cats (▶ see Chap. 6). Nasal lymphomas are rare in dogs. Nasal cavity tumors in other species are very rare, except for the retrovirus-induced enzootic nasal tumor (ENT) of sheep.

14.1.1 Canine Nasal Cavity Tumor

Box 14.1. Canine Nasal Cavity Tumors in Six Facts

1. The term "canine nasal cavity tumors" summarizes several mostly malignant tumor types
2. All tumor types show invasive growth and metastasis in advanced stages
3. Clinical appearance may resemble nonneoplastic rhinitis
4. Radiographs, computed tomography (CT), and magnetic resonance imaging (MRI) are necessary for staging
5. Biopsy or histopathology is required for final diagnosis
6. Radiotherapy is the treatment of choice

▪ Epidemiology and Pathogenesis

Nasal cavity tumors are rather rare tumors in the dog. They may occur at any age but a peak of first diagnosis is observed at the *age* of 10 years. Sarcomas occur earlier (around 5–7 years of age). There is a minimal *gender* predisposition for males and probably a *breed* predisposition for dolichocephalic dogs. Prolonged *exposure to air pollutants* like fumes and exhaust gases may contribute to the development of the tumors, but the available data are insufficient to prove a correlation. In the dog, approximately two-thirds are nasal *epithelial tumors* like anaplastic carcinomas, adenocarcinomas, and squamous cell carcinomas (SCC). *Mesenchymal sarcomas* are less common. Nasal lymphomas are rare in the dog, in contrast to the cat. *Benign tumors* like polyps may occur but are less common.

Aberrant expression of *p53* and *growth factor receptors* has been detected in different epithelial nasal cavity tumors and is believed to be involved in their carcinogenesis. However, the exact mechanisms of carcinogenesis in the nasal cavity are unknown.

▪ Clinical Appearance

The *clinical signs* for nasal cavity tumors are unspecific and initially resemble rhinitis. *Mucopurulent nasal discharge, epistaxis, and facial deformations* are the most common observation. Treatment of secondary inflammation with antibiotics or anti-inflammatories may lead to a short-term improvement of clinical signs. Malignant nasal tumors of all histologic types are *invasive*. Final stage nasal tumors *metastasize* in *up to 50 % of the cases*. Metastases are most common in the regional lymph nodes or the lung.

Imaging and histology are required for accurate diagnosis of nasal cavity tumors. *Radiography* is able to sensitively diagnose advanced tumors. Smaller tumors, however, have a better chance to be diagnosed with *computed tomography* (*CT*) *or magnetic resonance imaging* (*MRI*) due to the better resolution of the nasal cavity structures in cross-sectional images. Cytology or histology is required to distinguish between nasal cavity tumors and granulomas, which appear similar in X-ray, CT, or MRI. (◘ Table 14.1) have proposed a *staging system* for nasal cavity tumors based on diagnostic imaging.

Rhinoscopy is sometimes helpful to evaluate the extent of the tumor and can show foreign bodies in granulomatous rhinitis. It should be performed after diagnostic imaging as it often induces severe hemorrhage or requires flushing of the nasal cavity, both of which alter CT, MRI, or radiographic findings.

▪ Cytology and Histopathology

Tumor cells can be obtained by *punch biopsies, fine-needle aspiration, curettages, and nasal lavages*. Blind biopsies have the same diagnostic

Table 14.1 Staging system for canine nasal cavity tumors

Stage	Features	Survival time (months)
1	Unilateral with no bone involvement	24
2	Any tumor with bone involvement	14
3	Extension to the orbit or subcutis	16
4	Lysis of the cribriform plate	7

value as rhinoscopy-guided biopsies. Repeated biopsies are frequently required for definitive diagnosis. Biopsy of the nasal cavity should be performed under general anesthesia, and patients should be intubated due to the potential for massive bleeding (and subsequent aspiration). Biopsy devices should not be introduced deeper into the nasal cavity than the medial canthus of the eye.

Cytology of samples obtained by imprints of biopsies, Cytobrush, or fine-needle aspirates is often diagnostic (>80 % of cases), especially for epithelial tumors which exhibit characteristic proliferative or even pleomorphic tumor cells (Figs. 14.1 and 14.2). Cytological specimens prepared from nasal flushes are less diagnostic (only 50 %) as the number of tumor cells contained in the fluid is relatively low in comparison. Secondary inflammation and failure to target the main tumor mass can lead to a false negative diagnosis of rhinitis. In cases with a low number of tumor cells or only mild signs of malignancy, it might be difficult to differentiate neoplasia from dysplasia.

Up to one-quarter of nasal cavity, tumors test positive on *lymph node cytology* for metastatic cells, most often with carcinomas.

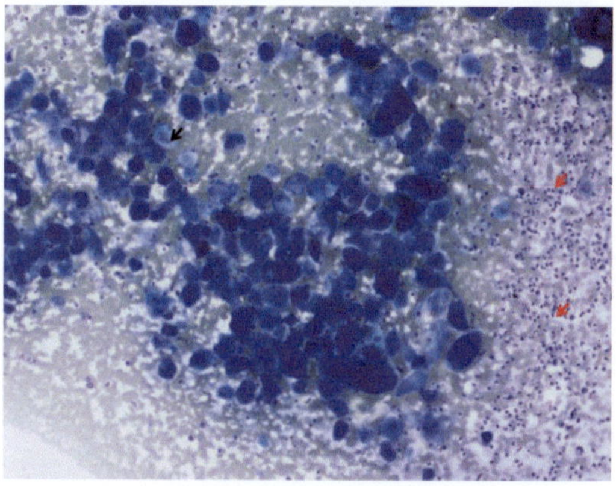

Fig. 14.1 Cytology, nasal squamous cell carcinoma, dog, May-Grünwald-Giemsa, 100×. Note the round to polygonal, turquoise to deeply basophilic cells with central round to oval nuclei and moderate to marked anisocytosis, anisokaryosis and pleomorphism. There is a marked focal purulent inflammation (*red arrows*) (Photo with permission of Dr. N. Bauer, Faculty of Veterinary Medicine, Justus Liebig University, Giessen, Germany)

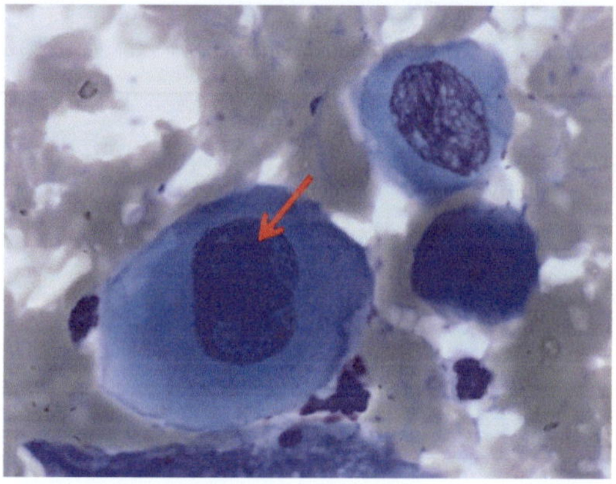

Fig. 14.2 Cytology, nasal squamous cell carcinoma, dog (same case as in Fig. 14.1.) May-Grünwald-Giemsa, 1000×. Note the binucleated cell with large macronucleoli (*red arrows*) and the moderate to marked anisocytosis, anisokaryosis, and pleomorphism of cells (Photo with permission from Dr. N. Bauer, Faculty of Veterinary Medicine, Justus Liebig University, Giessen, Germany)

Therapy

Therapy of nasal cavity tumors generally aims at *local disease control.* If epistaxis is present, mean survival times are as low as 3–5 months without treatment after initial diagnosis.

Surgical treatment with rhinotomy is associated with a high rate of nonneoplastic morbidity in dogs and therefore does not significantly increase the survival time. However, dogs with small, well-circumscribed, unilateral tumors may be good candidates for exclusive surgical treatment. Survival can be further prolonged with radiotherapy and additional surgical excision of surviving tumor cells.

Radiotherapy is the treatment of choice, although there are also contradictory studies that challenge the general efficacy of radiotherapy and its superiority to surgery. Other studies show that radiotherapy *increases median survival* from 3 months in untreated dogs *to more than 12 months* in treated dogs and is associated with a 2-year survival of up to 40 % of dogs. Radiotherapy is associated with side effects like stomatitis, rhinitis, keratoconjunctivitis, and skin desquamation. Radiation of the eye, which is unavoidable in treating the nasal cavity, damages orbital structures and can cause blindness. Radiotherapy is mostly not curative.

Chemotherapy is rarely used as a sole treatment and its efficacy in tumors of the nasal cavity is not well studied. Adjunctive protocols using doxorubicin, cisplatin, and piroxicam have been effectively applied in canines. The use of cisplatin as a radiosensitizer has been shown to slightly increase survival times.

■ Prognostic Factors and Markers

Diverse prognostic factors have been identified for canine nasal cavity tumors and are presented in Box 14.2.

Box 14.2. Negative Prognostic Factors for Canine Nasal Cavity Tumors

- Age over 10 years
- Epistaxis
- Higher tumor stage
- Metastatic spread
- Facial deformation
- Histologic type (anaplastic carcinoma, squamous cell carcinoma > adenocarcinoma > mesenchymal tumors)

14.1.2 Feline Nasal Cavity Tumors

Box 14.3. Feline Nasal Cavity Tumors in Four Facts

1. Mostly invasively growing
2. Mostly lymphoma
3. Radiotherapy is the treatment of choice
4. Combined radiotherapy and chemotherapy are efficient for nasal lymphoma

■ Epidemiology and Pathogenesis

Feline nasal cavity (nonlymphoid) tumors are less common than in the dog but if present are more often malignant. They occur at an average *age* of 9–10 years. Studies on the etiology and molecular mechanisms of feline nasal cavity tumor carcinogenesis are not available. There is a slight *breed* predisposition for Siamese and dolichocephalic cats. *Lymphoma* is the most common nasal tumor in cats, followed by epithelial tumors, like carcinomas, adenocarcinomas, and squamous cell carcinomas. If negative for feline leukemia virus (FeLV), nasal lymphomas are usually restricted to the nasal cavity and not part of a multicentric tumor. Mesenchymal and benign tumors are rare in the cat.

■ Clinical Appearance

Clinical appearance resembles that of the dog, as described above. The tumors occur *more often in the caudal nasal cavity and grow invasively. Unlike in the dog, nasal cavity tumors only rarely metastasize in cats* even at advanced stages of the disease. Deviation of the nasal structures on *radiographs* indicates neoplasia, but this is not diagnostic as it may also be seen with chronic inflammatory disease. *Computed tomography (CT) and magnetic resonance imaging (MRI)* are the diagnostic methods of choice. Bone destruction and infiltration into the adjacent bony and soft tissue structures are indicative of neoplastic disease. *Cytology and histopathology* are necessary for final diagnosis.

■ Cytology and Histopathology

Repeated biopsies or cytology is required for definitive diagnosis due to failure to target the tumor directly. Intubation during biopsy taking is recommended due to potential massive bleeding after biopsy and the risk of blood aspiration.

Cytology of imprints obtained by nasal brushing or fine-needle aspirates is often diagnostic, especially for epithelial tumors due to the presence of proliferative or even pleomorphic epithelial tumor cells (◘ Fig. 14.3). Secondary inflammation and failure to target the main tumor mass may however lead to a false negative diagnosis of rhinitis or a false-positive diagnosis of lymphoma. Lymph node cytology is usually negative in cats with nasal cavity tumors at the time of first diagnosis.

Histopathology of biopsies is able to differentiate lymphomas, carcinomas, adenocarcinomas, squamous cell carcinomas, and mesenchymal tumors. There is little information on the correlation of the histologic type with survival times.

■ Therapy

Radiotherapy is the treatment of choice for feline nasal cavity tumors. It may increase survival time,

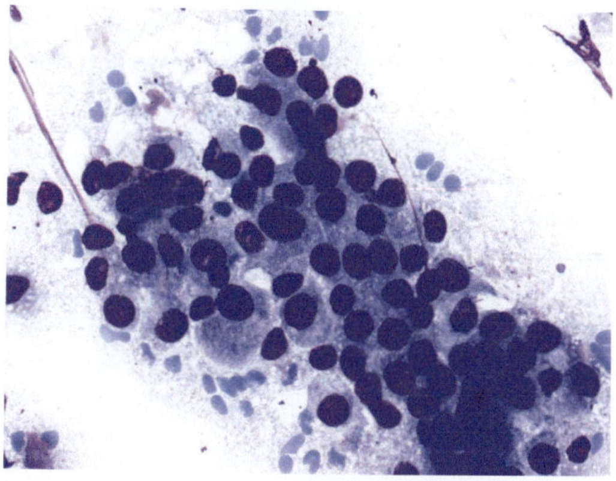

Fig. 14.3 Cytology, low grade nasal adenocarcinoma (as diagnosed by histopathology), cat, May-Grünwald-Giemsa, 200×. Tumor cells show only mild to moderate cellular pleomorphism and anisokaryosis

but prognosis for a 2-year survival is still very poor for non-lymphatic tumors. In contrast, *intranasal lymphomas* are also very radiosensitive, usually respond well to irradiation, and show survival times of up to 3 years after radiation.

A combination of *radiotherapy and chemotherapy is recommended for nasal lymphoma*. The common multi-agent protocols like COP (cyclophosphamide, vincristine, and prednisone) have a good response rate and increased survival in combination with radiotherapy. *Chemotherapy* alone is associated with median survival times of approximately 3 years.

14.1.3 Ovine and Caprine Enzootic Nasal Tumor

Box 14.4. Ovine and Caprine Enzootic Nasal Tumor Virus in Five Facts

1. Induced by betaretroviruses enzootic nasal tumor viruses 1 and 2 (ENTV-1, ENTV-2)
2. Expansively and invasively growing mass derived from the ethmoid turbinates
3. Metastasis extremely rare
4. Affected animals should be separated from the flock
5. No therapy available

Epidemiology and Pathogenesis

Tumors of the nasal cavity in sheep have been described on all continents except Australia and New Zealand. They are caused by the betaretroviruses *enzootic nasal tumor virus 1 (ENTV-1)* in sheep and ENTV-2 in goats. The disease does not usually present as an epidemic; several animals at a time are usually affected in a herd. However, transmission is through nasal secretions and the disease can spread. Due to the protracted course of the disease, clinical signs appear years after infection, most often in *adult animals*. There is no *breed* or *gender* predilection. The exact mechanisms of carcinogenesis are unknown but are likely similar to the closely related *Jaagsiekte sheep retrovirus*, the causative agent of pulmonary adenomatosis in sheep (discussed below). This virus is thought to induce pulmonary tumors by direct stimulation of cellular proliferation and transformation via the *ENV glycoprotein*. ENV appears to *directly activate several protein kinase signaling cascades* like phosphatidylinositol 3-kinase-AKT and the MEK-ERK pathway.

Clinical Appearance

As mentioned above, the course of disease is *slowly progressive*. Clinical signs of nasal tumors in sheep and goats include unilateral or bilateral *serous to mucopurulent nasal discharge*, dyspnea, open-mouth breathing, flared nostrils, respiratory stridor, and sneezing. In addition, facial deformation, exophthalmos, and lacrimation secondary to the expansive tumors are usually observed. Gradual weight loss over several months finally leads to death. The tumors are typically *invasive* but *rarely metastasize*. In addition to histopathology, diagnostics such as *immunohistochemistry* and/or *PCR* are required for a definitive diagnosis. If ENTV infection is confirmed, the animal should be separated from the flock to avoid further spread.

Pathology and Histopathology

Typical *macroscopic findings* in animals with ENTV are unilateral or bilateral white, firm, multinodular masses extending from the ethmoid turbinates. The masses fill most of the nasal cavity and compress the surrounding structures.

The *histologic appearance* is consistent with an adenoma or adenocarcinoma of the nasal respiratory mucosa with cuboidal or pseudostratified, non-ciliated epithelial cells. Histopathology cannot differentiate virus-induced tumors from rare, non-virally induced tumors of the nasal cavity. Viral infection can be confirmed with immunohistochemistry, PCR, or transmission electron microscopy.

▪ **Therapy**

There is *no described therapy* for ENTV in sheep and goats. Affected animals are usually euthanized for diagnostic pathology and to prevent further spread of the disease in the flock.

14.2 Tumors of the Lung

Lung tumors in dogs and cats are rare tumors of unknown etiology in dogs and cats; in sheep, they are mostly virus-induced. This is in contrast to the epidemiology in humans; human lung cancer, thought to be caused by carcinogens such as cigarette smoke, is the most common deadly cancer. A similar carcinogen is unknown in veterinary patients, which may explain the difference in epidemiology. Lung tumors in other domestic animals are very rare.

14.2.1 Canine Lung Tumors

Box 14.5. Canine Lung Tumors in Five Facts

1. No etiology or carcinogen known
2. Mostly malignant with a moderate to high metastatic rate
3. Clinical signs usually only at advanced stage of tumor development
4. CT superior sensitivity to radiographs
5. Surgery as the treatment of choice

14

▪ **Epidemiology and Pathogenesis**

Primary lung tumors are *rare in* dogs; when they occur they are usually found at the *age* of 10–11 years. Although an increasing number of mutations relevant for the development and treatment of human lung cancer are being found, none has been identified in canine lung tumors. However, an overexpression of the epithelial growth factor receptor (EGFR) has recently been identified as being positively correlated with a worse prognosis of primary canine lung tumors.

▪ **Clinical Appearance**

Lung tumors in the dog seem to grow slowly with *obvious clinical signs only at advanced stages* of tumor development. One-third of lung tumor diagnoses in dogs are incidental findings in thoracic radiographs made for other reasons (▪ Fig. 14.4). The other two-thirds of dogs diagnosed with lung tumors present with *chronic coughing, dyspnea, and lethargy*. In addition, lameness, swelling, and pain of the distal limbs are present in less than 5 % of dogs with pulmonary tumors. These are caused by *hypertrophic osteopathy*, a paraneoplastic periosteal bone formation at the distal limbs of dogs with thoracic masses of any kind. The mechanism of this paraneoplastic syndrome is unclear. Vagal nerve stimulation, cytokine secretions, and growth factor secretions have all been suggested as an underlying mechanism.

Thoracic radiographs are able to detect tumors of >1 cm in diameter. *Computed tomography* (*CT*) scans are more sensitive; they detect tumors with diameters of a few millimeters. The higher resolution of CT allows for improved detection and a better evaluation of tumor borders. *Bronchoscopy* is useful in the detection of tumors in the upper bronchi. However, lung tumors in the dog are most commonly located deeper in the respiratory tract and are not accessible by bronchoscopy. *Percutaneous biopsies or fine-needle aspirates* are required to definitively diagnose lung tumors. This requires *ultrasound or CT guidance* to reliably target the tumor during biopsy. A TNM staging system has been described by Owen et al. (1980, ▪ Table 14.2).

▪ **Cytology and Histopathology**

Cells derived from lung tumors by aspiration are usually *large polyhedral to round epithelial cells*

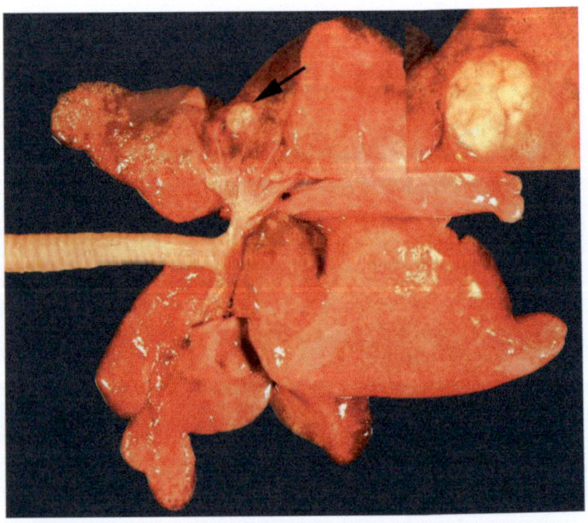

▪ **Fig. 14.4** Solitary pulmonary carcinoma in a dog. *Inset*: enlargement of the tumor (Photo with permission from Dr. M. von Deetzen, Institute of Veterinary Pathology, Freie Universität Berlin)

Table 14.2 TNM staging system for canine lung tumors (Owen et al. 1980)

Stage	Features
Primary tumors	
T1	Solitary tumors, unilateral with no bone involvement
T2	Multiple tumors
T3	Tumor/s with peripheral invasion
Regional lymph node	
N0	No metastasis
N1	Metastases in bronchial lymph nodes
N2	Metastases in distant lymph nodes
Distant metastases	
M1	Metastases
M2	No metastases

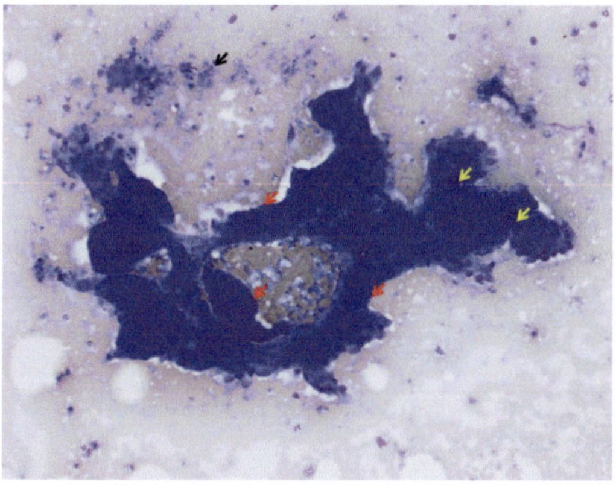

Fig. 14.5 Cytology, lung adenocarcinoma, dog, May-Grünwald-Giemsa, 100×. Note the large cluster of polygonal, deeply basophilic cells with tubular growth pattern (*red arrows*) intermixed with small amounts of calcified material (*yellow arrows*). There are small to moderate amounts of amorphous basophilic necrotic material (*black arrow*) (Photo with permission from Dr. N. Bauer, Faculty of Veterinary Medicine, Justus Liebig University, Giessen, Germany)

with a high nucleus to cytoplasm ratio and marked anisocytosis (Figs. 14.5 and 14.6). Occasionally, larger cell groups may show gland formation and production of secretory products.

Histologically, several types of lung tumors have been described, mostly based on general growth patterns such as bronchiolar or alveolar. At advanced stages, which is usually the case at the time of diagnosis, tumors usually lose their differentiation or contain areas with various growth patterns. A definitive diagnosis of a certain histologic type is therefore often not possible (with the exception of squamous cell carcinomas). This is usually not of clinical relevance. More clinically significant criteria include loss of differentiation in anaplastic carcinomas or necrosis and infiltration of the surrounding tissues. These are especially useful in assessing prognosis. For instance, dogs with well-differentiated tumors have an average survival time of up to 2 years, while dogs with anaplastic tumors have survival times of only a few days.

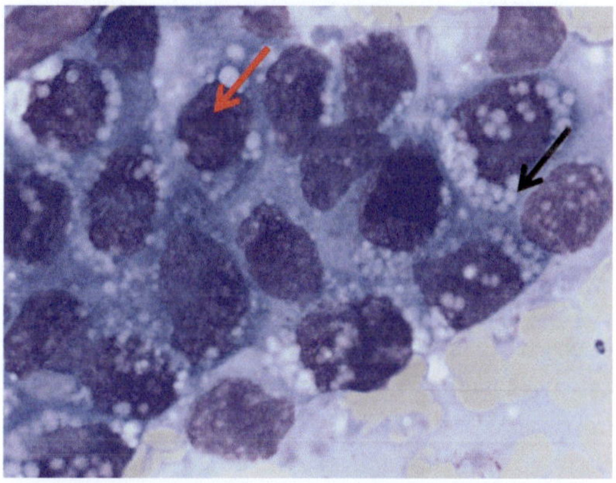

Fig. 14.6 Cytology, lung adenocarcinoma, dog (the same dog as in Fig. 14.5), May-Grünwald-Giemsa, 1000×. Note the cluster of polygonal cells with small to moderate amounts of basophilic cytoplasm containing multiple, clearly circumscribed vacuoles commonly seen in adenocarcinoma (*black arrow*). There is a mild to moderate anisocytosis, anisokaryosis, and pleomorphism. Several cells possess single prominent nucleoli (*red arrow*) (Photo with permission from Dr. N. Bauer, Faculty of Veterinary Medicine, Justus Liebig University, Giessen, Germany)

Therapy

Partial or complete lobectomy is the *surgical* treatment of choice for canine lung tumors. Intrapulmonary or systemically metastasized tumors would be a contraindication for surgery. Lobectomy of up to two lung lobes is usually well tolerated. Resection or at least fine-needle aspiration of the regional lymph node should always be performed for a better evaluation of prognosis. In general, survival time following surgery of primary lung tumors is short, except in clinical stage T1N0M0 (Table 14.2).

Information about *chemotherapy* as the sole or as adjunctive therapy to surgery is sparse.

Vincristine, doxorubicin, and cisplatin have been used with moderate success.

Radiotherapy is usually not applied to lung tumors due to side effects such as radiation-induced pneumonia and fibrosis.

▪ Prognostic Factors and Molecular Markers

Thyroid transcription factor 1 (TTF1) has been described as a specific and moderately sensitive immunohistochemical marker for canine primary lung tumors. Expression of TTF1 is lost in tumor metastases in distant organs.

14.2.2 Feline Lung Tumors

Box 14.6. Feline Lung Tumors in Three Facts

1. Rare, usually malignant tumors.
2. Occasionally metastasis to the distal limbs, regional lymph node or within the lung.
3. Lobectomy is the treatment of choice.

▪ Epidemiology and Pathogenesis

Primary lung tumors *are rare tumors of cats* and are usually diagnosed at the *age* of 10–12 years. No carcinogen or relevant mutation has been identified so far. The epidermal growth factor receptor (EGFR), K-ras, and the p53 gene, three genes with mutations in a subset of human lung cancer, have been analyzed recently. EGFR mutations were detected in 20 % of tumors while K-ras and p53 gene sequences contained no mutations in the few cases analyzed.

▪ Clinical Appearance

Clinically, *feline lung tumors* are described *aggressive* and *highly metastatic*. However, small, benign subclinical tumors are common incidental necropsy findings of old cats (▫ Fig. 14.7). Cats with lung tumors usually present with *weight loss*, *lethargy*, and *dyspnea*. Surprisingly, coughing is uncommon. Up to 10 % of the cats with primary lung tumors are initially presented due to lameness. In contrast to the dog, this is almost never caused by hypertrophic osteopathy of the distal limbs. *Instead*, a metastasis of primary lung tumors to the digits occurs, known as feline *lung-digit syndrome*. Cats with digital metastasis have a poor prognosis and usually only survive for a few

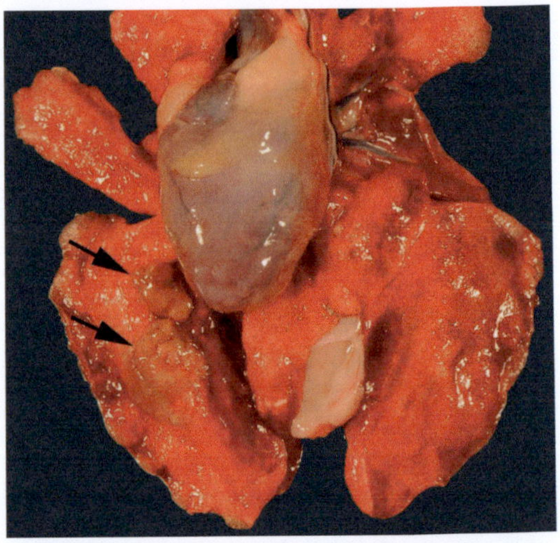

▫ **Fig. 14.7** Bifocal pulmonary carcinoma in a cat. *Arrows* is tumor (Photo with permission from Dr. P. Schlieben, Institute of Veterinary Pathology, Freie Universität Berlin)

months. Metastasis to the regional lymph node and within the lung is common; metastasis to other distant organs besides the digits is rare. Diagnostic imaging, staging, and therapy are the same as in the dog (described in the previous Sect. 14.2.1).

▪ Therapy

Surgery with partial or complete lobectomy is the *treatment of choice* for feline lung tumors. Contraindications are intrapulmonary or systemically metastasized tumors. Lobectomy of up to two lung lobes is usually well accepted. Resection or at least fine-needle aspiration of the regional lymph node should always be performed for a better evaluation of the prognosis for the animal.

Information about *chemotherapy* as the sole or adjunctive therapy to surgery is not available.

Radiotherapy is usually not applied for lung tumors due to the expected side effects like radiation induced pneumonia and fibrosis. The efficacy and safety of radiotherapy for primary lung tumors in cats however remains to be analyzed in clinical studies.

▪ Prognostic Factors and Molecular Markers

Clinical signs, pleural effusion, moderately and poorly differentiated tumors on histopathology, evidence of metastasis, and any stage beyond T1N0M0 are *negative prognostic indicators* for feline primary lung tumors. Immunohistochemical detection of *thyroid transcription factor 1* (*TTF1*) has been described as a specific marker for non-neoplastic thyroid and lung tissues and well-differentiated lung tumors in the cat. TTF1 expression is not found in poorly differentiated tumors, which questions the efficiency of this marker for malignant tumors.

14.2.3 Ovine Pulmonary Adenocarcinoma

Box 14.7. Ovine Pulmonary Adenocarcinoma in Five Facts

1. Induced by the Jaagsiekte sheep retrovirus (JSRV)
2. Viral ENV protein induces neoplastic transformation of type II pneumocytes
3. Weight loss, respiratory distress, and nasal discharge as the most common clinical symptoms
4. Wheelbarrow test induces massive nasal discharge (pathognomonic)
5. No treatment or vaccine available

▪ Epidemiology and Pathogenesis

Ovine pulmonary adenocarcinoma (*OPA*) is a contagious lung cancer in sheep induced by the *Jaagsiekte sheep retrovirus* (JSRV). The disease occurs worldwide with the exception of Australia, New Zealand and Iceland. It spreads mainly by contact with virus-containing respiratory secretions. The *incubation period* is several months, and the disease is usually seen in animals at the *age* of 2–4 years, but cases in younger animals have been reported. The highest *mortality rates* in flocks of sheep are reported during the first years after initial diagnosis of OPA. Gottorp and merino sheep may have a *breed* predisposition to develop the tumor. *Goats* can be infected with JRSV but rarely develop the tumor.

The *molecular mechanisms of JSRV-induced carcinogenesis* are incompletely understood. The classical retroviral mechanism of pathogenesis is insertional mutagenesis. However, OPA seems to function differently; the JSRV *envelope glycoprotein* (*ENV*) appears to induce cellular transformation by *direct activation of several protein kinase signaling cascades* like phosphatidylinositol 3-kinase-AKT and the MEK-ERK pathway. The ENV is also used for virus entry. The virus binds to the surface of several cell types but replicates mostly in type II pneumocytes and less frequently in the Clara cell of the lung. Another important feature of JRSV is the absence of a host immune response against the virus. This may be caused by the *immunologic tolerance* to the closely *related endogenous retrovirus* that is inherently integrated in the sheep genome and is in parts transcribed constantly.

▪ Clinical Appearance

Weight loss, despite normal food intake and *respiratory distress*, is the main symptom in sheep with OPA. Coughing is uncommon but may develop due to secondary bacterial pneumonia, which is also commonly the direct cause of death in animals with OPA. At the time of disease-associated death, almost 50 % of the lung may show neoplastic transformation (◘ Fig. 14.8). Massive amounts of white, frothy fluid are present in the air passages. The presence of 40–400 ml *nasal discharge* when the animal lowers its head or is lifted at the rear end ("wheelbarrow" *test*) is a pathognomonic sign. Both serological testing and PCR are of low sensitivity and specificity for the confirmation of OPA. *Ultrasonography* and more importantly *macroscopic and histologic pathology* are necessary for definitive diagnosis.

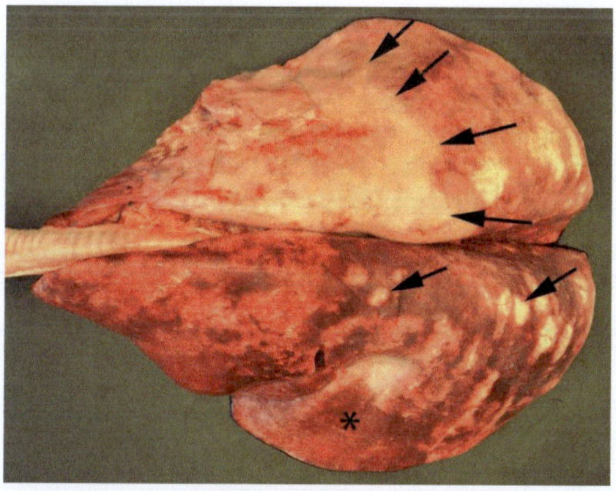

◘ **Fig. 14.8** Multifocal to coalescent ovine pulmonary adenocarcinoma (*arrows*) in a male goat. * means Normal lung (Photo with permission from Dr. A. Ostrowski, Institute of Veterinary Pathology, Freie Universität Berlin)

Pathology and Histopathology

At necropsy, affected lungs are heavy and wet with multifocal small, firm, gray nodules or large coalescing gray masses at lager stages. There is *excessive amount of clear, frothy, or mucoid exudate* on cut section and in the bronchi. The bronchial and mediastinal lymph nodes are often enlarged either due to secondary bacterial pneumonia or less commonly due to *metastasis* (<10 % of cases). Distant metastases are very rare. *Histologically*, there is a severe proliferation of columnar-shaped type II pneumocytes and Clara cells.

Therapy

Treatment or vaccines are not available for OPA. Thorough culling of affected animals is necessary to minimize virus spread in the flock, if clinical tests and ultrasonography are suspicious for OPA.

Suggested Reading

Alexander K, Joly H, Blond L, D'Anjou MA, Nadeau ME, Olive J, Beauchamp G (2012) A comparison of computed tomography, computed radiography, and film-screen radiography for the detection of canine pulmonary nodules. Vet Radiol Ultrasound Off J Am Coll Vet Radiol Int Vet Radiol Assoc 53:258–265

Armbrust LJ, Biller DS, Bamford A, Chun R, Garrett LD, Sanderson MW (2012) Comparison of three-view thoracic radiography and computed tomography for detection of pulmonary nodules in dogs with neoplasia. J Am Vet Med Assoc 240:1088–1094

Azizi S, Tajbakhsh E, Fathi F (2014) Ovine pulmonary adenocarcinoma in slaughtered sheep: a pathological and polymerase chain reaction study. J S Afr Vet Assoc 85:932

Ballegeer EA, Adams WM, Dubielzig RR, Paoloni MC, Klauer JM, Keuler NS (2010) Computed tomography characteristics of canine tracheobronchial lymph node metastasis. Vet Radiol Ultrasound Off J Am Coll Vet Radiol Int Vet Radiol Assoc 51:397–403

Barrett LE, Pollard RE, Zwingenberger A, Zierenberg-Ripoll A, Skorupski KA (2014) Radiographic characterization of primary lung tumors in 74 dogs. Vet Radiol Ultrasound Off J Am Coll Vet Radiol Int Vet Radiol Assoc 55:480–487

Bettini G, Marconato L, Morini M, Ferrari F (2009) Thyroid transcription factor-1 immunohistochemistry: diagnostic tool and malignancy marker in canine malignant lung tumours. Vet Comp Oncol 7:28–37

Cohn LA (2014) Canine nasal disease. Vet Clin North Am Small Anim Pract 44:75–89

Cousens C, Thonur L, Imlach S, Crawford J, Sales J, Griffiths DJ (2009) Jaagsiekte sheep retrovirus is present at high concentration in lung fluid produced by ovine pulmonary adenocarcinoma-affected sheep and can survive for several weeks at ambient temperatures. Res Vet Sci 87:154–156

Cousens C, Gibson L, Finlayson J, Pritchard I, Dagleish MP (2015) Prevalence of ovine pulmonary adenocarcinoma (Jaagsiekte) in a UK slaughterhouse sheep study. Vet Rec 176:413

D'Costa S, Yoon BI, Kim DY, Motsinger-Reif AA, Williams M, Kim Y (2012) Morphologic and molecular analysis of 39 spontaneous feline pulmonary carcinomas. Vet Pathol 49:971–978

De las Heras M, Garcia de Jalon JA, Sharp JM (1991) Pathology of enzootic intranasal tumor in thirty-eight goats. Vet Pathol 28:474–481

De las Heras M, Sharp JM, Ferrer LM, Garcia de Jalon JA, Cebrian LM (1993) Evidence for a type D-like retrovirus in enzootic nasal tumour of sheep. Vet Rec 132:441

De las Heras M, Garcia de Jalon JA, Minguijon E, Gray EW, Dewar P, Sharp JM (1995) Experimental transmission of enzootic intranasal tumors of goats. Vet Pathol 32:19–23

De las Heras M, Ortin A, Cousens C, Minguijon E, Sharp JM (2003) Enzootic nasal adenocarcinoma of sheep and goats. Curr Top Microbiol Immunol 275:201–223

Demko JL, Cohn LA (2007) Chronic nasal discharge in cats: 75 cases (1993-2004). J Am Vet Med Assoc 230:1032–1037

Elliot KM, Mayer MN (2009) Radiation therapy for tumors of the nasal cavity and paranasal sinuses in dogs. Can Vet J Rev Vet Can 50:309–312

Finck M, Ponce F, Guilbaud L, Chervier C, Floch F, Cadore JL, Chuzel T, Hugonnard M (2015) Computed tomography or rhinoscopy as the first-line procedure for suspected nasal tumor: a pilot study. Can Vet J Rev Vet Can 56:185–192

Fujiwara-Igarashi A, Fujimori T, Oka M, Nishimura Y, Hamamoto Y, Kazato Y, Sawada H, Yayoshi N, Hasegawa D, Fujita M (2014) Evaluation of outcomes and radiation complications in 65 cats with nasal tumours treated with palliative hypofractionated radiotherapy. Vet J 202:455–461

Goldfinch N, Argyle DJ (2012) Feline lung-digit syndrome: unusual metastatic patterns of primary lung tumours in cats. J Feline Med Surg 14:202–208

Gottfried SD, Popovitch CA, Goldschmidt MH, Schelling C (2000) Metastatic digital carcinoma in the cat: a retrospective study of 36 cats (1992-1998). J Am Anim Hosp Assoc 36:501–509

Griffiths DJ, Martineau HM, Cousens C (2010) Pathology and pathogenesis of ovine pulmonary adenocarcinoma. J Comp Pathol 142:260–283

Hahn KA, McEntee MF (1997) Primary lung tumors in cats: 86 cases (1979-1994). J Am Vet Med Assoc 211:1257–1260

Hahn KA, McEntee MF (1998) Prognosis factors for survival in cats after removal of a primary lung tumor: 21 cases (1979-1994). Vet Surg 27:307–311

Harris BJ, Lourenco BN, Dobson JM, Herrtage ME (2014) Diagnostic accuracy of three biopsy techniques in 117 dogs with intra-nasal neoplasia. J Small Anim Pract 55:219–224

Kim J, Kwon SY, Cena R, Park S, Oh J, Oui H, Cho KO, Min JJ, Choi J (2014) CT and PET-CT of a dog with multiple pulmonary adenocarcinoma. J Vet Med Sci Jpn Soc Vet Sci 76:615–620

Kuehn NF (2006) Nasal computed tomography. Clin Tech Small Anim Pract 21:55–59
Kujawa A, Olias P, Bottcher A, Klopfleisch R (2014) Thyroid transcription factor-1 is a specific marker of benign but not malignant feline lung tumours. J Comp Pathol 151:19–24
Lee JH, Lee JH, Yoon HY, Kim NH, Sur JH, Jeong SW (2012) Hypertrophic osteopathy associated with pulmonary adenosquamous carcinoma in a dog. J Vet Med Sci Jpn Soc Vet Sci 74:667–672
Little L, Patel R, Goldschmidt M (2007) Nasal and nasopharyngeal lymphoma in cats: 50 cases (1989-2005). Vet Pathol 44:885–892
Liu SL, Miller AD (2007) Oncogenic transformation by the jaagsiekte sheep retrovirus envelope protein. Oncogene 26:789–801
Malinowski C (2006) Canine and feline nasal neoplasia. Clin Tech Small Anim Pract 21:89–94
Maritato KC, Schertel ER, Kennedy SC, Dudley R, Lamm C, Barnhart M, Kass P (2014) Outcome and prognostic indicators in 20 cats with surgically treated primary lung tumors. J Feline Med Surg 16:979–984
Maruo T, Shida T, Fukuyama Y, Hosaka S, Noda M, Ito T, Sugiyama H, Ishikawa T, Madarame H (2011) Retrospective study of canine nasal tumor treated with hypofractionated radiotherapy. J Vet Med Sci Jpn Soc Vet Sci 73:193–197
Mayhew PD, Hunt GB, Steffey MA, Culp WT, Mayhew KN, Fuller M, Johnson LR, Pascoe PJ (2013) Evaluation of short-term outcome after lung lobectomy for resection of primary lung tumors via video-assisted thoracoscopic surgery or open thoracotomy in medium- to large-breed dogs. J Am Vet Med Assoc 243:681–688
McNiel EA, Ogilvie GK, Powers BE, Hutchison JM, Salman MD, Withrow SJ (1997) Evaluation of prognostic factors for dogs with primary lung tumors: 67 cases (1985-1992). J Am Vet Med Assoc 211:1422–1427
Mellanby RJ, Herrtage ME, Dobson JM (2002a) Long-term outcome of eight cats with non-lymphoproliferative nasal tumours treated by megavoltage radiotherapy. J Feline Med Surg 4:77–81
Mellanby RJ, Stevenson RK, Herrtage ME, White RA, Dobson JM (2002b) Long-term outcome of 56 dogs with nasal tumours treated with four doses of radiation at intervals of seven days. Vet Rec 151:253–257
Minguijon E, Gonzalez L, De las Heras M, Gomez N, Garcia-Goti M, Juste RA, Moreno B (2013) Pathological and aetiological studies in sheep exhibiting extrathoracic metastasis of ovine pulmonary adenocarcinoma (Jaagsiekte). J Comp Pathol 148:139–147
Ortin A, Perez de Villarreal M, Minguijon E, Cousens C, Sharp JM, De las Heras M (2004) Coexistence of enzootic nasal adenocarcinoma and jaagsiekte retrovirus infection in sheep. J Comp Pathol 131:253–258
Owen L. TNM classification of tumours in domestic animals. Geneva: World health organization; 1980
Polton GA, Brearley MJ, Powell SM, Burton CA (2008) Impact of primary tumour stage on survival in dogs with solitary lung tumours. J Small Anim Pract 49:66–71
Rassnick KM, Goldkamp CE, Erb HN, Scrivani PV, Njaa BL, Gieger TL, Turek MM, McNiel EA, Proulx DR, Chun R, Mauldin GE, Phillips BS, Kristal O (2006) Evaluation of factors associated with survival in dogs with untreated nasal carcinomas: 139 cases (1993-2003). J Am Vet Med Assoc 229:401–406
Reif JS, Bruns C, Lower KS (1998) Cancer of the nasal cavity and paranasal sinuses and exposure to environmental tobacco smoke in pet dogs. Am J Epidemiol 147:488–492
Sabattini S, Mancini FR, Marconato L, Bacci B, Rossi F, Vignoli M, Bettini G (2014) EGFR overexpression in canine primary lung cancer: pathogenetic implications and impact on survival. Vet Comp Oncol 12:237–248
Scott P, Collie D, McGorum B, Sargison N (2010) Relationship between thoracic auscultation and lung pathology detected by ultrasonography in sheep. Vet J 186:53–57
Sfiligoi G, Theon AP, Kent MS (2007) Response of nineteen cats with nasal lymphoma to radiation therapy and chemotherapy. Vet Radiol Ultrasound Off J Am Coll Vet Radiol Int Vet Radiol Assoc 48:388–393
Sones E, Smith A, Schleis S, Brawner W, Almond G, Taylor K, Haney S, Wypij J, Keyerleber M, Arthur J, Hamilton T, Lawrence J, Gieger T, Sellon R, Wright Z (2013) Survival times for canine intranasal sarcomas treated with radiation therapy: 86 cases (1996-2011). Vet Radiol Ultrasound Off J Am Coll Vet Radiol Int Vet Radiol Assoc 54:194–201
Stowe DM. A Case of Enzootic Nasal Adenocarcinoma in a Ewe. Case Reports in Veterinary Medicine 2012;2012:1–4
Walsh SR, Linnerth-Petrik NM, Yu DL, Foster RA, Menzies PI, Diaz-Mendez A, Chalmers HJ, Wootton SK (2013) Experimental transmission of enzootic nasal adenocarcinoma in sheep. Vet Res 44:66
Walsh SR, Stinson KJ, Menzies PI, Wootton SK (2014) Development of an ante-mortem diagnostic test for enzootic nasal tumor virus and detection of neutralizing antibodies in host serum. J Gen Virol 95:1843–1854
Wood EF, O'Brien RT, Young KM (1998) Ultrasound-guided fine-needle aspiration of focal parenchymal lesions of the lung in dogs and cats. J Vet Intern Med Am Coll Vet Intern Med 12:338–342
Yi G, Kaiyu W, Qigui Y, Zhongqiong Y, Yingdong Y, Defang C, Jinlu H (2010) Descriptive study of enzootic nasal adenocarcinoma in goats in southwestern China. Transbound Emerg Dis 57:197–200
Youssef G, Wallace WA, Dagleish MP, Cousens C, Griffiths DJ (2015) Ovine pulmonary adenocarcinoma: a large animal model for human lung cancer. ILAR J Natl Res Counc Inst Lab Anim Res 56:99–115

Vascular Tumors

Robert Klopfleisch

R. Klopfleisch (ed.), *Veterinary Oncology*, DOI 10.1007/978-3-319-41124-8_15

Vascular tumors develop from either the lymph or blood vessels. Hemangiosarcomas, which develop from blood vessels, are described for almost all animal species. They are most common in dogs and occasionally described in cats and horses. Lymphangiomas and lymphangiosarcomas are very rare tumors in all species and will not be covered here.

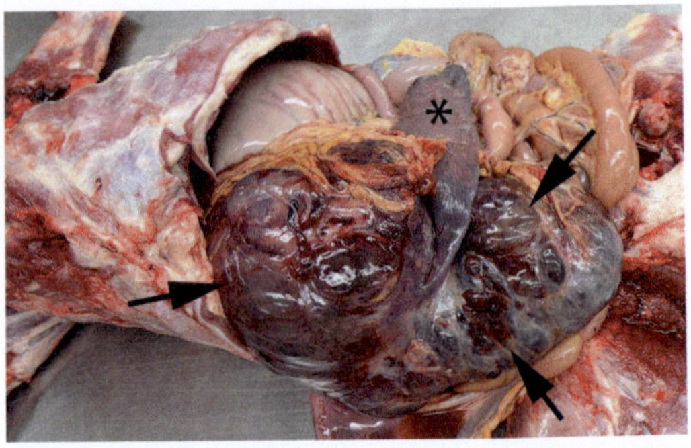

Fig. 15.1 Splenic hemangiosarcoma (*arrow*) in a dog (Photo with permission of A. Meyer, IDEXX, Ludwigshafen and the archive of the Institute of Veterinary Pathology, Freie Universität Berlin, Germany)

15.1 Canine Hemangiosarcomas

Box 15.1. Canine Hemangiosarcomas in Five Facts

1. Very common and highly malignant tumor in dogs
2. The spleen and right cardiac atrium most common sites of development
3. Metastatic rate of 80 %
4. Tumor rupture and hypovolemic shock most common cause of death
5. Palliative, extensive surgery as treatment of choice

Epidemiology and Pathogenesis

Hemangiosarcomas (HSA) are common and highly malignant tumors in dogs. They arise from primitive vascular endothelial precursor cells and represent almost 20 % of all mesenchymal tumors. HSA make up 50 % of *splenic neoplasms* and are common in the right cardiac atrium, but they can arise in any anatomical location in the body. HSA are the most common primary cardiac neoplasm of dogs (Figs. 15.1 and 15.2) and the most common metastatic neoplasm in the brain. Their *metastatic rate is 80 %* at first presentation. HSA most commonly metastasize to the liver and lung (Fig. 15.3). There is ongoing discussion about whether multicentric HSA are truly multicentric or whether they consist of a primary tumor with multiple metastases. HSA are tumors of middle *aged* to old dogs; the average age of dogs presenting with HSA is 10 years. A *breed* predisposition for German shepherds and golden retrievers has been found in most epidemiologic studies.

The etiology of the tumors is unclear in most aspects. However, *ultraviolet light* seems to influence carcinogenesis of HSA since nonpigmented, poorly haired skin is predisposed to developing these tumors. In addition, autocrine stimulation of tumor cells by *angiogenic growth factors* like vascular endothelial growth factor (VEGF) and basic fibroblast growth factor (bFGF) seems to at least be involved in tumor progression and growth. Increased gene expression associated with inflammation and angiogenesis has also been identified in HSA, but its explicit role in the initiation of the tumors is unclear. The benign form of hemovascular tumors, *hemangioma,* is less common and usually located in the subcutis.

Clinical Appearance

Clinical signs associated with HSA can be divided into those caused by local effect of the tumors and its metastases and those associated with general systemic effects.

The *local effects of HSA* very much depend on the anatomic tumor location. As previously mentioned, the most common anatomical sites for HSA in the dog are the spleen and the right cardiac atrium, but HSA may develop in any vascularized region of the body. Although HSA may have a *mass effect* and thus influence organ function, the most important associated clinical signs are usually based on *rupture* of the fragile, highly vascularized tumors. Thus, the most common clinical signs are *chronic mild* or *acute severe hemorrhage*. This may lead to hemoabdomen or hemopericardium with cardiac tamponade and life-threatening anemia, hypovolemia, and *hypotensive shock*. Rupture of tumors of the right atrium is also associated with clinical signs of right heart failure, including ascites and jugular pulse.

Anemia is a very common *systemic clinical sign* of dogs with HSA. The anemia may be regenerative

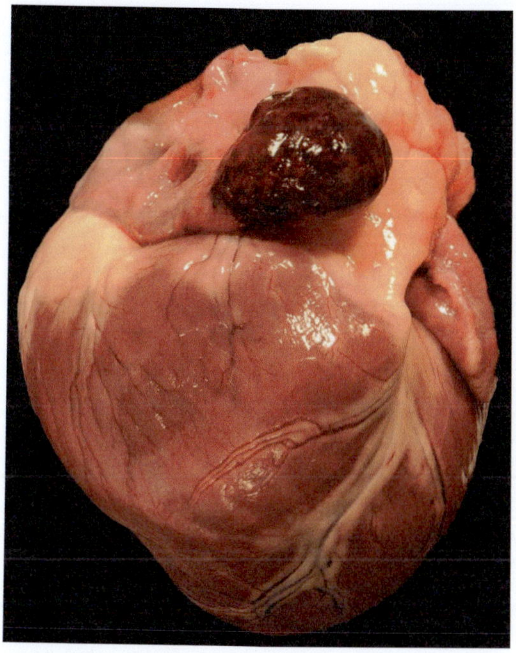

Fig. 15.2 Hemangiosarcoma of the right cardiac atrium in a dog (photo with permission of S. Binder, Institute of Veterinary Pathology, Freie Universität Berlin, Germany)

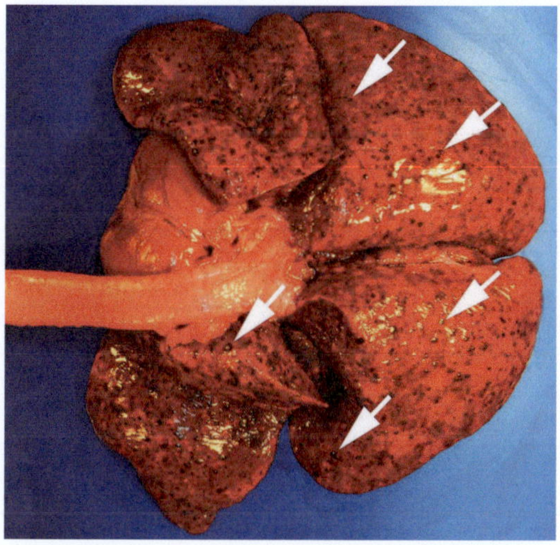

Fig. 15.3 Pulmonary metastases (*arrow*) of a hemangiosarcoma in a dog (Photo with permission of Dr. C. Holzhausen, Institute of Veterinary Pathology, Freie Universität Berlin, Germany)

or non-regenerative depending on the duration and grade of hemorrhage. In addition, *blood smears* of dogs with HSA often contain *schistocytes*. These malformed cells arise due to shear forces and microangiopathic hemolysis in the irregular-formed tumor vessels. *Thrombocytopenia* is the most common feature on clinical pathology of dogs with HSA. *Coagulation parameters are altered* in only approximately 50 % of dogs. These patients present with prolonged prothrombin time [PT] and activated partial thromboplastin time [APTT], hypofibrinogenemia, and increased levels of fibrin degradation products. Increased activation of the coagulation cascade due to distortion of the bloodstream in the tumor vessels and incomplete endothelial lining with constant exposure of subendothelial collagen is thought to cause the changes in coagulation parameters just mentioned.

Plasma concentrations of *serum levels of big endothelin-1 and VEGF* have been suggested as diagnostic markers for the detection of HSA in dogs.

Computed tomography (CT) of primary HSA and *thoracic radiographs* are helpful to evaluate pulmonary metastasis of HSA. *Echocardiography* and abdominal *ultrasound* are used to detect atrial HSA, splenic masses, and visceral metastasis in the abdomen. HSA can appear as cavernous or solid masses on ultrasound, depending on the blood content and diameter of intra-tumor vasculature.

A clinical staging system for HSA has been developed by Wood et al. (1998) (Table 15.1).

Cytology and Histopathology

HSA are solitary or multifocal mostly dark red, soft, occasionally fluctuating, moderately circumscribed, friable, and nonencapsulated masses on *gross pathology*. *Cytologic* preparations of HSA are rarely helpful due to *hemodilution* of the highly vascularized tumors. In addition, core needle biopsies from suspected visceral HSA are not recommended due to the risk of life-threatening hemorrhage. HSA tumor cells, when found, are characterized as polygonal to spindloid cells with cytoplasmic vacuoles. Due to the difficulties in obtaining and evaluating cytological preparation, morphologic diagnosis of HSA relies on *histopathology* of surgically excised tumors. However, histopathologic diagnosis may be difficult. Sections from different areas of the tumors must be analyzed since a high fraction of blood-filled spaces and tumor-associated hematomas can obscure the cavernous tumor. *Histologically*, HSA are composed of spindloid to polygonal or ovoid tumor cells. These cells usually form vascular channels or cavities at least in some parts of

Table 15.1 World Health Organization (WHO) staging for canine hemangiosarcomas (Wood et al. 1998)

Category/ stage	Description
Tumor (T)	
T0	No tumor
T1	Tumor <5 cm, restricted to one organ
T2	Tumor >5 cm or ruptured tumor
T3	Tumor >5 cm, invasion of adjacent structures
Lymph node (N)	
N0	No lymph node metastasis
N1	Regional lymph node involved
N2	Distant lymph nodes involved
Distant metastasis (M)	
M0	No metastasis
M1	Metastasis
Stage	
I	T0 or T1 with N0, M0
II	T2 with N0 or N1, M0
III	M1 with each T and N

the tumor. Solid tumor areas are often difficult to distinguish from poorly differentiated sarcomas. Immunohistochemistry for von *Willebrand factor or CD31* can be used to confirm the endothelial origin of tumor cells.

15

Therapy

Aggressive surgery is still the treatment of choice for canine HSA but is usually palliative and almost never curative. Splenic HSA requires a *splenectomy*. The major risk factor in surgical treatment of HSA is intraoperative rupture. Great care should be exercised in removing the spleen from the abdomen; appropriate treatments for hypotensive shock and a state of abnormal coagulation should be immediately available in case of rupture. Ventricular arrhythmia is a common side effect during the first few days after splenectomy, found in up to 25 % of dogs. Right atrium HSA can be treated with *pericardiectomy* as a palliative procedure. Removal of the pericardium does not include HSA resection; it is purely a preventative measure against the development of hemopericardium. The literature does include a few reports of atrial tumor resection and consequent reconstructive procedures. Surgical excision of *subcutaneous HSA* is more common; this procedure has a better prognosis with wide surgical margins of 2 cm.

Adjuvant chemotherapy is indicated due to the high metastatic rate of HSA. The most frequently described combination protocols include doxorubicin (DOX). These protocols may prolong survival, but most animals die due to metastatic disease within a few months. Non-adjuvant chemotherapy for non-resectable HSA appears to be an effective short-term treatment.

Radiation therapy is rarely utilized since treating metastasis is a more urgent concern than local tumor control in these cases and radiation has no significant impact on prolonging survival.

Prognostic Factors and Molecular Markers

Visceral HSA is more aggressive and has a poorer prognosis than cutaneous HSA. In general, prognosis of *splenic HSA* in dogs treated with surgery or surgery combined with adjuvant chemotherapy is poor. The median survival time of dogs treated with *surgery alone* is 3 months; the survival rate after 3 months is 33 %; after 12 months the survival rate is 10 %. *Doxorubicin-based adjuvant chemotherapy* may increase survival rate up to 30 % after 12 months and is associated with a median survival time between 5 and 9 months. *Cardiac HSA* also has a poor prognosis with average survival time ranging from 1 to 4 months. The presence of *necrosis* and a *high mitotic index* on histopathology is also associated with a poor prognosis.

Suggested Further Reading

(Alvarez et al. 2013; Bertazzolo et al. 2005; Dervisis et al. 2011; Fife et al. 2004; Frenz et al. 2014; Fukuda et al. 2014; Fukumoto et al. 2015; Hammond and Pesillo-Crosby 2008; Lamerato-Kozicki et al. 2006; Mullin et al. 2014; O'Brien 2007; Shiu et al. 2011; Smith 2003; Spangler and Kass 1997; Szivek et al. 2012; Teske et al. 2011;

Weisse et al. 2005; Wiley et al. 2010; Wood et al. 1998; Yamamoto et al. 2013)

15.2 Canine Perivascular Wall Tumors

Canine perivascular wall tumors (PWT), previously called hemangiopericytomas, derive from vascular mural cells. PWT are moderately invasive tumors with very low metastatic potential. Tumor size (>5 cm) and depth of invasion are positively correlated with recurrence. They are commonly included in the heterogeneous group of *soft tissue sarcomas (STS)*. ► See Sect. 4.1.3 for diagnosis, therapy, and prognosis of these tumors. The literature includes active discussion over whether STS with tumor cells whirling around small vessels or collagen bundles on histology should be classified as PWT or *peripheral nerve sheath tumors (PNST)*. While no consensus has been reached, it is safe to say that PWT can only be differentiated from PNST using immunohistochemistry of cell surface proteins and that most subcutaneous STS in the dog are PNST.

Suggested Reading

Alvarez FJ, Hosoya K, Lara-Garcia A, Kisseberth W, Couto G (2013) VAC protocol for treatment of dogs with stage III hemangiosarcoma. J Am Anim Hosp Assoc 49:370–377

Bertazzolo W, Dell'Orco M, Bonfanti U, Ghisleni G, Caniatti M, Masserdotti C, Antoniazzi E, Crippa L, Roccabianca P (2005) Canine angiosarcoma: cytologic, histologic, and immunohistochemical correlations. Vet Clin Pathol Am Soc Veter Clini Pathol 34:28–34

Dervisis NG, Dominguez PA, Newman RG, Cadile CD, Kitchell BE (2011) Treatment with DAV for advanced-stage hemangiosarcoma in dogs. J Am Anim Hosp Assoc 47:170–178

Fife WD, Samii VF, Drost WT, Mattoon JS, Hoshaw-Woodard S (2004) Comparison between malignant and nonmalignant splenic masses in dogs using contrast-enhanced computed tomography. Vet Radiol Ultrasound Off J Am College Veter Radiol Int Veter Radiol Ass 45:289–297

Frenz M, Kaup FJ, Neumann S (2014) Serum vascular endothelial growth factor in dogs with haemangiosarcoma and haematoma. Res Vet Sci 97:257–262

Fukuda S, Kobayashi T, Robertson ID, Oshima F, Fukazawa E, Nakano Y, Ono S, Thrall DE (2014) Computed tomographic features of canine nonparenchymal hemangiosarcoma. Vet Radiol Ultrasound Off J Am College Veter Radiol Int Veter Radiol Ass 55:374–379

Fukumoto S, Hanazono K, Miyasho T, Endo Y, Kadosawa T, Iwano H, Uchide T. Serum big endothelin-1 as a clinical marker for cardiopulmonary and neoplastic diseases in dogs. Life Sci 2014;118(2):329–32

Hammond TN, Pesillo-Crosby SA (2008) Prevalence of hemangiosarcoma in anemic dogs with a splenic mass and hemoperitoneum requiring a transfusion: 71 cases (2003–2005). J Am Vet Med Assoc 232:553–558

Kujawa A, Olias P, Bottcher A, Klopfleisch R. Thyroid transcription factor-1 is a specific marker of benign but not malignant feline lung tumours. Journal of comparative pathology 2014;151(1):19–24

Lamerato-Kozicki AR, Helm KM, Jubala CM, Cutter GC, Modiano JF (2006) Canine hemangiosarcoma originates from hematopoietic precursors with potential for endothelial differentiation. Exp Hematol 34:870–878

Mullins MN, Lana SE, Dernell WS, Ogilvie GK, Withrow SJ, Ehrhart EJ. Cyclooxygenase-2 expression in canine appendicular osteosarcomas. Journal of veterinary internal medicine/American College of Veterinary Internal Medicine 2004;18(6):859–65

O'Brien RT (2007) Improved detection of metastatic hepatic hemangiosarcoma nodules with contrast ultrasound in three dogs. Vet Radiol Ultrasound Off J Am College Veter Radiol Int Veter Radiol Ass 48:146–148

Shiu KB, Flory AB, Anderson CL, Wypij J, Saba C, Wilson H, Kurzman I, Chun R (2011) Predictors of outcome in dogs with subcutaneous or intramuscular hemangiosarcoma. J Am Vet Med Assoc 238:472–479

Smith AN (2003) Hemangiosarcoma in dogs and cats. Vet Clin North Am Small Anim Pract 33:533–552, vi

Spangler WL, Kass PH (1997) Pathologic factors affecting postsplenectomy survival in dogs. J Veter Intern Med Am College Veter Intern Med 11:166–171

Szivek A, Burns RE, Gericota B, Affolter VK, Kent MS, Rodriguez CO Jr, Skorupski KA (2012) Clinical outcome in 94 cases of dermal haemangiosarcoma in dogs treated with surgical excision: 1993-2007*. Vet Comp Oncol 10:65–73

Teske E, Rutteman GR, Kirpenstein J, Hirschberger J (2011) A randomized controlled study into the efficacy and toxicity of pegylated liposome encapsulated doxorubicin as an adjuvant therapy in dogs with splenic haemangiosarcoma. Vet Comp Oncol 9:283–289

Weisse C, Soares N, Beal MW, Steffey MA, Drobatz KJ, Henry CJ (2005) Survival times in dogs with right atrial hemangiosarcoma treated by means of surgical resection with or without adjuvant chemotherapy: 23 cases (1986–2000). J Am Vet Med Assoc 226:575–579

Wiley JL, Rook KA, Clifford CA, Gregor TP, Sorenmo KU (2010) Efficacy of doxorubicin-based chemotherapy for non-resectable canine subcutaneous haemangiosarcoma. Vet Comp Oncol 8:221–233

Wood CA, Moore AS, Gliatto JM, Ablin LA, Berg RJ, Rand WM (1998) Prognosis for dogs with stage I or II splenic hemangiosarcoma treated by splenectomy alone: 32 cases (1991–1993). J Am Anim Hosp Assoc 34:417–421

Yamamoto S, Hoshi K, Hirakawa A, Chimura S, Kobayashi M, Machida N (2013) Epidemiological, clinical and pathological features of primary cardiac hemangiosarcoma in dogs: a review of 51 cases. J Veter Med Sci Jap Soc Veter Sci 75:1433–1441

Ocular and Periocular Tumors

Robert Klopfleisch

R. Klopfleisch (ed.), *Veterinary Oncology*, DOI 10.1007/978-3-319-41124-8_16

Ocular and periocular tumors are uncommon in all species; when present they have severe consequences for vision and quality of life. Ocular tumors rarely metastasize to the regional lymph nodes or distant organs. However, particularly feline ocular tumors may have an invasive growth pattern into adjacent structures in the orbita. Surgery is the treatment of choice for all ocular and periocular tumors, while radiotherapy and chemotherapy are of minor importance. Melanomas, squamous cell carcinomas, and feline ocular posttraumatic sarcomas are the most common (peri) ocular tumors in veterinary oncology.

16.1 Canine Periocular Tumors of the Eyelid, Third Eyelid, Conjunctiva, and Limbus

Box 16.1. Canine Periocular Tumors in Four Facts

1. Usually meibomian gland adenomas, papillomas, or melanomas
2. Mostly benign tumors except for the more invasive conjunctival melanomas and rare third eyelid adenocarcinomas
3. May interfere with general physiology of the eye and vision
4. Surgery is the treatment of choice

▪ Epidemiology and Pathogenesis

Meibomian (sebaceous) gland adenomas, viral papillomas, and *conjunctival* and *limbal melanomas* are the most common periocular tumors in the dog. There may be a *breed* predisposition for boxers, collies, and spaniels, but epidemiologic studies are contradictory in their results. Periocular tumors usually affect *old dogs* except for the rare *eyelid histiocytomas and viral papillomas in young dogs*. Pigmented eyelids and conjunctiva of Weimaraner and German shepherds may be predisposed for *eyelid melanomas*. *Adenocarcinomas of the third eyelid gland* are rare malignant tumors with metastasis to regional lymph nodes in very few cases.

▪ Clinical Signs

The vast majority of canine periocular tumors show a *mostly benign biological behavior*. Even the few malignant tumors, *conjunctival melanomas* (in contrast to the usually benign limbal melanomas) and *adenocarcinomas of the third eyelid*, grow invasively but do not metastasize. Histiocytomas and viral papillomas of young dogs usually regress spontaneously within a few weeks of first appearance, similar to cutaneous histiocytomas. *Clinical signs* are usually based on the mass effect of the tumors and its interference with the normal physiology of nictitating and moistening and with the general integrity of the mucosal surfaces and immune barriers. Tumors may be ulcerated with a rough surface and thus lead to dominant clinical signs of *inflammation, epiphora, mucopurulent discharge*, protrusion of the third eyelid, and corneal neovascularization. Neoplasia is thus a differential diagnosis for chronic, refractory conjunctivitis and blepharitis.

Fluorescein stain, careful palpation, and inspection of ocular and periocular structures are usually sufficient for a tentative diagnosis of neoplastic disease. Melanomas may be pigmented but amelanotic melanomas are not uncommon. Fine needle aspiration (FNA) or incisional biopsies, ultrasound, or even computed tomography (CT) and magnetic resonance imaging (MRI) may help in planning the therapeutic approach for larger tumors.

▪ Cytology and Histopathology

Cytology using fine needle aspiration (FNA) is an uncommon diagnostic tool for periocular tumors. If performed, cytology may help in the diagnosis of periocular meibomian adenomas, melanomas, third eyelid gland tumors, histiocytomas, and papillomas. *Postsurgical histopathology of excisional biopsies* is by far the more common tool for definitive diagnosis of periocular tumors. *Melanomas* often contain pigmented epithelioid to spindloid cells, but immunohistochemistry for S100 or Melan A is occasionally required to confirm the diagnosis. *Meibomian gland adenomas* are usually composed of nests and cords of epithelial cells with occasional sebaceous differentiation or squamous epithelial differentiation and thus may resemble squamous cell carcinomas (SCC) in some cases. *Third eyelid gland tumors* are usually well differentiated, expansively growing adenomas and only occasionally show signs of invasive growth into the adjacent stromal structures.

▪ Therapy

Surgical excision is the treatment of choice for canine periocular tumors. Since most of periocular tumors are slow growing, surgery can be carefully planned, and tumors can be extensively observed for their clinical behavior. However, all periocular tumors are a threat to vision, ocular comfort, and quality of life and should be excised immediately if ocular structures become irritated and inflamed or eyelid function is impaired. *Cryosurgery* using liquid nitrogen and conservative surgery are increasingly the treatment of choice for periocular tumors.

The eyelids in particular and periocular structures in general are functionally very sensitive structures. *Tumors involving less than one third of the length of the eyelid* may be excised using a V-plasty or four-sided excision. If the tumors are larger than one third of the length of the eyelid, advanced blepharoplasty and surgical skills are required for preservation of eyelid function. *Presurgical tumor shrinkage* using systemic or local chemotherapy or radiation therapy may be recommended to minimize the fraction of the eyelid to be removed. Superficial conjunctival tumors can be treated with *superficial keratectomy or sclerectomy*, but if the tumor has progressed, they may require enucleation of the entire globe. Resection of the complete third eyelid is a rather simple procedure but is often associated with postsurgical complications like chronic ocular drying and keratitis.

The *prognosis* for canine eyelid tumors is excellent with <15 % recurrence rate; metastasis is very rare. The prognosis for tumors of the third eyelid and the conjunctiva is good, but recurrence rates of conjunctival and limbal melanomas and tumors of the third eyelid are significantly higher than for eyelid tumors.

Suggested Further Readings

(Aquino 2007, 2008; Bernays et al. 1999; Bussieres et al. 2005; Dees et al. 2015; Donaldson et al. 2006a, b; Featherstone et al. 2009; Finn et al. 2008; Hagard 2005; Lopes et al. 2010; Romkes et al. 2014)

16.2 Canine Ocular Tumors

Box 16.2. Canine Ocular Tumors in Three Facts

1. Usually benign tumors without metastasis
2. Mostly melanomas and ciliary body adenomas
3. Enucleation as treatment of choice

Epidemiology and Pathogenesis

Melanomas are the most common primary ocular tumor of the dog. The median *age* of affected dogs is 7 years. There is no *breed* or *gender* predilection for the development of ocular melanomas. Melanomas usually develop in the anterior uvea and the iris. More than 90 % of ocular melanomas are *benign with slow and expansive growth*. Less than 5 % of the tumors metastasize hematogenically. Malignant tumors tend to be less pigmented than benign tumors.

Ciliary body adenomas are the second most common primary canine intraocular tumors. They arise from the nonpigmented inner layer of the ciliary epithelium or the pigmented or nonpigmented epithelial cells of the iris or ciliary body. There is a slight *breed* predisposition for German shepherds and American cocker spaniel. Metastasis is extremely rare.

Clinical Signs

A *visible mass* are less common primary clinical signs for ocular tumors. Most primary ocular tumors are either incidental findings during ophthalmologic examination or dogs are initially presented with glaucoma, hyphema, and uveitis. *Transillumination and ultrasonography* are helpful for the diagnosis of melanomas but are usually not sufficiently specific for the differentiation from other masses such as hematomas. Fine needle aspiration (FNA) may significantly increase the specificity of the diagnosis but is associated with high risks of damaging the globe due to hemorrhage and infection.

Cytology and Histopathology

Cytology using fine needle aspiration (FNA) is a rather uncommon tool for diagnosing ocular tumors. If performed, cytology may help in the diagnosis of ocular melanomas due to the presence of pigmented cells. However, ciliary body adenomas can also contain pigmented cells and cannot be differentiated from melanomas on cytology alone.

Histopathology is an accurate tool for diagnosing ocular melanomas. Melanomas usually arise at the iris root or the ciliary body and contain lightly pigmented spindle cells and few more intensely pigmented plump melanocytes. A mitotic index >3 per 10 HPF indicates malignancy. A rare subtype of *choroidal melanoma* arises from the subretinal choroidea. *Ciliary body adenomas* usually contain well-differentiated, cuboidal to columnar cells arranged in papillary, tubular, or solid patterns. They are occasionally cystic and may contain areas of hemorrhage or necrosis

▪ **Therapy**

Surgical enucleation is the treatment of choice for canine ocular tumors. *Sector iridectomy*, when performed by a specialist, is also a good palliative treatment for these tumors if the volume is smaller than one quarter of the globe. However, this is not a curative treatment and the long-term results are unsatisfactory. Recently, *transscleral or transcorneal laser therapy* has been suggested as an efficient method of treating the tumor and avoiding enucleation. *Radiation therapy* is increasingly used for the treatment of canine ocular tumors but is associated with several ocular side effects.

▪ **Suggested Further Readings**

(Beckwith-Cohen et al. 2015; Finn et al. 2008; Giuliano et al. 1999; Maggio et al. 2013; Pinard et al. 2012; Wilcock and Peiffer 1986; Willis and Wilkie 2001)

16.3 Feline Periocular Tumors of the Eyelid, Third Eyelid, Conjunctiva, and Limbus

Box 16.3. Feline Periocular Tumors in Three Facts

1. Mostly squamous cell carcinomas and less often melanoma
2. Usually malignant with invasive growth but rare metastases
3. Early surgical excision as treatment of choice

▪ **Epidemiology and Pathogenesis**

Squamous cell carcinomas (SCC) are the only common tumor of the feline eyelids and third eyelid, making feline periocular tumors malignant in most cases. This is in strong contrast to canine periocular tumors, which are mostly benign. Feline periocular SCC usually develop in *lightly colored or white eyelids* and are thought to be *induced by ultraviolet light*. They often show *invasive growth but metastasis is rare. Feline conjunctival melanomas* are also often malignant with invasive behavior but rarely metastasize. *Limbal melanomas* are usually benign.

▪ **Clinical Signs**

Feline periocular tumors are usually clinically *malignant tumors* with the exception of the slowly growing, noninvasive limbal melanomas. *Clinical signs* are usually based on the mass effect of the tumors and its interference with the normal physiology of nictitating and moistening and with the general integrity of the mucosal surfaces and immune barriers. Tumors may be ulcerated with a rough surface and thus lead to dominant clinical signs of *inflammation, epiphora, mucopurulent discharge, protrusion of the third eyelid*, and corneal neovascularization.

Fluorescein stain, careful palpation, and inspection of ocular and periocular structures are usually sufficient for a tentative diagnosis of neoplastic disease. Melanomas may be pigmented but amelanotic melanomas are not uncommon. Fine needle aspiration or incisional biopsies, ultrasound, or even computed tomography (CT) and magnetic resonance imaging (MRI) may help in planning the therapeutic approach for larger tumors.

▪ **Cytology and Histopathology**

Cytology using fine needle aspiration (FNA) is an uncommon diagnostic tool for periocular tumors. If performed, cytology may help in the diagnosis of periocular melanomas or squamous cell carcinomas by identifying the presence of either pigmented or squamated cells, respectively. *Postsurgical histopathology of excisional biopsies* is by far the more common tool for definitive diagnosis of periocular tumors. *Melanomas* often contain pigmented epithelioid to spindloid cells, but immunohistochemistry for S100 or Melan A is occasionally required to confirm the diagnosis. SCC are composed of nests and cords of epithelial cells with occasional squamation of epithelial cells and presence of abundant secondary inflammation.

▪ **Therapy**

Surgical excision is the treatment of choice for feline periocular tumors. Since most periocular tumors are malignant, surgery should be performed promptly. *Cryosurgery* using liquid nitrogen and conservative surgery are increasingly the treatment of choice for periocular tumors. The eyelids in particular and periocular structures in general are functionally very sensitive structures. Tumors involving less than one third of the length of the eyelid may be excised using a *V-plasty or four-sided excision*. If the tumors are larger than one third of the length of the eyelid, advanced blepharoplasty is required to preserve eyelid function; this requires advanced surgical skills and referral to a specialty hospital. *Presurgical shrinkage* of the tumor using systemic or local chemotherapy or radiation therapy is recommended to minimize the fraction of the eyelid to be removed. Superficial conjunctival limbal melanomas may be treated by superficial keratectomy or sclerectomy but in progressed tumor states may require enucleation of the entire globe. Resection of the complete third eyelid is a rather simple procedure but is often associated with postsurgical complications like chronic ocular drying and keratitis.

Prognosis and Molecular Markers

The prognosis for feline periocular tumors is *worse than for canine tumors*; felines have a higher recurrence rate and a higher fraction of tumors requiring enucleation of the complete globe. However, when treated with sufficient surgical care, periocular tumors in the cat are associated with long survival times.

Suggested Further Readings

(Aquino 2007, 2008; Dees et al. 2015; Finn et al. 2008; Hagard 2005; Schobert et al. 2010; van der Woerdt 2004)

16.4 Feline Ocular Tumors

Box 16.4. Feline Ocular Tumors in Five Facts

1. Diffuse iris melanomas most common
2. Melanomas with slow growth but >50 % metastatic rate
3. Feline ocular posttraumatic sarcomas second most common tumor
4. Induced by trauma, invasively growing, rarely metastasizing
5. Early enucleation as treatment of choice for both tumor types

Epidemiology and Pathogenesis

Feline diffuse iris melanomas make up 50 % of primary ocular tumors in cats and are the most common ocular tumor in this species. The median *age* of affected cats is >9 years. There is no *breed* or *gender* predilection for the development of ocular melanomas. Feline ocular melanoma has a metastatic rate of >50 %. However, these metastases are slow growing and usually take 1–3 years to develop after enucleation.

Feline ocular posttraumatic sarcoma is the second most common feline ocular tumor but is very rare. The tumor develops in cats of all ages *after ocular trauma, including surgery, after a latency period of anywhere up to 7 years*. There is no *breed* predisposition, but a *gender* predisposition for males may be due to an increased risk of fighting wounds related to their socially more aggressive behavior. Damage to the lens and chronic uveitis are often associated with this tumor, and *the epithelial cells of the lens are likely the cell of origin*. Chronic inflammation is thought to support neoplastic transformation of a pluripotent cell, similar to the hypothesized etiology of feline injection site sarcomas. The tumors have a *severely invasive biologic behavior* with infiltration of the choroid, the retina, and the optic nerve. Metastasis is rare.

Clinical Signs

Typically the first *clinical signs observed in cats with diffuse iris melanoma are slowly progressing changes in the pigmentation of the iris*. Occasionally these may develop into or very rarely contain pigmented or amelanotic small masses. At later stages of progression, secondary glaucoma and typical signs of chronic anterior uveitis with iridal hyperpigmentation develop. The diagnosis of melanomas is based on the detection of progression of iridal thickening or irregularity of the iris surface.

Feline ocular posttraumatic sarcomas most commonly present with *white or red discoloration of the eye and changes in the shape of the globe*. Glaucoma, signs of uveitis, and corneal ulceration also commonly develop in these patients. Definitive diagnosis of these tumors is however difficult unless an actual mass can be visualized since most clinical features of the tumors are also found in feline eyes with chronic uveitis.

Cytology and Histopathology

Fine needle aspirates (FNA) are of uncertain value for the diagnosis of diffuse iris melanomas and ocular posttraumatic sarcomas in cats.

Histopathologically, diffuse iris melanomas are initially characterized by pleomorphic cells varying from spindle to more malignant multinucleated epithelioid cells at late stages of tumor development. Diffuse iridal melanomas infiltrate the stroma of the iris, the ciliary cleft, the overlying sclera, the peripheral cornea, and the ciliary body. Posttraumatic sarcomas present histopathologically as spindle cell tumors with areas of inflammation.

Therapy

Enucleation is the treatment of choice for feline iris melanoma. Due to the high metastatic rate of these tumors, immediate surgery after first diagnosis is often recommended and is associated with *survival times of up to 5 years*. If the tumor has invaded the ciliary body and the sclera, survival times are reduced to 1.5 years. Some authors recommend against enucleation prior to onset of glaucoma, signs of inflammation, and loss of vision because the positive effects of early enucleation are unproven, and most iris melanomas usually progress slowly and only develop clinical signs years later. Focal laser ablation treatment of hyperpigmented foci with preservation of vision has been described, but long-term efficacy has not been analyzed.

Enucleation is the treatment of choice for feline ocular posttraumatic sarcomas. Due to their invasive behavior, early enucleation is indicated. Enucleation at advanced tumor stages is often associated with orbital tumor recurrence. Prophylactic enucleation of traumatized or chronically inflamed globes has therefore been suggested. The optic nerve should be removed as extensively as possible, since the tumor commonly progresses from the globe into the orbita via this pathway. The *prognosis for feline ocular posttraumatic sarcomas is guarded* especially if the tumor has invaded the optic nerve. Local invasion of the orbita is usually observed within a few months and is associated with high mortality rates. Metastasis is rarely observed.

Radiation therapy is increasingly used for the treatment of feline ocular tumors but is associated with several ocular side effects.

Suggested Further Readings

(Finn et al. 2008; Grahn et al. 2006; Kalishman et al. 1998; Pinard et al. 2012; Willis and Wilkie 2001; Zeiss et al. 2003)

Suggested Reading

Aquino SM (2007) Management of eyelid neoplasms in the dog and cat. Clin Tech Small Anim Pract 22:46–54

Aquino SM (2008) Surgery of the eyelids. Top Companion Anim Med 23:10–22

Beckwith-Cohen B, Bentley E, Dubielzig RR (2015) Outcome of iridociliary epithelial tumour biopsies in dogs: a retrospective study. Vet Rec 176:147

Bernays ME, Flemming D, Peiffer RL Jr (1999) Primary corneal papilloma and squamous cell carcinoma associated with pigmentary keratitis in four dogs. J Am Vet Med Assoc 214:215–217, 204

Bussieres M, Krohne SG, Stiles J, Townsend WM (2005) The use of carbon dioxide laser for the ablation of meibomian gland adenomas in dogs. J Am Anim Hosp Assoc 41:227–234

Dees DD, Schobert CS, Dubielzig RR, Stein TJ (2016) Third eyelid gland neoplasms of dogs and cats: a retrospective histopathologic study of 145 cases. Vet Ophthalmol 19(2):138–143

Donaldson D, Sansom J, Adams V (2006a) Canine limbal melanoma: 30 cases (1992–2004). Part 2. Treatment with lamellar resection and adjunctive strontium-90beta plesiotherapy – efficacy and morbidity. Vet Ophthalmol 9:179–185

Donaldson D, Sansom J, Scase T, Adams V, Mellersh C (2006b) Canine limbal melanoma: 30 cases (1992–2004). Part 1. Signalment, clinical and histological features and pedigree analysis. Vet Ophthalmol 9:115–119

Featherstone HJ, Renwick P, Heinrich CL, Manning S (2009) Efficacy of lamellar resection, cryotherapy, and adjunctive grafting for the treatment of canine limbal melanoma. Vet Ophthalmol 12(Suppl 1):65–72

Finn M, Krohne S, Stiles J (2008) Ocular melanocytic neoplasia. Compendium 30:19–25; quiz 26

Giuliano EA, Chappell R, Fischer B, Dubielzig RR (1999) A matched observational study of canine survival with primary intraocular melanocytic neoplasia. Vet Ophthalmol 2:185–190

Grahn BH, Peiffer RL, Cullen CL, Haines DM (2006) Classification of feline intraocular neoplasms based on morphology, histochemical staining, and immunohistochemical labeling. Vet Ophthalmol 9:395–403

Hagard GM (2005) Eyelid reconstruction using a split eyelid flap after excision of a palpebral tumour in a Persian cat. J Small Anim Pract 46:389–392

Kalishman JB, Chappell R, Flood LA, Dubielzig RR (1998) A matched observational study of survival in cats with enucleation due to diffuse iris melanoma. Vet Ophthalmol 1:25–29

Lopes RA, Cardoso TC, Luvizotto MC, de Andrade AL (2010) Occurrence and expression of p53 suppressor gene and c-Myc oncogene in dog eyelid tumors. Vet Ophthalmol 13:69–75

Maggio F, Pizzirani S, Pena T, Leiva M, Pirie CG (2013) Surgical treatment of epibulbar melanocytomas by complete excision and homologous corneoscleral grafting in dogs: 11 cases. Vet Ophthalmol 16:56–64

Pinard CL, Mutsaers AJ, Mayer MN, Woods JP (2012) Retrospective study and review of ocular radiation side effects following external-beam Cobalt-60 radiation therapy in 37 dogs and 12 cats. Can Veter J La Revue Veter Canadienne 53:1301–1307

Romkes G, Klopfleisch R, Eule JC (2014) Evaluation of one- vs. two-layered closure after wedge excision of 43 eyelid tumors in dogs. Vet Ophthalmol 17:32–40

Schobert CS, Labelle P, Dubielzig RR (2010) Feline conjunctival melanoma: histopathological characteristics and clinical outcomes. Vet Ophthalmol 13:43–46

van der Woerdt A (2004) Adnexal surgery in dogs and cats. Vet Ophthalmol 7:284–290

Wilcock BP, Peiffer RL Jr (1986) Morphology and behavior of primary ocular melanomas in 91 dogs. Vet Pathol 23:418–424

Willis AM, Wilkie DA (2001) Ocular oncology. Clin Tech Small Anim Pract 16:77–85

Zeiss CJ, Johnson EM, Dubielzig RR (2003) Feline intraocular tumors may arise from transformation of lens epithelium. Vet Pathol 40:355–362

Thymomas

Robert Klopfleisch

R. Klopfleisch (ed.), *Veterinary Oncology*, DOI 10.1007/978-3-319-41124-8_17

Thymomas are neoplasms of the thymic epithelial cells. They are heterogeneous tumors that include and are sometimes dominated by well-differentiated, nonneoplastic lymphocytes. Well-differentiated lymphoma is a primary differential diagnosis for these tumors. Thymomas are rare tumors in all species. Most reports of thymomas in veterinary medicine are in dogs and cats. Rabbits are also commonly affected (▶ see Chap. 19), and some reports state that thymomas are one of the most common tumors in older goats.

17.1 Canine Thymomas

Box 17.1. Canine Thymomas in Six Facts

1. Rather rare tumor of dogs
2. Benign growth pattern but clinically malignant due to thoracic mass effect
3. Dyspnea, cranial edema, and cardiac insufficiency as the most common clinical signs
4. Several paraneoplastic syndromes including dermatitis and myasthenia gravis
5. Cytological/histopathologic diagnosis difficult due to lymphocyte dominance in the tumor
6. Surgery as the treatment of choice and associated with a good prognosis

▪ Epidemiology and Pathogenesis

Thymomas are rare tumors in dogs but are one of the most common tumors of the cranial mediastinum. They derive from thymic epithelial cells, usually have a *slow and expansive* growth, and only *rarely metastasize*. Nevertheless, due to their delicate location in close proximity to the heart and to the nerves and vessels in the cranial mediastinum, thymomas are often difficult to resect and are a *fatal and clinically malignant disease*. They occur in dogs at a median *age* of 9 years. There is no *gender* or *breed* predisposition. The causes and mechanism of thymoma development in dogs or any other animal species are unknown.

17

▪ Clinical Appearance

Common *clinical signs* in dogs with thymomas are usually related to the mass effect in the thorax. Compression atelectasis of the lung may be associated with *dyspnea, tachypnea, and coughing*. Compression of the cranial vena cava or any other veins draining the cranial region of the body may occasionally be associated with edema of the head and the front limbs. Finally, displacement and encasement of the heart may lead to *moderate cardiac insufficiency*. Exophthalmos is a very common finding in rabbits with mediastinal masses.

Thymomas are associated with several *paraneoplastic syndromes*, which occur in more than 50 % of affected dogs. *Thymoma-associated myasthenia gravis*, an antibody-based autoimmunity against acetylcholine receptors, is the most common paraneoplastic syndrome and may be present in 20–40 % of dogs with thymomas. The exact molecular mechanisms of the syndrome are unknown, but a lack of myoid cells in thymomas is suspected, but the exact mechanism is unclear. It is associated with paralysis of the esophagus and leads to megaesophagus, regurgitation, and aspiration pneumonia. *Thymoma-associated exfoliative dermatitis* is more often found in affected cats but has been described in some dogs. It is characterized by a diffuse severe cutaneous erythema and exfoliation (large scales). Again, the underlying molecular mechanisms of the disease are unclear. Finally, autoimmune polymyositis, anemia due to immune-mediated hemolysis, and hypercalcemia due to secretion of parathormone-related peptide have occasionally been described in dogs with thymomas.

Blood work is usually unremarkable in dogs with thymomas.

Thoracic radiographs and particularly *computed tomography (CT)* are usually helpful to identify cranial masses and to evaluate the extent of replacement and invasion of the surrounding structures (◘ Fig. 17.1). *Ultrasound* is also commonly used to identify and confirm mediastinal masses. Final diagnosis requires *ultrasound- or CT-guided fine needle aspiration* or biopsy.

▪ Cytology and Histopathology

Cytology of *fine needle aspirates* of the tumor mass and pleural fluids obtained by *thoracocentesis* usually contain a high fraction of small,

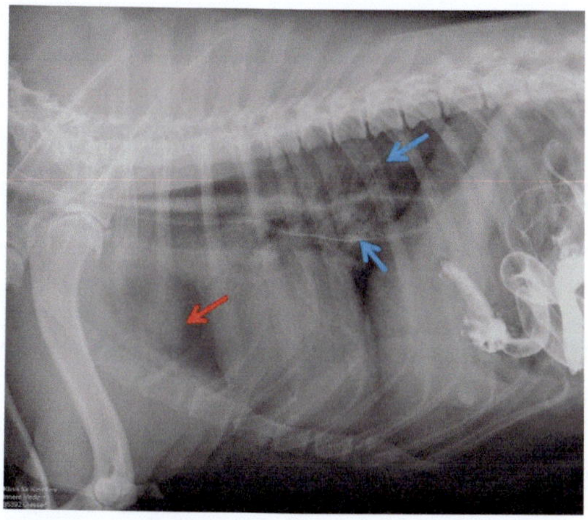

■ **Fig. 17.1** Thoracic radiograph, right lateral recumbency, thymoma (*red arrow*), and megaesophagus (*blue arrow*) due to subsequent myasthenia gravis (With permission of Dr. N. Bauer, Faculty of Veterinary Medicine, Justus Liebig University, Giessen, Germany)

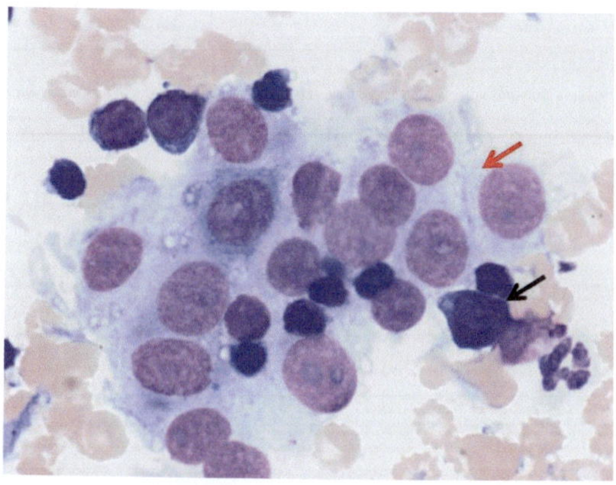

■ **Fig. 17.2** Cytology, thymoma dog (the same dog as in ■ Fig. 17.1), May-Grünwald-Giemsa, 1000×. Note the small cluster of slightly spindle-shaped to polygonal epithelial cells (*red arrow*) surrounded by small- to medium-sized mature lymphocytes (*black arrow*) (With permission of Dr. N. Bauer, Faculty of Veterinary Medicine, Justus Liebig University, Giessen, Germany)

mature, well-differentiated lymphocytes, and fewer medium-sized lymphocytes interspersed between a few neoplastic thymoma cells (■ Fig. 17.2). The lymphocytes often cover the actual epithelial spindloid and occasionally plump polygonal epithelial tumor cells. Well-differentiated mast cells and macrophages can also be present. *Cytological preparations may be misdiagnosed as a well-differentiated lymphoma.*

A homogenous population of one type of lymphocyte and the absence of other cell types are indicative of lymphoma, while a mixed cellular population is suggestive of thymoma even in the *absence of epithelial cells.*

Histopathology of biopsies or surgically excised tumors can be a good diagnostic tool. Diagnosis is often complicated by the presence of numerous well-differentiated lymphocytes covering the actual tumor cells. *Hassall's corpuscles*, concentric eosinophilic masses, are specific structures of thymic tissues and are usually also present in thymomas. *Immunohistochemical detection of cytokeratin* improves the detection and evaluation of cellular morphology of the positive tumor cells.

■ Therapy

Surgery is the most commonly used treatment modality for canine thymomas. Radiographs and CT must be used to determine how resectable the tumor is, but a lot depends on the skills and experience of the surgeon. In the few studies available, it is stated that surgical excision is associated with median survival times of 2–3 years in almost 50 % of patients. There is a 20 % recurrence rate, but secondary surgery is associated with a *good prognosis*.

Prednisone and doxorubicin are used as *primary and adjuvant chemotherapy*; chemotherapy is associated with partial remission and shrinking of the tumor. Shrinkage is however thought to be caused by a reduction of the non-neoplastic lymphocyte population in the tumor rather than directly targeting the thymoma cells.

Radiation therapy may also be associated with a partial or complete response and survival times of up to 8 months, but more studies are required to confirm its efficacy.

■ Prognostic Factors and Molecular Markers

The prognosis for canine thymomas very much depends on resectability and surgical treatment. Complete resection is associated with a good prognosis for long-term survival. Vascular invasion is negatively correlated with prognosis, whereas the amount of lymphocytic infiltrate is positively correlated with prognosis.

Studies do not show a correlation between survival time and hypercalcemia and the presence of myasthenia gravis or megaesophagus at the time of thymoma diagnosis, histopathological thymoma subtype, or tumor development at a later date.

▪ Suggested Further Reading

(Aronsohn et al. 1984; Atwater et al. 1994; Day 1997; Hunt et al. 1997; Hylands 2006; Marx et al. 2015; Moffet 2007; Robat et al. 2013; Smith et al. 2001; Tepper et al. 2011; Turek 2003; Yoon et al. 2004; Zitz et al. 2008)

17.2 Feline Thymomas

Box 17.2. Feline Thymomas in Six Facts

1. Rather rare tumor of cats
2. Benign growth pattern but clinically malignant due to thoracic mass effect
3. Dyspnea, cranial edema, and cardiac insufficiency as the most common clinical signs
4. Paraneoplastic syndromes less common than in the dog
5. Cytological/histopathologic diagnosis difficult due to lymphocyte dominance in the tumor
6. Surgery as the treatment of choice and associated with a good prognosis

▪ Epidemiology and Pathogenesis

Thymomas are very rare tumors of the cranial mediastinum. Mediastinal lymphomas by far outnumber thymomas in the cat (▶ see Chap. 6). There is significantly less literature on feline thymomas than on canine thymomas, but they seem to be similar in most aspects of their biology, clinical signs, and response to treatment. Feline thymomas derive from *thymic epithelial cells*, usually have a slow and expansive growth, and only *rarely metastasize*. Nevertheless, due to their delicate location in close proximity to the heart and to the nerves and vessels in the cranial mediastinum, thymomas are often difficult to resect and are a *fatal and clinically malignant disease*. They occur in cats at a median *age* of 10 years. There is no *gender* or *breed* predisposition. The causes and mechanism of thymoma development in cats or any other animal species are unknown.

▪ Clinical Appearance

The common *clinical signs* in cats are in almost all aspects similar to those in dogs with the exception of the incidence of paraneoplastic syndromes. Clinical signs are usually related to the mass effect in the thorax. Compression atelectasis of the lung may be associated with *dyspnea, tachypnea, and coughing*. Compression of the cranial vena cava or any other veins draining the cranial region of the body may be associated with edema of the head and the front limbs. Finally, displacement and encasement of the heart may lead to *moderate cardiac insufficiency*.

Thymomas are associated with several *paraneoplastic syndromes*. *Thymoma-associated myasthenia gravis*, an antibody-based autoimmunity against acetylcholine receptors, is occasionally described as a paraneoplastic syndrome in cats. The exact molecular mechanisms of the syndrome are unknown. It is associated with paralysis of the esophagus and leads to megaesophagus, regurgitation and aspiration pneumonia, and generalized weakness. *Thymoma-associated exfoliative dermatitis* (▫ Fig. 17.3) is rare but has been well described in the literature. It is characterized by a diffuse severe non-pruritic, cutaneous erythema and exfoliation (large scales). Again, the underlying molecular mechanisms of the disease are unclear.

Blood work is usually unremarkable in cats with thymomas.

Thoracic radiographs and particularly *computed tomography (CT)* are usually helpful to identify cranial masses and to evaluate the extent

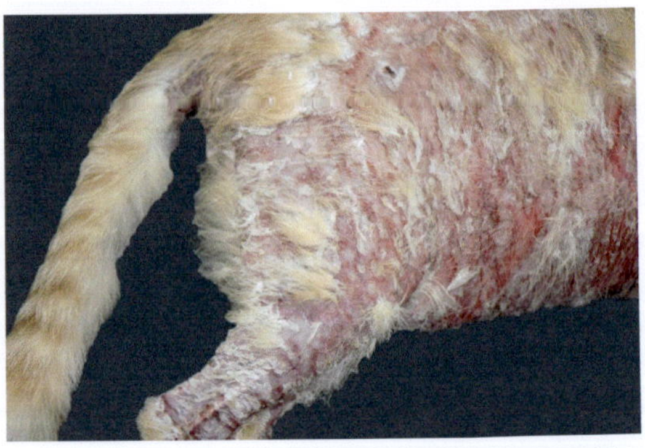

▫ **Fig. 17.3** Exfoliative dermatitis in a cat with a thymoma

of replacement and invasion of the surrounding structures. *Ultrasound* is also commonly used to identify and confirm mediastinal masses. Final diagnosis requires *ultrasound- or CT-guided fine needle aspiration* or biopsy.

▪ Cytology and Histopathology

Cytology of *fine needle aspirates* of the tumor mass and pleural fluids obtained by *thoracocentesis* usually contains a high fraction of small mature, well-differentiated lymphocytes, and a few well-differentiated mast cells and macrophages interspersed between a few neoplastic thymoma cells. The lymphocytes often cover the actual epithelial spindloid and occasionally plump polygonal epithelial tumor cells. Cytological preparations are may be misdiagnosed as well-differentiated lymphomas. A homogenous population of one type of lymphocyte and the absence of other cell types are indicative of lymphoma. A heterogeneous cellular population is suggestive of thymoma.

Histopathology of biopsies or surgically excised tumors can be a good diagnostic tool. Diagnosis is often complicated by the presence of numerous well-differentiated lymphocytes covering the actual tumor cells. *Hassall's corpuscles*, concentric eosinophilic masses, are specific structures of thymic tissues and are usually also present in thymomas. There is an uncommon, feline-specific cystic thymoma subtype, which is associated with a better prognosis than solid thymomas. *Immunohistochemical detection of cytokeratin* improves the detection and evaluation of cellular morphology of the positive tumor cells.

▪ Therapy

Surgery is the most commonly used treatment modality for feline thymomas. Radiographs and CT must be used to determine how resectable the tumor is, and success very much depends on the skills and experience of the surgeon. In the few studies available, it is stated that surgical excision is associated with survival rates of 89 % at 1 year and 75 % at 3 years and a median survival of 5 years.

Prednisone and doxorubicin have been tested as *primary and adjuvant chemotherapy* in a few studies and may be associated with partial remission and shrinking of the tumor. Shrinkage is thought to be caused by a reduction of the non-neoplastic lymphocyte population in the tumor rather than directly targeting the thymoma cells.

Radiation therapy may also be associated with a partial or complete response and survival times of up to 2 years, but more studies are required to confirm its efficacy.

▪ Prognostic Factors and Molecular Markers

The *prognosis* for feline thymoma very much depends on the resectability and surgical treatment. Complete resection is associated with a good prognosis for long-term survival. Vascular invasion is negatively correlated with prognosis, whereas the amount of lymphocytic infiltrate is positively correlated with prognosis. The recurrence and presence of paraneoplastic syndromes have no influence on prognosis.

▪ Suggested Further Reading

(Cavalcanti et al. 2014; Day 1997; Hill et al. 2013; Patnaik et al. 2003; Shilo et al. 2011; Singh et al. 2010; Smith et al. 2001; Spadavecchia and Jaggy 2008; Turek 2003; Yoon et al. 2004; Zitz et al. 2008)

17.3 Thymomas of Goats

Box 17.3. Thymomas of Goats in Three Facts

1. Common tumor in old goats
2. Benign growth, often incidental necropsy finding
3. No reported treatment modality in this species

▪ Epidemiology and Pathology

Thymomas in the goat are tumors of thymic epithelial cells. The few epidemiologic studies on tumors in goats indicate that thymoma may be the *third most common tumor* in this species after lymphoma and squamous cell carcinomas. There seems to be a predisposition for dairy goats. Up to 25 % of all tumors in *Saanen goats* are thymomas, suggesting a *breed disposition* for these animals. Thymomas are usually a tumor of middle-aged to old goats, appearing at an *age* of 4–10 years. Thymomas in the goat are usually *incidental find-*

ings found on necropsy. Clinical signs including *dyspnea* or esophageal compression with *megaesophagus* and regurgitation have been described in a few rare cases. Caprine thymomas are usually slowly and *expansively growing tumors*. Metastatic thymic carcinoma has been described in one case report in a goat with pulmonary metastases. *Cytologically and histopathologically*, the cytokeratin-positive cells are often hidden by abundant mature lymphocytes. There are no reports on treatment modalities or prognostic factors for caprine thymomas.

Suggested Further Reading

(Braun et al. 2009; Hadlow 1978; Lohr 2013; Olchowy et al. 1996; Parish et al. 1996; Rostkowski et al. 1985)

Suggested Reading

Aronsohn MG, Schunk KL, Carpenter JL, King NW (1984) Clinical and pathologic features of thymoma in 15 dogs. J Am Vet Med Assoc 184:1355–1362

Atwater SW, Powers BE, Park RD, Straw RC, Ogilvie GK, Withrow SJ (1994) Thymoma in dogs: 23 cases (1980–1991). J Am Vet Med Assoc 205:1007–1013

Braun U, Steininger K, Irmer M, Hagen R, Ohlerth S, Ruhl S, Ossent P (2009) Ultrasonographic and computed tomographic findings in a goat with mediastinal lymphocytic thymoma. Schweiz Arch Tierheilkd 151:332–335

Cavalcanti JV, Moura MP, Monteiro FO (2014) Thymoma associated with exfoliative dermatitis in a cat. J Feline Med Surg 16:1020–1023

Day MJ (1997) Review of thymic pathology in 30 cats and 36 dogs. J Small Anim Pract 38:393–403

Hadlow WJ (1978) High prevalence of thymoma in the dairy goat. Report of seventeen cases. Veter Pathol 15:153–169

Hill PB, Brain P, Collins D, Fearnside S, Olivry T (2013) Putative paraneoplastic pemphigus and myasthenia gravis in a cat with a lymphocytic thymoma. Vet Dermatol 24:646–649, e163–644

Hunt GB, Churcher RK, Church DB, Mahoney P (1997) Excision of a locally invasive thymoma causing cranial vena caval syndrome in a dog. J Am Vet Med Assoc 210:1628–1630

Hylands R (2006) Veterinary diagnostic imaging. Thymoma. Can Veter J La revue veterinaire canadienne 47:593–596

Lohr CV (2013) One hundred two tumors in 100 goats (1987–2011). Vet Pathol 50:668–675

Marx A, Porubsky S, Belharazem D, Saruhan-Direskeneli G, Schalke B, Strobel P, Weis CA (2015) Thymoma related myasthenia gravis in humans and potential animal models. Exp Neurol 270:55–65

Moffet AC (2007) Metastatic thymoma and acquired generalized myasthenia gravis in a beagle. Can Veter J La revue veterinaire canadienne 48:91–93

Olchowy TW, Toal RL, Brenneman KA, Slauson DO, McEntee MF (1996) Metastatic thymoma in a goat. Can Veter J La revue veterinaire canadienne 37:165–167

Parish SM, Middleton JR, Baldwin TJ (1996) Clinical megaoesophagus in a goat with thymoma. Vet Rec 139:94

Patnaik AK, Lieberman PH, Erlandson RA, Antonescu C (2003) Feline cystic thymoma: a clinicopathologic, immunohistologic, and electron microscopic study of 14 cases. J Feline Med Surg 5:27–35

Robat CS, Cesario L, Gaeta R, Miller M, Schrempp D, Chun R (2013) Clinical features, treatment options, and outcome in dogs with thymoma: 116 cases (1999–2010). J Am Vet Med Assoc 243:1448–1454

Rostkowski CM, Stirtzinger T, Baird JD (1985) Congestive heart failure associated with thymoma in two nubian goats. Can Veter J La revue veterinaire canadienne 26:267–269

Shilo Y, Pypendop BH, Barter LS, Epstein SE (2011) Thymoma removal in a cat with acquired myasthenia gravis: a case report and literature review of anesthetic techniques. Vet Anaesth Analg 38:603–613

Singh A, Boston SE, Poma R (2010) Thymoma-associated exfoliative dermatitis with post-thymectomy myasthenia gravis in a cat. Can Veter J La revue veterinaire canadienne 51:757–760

Smith AN, Wright JC, Brawner WR Jr, LaRue SM, Fineman L, Hogge GS, Kitchell BE, Hohenhaus AE, Burk RL, Dhaliwal RS, Duda LE (2001) Radiation therapy in the treatment of canine and feline thymomas: a retrospective study (1985–1999). J Am Anim Hosp Assoc 37:489–496

Spadavecchia C, Jaggy A (2008) Thymectomy in a cat with myasthenia gravis: a case report focusing on perianaesthetic management. Schweiz Arch Tierheilkd 150:515–518

Tepper LC, Spiegel IB, Davis GJ (2011) Diagnosis of erythema multiforme associated with thymoma in a dog and treated with thymectomy. J Am Anim Hosp Assoc 47:e19–e25

Turek MM (2003) Cutaneous paraneoplastic syndromes in dogs and cats: a review of the literature. Vet Dermatol 14:279–296

Yoon J, Feeney DA, Cronk DE, Anderson KL, Ziegler LE (2004) Computed tomographic evaluation of canine and feline mediastinal masses in 14 patients. Vet Radiol Ultrasound Off J Am College Veter Radiol Int Veter Radiol Asso 45:542–546

Zitz JC, Birchard SJ, Couto GC, Samii VF, Weisbrode SE, Young GS (2008) Results of excision of thymoma in cats and dogs: 20 cases (1984–2005). J Am Vet Med Assoc 232:1186–1192

Mesotheliomas

Robert Klopfleisch

R. Klopfleisch (ed.), *Veterinary Oncology*, DOI 10.1007/978-3-319-41124-8_18

Mesotheliomas are tumors of the mesothelial cells of the pleura, peritoneum, pericardium, and occasionally of the tunica vaginalis. The mesothelium is derived from the mesoderm, but mesothelial cells have several morphologic and biochemical features of epithelial cells. Mesotheliomas may thus be composed of varied cell types; these include epithelial cytokeratin-positive cells, mesenchymal vimentin-positive cells, and cells expressing both immunohistochemical markers. Mesotheliomas are one of the most common tumors in cattle but are rare in cats, dogs, horses, or other species.

18.1 Canine Mesotheliomas

Box 18.1. Canine Mesotheliomas in Five Facts

1. Tumor of the pleura, peritoneum, pericardium, or tunica vaginalis of older dogs
2. Always malignant due to rapid growth and widespread contact metastases
3. Difficult clinical diagnosis due to plane or micronodular tumor growth
4. Clinical signs usually effusions
5. Effusion drainage, cytoreduction, and intracavitary chemotherapy are palliative not curative

Epidemiology and Pathogenesis

Mesotheliomas are rare tumors of older dogs. They occur at an average *age* of 9 years but can occasionally be seen in younger dogs. There may be a slight *gender* predisposition for males. There is no known breed predisposition. Mesotheliomas are characterized by a multifocal to diffuse multinodular plane growth pattern, what makes their visualization by imaging technologies difficult. They are *always malignant* due to a fast growth rate with invasion of adjacent tissues and *metastases*; metastases are usually contained within the affected body cavity.

Development of human mesotheliomas is strongly associated with *asbestos exposure*. This may also be true for dogs. Asbestos exposure and development of mesothelioma in owners is a risk factor for concurrent disease in dogs. The lungs of dogs with mesotheliomas also contain asbestos fibers significantly more often than healthy dogs. Disease in dogs can be considered an indicator for risk of disease development in humans living in the same environment. A*sbestos is believed to directly induce DNA damage* after phagocytosis by phagocytic mesothelial cells. In humans, it has been shown that some forms of asbestos mechanically disrupt the spindle apparatus during mitosis. In addition, asbestos induces a secretion of *inflammatory cytokines* and *proproliferative growth factors*, which may further support the proliferation and transformation of cells in contact with asbestos fibers.

Clinical Signs

Clinical signs associated with mesotheliomas depend on the location of the tumor but are usually due to *effusions in the affected body cavity*. The most common clinical findings are hydrothorax with dyspnea, ascites, and pericardial effusions with cardiac tamponade and cardiac insufficiency. Blood work is usually unremarkable in these dogs.

Radiographs and ultrasound usually detect pleural, pericardial, or abdominal effusions. Due to the plane growth of these tumors, *actual tumor masses are not usually detected*. Clinical diagnosis of mesothelioma is very difficult, even after cytological analysis. A recent report on a single case of canine mesothelioma suggests that MRI may be the most specific method for detecting mesotheliomas

Cytology and Histopathology

Definitive *cytological diagnosis* of mesotheliomas requires advanced cytological skills and is not possible in all cases. Fluids obtained from affected body cavities usually contain abundant inflammatory cells and erythrocytes; mesothelioma cells are found less often. When found, mesothelioma cells are single or located in small groups and have an epithelioid shape with bluish and vacuolated cytoplasm. They may be anisokaryotic and pleomorphic. These same features are however also found in reactive, hypertrophic mesothelial cells in cases of pleuritis and peritonitis. Final diagnosis of mesothelioma requires *histopathology* and immunohistochemistry. Histopathology alone is usually diagnostic. In some cases though, it is not possible to exclude the differential diagnoses of chronic proliferative serositis or adenocarcinoma. Asbestos fibers are occasionally detectable as ferruginous bodies, fibers coated with ferritin and amorphous protein. Immunohistochemical detection of *parallel expression of cytokeratin and vimentin* is helpful in these cases. However, anaplastic carcinomas, melanomas, and renal carcinomas may also express both markers. Detection of *acid mucins* by alcian blue staining and *electron microscope-based detection* of numerous desmosomes and long slender microvilli with bundles of tonofilaments are other relatively specific markers of mesotheliomas.

■ Therapy

The *main goal of therapy of mesotheliomas is palliative care* and prolonging survival times. There is no cure.

The simplest but often most effective forms of treatment are *thoraco- or pericardiocentesis* or drainage of abdominal fluids. This usually alleviates clinical signs for up to several months but has to be repeated for the rest of the dog's life.

Surgery is used for cytoreduction especially by pericardiectomy. This may increase quality of life and is associated with survival times of several months. Adjuvant chemotherapy after surgery can further increase survival times up to 14 months.

Non-adjuvant intravenous chemotherapy using doxorubicin and cisplatin may be efficient for short-term partial or complete remission but is not effective for long-term disease control. *Intracavitary chemotherapy* using cisplatin or carboplatin alone or in combination with mitoxantrone has been used as an alternative to systemic chemotherapy. It is more effective and usually better tolerated and is associated with survival times of up to 2 years. Cisplatin for intracavitary application has to be diluted in isotonic sodium chloride.

Studies on the efficacy of *radiation therapy* for the treatment of mesotheliomas are not available.

■ Suggested Further Readings

(Charney et al. 2005; Dunning et al. 1998; Echandi et al. 2007; Gallach and Mai 2013; Glickman et al. 1983; Kerstetter et al. 1997; Liptak and Brebner 2006; MacDonald et al. 2009; Moore et al. 1991; Reetz et al. 2012; Seo et al. 2007; Spugnini et al. 2008; Stepien et al. 2000)

18.2 Feline Mesotheliomas

Box 18.2. Feline Mesotheliomas in Five Facts

1. Tumor of the pleura, peritoneum, pericardium, or tunica vaginalis of older cats
2. Always malignant due to rapid growth and widespread contact metastases
3. Difficult clinical diagnosis due to plane or micronodular tumor growth
4. Clinical signs of body cavity effusions
5. Effusion drainage, cytoreduction, and intracavitary palliative but not curative

According to the current knowledge, in most aspects, *feline mesotheliomas* behave biologically and clinically in their response to treatments *similar to canine mesotheliomas*. Below only the difference of feline from canine mesotheliomas are briefly described (for complete information, see ▶ Sect. 18.1). In contrast to dogs, there are no studies on the correlation between feline mesotheliomas and exposure to asbestos or the incidence of mesotheliomas in the owner. Intracavitary application of carboplatin in cats with pleural mesotheliomas is associated with survival times between 4 and 6 months (◻ Fig. 18.1).

■ Suggested Further Readings

(Bacci et al. 2006; Sparkes et al. 2005; Spugnini et al. 2008)

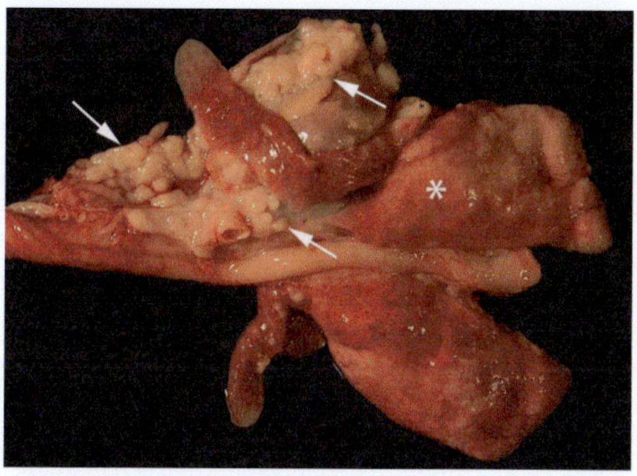

◻ **Fig. 18.1** Pleural mesothelioma (*arrows*) in a cat (* = unaffected lung) (Photo: with permission of A. Weiss, PhD, CVUA-MEL, Münster, Germany and the Archive of the Institute of Veterinary Pathology, Freie Universität Berlin)

18.3 Bovine Mesotheliomas

Mesotheliomas are common but still rare bovine tumors with *two age peaks* of appearance: *congenital mesotheliomas* in calves and *acquired mesotheliomas in aged cattle*. Congenital bovine mesotheliomas develop in few weeks old calves, and most are located commonly on the peritoneal and less commonly on the pleural or pericardial serosa. Intralesional *asbestos fibers* or an association with asbestos exposure of the calf or the mother has not been confirmed so far. *Clinical signs* are mostly due to body cavity effusions, abdominal extension ascites, and cachexia. Histopathology is usually required for ultimate diagnosis and is usually performed postmortem. Bovine mesotheliomas are *always malignant* and usually develop widespread contact metastases (Figs. 18.2 and 18.3). There are *no therapeutic modalities* described, and animals inevitably die or are euthanized due to the neoplasia.

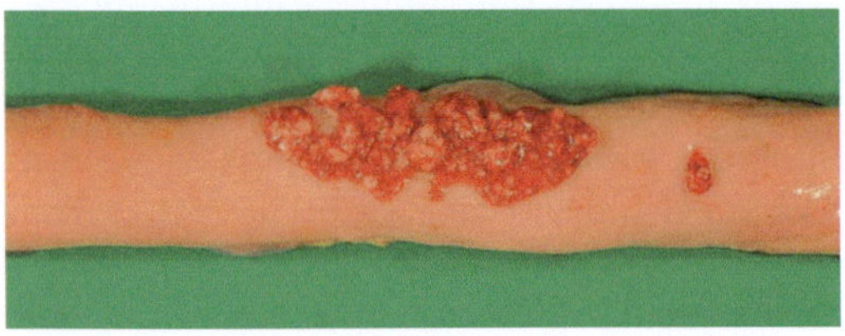

Fig. 18.2 Pleural (periesophageal) mesothelioma in a cow (Photo: with permission of M. Bothe, PhD, Fresenius Medical Care, Bad Homburg, Germany and the Archive of the Institute of Veterinary Pathology, Freie Universität Berlin)

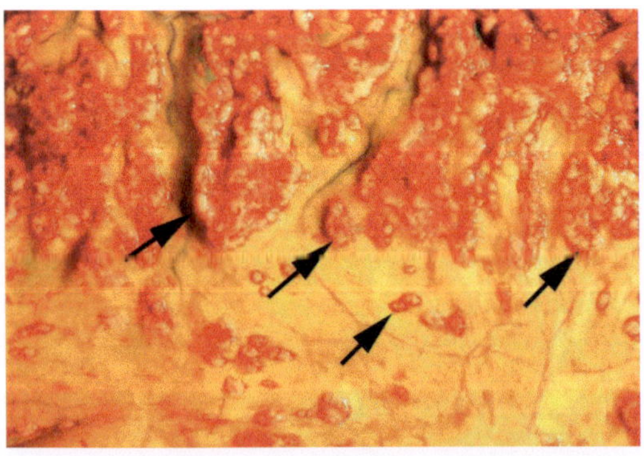

Fig. 18.3 Peritoneal mesothelioma (*arrows*) in a cow (Photo: with permission of M. Bothe, PhD, Fresenius Medical Care, Bad Homburg, Germany and the Archive of the Institute of Veterinary Pathology, Freie Universität Berlin)

Suggested Further Reading

(Baskerville 1967; Magnusson and Veit 1987; Misdorp 2002a, b; Schamber et al. 1982; Takasu et al. 2006)

Suggested Reading

Bacci B, Morandi F, De Meo M, Marcato PS (2006) Ten cases of feline mesothelioma: an immunohistochemical and ultrastructural study. J Comp Pathol 134:347–354

Baskerville A (1967) Mesothelioma in the calf. Pathol Vet 4:149–156

Charney SC, Bergman PJ, McKnight JA, Farrelly J, Novosad CA, Leibman NF, Camps-Palau MA (2005) Evaluation of intracavitary mitoxantrone and carboplatin for treatment of carcinomatosis, sarcomatosis and mesothelioma, with or without malignant effusions: a retrospective analysis of 12 cases (1997–2002)*. Vet Comp Oncol 3:171–181

Dunning D, Monnet E, Orton EC, Salman MD (1998) Analysis of prognostic indicators for dogs with pericardial effusion: 46 cases (1985–1996). J Am Vet Med Assoc 212:1276–1280

Echandi RL, Morandi F, Newman SJ, Holford A (2007) Imaging diagnosis – canine thoracic mesothelioma. Vet Radiol Ultrasound Off J Am College Veter Radiol Int Veter Radiol Ass 48:243–245

Gallach RG, Mai W (2013) Cardiac MRI findings in a dog with a diffuse pericardial mesothelioma and pericardial effusion. J Am Anim Hosp Assoc 49:398–402

Glickman LT, Domanski LM, Maguire TG (1983) Mesothelioma in pet dogs associated with exposure of their owners to asbestos. Environ Res 32:305–313

Kerstetter KK, Krahwinkel DJ Jr, Millis DL, Hahn K (1997) Pericardiectomy in dogs: 22 cases (1978–1994). J Am Vet Med Assoc 211:736–740

Liptak JM, Brebner NS (2006) Hemidiaphragmatic reconstruction with a transversus abdominis muscle flap after resection of a solitary diaphragmatic mesothelioma in a dog. J Am Vet Med Assoc 228:1204–1208

MacDonald KA, Cagney O, Magne ML (2009) Echocardiographic and clinicopathologic characterization of pericardial effusion in dogs: 107 cases (1985–2006). J Am Vet Med Assoc 235:1456–1461

Magnusson RA, Veit HP (1987) Mesothelioma in a calf. J Am Vet Med Assoc 191:233–234

Misdorp W (2002a) Congenital tumours and tumour-like lesions in domestic animals. 1. Cattle. A review. Vet Q 24:1–11

Misdorp W (2002b) Tumours in calves: comparative aspects. J Comp Pathol 127:96–105

Moore AS, Kirk C, Cardona A (1991) Intracavitary cisplatin chemotherapy experience with six dogs. J Veter Intern Med Am College Veter Intern 5:227–231

Reetz JA, Buza EL, Krick EL (2012) CT features of pleural masses and nodules. Vet Radiol Ultrasound Off J Am College Veter Radiol Int Veter Radiol Ass 53:121–127

Schamber GJ, Olson C, Witt LE (1982) Neoplasms in calves (Bos taurus). Vet Pathol 19:629–637

Seo KW, Choi US, Jung YC, Hong SJ, Byeun YE, Kang MS, Pachrin B, Kim WH, Hwang CY, Kim DY, Youn HY, Lee CW (2007) Palliative intravenous cisplatin treatment for concurrent peritoneal and pleural mesothelioma in a dog. J Veter Med Sci Jap Soc Veter Sci 69:201–204

Sparkes A, Murphy S, McConnell F, Smith K, Blunden AS, Papasouliotis K, Vanthournout D (2005) Palliative intracavitary carboplatin therapy in a cat with suspected pleural mesothelioma. J Feline Med Surg 7:313–316

Spugnini EP, Crispi S, Scarabello A, Caruso G, Citro G, Baldi A (2008) Piroxicam and intracavitary platinum-based chemotherapy for the treatment of advanced mesothelioma in pets: preliminary observations. J Exp Clini Cancer Res CR 27:6

Stepien RL, Whitley NT, Dubielzig RR (2000) Idiopathic or mesothelioma-related pericardial effusion: clinical findings and survival in 17 dogs studied retrospectively. J Small Anim Pract 41:342–347

Takasu M, Shirota K, Uchida N, Iguchi T, Nishii N, Ohba Y, Maeda S, Miyazawa K, Murase T, Kitagawa H (2006) Pericardial mesothelioma in a neonatal calf. J Veter Med Sci Jap Soc Veter Sci 68:519–521

Tumors of Mice, Rats, Rabbits, and Guinea Pigs

Olivia Kershaw

R. Klopfleisch (ed.), *Veterinary Oncology*, DOI 10.1007/978-3-319-41124-8_19

19.1 Common Tumors in Mice

19.1.1 Introduction

Most laboratory mice are prone to develop neoplasia. To investigate the genetic basis of cancer was one of the reasons that originally prompted the use of laboratory mice. With the development of genetically engineered mice, this trend was accelerated. Numerous of the most important inbred strains of mice were established because of their predisposition towards particular neoplasia. Besides the genetic impact due to homogeneity, the presence of numerous retroviral elements in the mouse genome makes neoplasia a common condition in mice. With the development of more and more mouse strains and substrains, the data turn out to be imprecise. Initiatives to not lose the overview were the establishment of systematic databases like the Mouse Tumor Biology database (MTB, http://tumor.informatics.jax.org/mtbwi/index.do) (Begley et al. 2007, 2012a, b; Krupke et al. 2008) and Pathbase (http://www.pathbase.net/) (Schofield et al. 2004a, b, 2010).

19.1.2 Hematopoietic Neoplasia of Mice

Box 19.1. Murine Hematopoietic Tumors in Five Facts

1. Very common
2. Females > males
3. Marked strain predispositions
4. Young and aged mice affected
5. Short disease course common

Epidemiology and Pathogenesis

The most important causes for hematopoietic neoplasia in mice are retroviruses (Taddesse-Heath et al. 2000), irradiation (Boorman et al. 2000), and diverse chemicals (Gold et al. 2001). Additionally, numerous mouse strains were genetically engineered to develop hematopoietic neoplasia (Kogan et al. 2002; Morse et al. 2002). In general, incidences in females are higher than in males.

19

Clinical Appearance

Generally, progression of disease is rapid and mice become “ill” with reduced general condition. Often tumors are can be identified externally, especially if lymph nodes are involved or organomegaly is present. Hematopoietic neoplasia arises in various locations, often with multiple organ involvement. Gross findings often give a first hint regarding the specific origin of neoplastic cells (■ see Table 19.1).

Cytology and Histopathology

Cytology of hematopoietic tumors is in general possible and often leads to the diagnosis of a round cell tumor. Because of the mostly short course of disease, cytology is however seldom applied. The cytological and histological features these tumors are similar to tumors in other species (see Chap. 6). Tumors are often highly invasive with severe displacement of preexisting tissues. Immunophenotyping using various markers and techniques (e.g., cytochemical stains, immunohistochemical stains, flow cytometric immunophenotyping) can be applied to finally characterize the specific cell of origin.

Therapy

With the exception of experimental settings, therapy is *unusual.*

Suggested Reading

(Begley et al. 2012a, b)

19.1.2.1 Lymphoid (B and T Cell) Tumors of Mice

Epidemiology and Pathogenesis

Lymphoid neoplasias are common but have varying incidences depending on strain, stock, sex, and age (Ward 2006). In general, two disease patterns can be differentiated. Tumors develop early with high mortality and short survival or late in aged mice. Typically, thymic T-cell lymphomas arise early, while aged mice develop B-cell lymphomas especially from the spleen, Peyer's patches, or mesenteric lymph nodes (Ward 2006).

Table 19.1 Gross necropsy classification of mouse hematopoietic tumors (Cardiff et al. 2000)

Gross distribution	T-cell lymphomas	B-cell lymphomas	Histiocytic sarcoma	Myeloid leukemia
Systemic (generalized)	Common	Rare	Rare	Rare
Thymic	*Primarily*	Rare	Rare	Rare
Spleen	Rare	*Common*–follicular or marginal zone	Occasionally – red pulp origin	*Common*
Peyer's patches	Rare	*Common*	Occasional	Rare
Mesenteric lymph nodes	Rare	*Common*	Occasional	Rare
Liver	Rare	Rare	*Common*	Rare
Uterus	Rare	Rare	*Common*	Rare
Peritoneum	Rare	Rare	*Common*	Rare
Skin	Rare	Rare	Occasional	Rare
Bone marrow	Rare	Rare	Rare	Occasional

▪ Clinical Appearance

B-cell tumors typically arise in the spleen, Peyer's patches (◘ Figs. 19.1 and 19.2), or mesenteric lymph nodes, but may appear also in other locations. T-cell tumors primarily arise in the thymus (◘ see Fig. 19.3).

Histopathology maybe useful for further classification but is only of minor relevance clinically. Tumor cells can be characterized by location within lymphoid structures, cell and/or nuclear size and form. If needed, immunophenotyping can be applied for specific classification according to the proposed classification of mouse B and T cell neoplasia (Box 19.2 and 19.3).

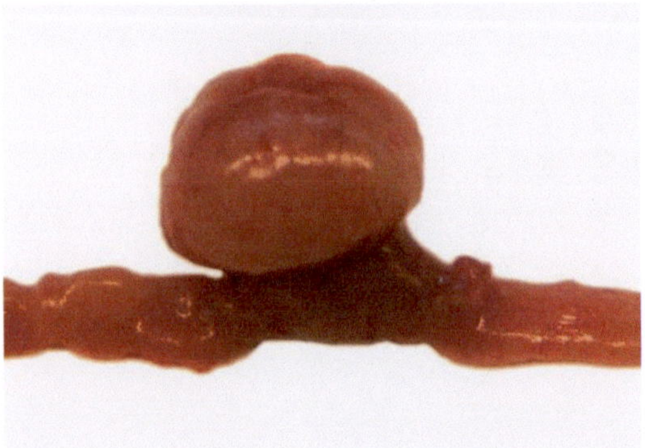

◘ **Fig. 19.1** Intestinal lymphoma in a Peyer's patch of a mouse (With permission of Kristina Dietert, Freie Universität Berlin)

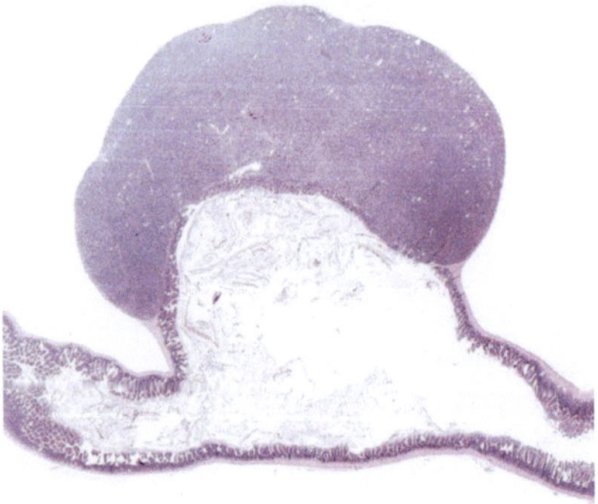

◘ **Fig. 19.2** Histology of an intestinal lymphoma of the Peyer's patch in a mouse

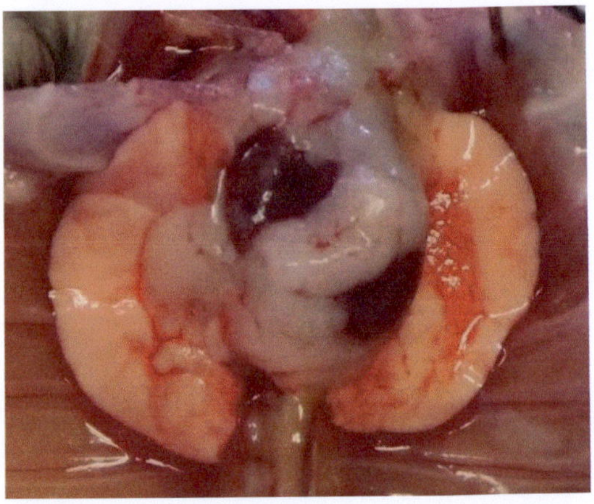

◘ **Fig. 19.3** Severely enlarged thymus with a thymic lymphoma in a mouse (With permission of Kristina Dietert, Freie Universität Berlin)

Box 19.2. Proposed Classification of Mouse B-cell Neoplasms (Morse et al. 2002)

1. Precursor B-cell neoplasm
   (a) Precursor B-cell lymphoblastic lymphoma/leukemia
2. Mature B-cell neoplasm
   (a) Small B-cell lymphoma
   (b) Splenic marginal zone B-cell lymphoma
   (c) Follicular B-cell lymphoma
   (d) Diffuse large B-cell lymphoma
      Morphologic variants
         Centroblastic
         Immunoblastic
         Histiocyte associated
      Subtypes
      Primary mediastinal (thymic) diffuse large B-cell lymphoma
   (e) Classic Burkitt lymphoma
   (f) Burkitt-like lymphoma (including mature B-cell lymphomas with lymphoblastic morphology)
   (g) Plasma cell neoplasms
      Plasmocytoma
      Extraosseous plasmacytoma
      Anaplastoc plasamcytoma
   (h) B-natural killer cell lymphoma

Box 19.3. Proposed Classification of Mcouse T-cell Neoplasms (Morse et al. 2002)

1. Precursor T-cell neoplasm
   (a) Precursor T-cell lymphoblastic lymphoma/leukemia
2. Mature B-cell neoplasm
   (a) Small T-cell lymphoma
   (b) T-natural killer cell lymphoma
3. T-cell neoplasm, character undetermined
   (c) Large cell anaplastic lymphoma

▪ **Suggested Reading**

(Ward 2006)

19.1.2.2 Non-lymphoid Tumors of Mice

▪ **Epidemiology and Pathogenesis**

The most common and important non-lymphoid tumor of mice is the *histiocytic sarcoma*, arising from phagocytic cells. Some strains are overrepresented and in general the tumor occurs in aged mice. Myeloid leukemia occurs occasionally in aged mice of some strains.

▪ **Clinical Appearance**

Histiocytic sarcomas are characterized by organomegaly especially affecting the spleen and often nodular involvement of other organs like liver, uterus, or kidneys. In myeloid leukemia, mice become ill with anemia and severe leukocytosis. Splenomegaly is often striking.

▪ **Histopathology**

Histopathology in cases of histiocytic sarcomas reveals often diffuse or nodular infiltrates by histiocytic to often fibrillary cells with usually abundant eosinophilic cytoplasm. Myeloid leukemia is characterized by diffuse infiltration of several organs by immature myeloid cells, occasionally with nuclear ring forms.

Box 19.4. Murine Nonlymphoid Hematopoietic Neoplasms and Related Disorders (Kogan et al. 2002)

1. Myeloid leukemias
   (a) Myeloid leukemias without maturation
   (b) Myeloid leukemias with maturation
   (c) Myeloproliferative-disease-like myeloid leukemia
   (d) Myelomonocytic leukemia
   (e) Megakaryocytic leukemia
   (f) Biphenotypic leukemia
2. Nonlymphoid Hematopoietic Sarcomas
   (a) Granulocytic sarcoma
   (b) Histiocytic sarcoma
   (c) Mast cell sarcoma
3. Myeloid Dysplasias
   (a) Myelodysplastic syndrome
   (b) Cytopenia with increased blasts
4. Myeloid Proliferations
   (a) Myeloproliferation
   (b) Myeloproliferative disease

▪ **Suggested Reading**

(Kogan et al. 2002)

19.1.3 Pulmonary Tumors of Mice

Box 19.5. Murine Pulmonary Tumors in Six Facts

1. Common
2. Incidence depended on mouse strain, viral infections, and others
3. Mostly arise from pneumocytes type II
4. Adenomas > adenocarcinomas
5. Often incidental finding
6. Called "pulmonary" adenoma / adenocarcinoma

▪ **Epidemiology and Pathogenesis**

Pulmonary tumors are among the most common murine neoplasia. In some strains, the prevalence reaches 100 % at the age of 4 months. Cell of origin is believed to be the pneumocytes type II. *K-ras* activation is an important trigger with increases tumors incidences in mice according to their *K-ras* allele status. For harmonization with human tumor nomenclature, the tumors are now called simply "pulmonary" instead of "bronchiolo-alveolar", "bronchiolar", or "alveolar".

■ **Clinical Appearance**

Tumors are often an incidental finding and present as small discrete nodules in the lungs that compress surrounding tissue. In cases of large or malignant tumors, local invasion with metastasis to the pleura may lead to respiratory symptoms.

■ **Histopathology**

Histopathology of adenomas is dominated by often well-differentiated cuboidal to columnar cells without cilia and often formation of papillary or tubular structures. In malignant tumors, local invasion is often detectable and cells tend to become pleomorphic.

■ **Suggested Reading**

(Renne et al. 2009)

19.1.4 Mammary Tumors of Mice

Box 19.6. Murine Mammary Tumors in Six Facts

1. Common
2. Incidence depended on mouse strain, number of pregnancies, stress, and others
3. May be induced by retroviral infection (MMTV)
4. Occur almost everywhere
5. Pulmonary metastasis common
6. Progression: hyperplasia, adenomas, adenocarcinomas

■ **Epidemiology and Pathogenesis**

Mammary tumors are common in mice, and mammary *carcinomas* are the most common in C3H mice. Besides spontaneous mutation, they are often induced by *retroviurs infection* with the mouse mammary tumor virus (MMTV). Tumor incidences are influenced by sex, hormonal status, age, and environment besides genetics and viral infection. Tumor progression includes hyperplasia, adenomas, and finally carcinomas.

■ **Clinical Appearance**

Tumors can be located on almost any location of the body as subcutaneous, well-circumscribed, firm, and sometimes multi-lobulated nodules. Large tumors may become partially necrotic with associated hemorrhages. Although local invasion is often not detectable, metastatic nodules may be present in the lung.

■ **Histopathology**

Histopathology can be variable with a wide spectrum of differentiation which is used for classification (◘ Table 19.2).

◘ **Table 19.2** Classification of mammary tumors according to their differentiation Cardiff et al. (2000)

Class	Histopathological features
Glandular	Tumor is composed of glands
Acinar	Tumor is composed of small glandular clusters with small lumens. While this is a subclass of glandular, it is very characteristic of MMTV-induced tumors
Cribriform	Tumor is composed of sheets or nests of cells forming lumens with round, punched out spaces
Papillary	Tumor has finger-like projections composed of epithelium covering a central fibrovascular core
Solid	Tumor is composed of solid sheets of epithelial cells with little or no glandular differentiation
Squamous	Tumors composed solely of squamous cells with or without keratinization, absence of glandular pattern
Fibroadenomas	Tumor is composed of a proliferation of both myxoid fibrous stroma and glands
Adenomyoepithelioma	Tumor is composed of myoepithelium and glands

19

Table 19.2 (continued)

Class	Histopathological features
Adenosquamous	Tumor has both glandular and squamous differentiation
Not Otherwise Specified (NOS)	Tumor does not have any of the other common descriptor patterns

■ **Therapy**

Surgery with margins as wide as possible is the treatment of choice. Ovariohysterectomy at time of surgical removal may enhance survival. Prognosis remains poor due to potential metastatic spread and recurrence.

■ **Suggested Reading**

(Cardiff et al. 2000; Rudmann et al. 2012)

19.1.5 Hepatocellular Tumors of Mice

Box 19.7. Murine Hepatocellular Tumors in Five Facts

1. Frequent in aged mice
2. Males > females
3. Incidence depended on mouse strain
4. *Helicobacter* spp. infection is associated with earlier onset and higher prevalence
5. Progression: foci of cellular alteration, adenomas, adenocarcinomas

■ **Epidemiology and Pathogenesis**

Hepatocellular adenomas and adenocarcinomas are the most common liver tumors with aged males being more often affected than females. They can be provoked by a variety of hepatocarcinogens. Infection with *Helicobacter* spp. is associated with earlier onset and higher prevalence. Besides hepatocellular tumors, cholangiocellular adenomas or adenocarcinomas arise only rarely.

■ **Clinical Appearance**

If mice become clinically apparent, they mostly only display unspecific reduced general condition. In case of large tumors, the abdomen may be distended. At necropsy, single or multiple nodules are present in the liver with variable sometimes liver-like color and consistency. Cholangiocellular tumors are often firm and gray to tan.

■ **Histopathology**

Histopathology of hepatocellular tumors is characterized by two growth patterns. Tumor cells form trabecula or grow solid with variable differentiation, which is not predictive regarding metastatic behavior. Anisokaryosis and anisocytosis are often striking, karyomegaly frequent. Adenomas and hepatocellular hyperplasia are often difficult to distinguish from each other and normal liver tissue.

■ **Suggested Reading**

(Thoolen et al. 2010)

19.1.6 Endocrine Tumors of Mice

Box 19.8. Murine Endocrine Tumors (Pituitary Adenomas) in Three Facts

1. Pituitary adenomas relatively common
2. Females > Males
3. Most tumors secrete prolactin

■ **Epidemiology and Pathogenesis**

Pituitary gland adenomas, mostly originating from the pars distalis, are the most frequent endocrine tumor in mice, with females being more often affected than males. The tumors are mainly benign but often secrete prolactin, thereby promote the development of mammary tumors. Sporadically, hyperplasia or adenoma formation is present in other endocrine organs like the adrenal or thyroid gland or the pancreatic islands of aged mice.

■ **Clinical Appearance**

Depending on the site of origin and a possible endocrine activity, secondary hormonal effects for example lactation in cases of prolactin secreting pituitary gland adenomas may appear. Especially space occupying tumors of the pituitary gland can lead to central nervous symptoms due to compression and atrophy of the brain. At necropsy, tumors often appear reddish due to hemorrhages (■ Fig. 19.4)

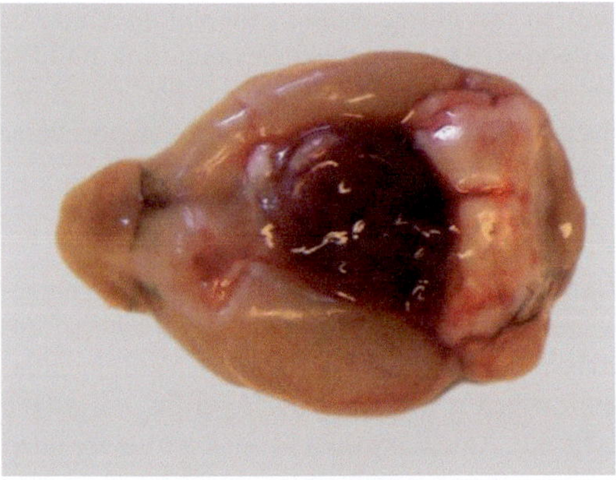

Fig. 19.4 Large pituitary gland adenoma in a mouse with extensive hemorrhage (With permission of Kristina Dietert at Freie Universität Berlin)

Histopathology

Histopathology reveals mainly benign tumors with nodular expansive growth and in general good differentiation. Pituitary gland tumors rarely become invasive.

Suggested Reading

(Boorman and Sills 1999; Hardisty and Boorman 1999; Mahler and Elwell 1999; Nyska and Maronpot 1999)

19.2 Tumors of Rats

19.2.1 Introduction

The incidence of spontaneous neoplasia is widely variable in the rat depending amongst others on strain, age, sex, and diet. The most common tumors are fibroadenomas while lymphocytic leukemia is the major life-limiting factor. Other important tumor locations are the Zymbal's gland, the thyroid, uterine endometrium, and mesenchymal tissues.

19.2.2 Hematopoietic Neoplasia of Rats

Box 19.9. Hematopoietic Tumors of Rats in Four Facts

1. Common
2. Females > males (LGL leukemia)
3. Strain predispositions
4. Major cause of death in aging rats

19.2.2.1 Large Granular Lymphocytic (LGL) Leukemia

Epidemiology and Pathogenesis

LGL leukemias occur in all strains of rats, but are the major cause of death in aging F344 rats. The cell of origin is a lymphocytic cell with at least some natural killer cell characteristics. A link to retroviral infection could not be established although often proposed.

Clinical Appearance

Typically, rats with LGL leukemia become clinically apparent with *anemia*, *jaundice*, reduced general condition, and severe *leukocytosis* with up to 400,000/ml^3. Due to cytotoxic properties of the tumor cells, also thrombocytopenia, hemolytic anemia, and consecutive hemorrhages are common. At necropsy, splenomegaly and hepatomegaly are typical finding, often in combination with petechiation or intestinal bleeding.

Histopathology

Histopathology is dominated by intravascular leukocytosis and diffuse infiltration of parenchymal organs by large lymphocytes (see Fig. 19.5). The typical cytoplasmic *granules* are striking especially in *cytology*, which may be done from impression smears of affected organs.

Suggested Reading

(Boorman and Everitt 2006)

19.2.2.2 Histiocytic Sarcomas of Rats

Epidemiology and Pathogenesis

Histiocytic sarcomas are observed occasionally in all strains, but are especially frequent in SD rats. Both sexes of aged rats are affected almost equally.

Clinical Appearance

If clinical signs are present, they are mostly unspecific with reduced general condition. At necropsy, nodular masses are often present in several organs including the spleen, liver, and lymph nodes, but also serosal surfaces or the skin and subcutaneous tissues.

Histopathology

Histopathology reveals pleomorphic often spindled cells with abundant eosinophilic cytoplasm and large, vesiculated nuclei. Cells are arranged in sheets or occasionally palisading with multinucleated cells often being intermingled.

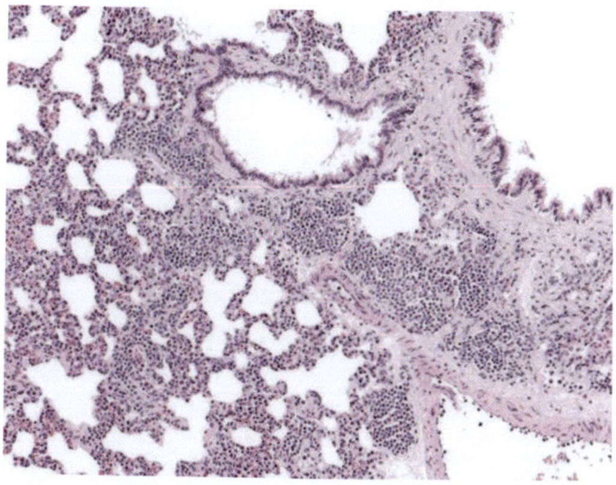

Fig. 19.5 Histologic picture of the lung from a rat with LGL leukemia. Capillaries and lymphatic vessels are tightly filled be mostly monomorphic large lymphoid cells (leukemia)

■ **Suggested Reading**

(Boorman and Everitt 2006)

19.2.3 Mammary Tumors of Rats

Box 19.10. Mammary Tumors of the Rat in Six Facts

1. Common
2. Mostly benign fibroadenomas
3. Strain predispositions
4. Incidence dependent on environmental (diet!) and hormonal factors
5. No viral genesis
6. Can be triggered by various carcinogens

■ **Epidemiology and Pathogenesis**

Mammary tumors are common in female, but occur occasionally in male rats also. Most tumors are benign *fibroadenomas* with mammary *carcinomas* being rare. With time, fibroadenomas may become very large and occasionally locally invasive, but malignant progression with metastasis is extremely rare.

■ **Clinical Appearance**

Due to the widespread distribution of mammary tissue, masses can be located on almost any location of the body as movable, well-circumscribed, firm, and often lobulated nodules. Large tumors may become superficially ulcerated and with restricted mobility.

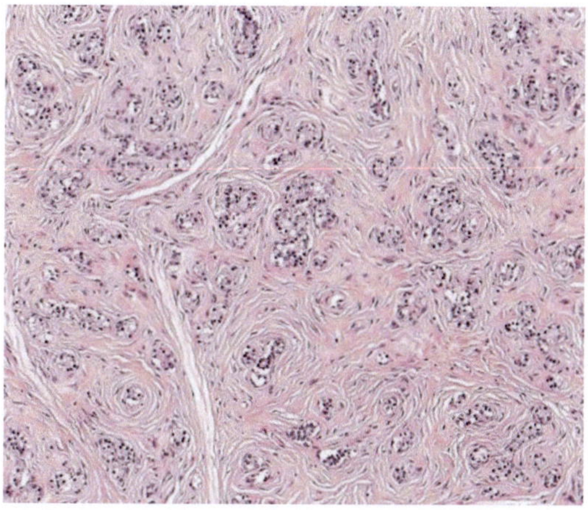

Fig. 19.6 Histologic picture of a fibroadenoma in rat. Small islands of epithelial cells are enclosed by abundant collagen rich connective tissue. HE-stain

■ **Histopathology**

Histopathology of fibroadenomas reveals the typical combination of abundant connective tissue enclosing small islands of well-differentiated epithelial tumor cells mostly arranged in small acinar structures (see Fig. 19.6). Malignant adenocarcinomas have been classified according to their growth pattern similar to murine tumors in several groups including “alveolar/tubular”, “cystic”, “papillary”, “scirrhous”, and “spindle cell”.

■ **Therapy**

Surgery is the treatment of choice and recommended especially in large tumors limiting mobility.

■ **Suggested Reading**

(Rudmann et al. 2012)

19.2.4 Pituitary Gland Tumors of Rats

Box 19.11. Pituitary Adenomas of Rats in Four Facts

1. Common especially in F344 and Wistar rats
2. Incidence dependent on environmental (diet!) and hormonal factors
3. Most tumors are benign
4. Often secretion of prolactin

Epidemiology and Pathogenesis

The majority of *pituitary gland tumors* are chromophobe adenomas originating from the pars distalis. Frequently they produce prolactin. Tumor frequency rises with age. In some strains like F344 and Wistar rats, these tumors are a major cause of death. *Malignant* tumors are rare.

Clinical Appearance

Lactation of affected older rats is a typical clinical finding due to frequent prolactin secretion by the tumors. Central nervous symptoms may dominate in cases of space occupying large masses.

Histopathology

Histopathology is mainly characterized by well-differentiated adenoid cells arranged in nests or cords sustained by extensively vascularized stroma. Often multiple nodules are detectable histologically, which are usually independent proliferations. Hemorrhages and consequential deposition of hemosiderin are frequent findings.

Therapy

Surgery is the treatment of choice and recommended especially in large, mobility-limiting mobility.

Suggested Reading

(Boorman and Everitt 2006)

19.3 Tumors of Rabbits

19.3.1 Introduction

Adenocarcinomas of the uterus are the most common and relevant tumor in rabbits especially due to its tendency to metastasize extensively. Other relevant tumors are lymphomas which often affect the gut associated lymphoid tissue which is the largest accumulation of lymphoid tissue in the rabbit at all. Mesenchymal, often myxoid tumors are also typical for rabbits, but they are mainly induced by poxviral infection with myxomatosis being the systemic variant of the infection.

19

19.3.2 Tumors of the Female Reproductive Tract of Rabbits

Box 19.12. Female Reproductive Tract Tumors of the Rabbit in Three Facts

1. Uterine adenocarcinomas most recognized tumor in aged female rabbits
2. May early spread to distant organs (lung)
3. Incidences of up to 80 % in aged rabbits

Epidemiology and Pathogenesis

Uterine adenocarcinomas are the most frequent tumor of rabbits (*Oryctolagus cuniculi*). The incidence increases with age. A predisposing hormonal effect by estrogens is discussed but study results are contradictory. There is no known breed predilection.

Clinical Appearance

Clinical signs affect especially *breeder rabbits* coming recognized with *reproductive disturbances* like reduced fertility, litter size, or increased stillbirths. At necropsy, the uterine horns are expanded by often multiple masses, which are ulcerated on their mucosal surface or have papilliform proliferations (Fig. 19.7).

Histopathology

Histopathology is often variable with proliferation of mostly cuboidal cells forming papillary, acinar,

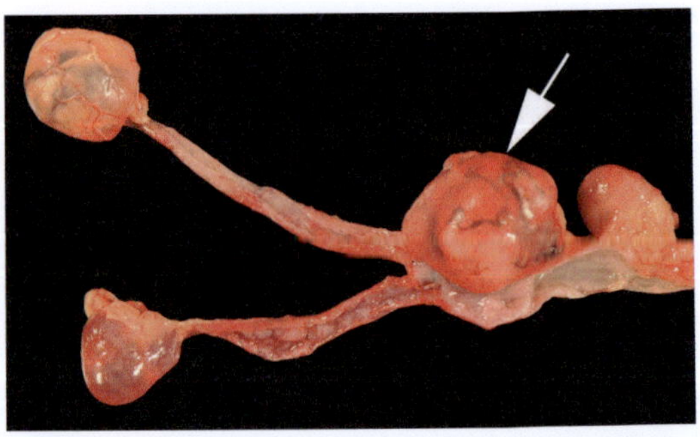

Fig. 19.7 Uterine adenocarcinoma (*white arrow*) of an rabbit

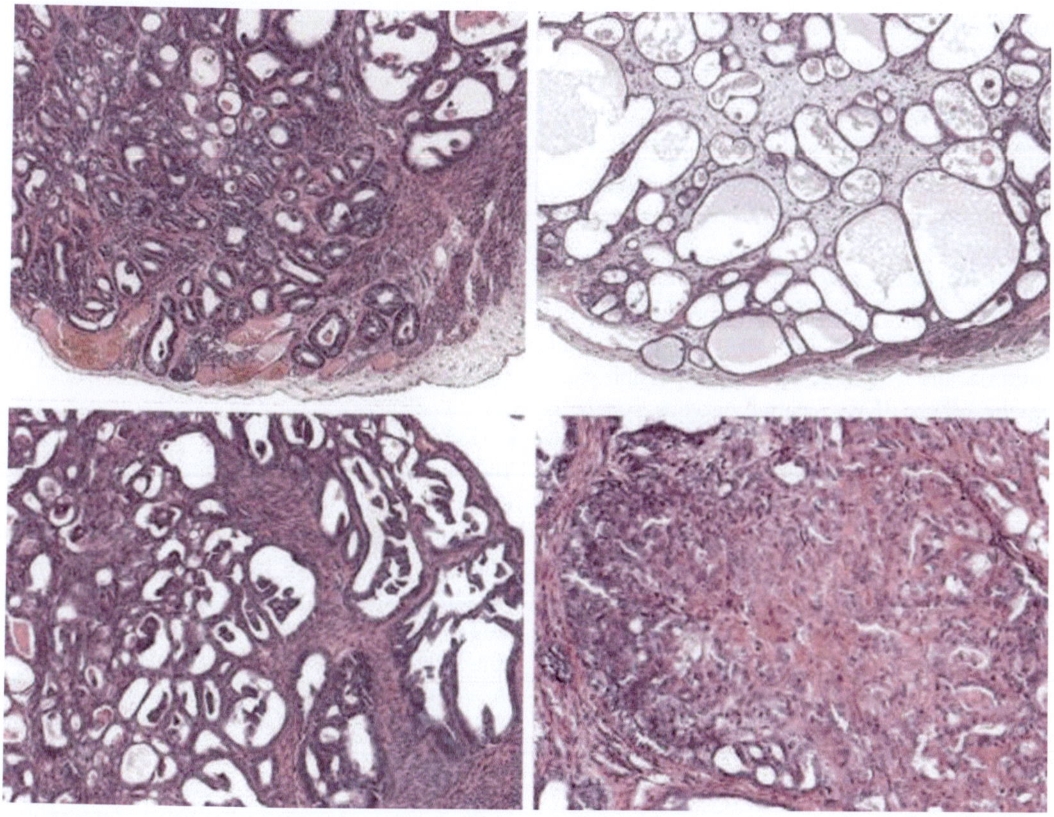

Fig. 19.8 Histologic picture of the variable differentiations of uterine adenocarcinomas in rabbits: acinar (*top left*), cystic (*top right*), papillary (*bottom left*) and solid (*bottom right*) growth patterns. HE-stain

or tubular structures or forming solid tumor areas. Invasion into surrounding uterine stroma and myometrial layers is common (Fig. 19.8). Metastases are detectable in numerous cases in regional lymph nodes, in the peritoneal cavity or especially the lung.

Therapy

Surgery is the treatment of choice although the time between clinical detection and death as a result from metastasis is variable ranging from 12 to 24 month.

Suggested Reading

(Tinkey et al. 1999)

19.3.3 Hematopoietic Neoplasia of Rabbits

19.3.3.1 Lymphomas/Leukemia of Rabbits

Box 19.13. Malignant Lymphomas/Leukemia of Rabbits in Four Facts

1. Second most common tumor in rabbits
2. Most common tumor in young or juvenile rabbits
3. Leukemia often associated with multiple organ involvement
4. Most affected organs are kidneys, liver, spleen, and lymph nodes

Epidemiology and Pathogenesis

Lymphomas/leukemia are the second most common tumors in rabbits and the most common tumors in *young or juvenile* rabbits. There is no known sex or breed predilection. Lymphomas may be aleukemic or leukemic, while leukemia is mostly associated with involvement of several organs.

Clinical Appearance

Clinical signs are mostly not specific with the exception of leukocytosis if present. Anemia, anorexia, and lymphadenopathy are possible signs among others. If the central nervous system is affected by neoplastic infiltrates sudden paralysis or neurological dysfunction may be overt. At necropsy, neoplastic nodules may be present in different locations; organomegaly and pale bone marrow are other possible signs. The combination of tan and superficial irregular kidneys with a thickened whitish cortex, an enlarged liver with diffuse small foci, splenomegaly, and lymphadenopathy is considered pathognomonic for lymphomas.

Histopathology

Histopathology identifies infiltrations of neoplastic lymphocytes in almost any organ with an often multicentric pattern. Commonly involved are parenchymal organs like liver, spleen, kidneys, lung, and lymphoid tissues of which the mucosa associated lymphoid tissue is the most often affected. Besides diffuse infiltration of preexisting tissue, also solid tumor nodules are detectable in virtually any location. Neoplastic cells are larger than mature lymphocytes and have scant cytoplasm. Mitotic figures are frequent and necrosis is often detectable as consequence of fast growth.

Suggested Reading

(Tinkey et al. 1999)

19.3.3.2 Thymomas of Rabbits

Box 19.14. Thymomas of Rabbits in Five Facts

1. A common tumor in rabbits
2. Benign growth but clinically malignant due to thoracic mass effect
3. Clinical signs usually consist of dyspnea, exercise intolerance, and exophthalmos
4. Paraneoplastic syndromes rarely observed
5. Surgery associated with high risk of perioperative mortality

Epidemiology and Pathogenesis

Thymomas are common tumors of rabbits, which make up to 10 % of all tumors in this species. They are the *most common tumor of the cranial mediastinum* and develop from thymic epithelial cells. They usually have a *slow growth rate*, mostly grow expansively, occasionally invasively but only *rarely metastasize* (■ Fig. 19.9). The *age* of affected rabbits varies from 1 to 4 years. There is no *gender* or *breed* predisposition. The causes and mechanism of thymomas development in rabbits or any other animal species are unknown.

Clinical Appearance

Thymomas in the rabbit are *often incidental findings* at necropsy in animals with other fatal diseases. If clinically relevant, thymomas are commonly associated with *tachy- or dyspnea*, *exercise intolerance*, and *exophthalmos*. Other less common clinical signs include inappetence, coughing, prolapse of the third eyelid, edema of the cranial body parts, and muffled heart sounds. *Exophthalmos* and edema of the cranial body parts are caused by compression of the cranial vena cava and accumulation of blood in the retrobulbar venous plexus or other veins of the cranial body, respectively.

Thymomas in rabbits are occasionally associated with two *paraneoplastic syndromes*. A few case reports identified *autoimmune hemolytic anemia* and/or thymoma-*associated exfoliative dermatitis*, which is characterized by patchy alopecia, scaling, and hyperkeratosis, in rabbits with thymomas. Often concurrent effusions (pleural effusion and/or hydropericard) are present.

Blood work is usually unremarkable in rabbits with thymomas. *Thoracic radiographs* are sufficient to identify cranial masses of appropriate size but are not specific to exclude the differential diagnoses of thymiclymphomas, abcessation, fibrosarcomas, or secondary metastatic tumors. *Ultrasound guided fine needle aspiration* or thoracocentesis are necessary to confirm the diagnosis but are often difficult to interpret due to the dominance of lymphocytes in the cell population.

Cytology and Histopathology

Fine needle aspirates and pleural fluids of rabbits with thymomas usually contain a mixed population of small mature to occasional large lymphocytes interspersed in between a few neoplastic thymoma cells. Macrophages may be also present especially if there are cystic

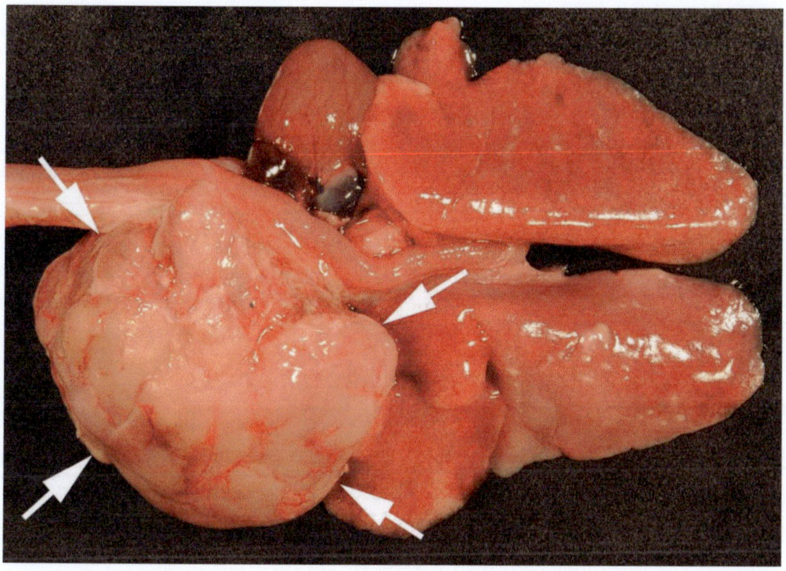

Fig. 19.9 Thymoma (*arrow*) in a rabbit (With permission of Robert Klopfleisch, Freie Universitaet Berlin)

areas. Often these lymphocytes severely outnumber and thus hide the actual epithelial spindloid and occasionally plump polygonal epithelial tumor cells. Cytological preparations may be thus misdiagnosed as a well-differentiated lymphoma rather than thymoma; however, a heterogenous cellular population is indicative of thymomas.

Histopathology of biopsies or surgically excised tumors often allows for the diagnosis but is nevertheless also often complicated by the presence of numerous well-differentiated lymphocytes which cover the actual tumor cells. *Hassall's corpuscles*, concentric eosinophilic masses, are specific structures of thymic tissues and are usually also present in thymomas. *Immunohistochemical detection of cytokeratin* maybe used to improve the detection and evaluation of cellular morphology of the cytokeratin-positive tumor cells.

- **Therapy**

Rabbits with clinically overt thymomas are *often euthanized* due to poor clinical conditions and the high demands on intra- and perioperative management of rabbits during and after surgery.

Surgery for complete excision or palliative cytoreduction is nevertheless the most commonly described used treatment modality for rabbits with thymomas. *Perioperative mortality is high.* However, if the animals survive surgery and the first few days thereafter survival times of 6 months or more have been reported.

A recent study reported that megavoltage *radiation therapy* may be a valuable, efficient, and safe method for the treatment of rabbits with thymomas. Only three of 19 treated animals died within the first 14 days after radiation and the remaining rabbits showed a median survival time of 727 days. A body weight of >1.5 kg was identified as a positive prognostic factor for survival after treatment.

Prednisone is commonly used as a medical treatment of thymomas in rabbits. The anecdotal reports available indicate a reduction in size during treatment and survival times of 5–9 months.

- **Suggested Further Reading**

(Andres et al. 2012; Florizoone 2005; Kunzel et al. 2012; Wagner et al. 2005; Tinkey et al. 1999)

19.4 Tumors of Guinea Pigs

19.4.1 Introduction

In general, tumor incidence in the guinea pig is low with an increase in animals older than 3 years. Pulmonary tumors are the largest group in aged animals, followed by tumors of the reproductive tract mammary gland and skin. Hematopoietic neoplasia is seen predominantly in younger guinea pigs less than 3 years of age.

19.4.2 Hematopoietic Neoplasia of Guinea Pigs

19.4.2.1 "Cavian Leukemia" of Guinea Pigs

Box 19.15. Leukemia of Guinea Pigs in Three Facts

1. Most common tumor in young guinea pigs (<3 years)
2. Retroviral infection suspected (Type C)
3. Most affected organs are liver, spleen, and lymph nodes

- **Epidemiology and Pathogenesis**

Leukemia is the most common tumor in young guinea pigs. Retroviral Type C particles are suspected to be involved in etiology because viral particles were detectable by electron microscopy in tumor cells.

- **Clinical Appearance**

Clinical symptoms are often unspecific, with lymphadenopathy and leukocytosis being indicative. Animals generally have severe leukocytosis with increased numbers of circulating blasts and variably additional lymphadenopathy. At necropsy, enlarged lymph nodes as well as hepato- and splenomegaly are typical.

- **Histopathology**

Histopathology is dominated by diffuse infiltrations of the liver, lung, spleen, kidney, and the gut-associated lymphoid and a wide spectrum of other tissues by neoplastic lymphocytes.

- **Suggested Reading**

(Williams 1999)

19.4.3 Tumors of the Respiratory Tract of Guinea Pigs

Box 19.16. Pulmonary Tumors of Guinea Pigs in Two Facts

1. Most common in aged guinea pigs
2. Mostly benign adenomas

- **Epidemiology and Pathogenesis**

Pulmonary tumors are most common tumor in aged guinea pigs with the most tumors being benign adenomas.

- **Clinical Appearance**

Tumors are often an incidental finding at necropsy and clinical signs rare. Large tumors may cause respiratory symptoms. At necropsy, small nodules are present in the lung parenchyma, which are well demarcated and often whitish.

- **Histopathology**

Histopathology reveals well-differentiated adenomas with well-differentiated cuboidal to columnar cells arranged in mostly papillary structures. Malignant tumors are rare.

- **Suggested Reading**

(Williams 1999)

19.4.4 Tumors of the Female Reproductive Tract of Guinea Pigs

Box 19.17. Female Reproductive Tract Tumors of the Guinea Pig in Three Facts

1. Mostly benign mesenchymal tumors of the uterus
2. Ovarian tumors are mostly teratomas
3. Malignant tumors are rare

- **Epidemiology and Pathogenesis**

Leiomyomas are the most frequent *uterine* tumor of guinea pigs with malignant variants being rare. Of the *ovarian* tumors *teratomas* are dominating, but also granulosa cell tumors or cystadenomas may occur.

- **Clinical Appearance**

Clinical signs may be obvious in breeder guinea pigs or in case of ovarian tumors with hormonal activity and eventual consequential changes of the skin.

- **Histopathology**

Histopathology reveals in case of *mesenchymal tumors* spindle cells arranged in stream, depending on the cell origin with more or less spindled or typical "cigar"-shaped nuclei. Teratomas are characterized by the presence of well-differentiated tissues of ecto-, meso-, and endodermal origin and often contain parts of osseous, dental, cutaneous, and nervous tissues.

- **Therapy**

Surgery is the treatment of choice.

- **Suggested Reading**

(Williams 1999)

19.4.5 Tumors of the Skin of Guinea Pigs

19.4.5.1 Tumors of the Mammary Gland of Guinea Pigs

Box 19.18. Mammary Tumors of the Guinea Pig in Three Facts

1. Mostly benign fibroadenomas
2. About one third are adenocarcinomas
3. High incidence of adenocarcinomas in male guinea pigs

- **Epidemiology and Pathogenesis**

Most mammary tumors in the guinea pig are benign *fibroadenomas. Adenocarcinomas* are rare and often of ductal origin. Male guinea pigs have a relatively high incidence of adenocarcinomas.

- **Clinical Appearance**

Mammary tumors appear as often well-circumscribed, firm, and lobulated nodules. Large tumors may become superficially ulcerated. At necropsy, lung metastases may be present in case malignant adenocarcinomas.

- **Histopathology**

Histopathology in case of *fibroadenomas* is characterized by a combination of connective tissue enclosing epithelial islands. Malignant adenocarcinomas can be variable regarding differentiation, simple, and mixed carcinomas occur.

- **Therapy**

Surgery is the treatment of choice, the prognosis is poor for malignant, metastatic tumors.

- **Suggested Reading**

(Williams 1999)

19.4.5.2 Trichofolliculomas of Guinea Pigs

Box 19.19. Trichofolliculomas of the Guinea Pig in Three Facts

1. Most common skin tumor in aged guinea pigs
2. Benign tumor arising in the pilosebaceous unit of the hair follicle
3. Expansile masses often located in the lumbosacral area

- **Epidemiology and Pathogenesis**

Trichofolliculomas are typical benign *hair follicle tumors* and are the most common skin tumor in guinea pigs, while this tumor is rare in other species.

- **Clinical Appearance**

Most tumors arise in the lumbosacral area and can reach remarkable size. Ulceration in case of large tumors is frequent. Tumors are well demarcated and firm, often displaying a central pore. Trauma can induce a severe inflammatory response due to abundant keratin in the lumen of these tumors.

- **Histopathology**

Histopathology reveals well-differentiated hair follicle epithelia forming arborized follicular structures radiating from a large central "primary" follicle (Fig. 19.10).

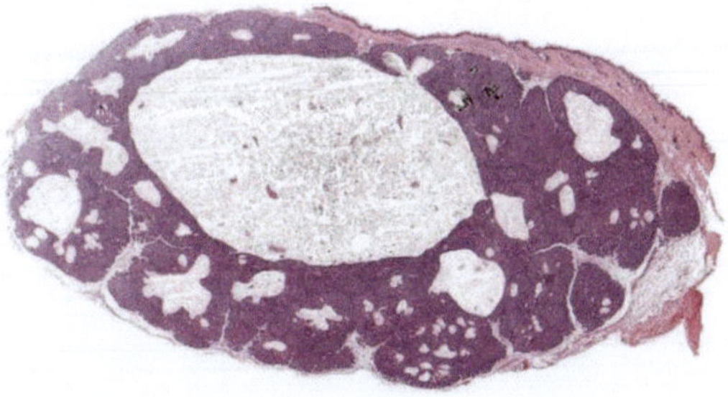

Fig. 19.10 Histologic picture of a trichofolliculoma in a guinea pig. Central cystic "primary"follicle with peripheral radiating smaller follicular structures. HE-stain

▪ **Therapy**

Surgery is the treatment of choice, prognosis is good.

▪ **Suggested Reading**

(Williams 1999)

Suggested Reading

Andres KM, Kent M, Siedlecki CT, Mayer J, Brandao J, Hawkins MG, Morrisey JK, Quesenberry K, Valli VE, Bennett RA (2012) The use of megavoltage radiation therapy in the treatment of thymomass in rabbits: 19 cases. Vet Comp Oncol 10:82–94

Begley DA, Krupke DM, Vincent MJ, Sundberg JP, Bult CJ, Eppig JT (2007) Mouse Tumor Biology Database (MTB): status update and future directions. Nucleic Acids Res 35:D638–D642

Begley DA, Krupke DM, Neuhauser SB, Richardson JE, Bult CJ, Eppig JT, Sundberg JP (2012a) The Mouse Tumor Biology Database (MTB): a central electronic resource for locating and integrating mouse tumor pathology data. Vet Pathol 49:218–223

Begley D, Sundberg BA, Berndt A, Eppig J, Schofield PN, Sundberg JP (2012b) Diversity of spontaneous neoplasms in commonly used inbred strains of laboratory mice. In: The laboratory mouse. Academic Press/Elsevier, London, pp 411–426

Boorman GA, Everitt JI (2006) Neoplastic disease. In: The laboratory rat, 2nd edn. Elsevier Academic Press, Amsterdam/Heidelberg, pp 479–511

Boorman GA, Sills RC (1999) Exocrine and Endocrine Pancreas. In: Pathology of the mouse: reference and atlas, 1st edn. Cache River Press, Saint Louis, pp 185–206

Boorman GA, Rafferty CN, Ward JM, Sills RC (2000) Leukemia and lymphomas incidence in rodents exposed to low-frequency magnetic fields. Radiat Res 153:627–636

Cardiff RD, Anver MR, Gusterson BA, Hennighausen L, Jensen RA, Merino MJ, Rehm S, Russo J, Tavassoli FA, Wakefield LM, Ward JM, Green JE (2000) The mammary pathology of genetically engineered mice: the consensus report and recommendations from the Annapolis meeting. Oncogene 19:968–988

Florizoone K (2005) Thymomas-associated exfoliative dermatitis in a rabbit. Vet Dermatol 16:281–284

Gold LS, Manley NB, Slone TH, Ward JM (2001) Compendium of chemical carcinogens by target organ: results of chronic bioassays in rats, mice, hamsters, dogs, and monkeys. Toxicol Pathol 29:639–652

Hardisty JF, Boorman GA (1999) Thyroid and parathyroid glands. In: Pathology of the mouse: reference and atlas, 1st edn. Cache River Press, Saint Louis, pp 537–554

Kogan SC, Ward JM, Anver MR, Berman JJ, Brayton C, Cardiff RD, Carter JS, de Coronado S, Downing JR, Fredrickson TN, Haines DC, Harris AW, Harris NL, Hiai H, Jaffe ES, MacLennan IC, Pandolfi PP, Pattengale PK, Perkins AS, Simpson RM, Tuttle MS, Wong JF, Morse HC 3rd (2002) Bethesda proposals for classification of nonlymphoid hematopoietic neoplasms in mice. Blood 100:238–245

Krupke DM, Begley DA, Sundberg JP, Bult CJ, Eppig JT (2008) The mouse tumor biology database. Nat Rev Cancer 8:459–465

Kunzel F, Hittmair KM, Hassan J, Dupre G, Russold E, Guija de Arespachochaga A, Fuchs-Baumgartinger A, Bilek A (2012) Thymomass in rabbits: clinical evaluation, diagnosis, and treatment. J Am Anim Hosp Assoc 48:97–104

Mahler JF, Elwell MR (1999) Pituitary gland. In: Pathology of the mouse: reference and atlas, 1st edn. Cache River Press, Saint Louis, pp 491–508

Morse HC 3rd, Anver MR, Fredrickson TN, Haines DC, Harris AW, Harris NL, Jaffe ES, Kogan SC, MacLennan IC, Pattengale PK, Ward JM (2002) Bethesda proposals for classification of lymphoid neoplasms in mice. Blood 100:246–258

Nyska A, Maronpot RR (1999) Adrenal gland. In: Pathology of the mouse: reference and atlas, 1st edn. Cache River Press, Saint Louis, pp 509–536

Renne R, Brix A, Harkema J, Herbert R, Kittel B, Lewis D, March T, Nagano K, Pino M, Rittinghausen S, Rosenbruch M, Tellier P, Wohrmann T (2009) Proliferative and nonproliferative lesions of the rat and mouse respiratory tract. Toxicol Pathol 37:5S–73S

Rudmann D, Cardiff R, Chouinard L, Goodman D, Kuttler K, Marxfeld H, Molinolo A, Treumann S, Yoshizawa K (2012) Proliferative and nonproliferative lesions of the rat and mouse mammary, Zymbal's, preputial, and clitoral glands. Toxicol Pathol 40:7S–39S

Schofield PN, Bard JB, Boniver J, Covelli V, Delvenne P, Ellender M, Engstrom W, Goessner W, Gruenberger M, Hoefler H, Hopewell JW, Mancuso M, Mothersill C, Quintanilla-Martinez L, Rozell B, Sariola H, Sundberg JP, Ward A (2004a) Pathbase: a new reference resource and database for laboratory mouse pathology. Radiat Prot Dosimetry 112:525–528

Schofield PN, Bard JB, Booth C, Boniver J, Covelli V, Delvenne P, Ellender M, Engstrom W, Goessner W, Gruenberger M, Hoefler H, Hopewell J, Mancuso M, Mothersill C, Potten CS, Quintanilla-Fend L, Rozell B, Sariola H, Sundberg JP, Ward A (2004b) Pathbase: a database of mutant mouse pathology. Nucleic Acids Res 32:D512–D515

Schofield PN, Gruenberger M, Sundberg JP (2010) Pathbase and the MPATH ontology. Community resources for mouse histopathology. Veterinary Pathol 47:1016–1020

Taddesse-Heath L, Chattopadhyay SK, Dillehay DL, Lander MR, Nagashfar Z, Morse HC 3rd, Hartley JW (2000) Lymphomass and high-level expression of murine leukemia viruses in CFW mice. J Virol 74:6832–6837

Thoolen B, Maronpot RR, Harada T, Nyska A, Rousseaux C, Nolte T, Malarkey DE, Kaufmann W, Kuttler K, Deschl U, Nakae D, Gregson R, Vinlove MP, Brix AE, Singh B, Belpoggi F, Ward JM (2010) Proliferative and nonproliferative lesions of the rat and mouse hepatobiliary system. Toxicol Pathol 38:5S–81S

Tinkey PT, Uthamanthil RK, Weisbroth SH (1999) Rabbit neoplasia. In: The laboratory rabbit, guinea pig, hamster, and other rodents. Academic Press/Elsevier, London, pp 448–501

Wagner F, Beinecke A, Fehr M, Brunkhorst N, Mischke R, Gruber AD (2005) Recurrent bilateral exophthalmos associated with metastatic thymic carcinomas in a pet rabbit. J Small Anim Pract 46:393–397

Ward JM (2006) Lymphomass and leukemias in mice. Exp Tox Pathol Off J Gesellschaft fur Toxikologische Pathologie 57:377–381

Williams BH (1999) Guinea pigs: non-infectious diseases. In: The laboratory rabbit, guinea pig, hamster, and other rodents. Academic Press/Elsevier, London, pp 685–704

Service Part

R. Klopfleisch (ed.), *Veterinary Oncology*, DOI 10.1007/978-3-319-41124-8

Index

L

M

N

O

U

V

W

MIX
Papier aus verantwortungsvollen Quellen
Paper from responsible sources
FSC® C105338

If you have any concerns about our products,
you can contact us on
ProductSafety@springernature.com

In case Publisher is established outside the EU,
the EU authorized representative is:
Springer Nature Customer Service Center GmbH
Europaplatz 3, 69115 Heidelberg, Germany

Printed by Libri Plureos GmbH
in Hamburg, Germany